The SAGES Manual of Colorectal Surgery

The SAGES University Masters Program Series
Editor-in-Chief: Brian Jacob

Patricia Sylla • Andreas M. Kaiser
Daniel Popowich
Editors

The SAGES Manual of Colorectal Surgery

SAGES University MASTERS PROGRAM

Springer

Editors
Patricia Sylla
Icahn School of Medicine at Mount Sinai Hospital
New York, NY
USA

Andreas M. Kaiser
Keck School of Medicine of USC
Los Angeles, CA
USA

Daniel Popowich
Icahn School of Medicine at Mount Sinai Hospital
New York, NY
USA

ISBN 978-3-030-24811-6 ISBN 978-3-030-24812-3 (eBook)
https://doi.org/10.1007/978-3-030-24812-3

This Springer imprint is published by the registered company Springer Nature Switzerland AG
The registered company address is: Gewerbestrasse 11, 6330 Cham, Switzerland

To Paul, for his unwavering support and shared passion for academic excellence.
Patricia Sylla, MD, FACS, FASCRS

With the hope that a seed put into the ground will grow into a promising harvest, I dedicate this book to the hard-working army of enthusiastic individuals who share my belief that learning remains a lifelong necessity. At some point, I may need to have the confidence to put my life in their skilled hands.
Andreas M. Kaiser, MD, FACS, FASCRS

To Charles Barkley: When I was in fifth grade and absolutely certain I was going to become a professional basketball player, you told me that I had no chance. You told me that I had a better chance of becoming a doctor. So that's what I did.

To my late grandfather, Dr. Irvin M. Gerson: I have hoped to model my life and career on the way he dedicated his to his patients and family.

Most importantly, to Cristina: your patience and loyal support while holding down the chaos at home have not gone unnoticed.
Daniel Popowich, MD

Preface

Nearly 30 years after its inception, laparoscopy has been established as the preferred surgical approach in the treatment of most benign and malignant colorectal conditions. Minimally invasive surgery (MIS) not only mitigates the adverse effects of surgical trauma, but when incorporated in standardized enhanced recovery programs, a laparoscopic approach significantly reduces opioid consumption and length of hospital stay and abbreviates recovery time relative to open surgery. Long-term benefits of MIS may not have been entirely captured yet but promises cost savings from reduced readmission and reoperation for adhesion- and hernia-related complications.

Over the past decade, the adoption of MIS in colon surgery among general surgeons has steadily increased through the implementation of the Fundamentals of Laparoscopic Surgery (FLS) curriculum and teaching and training in standardized techniques for various colorectal procedures. With the introduction of robotic surgery, the adoption of MIS for pelvic surgery and rectal resections in particular has steadily grown with decreasing conversion rates among surgeons beyond their learning curve. Other emerging minimally invasive techniques with potential clinical benefit include intracorporeal anastomosis and transrectal specimen extraction, which can be performed using standard laparoscopic or robotic approaches.

Acquisition of the fund of knowledge and technical skills required to perform high-quality MIS colorectal surgery is not without challenges. The implementation of standardized techniques for various procedures and development of a structured curriculum has been recognized as instrumental in educating and training the next generation of surgeons. The *SAGES Manual of Colorectal Surgery* provides essential didactic content for the SAGES University Masters Program Colorectal Surgery Curriculum. Surgeons seeking to complete the competency, proficiency, or mastery curriculum of the Masters Colorectal Pathway for a particular anchoring colorectal procedure will find relevant educational content in this SAGES Manual.

The editors have compiled a textbook with practical contributions from experts in the field. Each chapter provides detailed guidance on preoperative and periprocedural considerations for right and left elective and emergency colorectal resections, for both benign and malignant pathologies. Technical pearls and strategies to manage pitfalls and complications are also extensively reviewed along with detailed guidance for both laparoscopic and robotic procedures.

We are grateful to SAGES for its vision, leadership, and commitment to develop high-quality educational content to support practicing surgeons, fellows, and surgical residents in bridging the gap in adoption of MIS in colorectal surgery. We are extremely grateful to the members of the SAGES Colorectal Taskforce who have worked tirelessly on a very short timeline to provide expert content for this manual. Finally, we are thankful for this collaboration which has further strengthened our shared passion for surgical education and friendship. We are confident that *SAGES Manual of Colorectal Surgery* will provide a wealth of practical guidance to surgeons along their journey to progress from competency to mastery in various minimally invasive approaches to colorectal surgery.

Acknowledgments

We would like to thank Dr. Anthony D'Andrea for his assistance in editing the chapters. We would also like to thank Elizabeth Corra, Development Editor, for all of her expert guidance in completing this manual in a remarkably short period of time. Finally, we would like to thank Erin Schwartz from SAGES for her tireless support of and engagement with the Colorectal Task Force, which was instrumental to this project.

New York, NY, USA — Patricia Sylla
Los Angeles, CA, USA — Andreas M. Kaiser
New York, NY, USA — Daniel Popowich

Contents

Part VI Other Colorectal Resections and Advanced Techniques

Contributors

Alberto Arezzo, MD Department of Surgical Sciences, University of Torino, Torino, Italy

Ovunc Bardakcioglu, MD, FACS, FASCRS Division of Colorectal Surgery, Department of Surgery, University of Nevada at Las Vegas School of Medicine, Las Vegas, NV, USA

Anuradha R. Bhama, MD, FACS, FASCRS Department of Surgery, Division of Colorectal Surgery, Rush University Medical Center, Chicago, IL, USA

Marylise Boutros, MD Jewish General Hospital, Division of Colorectal Surgery, Montreal, QC, Canada

McGill University, Department of Surgery, Montreal, QC, Canada

Matthew T. Brady, MD Division of Colon and Rectal Surgery, Department of Surgery, University of California at Irvine, Orange, CA, USA

John Byrn, MD Division of Colorectal Surgery, Department of Surgery, University of Michigan, Ann Arbor, MI, USA

Lisa M. Cannon, MD University of Chicago, Chicago, IL, USA

Joseph C. Carmichael, MD Division of Colon and Rectal Surgery, Department of Surgery, University of California at Irvine, Orange, CA, USA

Antonio Caycedo-Marulanda, MD, MSc, FRCSC, FACS, FASCRS Health Sciences North, Department of General Surgery, Division of Colorectal Surgery, Northern Ontario School of Medicine, Sudbury, ON, Canada

Sami A. Chadi, MD, MSc, FRCSC, FACS Division of Surgical Oncology, Department of Surgery, University Health Network and Princess Margaret Hospital, Toronto, ON, Canada

University of Toronto, Department of Surgery, Toronto, ON, Canada

Melissa I. Chang, MD Saint Joseph Mercy Hospital Ann Arbor, Department of Surgery, Ypsilanti, MI, USA

Meagan Costedio, MD Department of Colorectal Surgery, Ahuja Medical Center of University Hospitals, Beachwood, OH, USA

Giovanni Dapri, MD, PhD, FACS Saint-Pierre University Hospital, European School of Laparoscopic Surgery, Department of Gastrointestinal Surgery, Brussels, Belgium

Digestive Clinic, Brussels, Belgium

Giovanna da Silva, MD Department of Colorectal Surgery, Cleveland Clinic Florida, Weston, FL, USA

Teresa deBeche-Adams, MD, FACS, FASCRS AdventHealth Orlando, Colorectal Surgery, Orlando, FL, USA

Conor P. Delaney, MD, MCh, PhD, FACS, FRCSI Digestive Disease and Surgery Institute, Cleveland Clinic, Cleveland, OH, USA

Samuel Eisenstein, MD University of California San Diego Health Systems, Department of Surgery, Division of Colon and Rectal Surgery, La Jolla, CA, USA

Fergal Fleming, MD, FRCSI Department of Colorectal Surgery, University of Rochester Medical Center, Rochester, NY, USA

James Fleshman, MD, FASCRS Baylor University Medical Center, Department of Surgery, Texas A & M Health Science Center, Dallas, TX, USA

Todd D. Francone, MD, MPH Newton/Wellesley Hospital, Newton, MA, USA

Massachusetts General Hospital, Boston, MA, USA

Tufts Medical University, Boston, MA, USA

Kelly A. Garrett, MD Weill Cornell Medicine/New York Presbyterian Hospital, Department of Surgery, Division of Colon and Rectal Surgery, New York, NY, USA

Alexander John Greenstein, MD, MPH Mount Sinai Hospital, Department of Surgery and Health Policy, New York, NY, USA

Ari Grinspan, MD Mount Sinai Hospital, The Dr. Henry D. Janowitz Division of Gastroenterology, New York, NY, USA

Icahn School of Medicine at Mount Sinai, The Dr. Henry D. Janowitz Division of Gastroenterology, New York, NY, USA

Alexis L. Grucela, MD New York University Langone Health, New York University, Department of Surgery, Division of Colon and Rectal Surgery, New York, NY, USA

Eric M. Haas, MD, FACS, FASCRS Division of Colon and Rectal Surgery, Houston Methodist Hospital, Department of Surgery, Houston, TX, USA

Alan E. Harzman, MD, FACS, FASCRS The Ohio State University, Department of Surgery, Columbus, OH, USA

Ohio State University Wexner Medical Center, Division of Colon and Rectal Surgery, Columbus, OH, USA

Alexander T. Hawkins, MD Vanderbilt University Medical Center, Department of General Surgery, Nashville, TN, USA

Dana M. Hayden, MD, MPH Division of Colon and Rectal Surgery, Rush University Medical Center, Department of General Surgery, Chicago, IL, USA

Amanda V. Hayman, MD, MPH, FACS, FASCRS The Oregon Clinic, Division of Gastrointestinal and Minimally Invasive Surgery, Oregon Health and Science University, Department of Surgery, Portland, OR, USA

Traci L. Hedrick, MD, MS University of Virginia Health System, Department of Surgery, Charlottesville, VA, USA

Stefan D. Holubar, MD, MS Department of Colon and Rectal Surgery, Cleveland Clinic Foundation, Cleveland, OH, USA

Syed Husain, MBBS, FACS, FASCRS Ohio State University Wexner Medical Center, Division of Colon and Rectal Surgery, Columbus, OH, USA

The Ohio State University, Department of Surgery, Columbus, OH, USA

Brian P. Jacob, MD Icahn School of Medicine at Mount Sinai, Department of Surgery, New York, NY, USA

Mehraneh D. Jafari, MD University of California, Irvine, Colon and Rectal Surgery, Orange, CA, USA

Daniel B. Jones, MD, MS Beth Israel Deaconess Medical Center; Harvard University Medical School, Boston, MA, USA

Deborah S. Keller, MS, MD Division of Colorectal Surgery, Department of Surgery, New York Presbyterian Hospital-Columbia University Medical Center, New York, NY, USA

Hermann Kessler, MD, PhD Cleveland Clinic, Department of Colorectal Surgery, Cleveland, OH, USA

David A. Kleiman, MD, MSc Division of Colon and Rectal Surgery, Lahey Hospital and Medical Center, Burlington, MA, USA

Tufts University School of Medicine, Boston, MA, USA

Kunal Kochar, MD, FACS University of Illinois at Chicago, Chicago, IL, USA

Advocate Lutheran General Hospital, Division of Colorectal Surgery, Park Ridge, IL, USA

Angela H. Kuhnen, MD, FACS, FASCRS Division of Colon and Rectal Surgery, Lahey Hospital and Medical Center, Burlington, MA, USA

Ron G. Landmann, MD, FACS, FASCRS Section of Colon and Rectal Surgery, Department of Surgical Oncology, Inflammatory Bowel Disease Center, Baptist-MD Anderson Cancer Center, Jacksonville, FL, USA

Steven A. Lee-Kong, MD New York Presbyterian Hospital, Columbia University, New York, NY, USA

Lawrence Lee, MD, PhD Department of Surgery, McGill University Health Centre, Montreal, QC, Canada

Jeremy M. Lipman, MD, FACS, FASCRS Cleveland Clinic, Lerner College of Medicine of Case Western Reserve University, Cleveland, OH, USA

Cleveland Clinic, Department of Colorectal Surgery, Cleveland, OH, USA

Peter W. Marcello, MD Lahey Hospital and Medical Center, Division of Colon and Rectal Surgery, Burlington, MA, USA

Slawomir Marecik, MD, FACS, FASCRS University of Illinois at Chicago, Chicago, IL, USA

Advocate Lutheran General Hospital, Division of Colorectal Surgery, Park Ridge, IL, USA

John H. Marks, MD Lankenau Medical Center, Department of Colon and Rectal Surgery, Wynnewood, PA, USA

Elisabeth C. McLemore, MD, FACS, FASCRS Kaiser Permanente Los Angeles Medical Center, Department of Surgery, Los Angeles, CA, USA

George Melich, MD, FRCSC Royal Columbian Hospital, Department of General Surgery, New Westminster, BC, Canada

University of British Columbia, Department of General Surgery, New Westminster, BC, Canada

Evangelos Messaris, MD, PhD Beth Israel Deaconess Medical Center, Department of Surgery, Harvard University Medical School, Boston, MA, USA

Marco Montorsi, MD Humanitas University, Humanitas Research Hospital, Rozzano, Italy

Matthew G. Mutch, MD Washington University School of Medicine, Department of Surgery, Section of Colon and Rectal Surgery, St. Louis, MO, USA

Garrett M. Nash, MD, MPH Department of Surgery, Memorial Sloan Kettering Cancer Center, Weill Cornell Medical College, New York, NY, USA

Izi Obokhare, MD, FACS, FICS Texas Tech University Health Sciences Center, Department of Surgery, Amarillo, TX, USA

Craig H. Olson, MD Clements University Hospital, University of Texas Southwestern, Dallas, TX, USA

Emmanouil Pappou, MD, PhD Department of Surgery, Memorial Sloan Kettering Cancer Center, Cornell University, New York, NY, USA

Ian M. Paquette, MD University of Cincinnati College of Medicine, Cincinnati, OH, USA

John J. Park, MD, FACS, FASCRS Chicago Medical School, Chicago, IL, USA

Advocate Lutheran General Hospital, Division of Colorectal Surgery, Park Ridge, IL, USA

Alessio Pigazzi, MD, PhD University of California, Irvine, Colon and Rectal Surgery, Orange, CA, USA

Barry Salky, MD, FACS Mount Sinai Hospital, Department of Surgery, New York, NY, USA

Julia T. Saraidaridis, MD, MMSC Lahey Hospital and Medical Center, Division of Colon and Rectal Surgery, Burlington, MA, USA

Linda Schultz, BS Society of American Gastrointestinal and Endoscopic Surgeons, Los Angeles, CA, USA

Virginia Oliva Shaffer, MD Emory University School of Medicine, Department of Surgery, Emory University Hospital, Atlanta, GA, USA

Mark Karam Soliman, MD, FACS, FASCRS Colon and Rectal Clinic of Florida, University of Florida, Orlando, FL, USA

Colorectal Surgery, AdventHealth Central Florida, Orlando, FL, USA

Emily Steinhagen, MD, FACS University Hospitals Cleveland Medical Center, Case Western Reserve University, Cleveland, OH, USA

Luca Stocchi, MD The Story-Garschina Chair in Colorectal Surgery, Cleveland Clinic Department of Colorectal Surgery, Digestive Disease and Surgery Institute, Cleveland, OH, USA

Konstantin Umanskiy, MD University of Chicago, Department of Surgery, Chicago, IL, USA

Elena Vikis, MD, FRCSC Royal Columbian Hospital, Department of General Surgery, New Westminster, BC, Canada

University of British Columbia, Department of General Surgery, New Westminster, BC, Canada

Martin R. Weiser, MD, FACS, FASCRS Department of Surgery, Stuart H.Q. Quan Chair in Colorectal Surgery, Vice Chair for Education and Faculty Development, Memorial Sloan Kettering Cancer Center, Cornell University, New York, NY, USA

Eric G. Weiss, MD, FACS, FASCRS, FACG Department of Colorectal Surgery, Cleveland Clinic Florida, Weston, FL, USA

Katerina Wells, MD, MPH Baylor University Medical Center, Department of Surgery, Texas A & M Health Science Center, Dallas, TX, USA

Steven D. Wexner, MD, PhD, FACS, FRCS, FRCS, FRCSI Cleveland Clinic Florida, Department of Colorectal Surgery, Weston, FL, USA

Cleveland Clinic Lerner College of Medicine of Case Western Reserve University, Cleveland, FL, USA

Charles E. Schmidt College of Medicine, Florida Atlantic University, Boca Raton, FL, USA

Herbert Wertheim College of Medicine, Florida International University, Miami, FL, USA

Mark H. Whiteford, MD The Oregon Clinic, PC, Gastrointestinal and Minimally Invasive Surgery Division, Providence Cancer Institute, Oregon Health and Science University, Portland, OR, USA

Albert M. Wolthuis, MD, PhD, FEBS, FASCRS, FACS University Hospital Leuven, Department of Abdominal Surgery, Catholic University Leuven, Leuven, Belgium

Heather Yeo, MD, MHS New York Presbyterian – Weill Cornell Medicine, Department of Surgery, New York, NY, USA

Tonia M. Young-Fadok, MD, MS, FACS, FASCRS Mayo Clinic College of Medicine, Division of Colon and Rectal Surgery, Phoenix, AZ, USA

Part I

Masters Program Anchoring Procedures

SAGES University MASTERS Program: Colorectal Pathway

1

Daniel B. Jones, Linda Schultz, and Brian P. Jacob

Introduction

The MASTERS Program organizes educational materials along clinical pathways into discrete blocks of content which will be accessible to surgeons at the SAGES annual meeting or logging into the online SAGES University (Fig. 1.1) [1]. The SAGES MASTERS Program currently includes 8 pathways: acute care, biliary, bariatrics, colorectal, foregut, hernia, flexible endoscopy, and robotic surgery (Fig. 1.2). Each pathway is divided into three levels of targeted performance: competency, proficiency, and mastery (Fig. 1.3). The levels originate from the Dreyfus model of skill acquisition [2], which has five stages: novice, advanced beginner, competency, proficiency, and expertise. The SAGES MASTERS Program is based on the three most advanced stages of skill acquisition: competency, proficiency, and expertise. Competency is defined as what a graduating general surgery chief resident or MIS fellow should be able to achieve; proficiency is what a surgeon approximately 3 years out from training should be able to accomplish; and mastery is what a more experienced surgeon should be able to accomplish after several years in practice.

Adapted with permission of Springer Nature from Jones, DB, Stefanidis D, Korndorffer JR, Dimick JB, Jacob BP, Schultz L, Scott DJ, SAGES University Masters Program: a structured curriculum for deliberate, lifelong learning. Surg Endoscopy, 2017;31(8):3061–71.

D. B. Jones (✉)
Beth Israel Deaconess Medical Center; Harvard University Medical School, Boston, MA, USA
e-mail: Djones1@bidmc.harvard.edu

L. Schultz
Society of American Gastrointestinal and Endoscopic Surgeons, Los Angeles, CA, USA
e-mail: linda@sages.org

B. P. Jacob
Icahn School of Medicine at Mount Sinai, Department of Surgery, New York, NY, USA

P. Sylla et al. (eds.), *The SAGES Manual of Colorectal Surgery*,
https://doi.org/10.1007/978-3-030-24812-3_1

Fig. 1.1 MASTERS Program logo

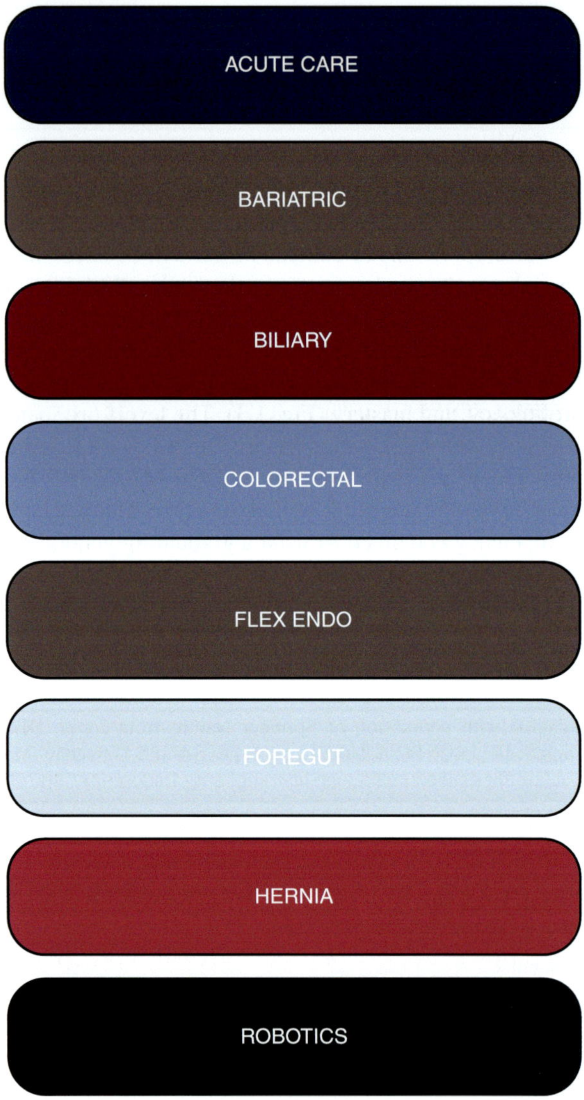

Fig. 1.2 MASTERS Program clinical pathways

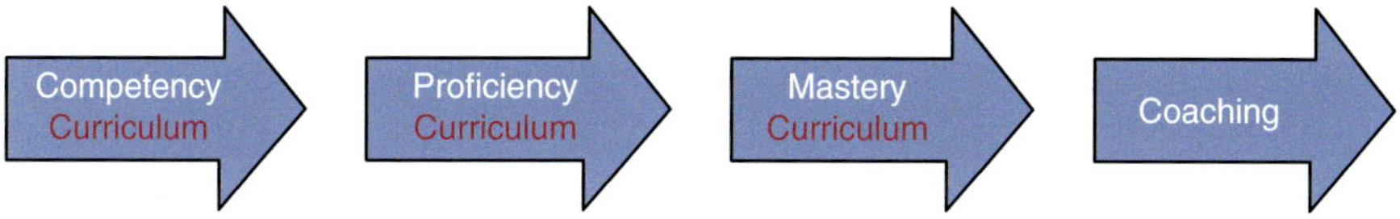

Fig. 1.3 MASTERS Program progression

Mastery is applicable to SAGES surgeons seeking in-depth knowledge in a pathway, including the following: areas of controversy, outcomes, best practice, and ability to mentor colleagues. Over time, with the utilization of coaching and participation in SAGES courses, this level should be obtainable by the majority of SAGES members. This edition of the SAGES Manual of Colorectal Surgery aligns with the current version of the new SAGES University MASTERS Program Colorectal Surgery Pathway (Table 1.1).

Colorectal Surgery Curriculum

The key elements of the Colorectal Surgery curriculum include core lectures for the pathway, which provide 45-minute general overview including basic anatomy, physiology, diagnostic work-up, and surgical management. As of 2018, all lecture contents of the annual SAGES meetings are labeled as follows: basic (100), intermediate (200), and advanced (300). This allows attendees to choose lectures that best fit their educational needs. Coding the content additionally facilitates online retrieval of specific educational material, with varying degrees of surgical complexity, ranging from introductory to revisional surgery.

SAGES identified the need to develop targeted complex content for its mastery level curriculum. The idea was that these 25-minute lectures would be focused on specific topics. It assumes that the attendee already has a good understanding of diseases and management from attending/watching competency and proficiency level lectures. Ideally, in order to supplement a chosen topic, the mastery lectures would also identify key prerequisite articles from *Surgical Endoscopy* and other journals, in addition to SAGES University videos. Many of these lectures will be forthcoming at future SAGES annual meetings.

The MASTERS Program has a self-assessment, multiple choice exam for each module to guide learner progression throughout the curriculum. Questions are submitted by core lecture speakers and SAGES annual meeting faculty. The goal of the questions is to use assessment for learning, with the assessment being criterion-referenced with the percent correct set at 80%. Learners will be able to review incorrect answers, review educational content, and retake the examination until a passing score is obtained.

In addition to this new edition of the SAGES Colorectal Surgery Manual, the MASTERS Program Colorectal Surgery curriculum taps much of the SAGES existing educational products including FLS®, FES™, FUSE™, SMART™, Top

Table 1.1 MASTERS Program colorectal curriculum outline

Curriculum elements	**Competency**
Anchoring procedure – Competency	2
Core lecture	1
Core MCE 70%	1
Annual meeting content	6
Guidelines	1
SA CME hours	6
Sentinel articles	2
Social media	2
SAGES top 21 video	1
FLS	12
Pearls	1
Credits	**35**
Curriculum elements	**Proficiency**
Anchoring procedure – Proficiency	2
Core lecture	1
Core MCE 70%	1
Annual meeting content	5
FUSE	12
Outcomes database enrollment	2
CME hours (SAGES or SAGES-endorsed)	6
Sentinel articles	2
Social media	2
SAGES top 21 video	1
Pearls	1
Credits	**35**
Curriculum elements	**Mastery**
Anchoring procedure – Mastery	2
Core lecture	1
CoreMCE 70%	1
Annual meeting content	6
Fundamentals of surgical coaching	4
Outcomes database reporting	2
CME credits (SAGES or SAGES-endorsed)	6
Sentinel articles	2
Serving as video assessment reviewer and Providing feedback (FSC)	4
Social media	7
SMART enhanced recovery	1
FES	9
Credits	**45**

21 videos, and Pearls (Fig. 1.4a–d). The Curriculum Task Force has placed the aforementioned modules along a continuum of the curriculum pathway. For example, FLS, in general, occurs during the Competency Curriculum, whereas the Fundamental Use of Surgical Energy (FUSE) is usually required during the Proficiency Curriculum. The Fundamentals of Laparoscopic Surgery (FLS) is a

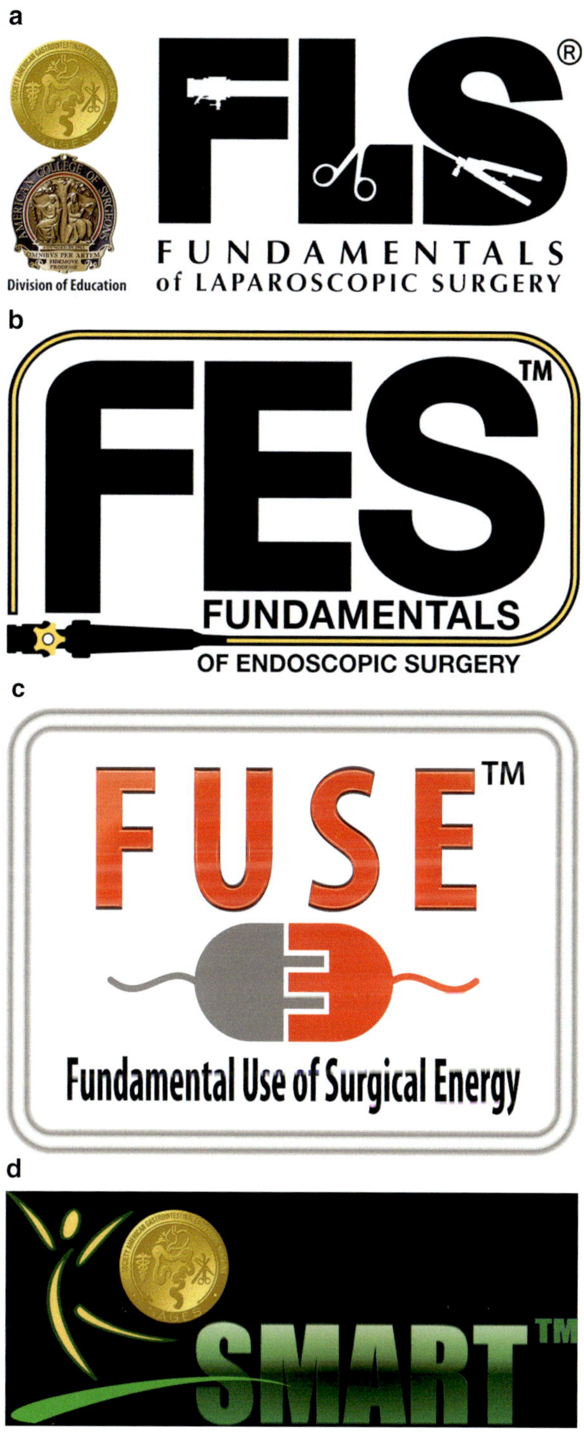

Fig. 1.4 (**a**–**d**) SAGES educational content: (**a**) FLS®; (**b**) FES™; (**c**) FUSE™; (**d**) SMART™. (Trademarks by SAGES)

multiple choice exam and a skills assessment conducted on a video box trainer. Tasks include peg transfer, cutting, intracorporeal and extracorporeal suturing, and knot tying. Since 2010, FLS has been required of all the US general surgery residents seeking to sit for the American Board of Surgery qualifying examinations. The Fundamentals of Endoscopic Surgery (FES) assesses endoscopic knowledge and technical skills in a simulator. FUSE teaches about the safe use of energy devices in the operating room and is available at FUSE.didactic.org. After, learners complete the self-paced modules, and they may take the certifying examination.

The SAGES Surgical Multimodal Accelerated Recovery Trajectory (SMART) Initiative combines minimally invasive surgical techniques with enhanced recovery pathways (ERPs) for perioperative care, with the goal of improving outcomes and patient satisfaction. Educational materials include a website with best practices, sample pathways, patient literature, and other resources such as videos, FAQs, and an implementation timeline. The materials assist surgeons and their surgical team with implementation of an ERP.

Top 21 videos are edited videos of the most commonly performed MIS operations and basic endoscopy. Cases are straightforward with quality video and clear anatomy.

Pearls are step-by-step video clips of ten operations. The authors show different variations for each step. The learner should have a fundamental understanding of the operation.

SAGES Guidelines provide evidence-based recommendations for surgeons and are developed by the SAGES Guidelines Committee following the Health and Medicine Division of the National Academies of Sciences, Engineering, and Medicine standards (formerly the Institute of Medicine) for guideline development [3]. Each clinical practice guideline has been systematically researched, reviewed, and revised by the SAGES Guidelines Committee and an appropriate multidisciplinary team. The strength of the provided recommendations is determined based on the quality of the available literature using the GRADE methodology [4]. SAGES Guidelines cover a wide range of topics relevant to the practice of SAGES surgeon members and are updated on a regular basis. Since the developed guidelines provide an appraisal of the available literature, their inclusion in the MASTERS Program was deemed necessary by the group.

The Curriculum Task Force identified the need to select required readings for the MASTERS Program based on key articles for the various curriculum procedures. Summaries of each of these articles follow the American College of Surgeons (ACS) Selected Readings format.

Facebook™ Groups

While there are many great platforms available to permit online collaboration by user-generated content, Facebook™ offers a unique, highly developed mobile platform that is ideal for global professional collaboration and daily continuing surgical education (Fig. 1.5a, b). These Facebook groups allow for video assessment, feedback, and coaching as a tool to improve practice.

Based on the anchoring procedures determined via group consensus (Table 1.2), participants in the MASTERS Program will submit video clips on closed Facebook groups, with other participants and/or SAGES members providing qualitative feedback. For example, for the colorectal competency pathway, surgeons would submit the critical steps during a laparoscopic right colectomy such as identification of the duodenum or mobilization of the ileocolic vessels. Using crowdsourcing, other surgeons would comment and provide feedback.

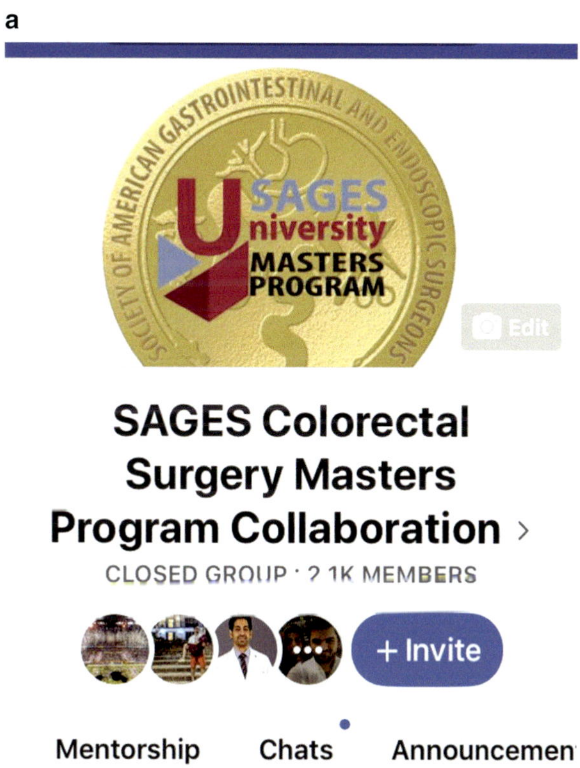

Fig. 1.5 (**a**, **b**) Colorectal Surgery Facebook™ Group. (Trademark by Facebook)

Fig. 1.5 Continued

b

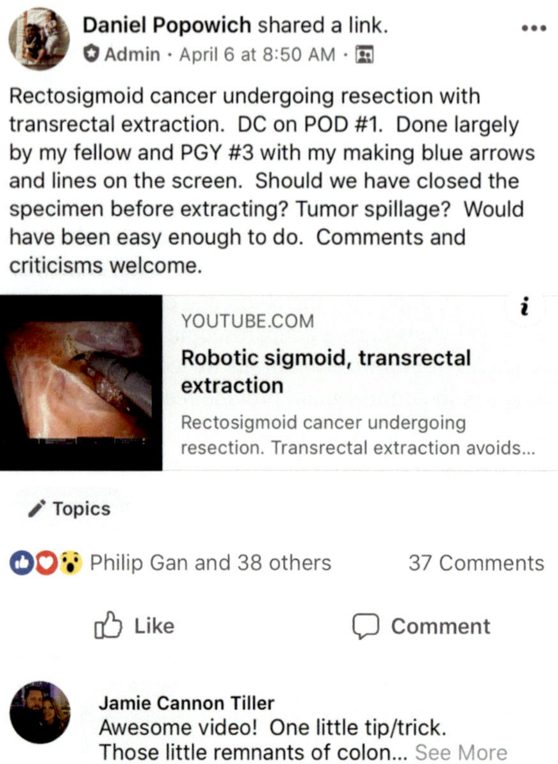

Table 1.2 Colorectal surgery anchoring procedures by pathway

Anchoring procedure by pathway	Level
Colorectal surgery	
Laparoscopic right colectomy	Competency
Laparoscopic simple left colectomy	Proficiency
Laparoscopic complex left colectomy	Mastery

Eight uniquely vetted membership-only closed Facebook groups were created for the MASTERS Program, including a group for bariatrics, hernia, colorectal, biliary, acute care, flexible endoscopy, robotics, and foregut. The Colorectal Surgery Facebook group is independent of the other groups and will be populated only by physicians, mostly surgeons or surgeons in training interested in colorectal surgery. The group provides an international platform for surgeons and healthcare providers interested in optimizing outcomes in a surgical specialty to collaborate, share, discuss, and post photos, videos, and anything related to a chosen specialty. By embracing social media as a collaborative forum, we can more effectively and transparently obtain immediate global feedback that can potentially improve patient outcomes, as well as the quality of care we provide, all while transforming the way a society's members interact.

For the first two levels of the MASTERS Colorectal Surgery Program, Competency, and Proficiency, participants will be required to post videos of the anchoring procedures and will receive qualitative feedback from other participants. However, for the mastery level, participants will submit unedited videos to be evaluated by an expert panel. A standardized video assessment tool, depending on the specific procedure, will be used. A benchmark will also be utilized to determine when the participant has achieved the mastery level for that procedure.

Once the participant has achieved mastery level, they will participate as a coach by providing feedback to participants in the first two levels. MASTERS Program participants will therefore need to learn the fundamental principles of surgical coaching. The key activities of coaching include goal setting, active listening, powerful inquiry, and constructive feedback [5, 6]. Importantly, peer coaching is much different than traditional education, where there is an expert and a learner. Peer coaching is a "co-learning" model where the coach is facilitating the development of the coachee by using inquiry (i.e., open-ended questions) in a noncompetitive manner.

Surgical coaching skills are a crucial part of the MASTERS curriculum. At the 2017 SAGES Annual Meeting, a postgraduate course on coaching skills was developed and video recorded. The goal is to develop a "coaching culture" within the SAGES MASTERS Program, wherein both participants and coaches are committed to lifelong learning and development.

The need for a more structured approach to the education of practicing surgeons as accomplished by the SAGES MASTERS Program is well recognized [7]. Since performance feedback usually stops after training completion and current approaches to MOC are suboptimal, the need for peer coaching has recently received increased attention in surgery [5, 6]. SAGES has recognized this need, and its MASTERS Program embraces social media for surgical education to help provide a free, mobile, and easy to use platform to surgeons globally. Access to the MASTERS Program groups enables surgeons at all levels to partake in the MASTERS Program curriculum and obtain feedback from peers, mentors, and experts. By creating surgeon-only private groups dedicated to this project, SAGES can now offer surgeons posting in these groups the ability to discuss preoperative, intraoperative (even during live feed), and postoperative issues with other SAGES colleagues and mentors. In addition, the platform permits transparent and responsive dialogue about technique, continuing the theme of deliberate, lifelong learning.

To accommodate the needs of this program, SAGES University is upgrading its web-based features. A new learning management system (LMS) will track progression and make access to SAGES University simple. Features of the new IT infrastructure will provide the ability to access a video or lecture on demand in relation to content, level of difficulty, and author. Once enrolled in the MASTERS Program, the LMS will track lectures, educational products, MCE, and other completed requirements. Participants will be able to see where they stand in relation to module completion, and SAGES will alert learners to relevant content they may be interested in pursuing. Until such time that the new LMS is up and running, it is hoped that the SAGES Manual will help guide learners through the MASTERS Program Curriculum.

Conclusion

The SAGES MASTERS Program Colorectal Surgery Pathway facilitates deliberate, focused postgraduate teaching and learning. The MASTERS Program certifies completion of the curriculum but is not meant to certify competency, proficiency, or mastery of surgeons. The MASTERS Program embraces the concept of continued learning after fellowship, and its curriculum is organized from basic principles to more complex content. The MASTERS Program is an innovative, voluntary curriculum that supports MOC and deliberate, lifelong learning.

References

1. Jones DB, Stefanidis D, Korndorffer JR, Dimick JB, Jacob BP, Schultz L, et al. SAGES University Masters Program: a structured curriculum for deliberate, lifelong learning. Surg Endoscopy. 2017;31(8):3061–71.
2. Dreyfus SE. The five-stage model of adult skill acquisition. Bull Sci Technol Soc. 2004;24:177–81.
3. Graham R, Mancher M, Miller Woman D, Greenfield S, Steinberg E, Institute of Medicine (US) Committee on Standards for Developing Trustworthy Clinical Practice Guidelines. Clinical practice guidelines we can trust. Washington, D.C.: National Academies Press (US); 2011.
4. Guyatt GH, Oxman AD, Vist GE, Kunz R, Falck-Ytter Y, Alonso-Coello P, et al. GRADE: an emerging consensus on rating quality of evidence and strength of recommendations. BMJ. 2008;336:924–6.
5. Greenberg CC, Ghousseini HN, Pavuluri Quamme SR, Beasley HL, Wiegmann DA. Surgical coaching for individual performance improvement. Ann Surg. 2015;261:32–4.
6. Greenberg CC, Dombrowski J, Dimick JB. Video-based surgical coaching: an emerging approach to performance improvement. JAMA Surg. 2016;151:282–3.
7. Sachdeva AK. Acquiring skills in new procedures and technology: the challenge and the opportunity. Arch Surg. 2005;140:387–9.

Masters Program Colorectal Pathway: Laparoscopic Right Colectomy for Benign Disease

2

Tonia M. Young-Fadok

Introduction and Rationale

Being able to perform mobilization, resection, and reestablishment of bowel continuity for right colectomy is an essential set of skills for all general surgeons who perform colon and rectal procedures [1].

In basic terms, laparoscopic colorectal surgery can be broken down into three anatomic building blocks: mobilization of the right colon; mobilization of the left/sigmoid colon; and mobilization with transection of the rectum. Completion of each of these blocks results in that segment of the colon or rectum becoming a mobile midline structure which can then be exteriorized through a periumbilical or other suitable incision.

Of these three essential building blocks, right colectomy is widely considered to be technically the easiest to learn, and the procedure has the best safety profile in terms of having the lowest anastomotic leak rate compared with either sigmoid resection or rectal resection. This chapter focuses on right colectomy for benign disease in order to establish basic principles. The presumption is that benign disease is easy for the novice laparoscopic surgeon and safe for the patient [2]. The provisos are that the two commonest indications (polyp and Crohn's disease) are not complex examples of the cases for those early in the learning curve, i.e., that a right colon polyp is not clinically suspicious for a malignancy or that ileocolic Crohn's disease is not associated with fistulas or a phlegmon. Much less common examples of benign right-sided disease include diverticular disease and cecal volvulus.

T. M. Young-Fadok (✉)
Mayo Clinic College of Medicine, Division of Colon and Rectal Surgery, Phoenix, AZ, USA
e-mail: Youngfadok.tonia@mayo.edu

P. Sylla et al. (eds.), *The SAGES Manual of Colorectal Surgery*,
https://doi.org/10.1007/978-3-030-24812-3_2

Indications and Contraindications

The commonest indication for right colon resection is neoplasia of the right colon, which includes right colon cancer and right-sided polyps. Resection of the right colon for known malignancy is covered in a separate chapter. Although polyps of the right colon that are too large to be resected endoscopically should also be considered to harbor a risk of cancer and an oncologic resection should be performed, polyps thought to be at low risk for harboring malignancy are generally felt to be a safe model for the novice laparoscopic surgeon.

The next commonest indication is ileocolic Crohn's disease [3]. Early in the learning curve, it is wise to avoid complex Crohn's disease with multiple fistulas or a tethered phlegmon, but simple ileocolic disease is an excellent model for early experience. Knowledge of how to mobilize the right colon and transect the mesentery is also necessary for more extensive colorectal procedures including total colectomy or proctocolectomy for indications such as Crohn's colitis, ulcerative colitis, colonic polyposis syndromes, and colonic inertia.

Other general contraindications to a laparoscopic approach, not related to the specific procedure, also apply, such as marked colonic or small-bowel distention precluding attainment of an adequate pneumoperitoneum; levels of obesity that can also prevent an adequate working space; hemodynamic instability; and intestinal perforation with multiloculated pus or fecal peritonitis. A relative contraindication, dependent on the experience of the surgeon, is advanced tumor with involvement of adjacent organs requiring en bloc resection.

Principles and Quality Benchmarks

Whatever the indication for right colectomy, establishment of the landmarks is critical for a safe procedure. Mobilization of the right colon is the simplest of the three building blocks described above. It introduces skills such as recognition of the retroperitoneal plane and identification of the right ureter, inferior vena cava (IVC), and duodenum and incorporates decision-making regarding delineation of the vasculature and where it should be divided.

The primary distinction between resection for benign disease and resection for malignant disease is that oncologic principles are not in force. For right colon cancer, an oncologic operation requires specific margins of bowel resection, high ligation of the vascular pedicles, and an intact mesenteric envelope to ensure adequate lymph node harvest. In benign disease, e.g., Crohn's ileocolitis, resection margins are determined by the extent of disease, and transection of the mesentery can be a "division of convenience," i.e., dividing the colon where the division is most easily achieved without the potential additional dissection and exposure required for proximal ligation of vascular pedicles.

Another principle in oncologic resection is maintenance of an intact mesentery and standard extent of lymphadenectomy to meet current guidelines for lymph node harvest, and this is captured in the concept of complete mesocolic excision (CME).

During mobilization of the colon, this means in essence remaining in the correct embryologically defined anatomical plane that separates the retroperitoneum from the colon. This is a bloodless plane, and staying in this plane protects the ureter, inferior vena cava (IVC), and duodenum. It is therefore recommended to use this dissection plane also for benign disease, even though there is no oncologic necessity as in a cancer case.

There are no benchmarks specific to the performance of right colectomy for benign disease. However, resection margins for large polyps with a risk of cancer should be identical to a cancer operation. In Crohn's disease the standard of care is to resect to macroscopically and palpably normal bowel.

Preoperative Planning, Patient Workup, and Optimization

As with all patients being considered for an operation, the diagnosis should be reviewed and confirmed. If necessary, further expert opinions should be sought regarding the need for resection, e.g., the role of an adjusted medication regimen in Crohn's disease, or repeated colonoscopic evaluation of a large polyp if the Paris classification were not reported on the original procedure. The location of pathology should be confirmed as far as possible preoperatively, with tattooing, CT imaging, etc. to avoid the need for intraoperative colonoscopy unless the latter is considered part of the procedure (e.g., combined endoscopic resection/laparoscopic visualization of a polyp).

All patients undergoing elective resection of the colon should undergo a general workup to optimize their condition for an operation in addition to the appropriate workup for the specific disease entity. It is now standard of care that specific entities are addressed or corrected for preoperative patient optimization: anemia, poor blood sugar control, malnutrition, smoking, and excessive alcohol use. If time allows, consideration should also be given to preconditioning of the deconditioned patient. The reader is also referred to the relevant chapters on checklist for patients in preparation for laparoscopic colorectal surgery (Chap. 9) and enhanced recovery protocols in colorectal surgery (Chaps. 7 and 8) [4].

Operative Setup

Operating Room Setup

Careful placement of the video screens, insufflator, and light source is required to maximize access to the abdomen and minimize entanglement of cords (Fig. 2.1). The primary view screen is generally on the right side of the patient, with the subsidiary screen on the left. Some ORs will have ceiling-mounted booms that carry the equipment and make this planning simpler. In ORs with cart-mounted equipment, one must anticipate that the surgeon and camera assistant will both need to be on the left side of the patient, facing the right colon, and the bank of equipment needs to be

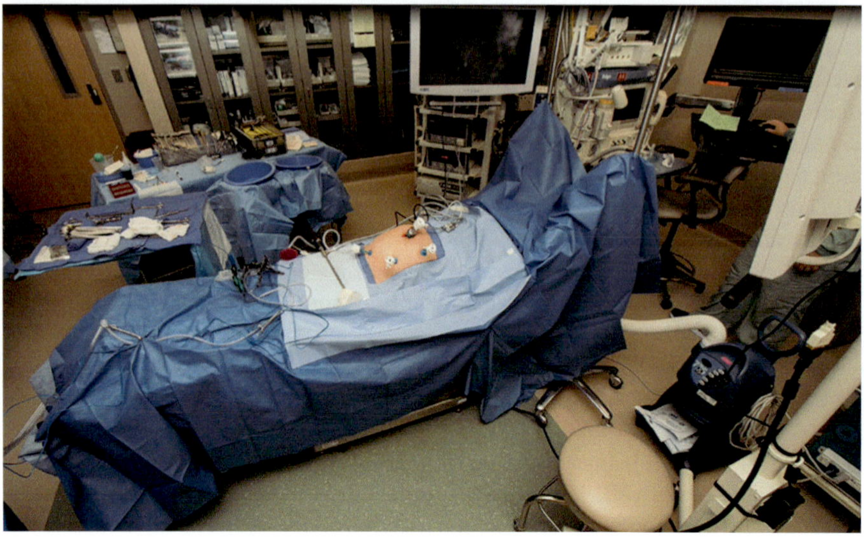

Fig. 2.1 Operating room setup

able to move between the patient's hip and shoulder in order to maintain the desirable straight line between the surgeon's hands, operative site, and screen, as this helps to minimize surgeon fatigue.

Patient Positioning

Steep position changes are often necessary to facilitate exposure and move small bowel out of the operative field, and it is imperative to prevent slipping. The patient is usually placed in the supine position, on egg crate foam secured to the OR table, or other mechanism to prevent the patient moving during steep position changes. A draw sheet is placed beneath the patient, and behind the foam to maximize patient contact with the foam, to then allow the sheet to be wrapped around the patient's arms to align them alongside the patient after padding of the hands. Alternatively, a combined synchronous position with the patient in low stirrups can be considered to allow for the surgeon to be positioned between the legs to facilitate access during mobilization of the hepatic flexure. This is helpful when mobilization of the hepatic flexure is more complex than usual (phlegmon/large mass at the hepatic flexure, obesity) or if intraoperative endoscopy is anticipated. In this case, the patient's thighs should be flat and aligned with the patient's abdomen to prevent interference of the patient's knees during the use of lower abdominal trocars. During the main portion of the case, both surgeon and assistant will need to be on the left side of the patient, facing the right colon. Preferably, both arms are tucked at the patient's sides, or at least the left arm should be tucked alongside the patient.

Operative Technique: Surgical Steps

There are, quite simply, two approaches to the right colon. One either chooses lateral-to-medial [5] or medial-to-lateral. Multiple other approaches have been described including inferior upwards and top-down from the hepatic flexure. This does not change the fact that there are basically two approaches. The lateral-to-medial approach uses the right lateral peritoneal reflection as a marker for entering the correct retroperitoneal plane. The medial-to-lateral approach starts by isolating the base of the ileocolic pedicle and using this as an entry into the retroperitoneal plane.

This chapter will focus on the technique of extracorporeal creation of the anastomosis following resection. The techniques for intracorporeal anastomosis are covered in a separate chapter.

Trocar Placement

Insertion of trocars should be adapted to the case.

In the most simple cases, i.e., limited ileocolic resection in the patient with BMI <30, it is possible to fully mobilize the right colon and exteriorize it through a periumbilical incision, without needing to divide either the mesentery or the bowel intracorporeally. A triangular configuration, facing the right colon, uses umbilical, suprapubic, and left lower quadrant port sites.

In the event that the case is not simple, requiring an additional port either to divide the mesentery or to mobilize a phlegmon, an additional fourth trocar is placed (Fig. 2.2). This can be positioned in the right lower quadrant or the left upper quadrant, where an instrument through this port is generally deployed by the camera holder.

Mobilization of the Right Colon

Lateral-to-Medial Dissection (Table 2.1)

The main aim of this approach is full mobilization of the right colon to the midline. This makes the right colon a midline structure and allows choices regarding ligation of the vasculature and transection of the mesentery [6].

Classically in this approach, the patient is first placed in Trendelenburg position with the right side inclined up. The right lateral peritoneal reflection alongside the cecum and ascending colon is identified and scored. My preference is for an electrocautery device rather than a bipolar device which when used inappropriately can enter a nonanatomic plane. Once the correct retroperitoneal plane is identified, the cecum is gently swept medially, and the ureter is identified and protected (Fig. 2.3a, b). With the cecum under tension, which means retracting it medially and cephalad, the medial peritoneal reflection alongside the distal terminal ileum can be entered, and the terminal ileal mesentery can be mobilized off of the retroperitoneum.

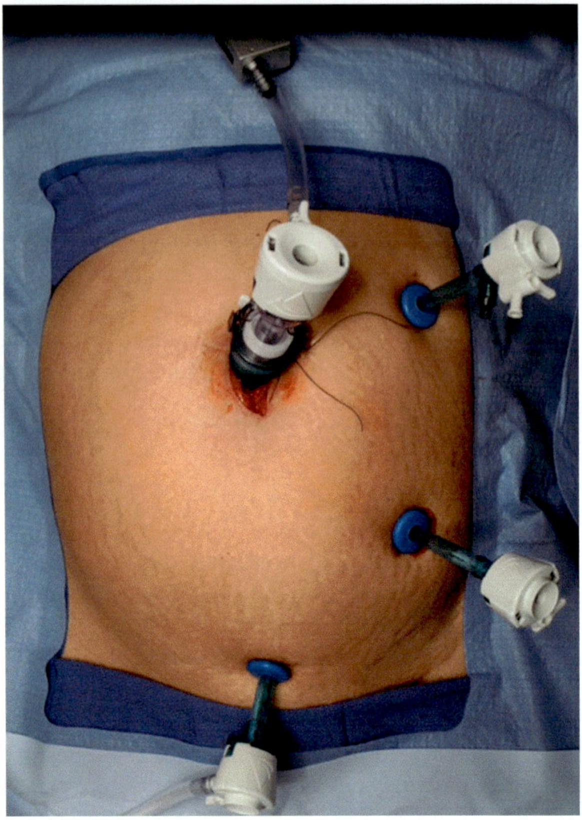

Fig. 2.2 Trocar placement

The right lateral peritoneum alongside the ascending colon is exposed by retracting the ascending colon towards the midline. The anterior surface of Gerota's fascia should remain intact (Figs. 2.4 and 2.5). The dissection can be continued towards the liver (Fig. 2.6). In a patient with a BMI <30, the ascending colon can be mobilized to the midline, releasing its attachments from the duodenum and allowing visualization of the mesenteric window cephalad to the ileocolic pedicle (Fig. 2.7). In patients of higher BMI, this particular view may not be visible until the mobilization of the hepatic flexure is completed.

The operative table should then be placed in reverse Trendelenburg still with the OR table inclined right side up. The hepatocolic attachments at the hepatic flexure should be identified. These can be better delineated by gently lifting them up noting the movement of the superficial tissues over the underlying retroperitoneal plane. This will help to identify the plane of transection which can be developed between the retroperitoneal plane and the hepatocolic attachments (Fig. 2.8). These attachments often have small blood vessels, and here a vessel sealing device can be helpful (Fig. 2.9).

Table 2.1 Steps for lateral-to-medial right colectomy

Step	Patient position
Survey of peritoneal cavity	Neutral
Mobilize cecum and ascending colon 1. Identify RLQ landmarks: Cecum, right ureter 2. Incise peritoneum around base of cecum and mobilize cecum medially 3. Incise right lateral peritoneal reflection, mobilize ascending colon medially 4. Confirm identification of right ureter, IVC, inferior portion of duodenum	Trendelenburg, right side inclined up
Mobilize hepatic flexure 1. Elevate hepatocolic attachments and identify duodenum 2. Divide hepatocolic attachments 3. Join dissection with the lateral dissection already performed 4. Divide right branch of middle colic vessels if required	Reverse Trendelenburg, right side inclined up
Transection of mesentery 1. Place mobilized right colon back in anatomic position and elevate to expose base of ileocolic pedicle 2. Open mesenteric windows cephalad and caudad 3. Identified duodenum via cephalad window 4. Divide vascular pedicle 5. Divide remaining mesentery 6. Divide R branch of middle colic vessels if not already done and required	Neutral horizontal position, right side inclined up
Exteriorization and anastomosis 1. Deflate pneumoperitoneum via trocars 2. Extract colon via chosen extraction site using wound protector 3. Resect and create anastomosis per preferred technique 4. Return anastomosis to abdominal cavity 5. Remove ports and check for hemostasis	Neutral

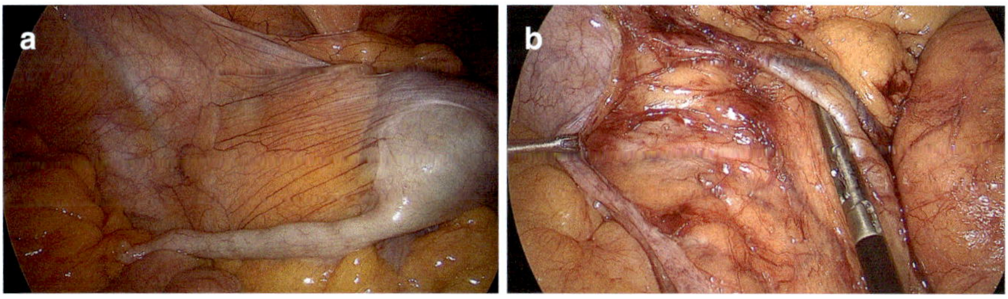

Fig. 2.3 (**a**) Cecum, and right ureter covered by peritoneum. (**b**) Cecum, and right ureter exposed after peritoneum incised

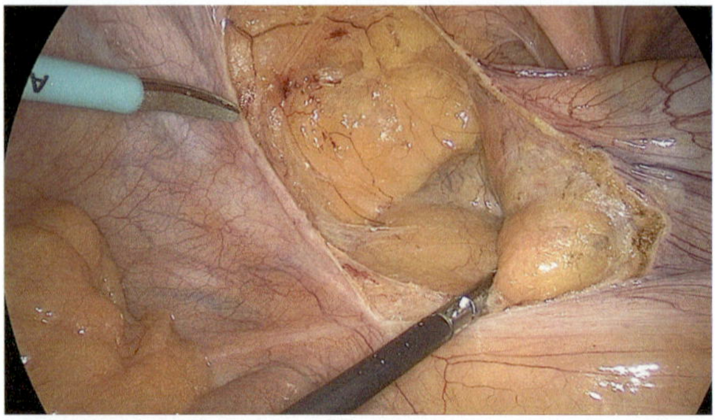

Fig. 2.4 Gerota's fascia inferior portion

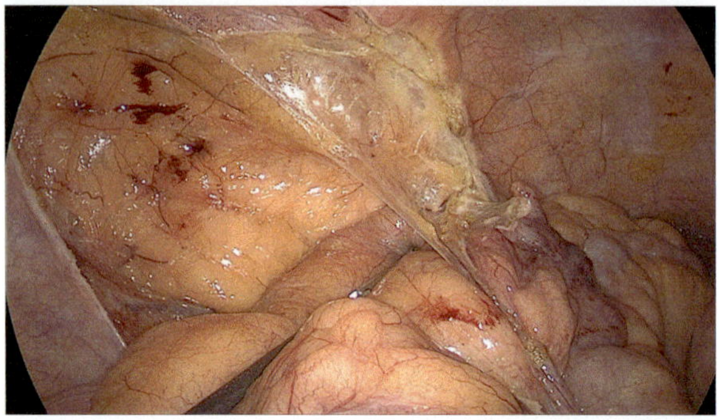

Fig. 2.5 Gerota's fascia mid portion

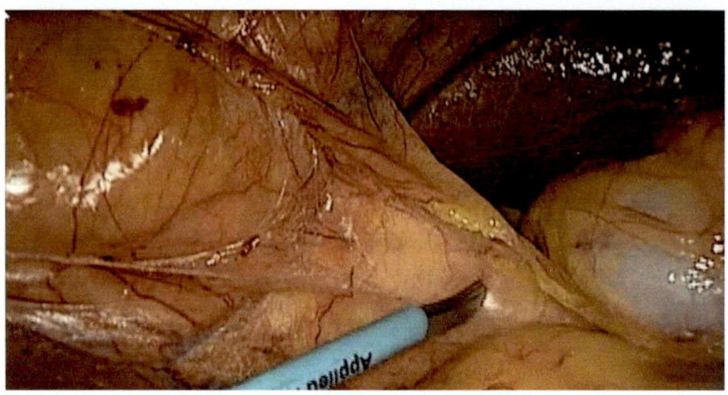

Fig. 2.6 Right lateral peritoneal reflection at hepatic flexure

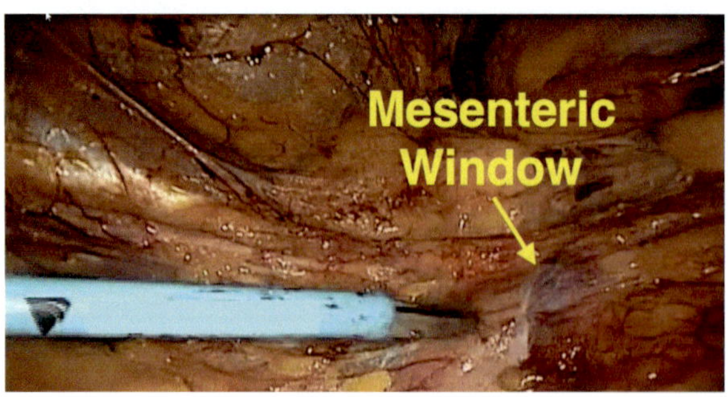

Fig. 2.7 Mesenteric window cephalad to the ileocolic pedicle

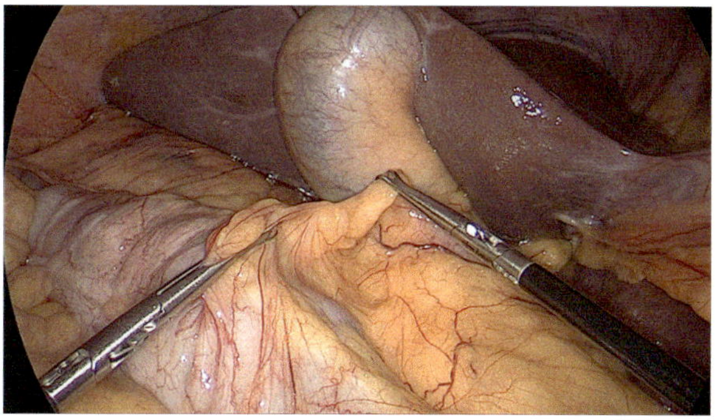

Fig. 2.8 Developing the plane beneath the hepatocolic attachments

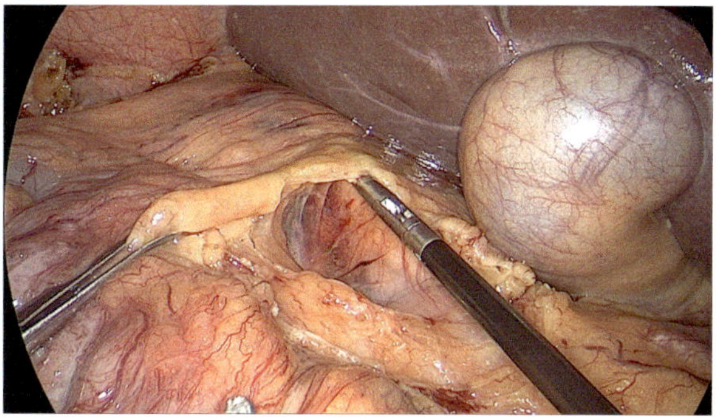

Fig. 2.9 Division of hepatocolic attachments

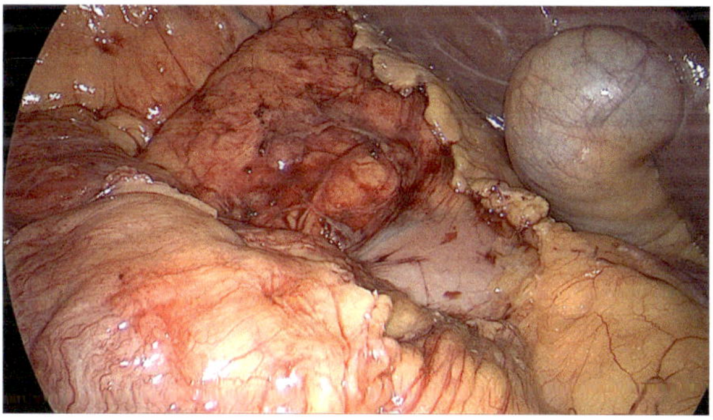

Fig. 2.10 Duodenum at hepatic flexure

It is helpful to determine the most medial desired point of mobilization of the transverse colon and start by elevating the hepatic colic attachments here. The plane can be entered and the hepatic colic attachments divided, working laterally towards the dissection which has already been done from the lateral aspect. During this dissection, the duodenum should be identified and protected (Fig. 2.10).

For a right colon cancer, at this point the base of the ileocolic pedicle and the right branch of the middle colic vessels can be clearly delineated, and the association of the latter with the pancreatic inferior margin can likewise be confirmed (Fig. 2.11) [6]. The right branch of the middle colic artery can be divided at this

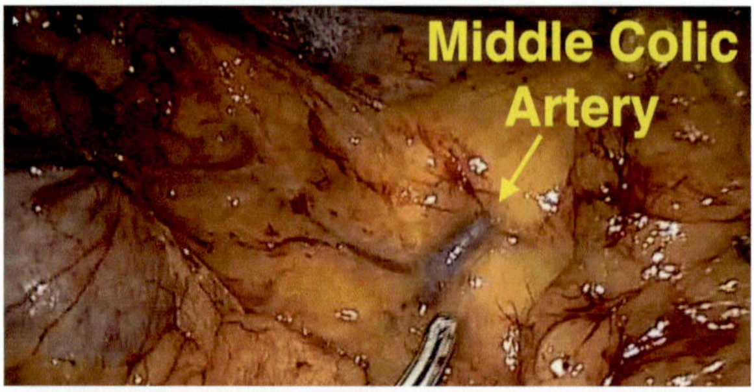

Fig. 2.11 Base of the middle colic artery and duodenum

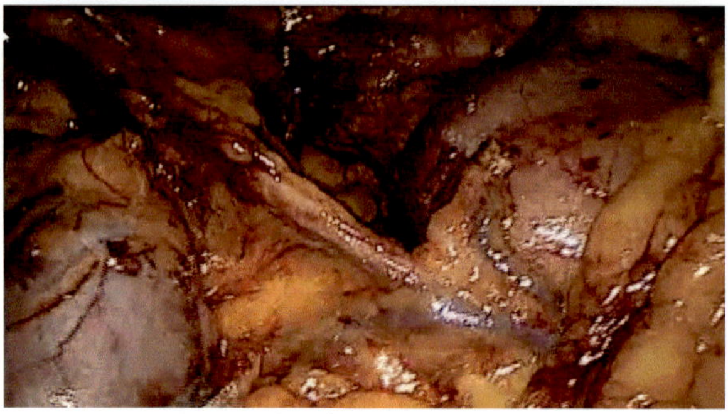

Fig. 2.12 Right branch of middle colic artery

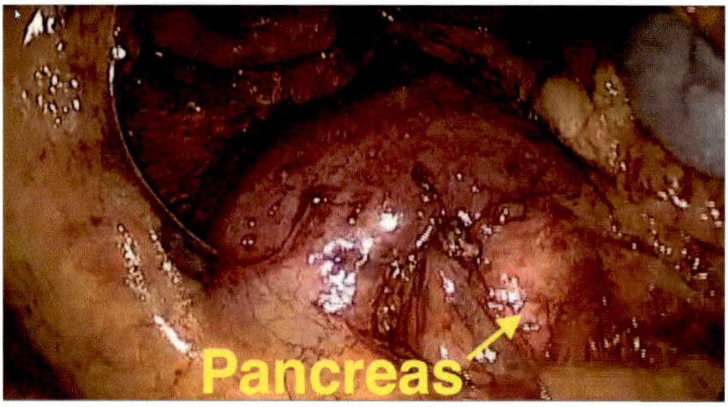

Fig. 2.13 Duodenum and pancreas seen through cephalad mesenteric window

point, with the patient still in reverse Trendelenburg while viewing the hepatic flexure from above (Fig. 2.12).

The patient can then be placed in a neutral horizontal position while still maintaining the right side inclined upwards. The fat pad at the ileocolic pedicle is placed under tension and elevated after laying the colon back in its normal anatomic position, which allows visualization of the entire medial aspect of the mesentery. The remaining peritoneum of the mesenteric windows cephalad and caudad to the base of the ileocolic pedicle is scored, and the base of the ileocolic pedicle is isolated. After confirming the position of the duodenum through the cephalad window (Fig. 2.13), the ileocolic pedicle may be divided at the level of the lateral border of the duodenum. In benign disease, high ligation near the origin of the superior mesenteric vein (SMV) is not indicated.

Proponents of this approach indicate the ease of identifying the correct retroperitoneal plane and the ability to mobilize the right colon to the midline.

Medial-to-Lateral Dissection (Table 2.2)

The first step is putting the ileocolic pedicle under tension by grasping the fat pad on the medial aspect of the mesentery adjacent to the ileocecal junction (Fig. 2.14). This exposes the two mesenteric windows, one cephalad above the ileocolic pedicle and the other caudad and inferior to the ileocolic pedicle. In patients with BMI <30,

Table 2.2 Steps for medial-to-lateral right colectomy

Step	Patient position
Survey of peritoneal cavity	Neutral
Isolate and divide ileocolic pedicle	Neutral horizontal position, right side inclined up
1. Place ileocolic pedicle under tension	
2. Identify mesenteric widows cephalad and caudad	
3. Score peritoneum over base of pedicle	
4. Identify retroperitoneum and isolate base of pedicle (and right colic if present)	
5. Divide pedicle	
Mobilize cecum and ascending colon	Neutral horizontal position, right side inclined up
1. Continue dissection in retroperitoneal plane to peritoneal attachments laterally, inferiorly, and superiorly	
2. Confirm identification of gonadal vessels, right ureter, IVC, inferior portion of duodenum	
3. Divide remaining mesentery	
4. Divide inferior and lateral peritoneal attachments	
Mobilize hepatic flexure	Reverse Trendelenburg, right side inclined up
1. Divide remaining hepatocolic attachments and identify duodenum	
2. Isolate and divide right branch of middle colic vessels if required	
Exteriorization and anastomosis	Neutral
1. Deflate pneumoperitoneum via trocars	
2. Extract colon via chosen extraction site using wound protector	
3. Resect and create anastomosis per preferred technique	
4. Return anastomosis to abdominal cavity	
5. Remove ports and check for hemostasis	

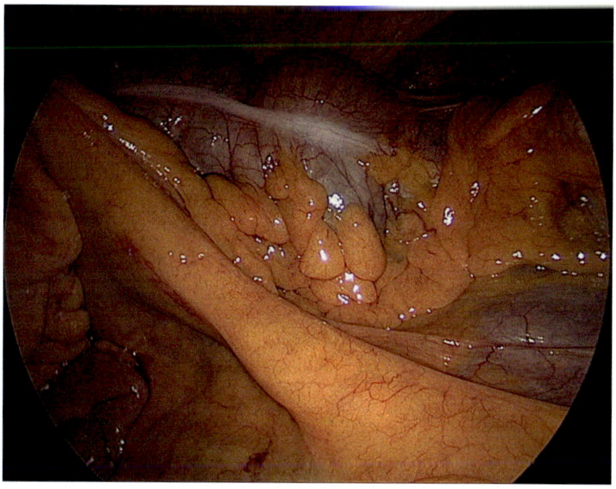

Fig. 2.14 Exposure of the medial aspect of the ascending colon mesentery and the base of the ileocolic pedicle

the duodenum can be visualized through the cephalad mesenteric window, and a transverse line of dissection can be estimated across the base of the ileocolic pedicle, in line with the lateral margin of the duodenum (Fig. 2.15). In the heavier patient (BMI >30), the anatomy is often difficult to discern. After a transverse scoring incision is made across the medial peritoneum of the right colon, over the estimated base of the ileocolic pedicle; careful dissection is employed to achieve two aims: isolation of the base of the ileocolic pedicle and identification of the retroperitoneal plane by using gentle sweeping actions to elevate the posterior aspect of the mesentery off the retroperitoneum. Once the base of the ileocolic pedicle is identified, the vein and artery can be dissected separately and divided using an electrocautery device (Fig. 2.16). For benign disease, the artery and vein can often be divided together using an advanced energy or stapling device. Many surgeons also prefer the addition of an endoloop to confirm control of the vascular supply.

Dissection then continues in the correct retroperitoneal plane, sweeping the right ureter, IVC, gonadal vessel, and duodenum posteriorly while elevating the right colon and extending the plane of dissection to the right lateral peritoneal reflection. The mesenteric transection is carried towards the chosen proximal margin in the distal ileum and also towards the chosen distal resection margin in the colon. Full mobilization is extended laterally to the right lateral peritoneal reflection which is then also divided. As entry into this plane is somewhat by trial and error, without the landmark provided by the right lateral peritoneal reflection, videos of this approach tend to have a more bloody exposure, other than in expert hands. In patients with

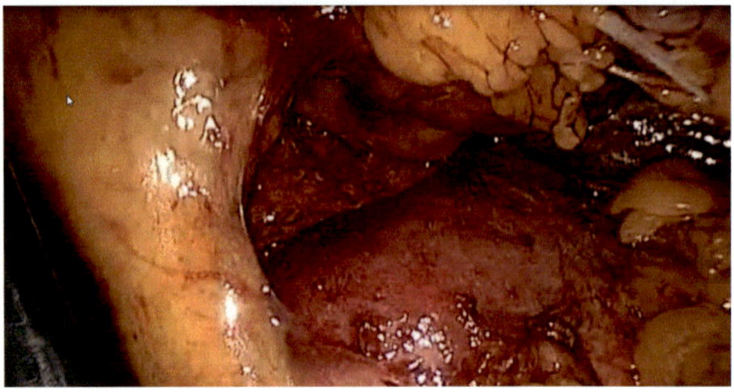

Fig. 2.15 Duodenum seen after opening mesenteric window cephalad to the base of the ileocolic pedicle

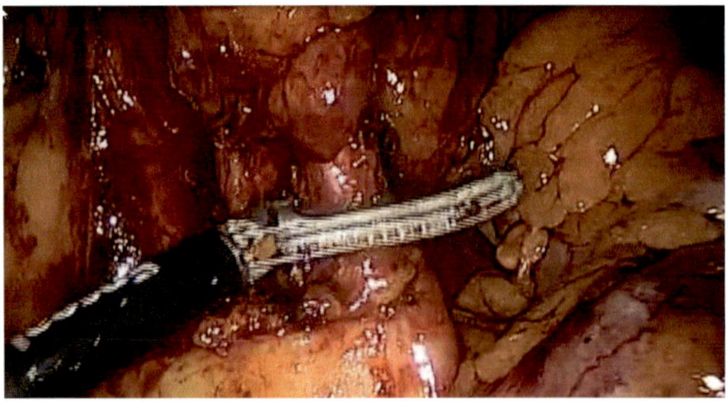

Fig. 2.16 Division of ileocolic artery

Crohn's disease, division of the mesentery can be challenging due to marked thickening and also friability if steroids have been used. Transection of the mesentery may be safer near the base of the ileocolic pedicle where mesenteric thickening is less prominent, or the mesentery may be more safely approached extracorporeally after exteriorization of the mobilized right colon.

Proponents of this approach indicate early vascular control as an important feature. The lymph node harvest may be greater [7] although the oncologic significance of more than 12 lymph nodes is as yet unclear.

Top-Down Approach

This approach is a variant of the lateral-to-medial approach described above except that it starts at the hepatic flexure rather than at the cecum. This is slightly more technically challenging than starting at the cecum, as there is no peritoneal reflection. This is an attractive option when inflammation from ileocolic Crohn's disease or a desmoplastic reaction from a cecal cancer obscures the retrocecal plane.

Transection and Anastomosis of the Right Colon

Decisions regarding transection margins, and intra- versus extracorporeal anastomosis, are often decided ahead of time based on the patient's underlying diagnosis and pathology. It is important, however, to be able to adjust the operative approach as indicated by intraoperative findings. In the case of ileocolic Crohn's disease, the distal transection margin is generally somewhere in the ascending colon, as determined by the extent of disease. Mobilization of the hepatic flexure is still helpful, not to obtain margins but in order to obtain adequate length to perform a long side-to-side anastomosis if that is the preferred method.

For the novice and intermediate surgeon, laparoscopic mobilization is the minimum necessary to make the distal ileum, right colon, and proximal transverse colon a mobile section of bowel that, in a patient of BMI <25–30, can be exteriorized through a periumbilical incision with the resection and anastomosis performed extracorporeally. Patients with a higher BMI should have the vascular pedicle and mesentery divided intracorporeally, and this allows the anastomosis to be performed extra- or intracorporeally without tension and pulling on the middle colic vessels. Intracorporeal anastomosis, addressed in a separate chapter, requires more advanced skills [8–10].

With regard to extraction incisions, the easiest incision to use is a periumbilical incision. This requires only mobilization of the right colon to the midline, at which point it is now a midline structure and can be easily exteriorized. However, this incision is associated with a higher subsequent incisional hernia rate [11]. Transection of the mesentery and vasculature intracorporeally allow additional choices in terms of an extraction incision, and a right lower quadrant or even a Pfannenstiel incision can be employed. Use of a wound protector may reduce the risk of surgical site infection. Transrectal extraction has been described for specific distal colonic and rectal procedures, but is not advocated for right-sided procedures and requires intracorporeal anastomosis.

Pitfalls and Troubleshooting

Troubleshooting is the forethought given to avoiding pitfalls! Difficulties can potentially be anticipated in certain settings: uncertain location of lesion, obesity, and inflammation.

A common error with both lateral and medial approaches is straying from the correct retroperitoneal plane, which can disrupt either the complete mesenteric excision plane by being too superficial or dissect too deeply into the retroperitoneum risking injury to the right ureter, inferior vena cava, or duodenum. With the lateral approach, being both too lateral and too deep can incur the risk of undermining the right kidney.

A bulky mass or extensive inflammation should prompt a very close look on CT scan at the relationship to the ureter, and consideration should be given to placement of ureteral stents to assist intraoperative identification of the ureter.

While T4 malignancies and large Crohn's phlegmons can be approached laparoscopically by an experienced surgeon, these are not cases for the novice laparoscopic surgeon and should prompt conversion if they were not anticipated preoperatively. Other indications for conversion are inability to find the correct tissue planes, concern regarding injury to the ureter, IVC or duodenum, and uncontrolled bleeding. Failure to make progress with the procedure is also an indication to convert.

Learning curves are a popular way of conveying the potential difficulty of learning a procedure. For a straightforward right colectomy, in the absence of complex anatomy or pathology, a trainee who is capable of performing a laparoscopic cholecystectomy should be able to develop the skills for right colectomy, as described here with extracorporeal anastomosis, within 5–10 cases. More complex techniques, such as single-incision right colectomy [12], intracorporeal anastomosis, and complete mesorectal excision, have longer learning curves which are yet to be defined.

Outcomes

Most level 1 evidence for the role of laparoscopy in colorectal surgery has focused on randomized controlled trials (RCTs) for colon cancer and subsequently for rectal cancer. There is less evidence for benign disease. For example, a Cochrane review found only two RCTs for ileocolic Crohn's disease, involving 120 patients, and concluded that there was no significant difference in perioperative outcomes and long-term reoperation rates for disease-related or non-disease-related complications of Crohn's disease. Multiple cohort studies exist, however, that cumulatively support the benefits of a laparoscopic approach, to the point where RCTs became untenable from the perspective of assuming equipoise. In other words, repeated, consistent, believable evidence from reliable experts led to the situation whereby it would not be possible to devise a RCT where the investigator truly believed that it was unknown whether either arm of a laparoscopic vs open RCT would show improved outcomes.

Table 2.3 Short and long term advantages of laparoscopy

Short-term advantages	Long-term advantages
Reduced time to bowel function Reduced pain Less opioid use Shorter length of hospital stay Less pulmonary impact Decreased costs	Fewer/smaller incisional hernias Reduced incidence of small bowel obstruction

Laparoscopic approaches gained acceptance with reported advantages of faster return to normal activity and diet, reduced hospital stay, reduced postoperative pain, and better cosmesis. Longer-term, laparoscopic surgery has shown smaller abdominal fascial wounds, lower incidence of hernias, and decreased rates of small bowel obstruction from adhesions (Table 2.3).

Although evidence accumulated re. potential improved outcomes from laparoscopy, there also came concerns related to the loss of tactile evaluation of the bowel, i.e., missing occult segments of Crohn's disease and inability to palpate a polyp which would not have visible serosal manifestations. These issues are usually addressed by the exhortation to define anatomy preoperatively, e.g., CT enterography to elicit evidence of proximal small bowel disease in Crohn's, and use of tattooing, CT colonography, and intraoperative endoscopy to localize polyps.

Conclusions

Laparoscopic right colectomy for benign disease is a good starting point for those learning the skills necessary for minimally invasive colorectal surgery, including not just trainees but also surgeons already experienced in open colorectal procedures but wishing to develop laparoscopic skills. Operative planning, OR setup, patient positioning, and trocar placement are important components of a successful operation that also recognizes correct tissue planes, resection margins, anastomotic technique, and specimen retrieval.

References

1. Champagne BJ, Steele SR, Hendren SK, Bakaki PM, Roberts PL, Delaney CP, et al. The American Society of Colon and Rectal Surgeons Assessment Tool for performance of laparoscopic colectomy. Dis Colon Rectum. 2017;60(7):738–44.
2. Homma S, Kawamata F, Yoshida T, Ohno Y, Ichikawa N, Shibasaki S, et al. The balance between surgical resident education and patient safety in laparoscopic colorectal surgery: surgical resident's performance has no negative impact. Surg Laparosc Endosc Percutan Tech. 2017;27(4):295–300.
3. Dasari BVM, McKay D, Gardiner K. Laparoscopic versus open surgery for small bowel Crohn's disease. Cochrane Database Syst Rev. 2011;(1):CD006956.
4. Gustafsson UO, Scott MJ, Hubner M, Nygren J, Demartines N, Francis N, et al. Guidelines for perioperative care in elective colorectal surgery: Enhanced Recovery After Surgery (ERAS®) Society Recommendations. World J Surg. 2019;43(3):659–95.

5. Young-Fadok TM. Video podium presentation, SAGES Annual Meeting 2018. Session: masters colorectal: MIS approaches to the right colon. Laparoscopic lateral-to-medial dissection – a safer approach? [Internet]. Available from: https://www.youtube.com/watch?v=zAz_XdSceh8
6. Lee SJ, Park SC, Kim MJ, Sohn DK, Oh JH. Vascular anatomy in laparoscopic colectomy for right colon cancer. Dis Colon Rectum. 2016;59(8):718–24.
7. Honaker M, Scouten S, Sacksner J, Ziegler M, Wasvary H. A medial to lateral approach offers a superior lymph node harvest for laparoscopic right colectomy. Int J Colorectal Disease. 2016;31(3):631–4.
8. Biondi A, Santocchi P, Pennestri F, Santullo F, D'Ugo D, Persiani R. Totally laparoscopic right colectomy versus laparoscopically assisted right colectomy: a propensity score analysis. Surg Endosc. 2017;31(12):5275–82.
9. Martinek L, You K, Giuratrabocchetta S, Gachabayov M, Lee K, Bergamaschi R. Does laparoscopic intracorporeal ileocolic anastomosis decreases surgical site infection rate? A propensity score-matched cohort study. Intl J Colorectal Dis. 2018;33(3):291–8.
10. Milone M, Elmore U, Di Salvo E, Delrio P, Bucci L, Ferulano GP, et al. Intracorporeal versus extracorporeal anastomosis. Results from a multicentre comparative study on 512 right-sided colorectal cancers. Surg Endosc. 2015;29(8):2314–20.
11. Pares D, Shamali A, Stefan S, Flashman K, O'Leary D, Conti J, et al. Predictive factors for extraction site hernia after laparoscopic right colectomy. Int J Colorectal Disease. 2016;31(7):1323–8.
12. Haas EM, Nieto J, Ragupathi M, Aminian A, Patel CB. Critical appraisal of learning curve for single incision laparoscopic right colectomy. Surg Endosc. 2013;27(12):4499–503.

Masters Program Colorectal Pathway: Laparoscopic Left and Sigmoid Colectomy for Benign Disease

3

Julia T. Saraidaridis and Peter W. Marcello

Introduction and Rationale

Laparoscopic colectomy was first described in the early 1990s. The first randomized trials evaluating laparoscopic colectomy versus open surgery were in patients with malignant disease. These trials demonstrated less blood loss, earlier recovery of bowel function, less need for narcotics, and a shorter length of stay for patients who had procedures performed laparoscopically [1–5]. Because of the inflammatory nature of most benign conditions prompting colectomy, there was some hesitation regarding the feasibility of a laparoscopic approach for these indications. Slowly, data evaluating laparoscopic sigmoid colectomy in patients with diverticulitis accumulated [6–10]. These studies demonstrated that laparoscopic left or sigmoid colectomy is possible in patients with diverticular disease with an increased operative time compared to open surgery, a decreased length of stay, and a decreased complication profile. They also demonstrated that conversion is less for surgeons who utilized a hand-assisted laparoscopic approach. Using these two approaches, straight laparoscopy and hand-assisted laparoscopy, most patients with diverticular disease requiring sigmoid colectomy can undergo surgery in a minimally invasive fashion. This chapter details the indications, operative technique, and outcomes of studies evaluating laparoscopic and hand-assisted laparoscopic (HAL) sigmoid and left colectomy for benign disease.

J. T. Saraidaridis (✉) · P. W. Marcello
Lahey Hospital and Medical Center, Division of Colon and Rectal Surgery, Burlington, MA, USA
e-mail: julia.t.saraidaridis@lahey.org; peter.w.marcello@lahey.org

P. Sylla et al. (eds.), *The SAGES Manual of Colorectal Surgery*,
https://doi.org/10.1007/978-3-030-24812-3_3

Indications and Contraindications

The most common benign condition that prompts left or sigmoid colectomy is the many manifestations of diverticulitis including recurrent disease, smoldering disease, colovesical/colovaginal fistula, or stricture. Other benign conditions prompting an elective left or sigmoid colectomy include Crohn's colitis, ischemic colitis, endometriosis, or diverticular bleeding. As diverticulitis is the most commonly seen disorder requiring left or sigmoid colectomy in benign disease, this chapter will focus on this indication.

In the past, the inflammation and scarring associated with the chronic manifestations of diverticular disease prompted many surgeons to shy away from minimally invasive approaches. However, increasing experience with both hand-assisted laparoscopy and straight laparoscopy has prompted minimally invasive techniques to be the mainstay of treating this condition. In our practice, for repeated attacks of uncomplicated diverticulitis, we proceed with a straight laparoscopic approach with a planned extraction through a small Pfannenstiel incision. For patients with a body mass index greater than 30 kg/m^2, the size of the extraction site for a straight laparoscopic case is relatively similar to a hand-assisted incision. So, for this reason, for morbidly obese patients, we utilize a hand-assisted approach. Additionally, for any patient with a history of complicated diverticulitis including abscess, phlegmon, or fistula, a hand-assisted laparoscopic approach can be particularly helpful to facilitate blunt dissection and identify the correct surgical planes.

There are very few contraindications to approaching benign conditions of the left and sigmoid colon using a laparoscopic approach. Contraindications include patients who are unable to tolerate laparoscopy or steep changes in operating room table positioning. A relative contraindication is the presence of dense or extensive adhesions associated with a prior history of open laparotomy in the past. With experience, however, most laparoscopic surgeons will attempt a laparoscopic approach, even in the setting of previous open surgery. Extreme caution should be taken when entering the reoperative abdomen in order to avoid an injury, especially in the setting of prior peritonitis, prior intraabdominal bleeding, or previous mesh placement, which may result in formation of dense adhesions. If the abdomen proves to be hostile, conversion to an open procedure should quickly be decided.

Principles and Quality Benchmarks of the Approach/Technique

The principles of resection for diverticular disease are the same in laparoscopic approaches as they are in open approaches: isolation and ligation of the sigmoid pedicle, mobilization of the left and sigmoid colon including takedown of the splenic flexure, proximal transection, distal transection at the proximal rectum, and anastomosis. For diverticular disease, there are additional parameters including the performance of an adequate colon resection to minimize recurrence of disease and an attempt to decrease the risk of common complications of sigmoid resection. In our practice, to assist in reducing the risk of recurrence of diverticular disease, all prior

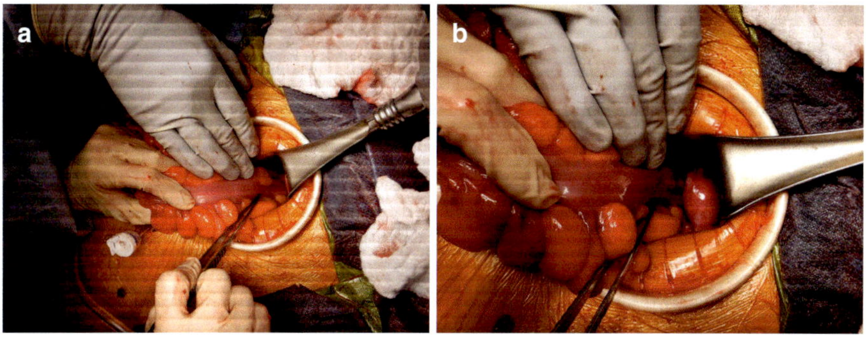

Fig. 3.1 (**a**, **b**) Splaying of the taeniae

CT scans are evaluated to assess the proximal extent of disease. Any portion of the bowel that has been involved in previous inflammation/diverticulitis attacks is included in the planned resection. Once in the operating room, prior to initiating the mobilization of the bowel, the bowel is palpated to assess for chronic thickening or acute inflammation. The proximal transection margin does not need to be so proximal so as to include all diverticula, it just needs to be proximal enough to include all areas of previous inflammation. It should also be on soft, pliable bowel with soft pliable mesentery. The planned proximal colon transection can be marked (using an ink pen tip, clip, or cautery) at the start of the operation. This will ensure that the appropriate proximal margin is achieved which can be more challenging to determine once the colon and its mesentery are fully mobilized. The distal transection margin should be on the proximal rectum. This is identified by the splaying of the taeniae (Fig. 3.1a, b). A colorectal rather than a colosigmoid anastomosis is believed to be the single most important factor in decreasing the chance of recurrent diverticular disease [11, 12].

In addition to providing an adequate resection, a principle of left/sigmoid resection for benign disease is to avoid a high ligation of the sigmoid pedicle. The avoidance of a high ligation decreases the risk of ureteral injury and hypogastric nerve injury. Some studies have indicated that avoiding a high ligation of the pedicle decreases the chance of anastomotic leak [13]. Other studies have not confirmed this association [14]. However, in our practice for benign disease, we preserve the sigmoid pedicle given this concern.

Preoperative Planning, Patient Work-Up, and Optimization

In the planning of a minimally invasive approach to surgical resection for diverticulitis, a number of factors must be considered preoperatively. For those patients whom have not had a colonoscopy in the 2 years prior to resection, repeat endoscopic evaluation is warranted. Some of our surgeons will perform an on-table colonoscopy on the day of surgery in order to avoid repeating a bowel preparation. For patients with complicated diverticulitis, additional factors must be taken into account preoperatively. Patients with residual diverticular abscess and/or fistula will keep their percutaneous drain up until the time of surgery. The drain will be prepped into the field and then removed once the abdomen has been entered. For those patients with suspected colovesical fistula, cystoscopy and ureteral stent placement are usually performed just prior to surgery. If the fistula takedown results in a bladder defect, it should be repaired with sutures. In regard to ureteral stent usage in the absence of colovesical fistula, the decision to place stents prophylactically is up to the individual surgeon. In general, when significant inflammation and/or residual phlegmon, abscess, or fistula is anticipated, left-sided stents are usually placed prophylactically to minimize the risk of an unrecognized ureteral injury.

All prior abdominal scars should be evaluated as potential extraction sites. Patients are educated about enhanced recovery pathways including non-opioid pain relief alternatives, early ambulation, and early resumption of diet. All of our patients undergoing elective colon surgery undergo mechanical and antibiotic bowel preparation the day before surgery. Please refer to the chapters on enhanced recovery protocol in colorectal surgery for more details on this topic (Chaps. 7 and 8).

Operative Setup

Patients are placed on a bean bag in a modified lithotomy position on a split-leg table. The arms are tucked at the sides and surrounded by foam padding and an inflated bean bag. The chest is wrapped circumferentially three times with three-inch silk tape affixing them to the table. The legs are split with the buttock at the bottom of the table to allow for trans-anal access, and then the legs are secured in place with Velcro straps. Patients are given subcutaneous heparin, and sequential compression devices are applied for deep venous thrombosis prophylaxis. Antibiotics are administered less than 1 hour prior to surgical incision. We use both monopolar cautery and the bipolar vessel sealer as our energy sources. Both of these instruments are placed on the field at the initiation of the case. A CO_2 colonoscope is available as needed for the procedure. Most cases are initiated with a colonoscopic evaluation of the colon. The Foley catheter is placed after colonoscopy in women to avoid risk of urinary tract infection as our group found that there was contamination of the catheter from colonoscopy if it had been placed pre-procedure. The catheter is draped over the leg to reduce contamination from the passage of staplers and endoscopes trans-anally.

Operative Technique

Port Placement

For straight laparoscopic procedures, a 12 mm Hassan port is placed in the umbilicus. 5 mm ports are placed in the right upper quadrant, the right lower quadrant, and the left lower quadrant (Fig. 3.2). Extraction is most often performed through a small Pfannenstiel incision or via an extension of the Hassan port site.

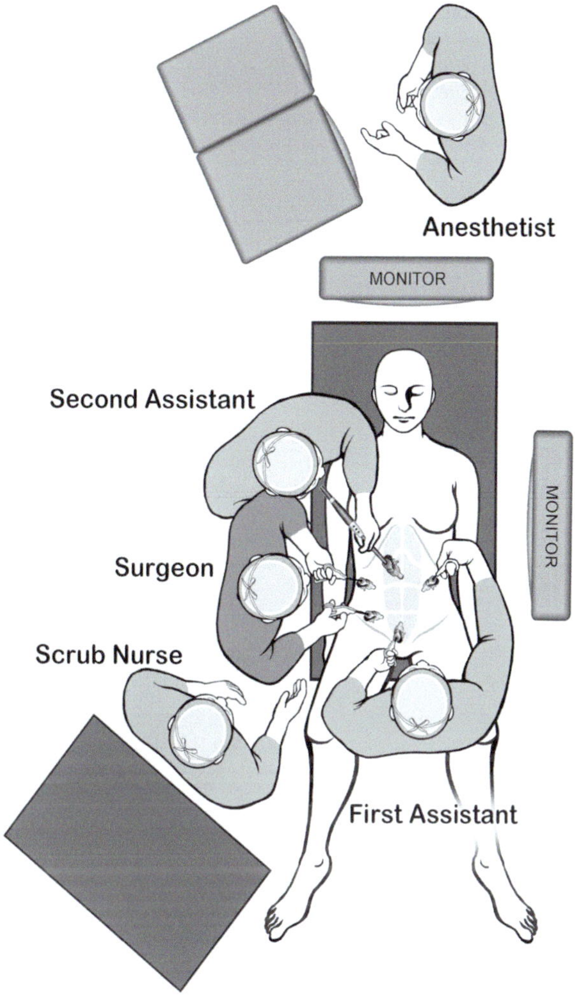

Fig. 3.2 Room setup for laparoscopic sigmoid colectomy. (Used with permission of Springer Nature from Leroy et al. [26])

For a hand-assisted approach, the operation begins with the creation of an incision for the hand-port. Early along the learning curve of hand-assisted, an 8 cm lower midline incision is recommended in the case that conversion is required. Once the surgeon is comfortable with a hand-assisted approach, a Pfannenstiel incision 2 cm above the pubis is the preferred approach. The incision is cosmetically pleasing, has an extremely low risk of incisional hernia, and is an excellent incision to work in the pelvis where further dissection or an anastomosis can be completed. The hand device is placed into the incision, and then three 5 mm trocars are placed in the left lateral, right lateral, and umbilical positions (Fig. 3.3). The trocars are placed with the hand inside the abdomen to protect the intestines from injury.

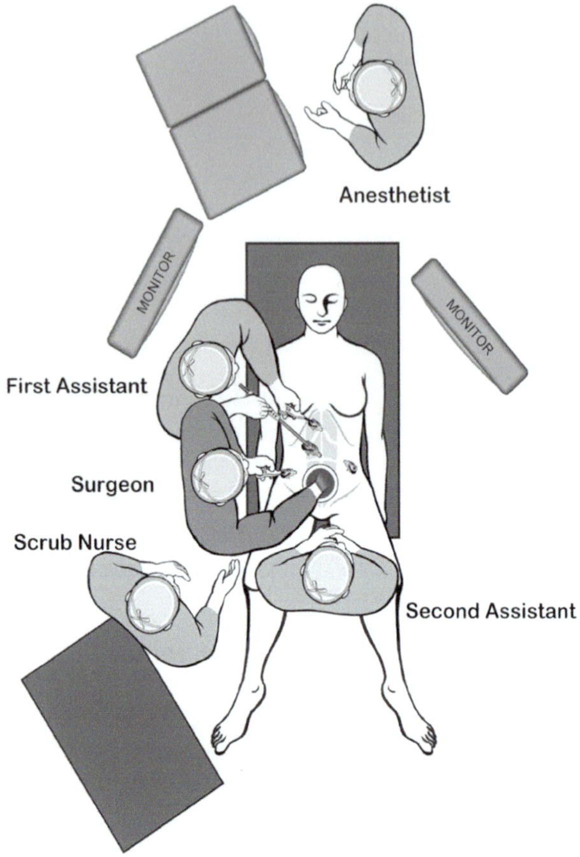

Fig. 3.3 Room setup for HAL sigmoid colectomy. (Used with permission of Springer Nature from Sonoda [25])

Following access to the abdomen, the procedural steps of the operation are performed in the same sequence whether the procedure is performed by straight laparoscopic or a hand-assisted laparoscopic approach.

Left/Sigmoid Colectomy

The surgeon and assistant stand on the patient's right side. The patient is placed in a mild Trendelenburg and left-side up position. In our practice, we perform a medial to lateral mobilization of the left/sigmoid colon. To do this, the omentum is lifted over the transverse colon, and the small bowel is moved out of the pelvis to the right upper quadrant (Fig. 3.4). The "bare area" of the left colon (the mesentery just lateral to the IMV between the left colic and first sigmoidal branches) is grasped and lifted. This mesentery is incised just lateral to the IMV, and a dissection begins between the left colon mesentery and Gerota's fascia. The gonadal vessels will be below with Gerota's fascia, and the dissection continues out to the lateral side wall. The left ureter is typically under the IMA pedicle and will not be seen unless

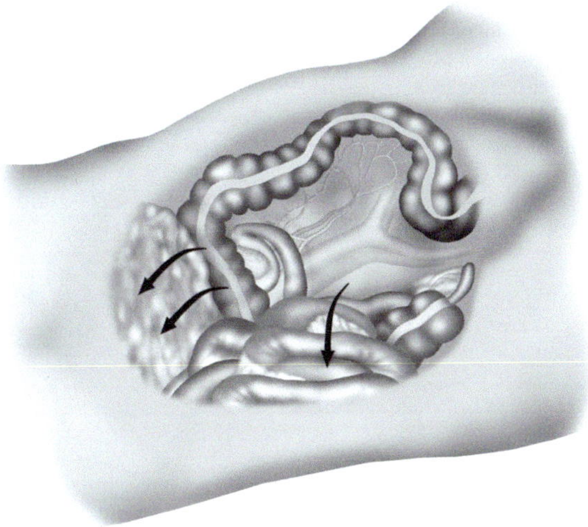

Fig. 3.4 The omentum is lifted over the transverse colon and the small bowel is moved to the right side of the abdomen. (Used with permission of Springer Nature from Leroy et al. [26])

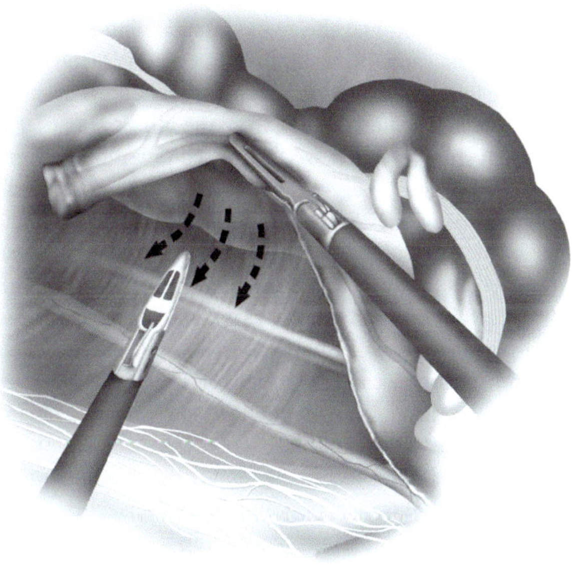

Fig. 3.5 Medial to lateral mobilization. (Used with permission of Springer Nature from Leroy et al. [26])

dissection is carried backwards toward the aorta. The first one or two sigmoid branches are then identified, isolated, and divided with the bipolar vessel sealer. The left colon is then mobilized from medial to lateral in a plane overlying Gerota's fascia (Fig. 3.5). This dissection extends out to the left pelvic sidewall, inferiorly into the upper retrorectal space, and superiorly up towards the splenic flexure.

After the medial to lateral mobilization has been performed, the lateral attachments starting with the white line of Toldt are divided (Fig. 3.6). This maneuver connects the medial dissection plane to the lateral dissection plane. Moving up towards the

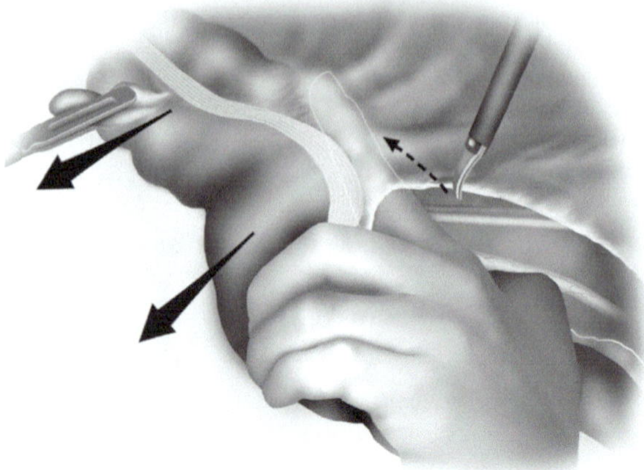

Fig. 3.6 Taking down the lateral attachments. (Used with permission of Springer Nature from Sonoda [25])

splenic flexure, the lateral aspects of the splenic flexure are divided. For this part of the procedure, the assistant moves to the area between the legs and holds the camera with his left hand and the hook cautery with his right hand through the left-sided trocar. In this same position, the omentum is taken off of the distal transverse colon allowing the splenic flexure to be approached from a medial direction. Then the distal transverse mesocolon is freed from the inferior boarder of the pancreas. At this point, the colon should be assessed for reach down to the proximal rectum. If the reach is adequate, the mesentery can be taken with a bipolar device up to but not crossing the marginal artery on the proximal transection margin (the rest of the mesentery will be ligated once the colon is exteriorized). For the distal transection margin, the mesentery can be taken up to the edge of colon laparoscopically. However, if the procedure is being performed with a hand-assisted, that portion of the case can be done via the hand-port in an open fashion. At that point, the bowel can be exteriorized (Fig. 3.7), and the specimen can be brought out through the hand-port (in the case of hand-assisted) or through an extraction site (straight laparoscopy). In the situation of straight laparoscopy, a small wound protector should be used to ease specimen extraction and to protect the wound from contamination.

The proximal transection and distal transection are completed via the extraction site. For straight laparoscopy, the anvil is placed in the proximal colon which is returned to the abdomen. The stapled colorectal anastomosis can be performed while under laparoscopic view (or in some cases through the wound directly if a Pfannenstiel or lower midline incision is used). It is critical to ensure that there are no twists in the proximal colon or the mesentery and that the small bowel is not trapped under the left colon mesentery before the stapler is fired. For hand-assisted cases the anastomosis can be performed through the hand-port site. The anvil is secured to the stapler and closed under direct visualization. However, prior to firing of the stapler, a pneumoperitoneum is reestablished to ensure that the proximal colon and its mesentery are not twisted, that the small bowel is not trapped under the left colon mesentery, and that there is no tension upon the anastomosis. In either

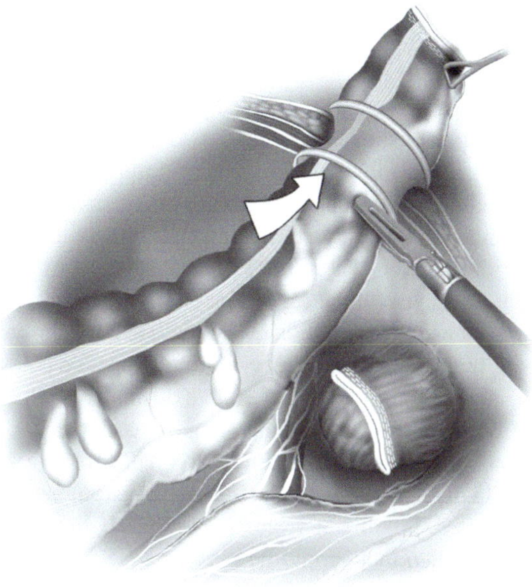

Fig. 3.7 Exteriorizing the sigmoid colon. (Used with permission of Springer Nature from Leroy et al. [26])

approach, the omentum is brought down over the small bowel and colon to an anatomical position. Following the anastomosis, air leak testing is performed with CO_2 colonoscopy, and the mucosa is examined for perfusion. The anastomosis may be reinforced with a few additional sutures depending upon the surgeon's preference. For cases without significant spillage or concern for colovesical fistula, no closed suction drain is left behind. For patients in whom a colovesical fistula repair was performed, a closed suction is placed in the pelvis.

Pitfalls and Troubleshooting

Some of the most common pitfalls in this operation are extensive scarring due to diverticular inflammation which distorts the anatomy, a lack of reach of the proximal colon into the pelvis, or a positive leak test. Extensive scarring from repeated episodes of uncomplicated diverticulitis or complicated diverticulitis with abscess/fistula can preclude a straight laparoscopic approach. This is where the hand-assisted approach can be the most helpful. The hand and fingers allow for safe blunt dissection. In addition, portions of the procedure can be performed via the hand-port in an open fashion, should the situation demand it. If the procedure cannot be performed in a straight laparoscopic fashion, or if failure to progress occurs, one should consider a hand-assisted approach prior to converting to a midline laparotomy. A meta-analysis of the three published RCTs comparing hand-assisted laparoscopic to conventional laparoscopic colorectal resection showed a significantly lower rate of conversion in the hand-assisted patients, while morbidity rates and outcomes were equivalent [15].

Another possible intraoperative difficulty in surgery for diverticulitis is extensive residual disease requiring more distal transection onto the patient's rectum. Usually, the goal is to keep the distal transection margin at the colorectal junction. However, in some scenarios such as a residual phlegmon/abscess involving the top of the rectum or a colovaginal fistula, it is necessary to dissect further distally onto the rectum than initially planned. In these scenarios, it is important to consider and warn the patient of potential functional consequences. More than 50% of patients who undergo low anterior resection for benign or malignant disease will develop signs and symptoms of low anterior resection syndrome. This is a defecatory dysfunction defined by urgency, frequent stools, incontinence, and incomplete emptying. These patients may require fiber supplementation and antidiarrheals to assist in improving quality of life. In more severe cases, biofeedback, sacral nerve stimulation, and colostomy can be considered.

Another common intraoperative difficulty is a lack of reach of the proximal transection margin to the rectum. This is particularly common if the patient's disease extends up into the descending colon. There is a stepwise approach to achieving more laxity to allow for a tension-free anastomosis. First, the bowel must be assessed for what is holding it from the pelvis. If the splenic flexure has not been fully released, then that should be performed. Second, the IMV and or left colic can be transected close to the inferior margin of the pancreas to allow further mobility. The transection margin must be assessed for viability after that maneuver. Here, every lateral 1 centimeter of division provides two additional centimeters of reach. Third, the rectum can be mobilized below Waldeyer's fascia, thereby straightening the rectum, which typically provides several additional centimeters of length. A final option is the Turnbull maneuver, wherein the distal transverse colon is brought down to the right of midline, through an ileal mesenteric defect [16]. All of these maneuvers can be performed via hand-assisted or straight laparoscopic methods.

Lastly, one of the most concerning pitfalls is a positive intraoperative leak test. If leaking is demonstrated, our recommendation is to either redo the anastomosis or, if an attempt at repair of the anastomosis is performed, strong consideration should be made for a diverting loop ileostomy. Data from our own institution demonstrate that out of 2360 patients who underwent left-sided anastomosis, 119 had a positive intraoperative leak test. Sixty-eight underwent suture repair alone, of which 9% had a clinical leak postoperatively. Fifty-one patients underwent either proximal diversion or reconstruction, and none of these patients had evidence of clinical leak postoperatively. Given these data, our strong recommendation is to either redo or divert the anastomosis in this clinical scenario. For all other patients, the decision to proceed with a diverting loop ileostomy to protect the colorectal anastomosis is based on three factors: the integrity and perfusion of the bowel, the degree of intraabdominal contamination, and the status of the patient. If following resection of the specimen the bowel is intact and well-perfused, the abdomen is free of infection, and the patient has remained hemodynamically stable during the case, there is no strict indication for a prophylactic diverting loop ileostomy. However, if any of those three factors are concerning, a diverting loop ileostomy should be strongly considered.

Outcomes

When considering laparoscopic approaches for patients with benign disease, there are two questions that need to be answered. The first is whether the laparoscopic or hand-assisted techniques are equivalent to an open surgical approach. In some ways, this is a difficult question to answer as, unlike cancer, there are not specific criteria of the surgical specimen that need to be obtained for the operation to be considered a success. Instead we have to rely on outcome measures like operative time, conversion rate, length of stay, and complications to assess whether the procedures are equivalent (or superior). The second question is which laparoscopic approach is appropriate (straight laparoscopic versus hand-assisted laparoscopy).

When laparoscopic colectomy was first introduced in the 1990s, diverticular disease-related complications were the last indications to be evaluated scientifically given the concerns of extensive scarring and/or inflammation as potentially precluding a minimally invasive approach. Following this initial hesitation, studies were conducted to compare laparoscopic versus open sigmoid colectomy for diverticulitis in the late 1990s/early 2000s (Table 3.1). Most studies found that the laparoscopic approach had longer operative times with conversion rates ranging from 6% to 20%. Length of stay was significantly shorter in the laparoscopic groups. With regard to complications, some studies found no differences between the groups, while other studies found that there were fewer complications with a laparoscopic approach. Even patients with complicated disease such as abscess or fistula were completed by a laparoscopic approach. This was detailed by Bartus and colleagues in 36 patients who underwent laparoscopic colovesical fistula takedown [17]. The conversion rate was higher for procedures involving fistula (25% versus 5%, p <0.001), but demonstrated that for many, the procedure could be performed successfully. Overall, for elective benign indications like diverticulitis, these studies demonstrated that a laparoscopic approach was possible and that it had a positive effect on the length of stay and extent of complication profile.

When comparing straight laparoscopic to hand-assisted approaches, there are a number of studies that evaluated colectomies for all indications (Table 3.2). Three of the studies are randomized controlled trials [18–20]. However, all three included a wide range of surgical indications and are not limited to left/sigmoid colectomy. Regardless, their findings can be extrapolated to the diverticular population. A meta-analysis of these three randomized controlled trials concluded that there was no difference in operating time between the straight laparoscopic and HAL patients. There was a lower conversion rate for HAL versus straight laparoscopic approaches.

Table 3.1 Laparoscopic approach versus open surgical approach for diverticulitis

Study	Date	Patient population	Operating room time (minutes)	Conversion	Length of stay (days)	Complications
Tuech et al. [21]	1993–1998	All diverticulitis: lap = 22, open = 24	Lap = 136 open = 234, $p = 0.001$	9%	Lap = 13.1 days, open = 20.2 days, $p = 0.003$	Morbidity: lap = 18%, open = 50%, $p = 0.02$
Dwivedi et al. [8]	1995–2000	All diverticulitis: lap = 66, open = 88	Lap = 212, open 143, $p < 0.05$	19.7%	Lap = 4.8 days, open = 8.8 days, $p < 0.05$	Not calculated in composite
Senagore et al. [7]	1999–2000	All diverticulitis: lap = 61, open = 71	Lap = 109, open = 101, p = NS	6.6%	Lap = 3.1 days, open = 6.8 days, $p < 0.05$	Pulmonary: lap = 1.6% open = 5.6%, $p < 0.05$ wound: lap = 0%, open 7%, $p < 0.05$
Klarenbeek et al. [6]	2002–2006	All diverticulitis lap = 54, open = 54	Lap = 183, open = 127 ($p = 0.0001$)	19.2%	Lap = 5 days, Open = 7 days, $p = 0.046$	Morbidity: lap = 42.3%, open 53.8%, $p = 0.239$
Raue et al. [10]	2005–2008	All diverticulitis: lap = 75, open = 68	Lap = 180, open 140, $p = 0.001$	9%	Lap = 9 days, open = 10 days, $p = 0.168$	Morbidity: lap = 37%, open = 40%, $p = 0.899$
Gervaz et al. [9]	2005–2009	All diverticulitis: lap = 59, open 54	Lap = 165, open = 110, $p < 0.0001$	Not stated in article	Lap = 5 days, open = 7 days, $p < 0.0001$	Morbidity: lap = 13.5%, open = 9%, $p = 0.56$

Table 3.2 Hand-assisted laparoscopic surgery versus laparoscopic surgery

Study	Date	Patient population	Operating room time	Conversion	Length of stay	Complications
HALS Study Group [18]	2000	All disease (multiple operations) lap =18, HAL = 22	Lap = 141, HAL = 152, $p = 0.58$	Lap = 13.6%, HAL = 22%, $p = 0.68$	Lap = 6.0, HAL = 7.0, $p = 0.25$	Complication: lap = 4.5%, HAL = 22%, p = NS
Anderson et al. [22]	2000–2005	All diverticular: open = 110, lap = 17, HAL = 98	Open = 111.6, lap = 153.0, HAL = 142.0, $p < 0.05$	Lap = 23.5% (conversion to HAL 17.6%) HAL = 6.1%, $p < 0.05$	Open = 7.9, lap = 5.1, HAL = 5.0, $p < 0.05$	Open = 28%, lap = 29.4%, HAL = 14.6%, $p < 0.05$
Targarona et al. [20]	2002	All disease: lap = 27, HAL = 27	Lap = 135, HAL 120, p = NS	Lap → HAL = 15%, lap → open = 7%, HAL → open = 7%, p = NS	Lap = 6 days, HAL = 6 days, p = NS	Morbidity: lap = 23%, HAL = 23%, p = NS
Marcello et al. [19]	2005–2006	All disease (sigmoid, total colectomy) lap = 48, HAL = 47	Lap = 208, HAL = 175, $p = 0.021$	Lap = 12.5%, HAL = 2%, $p = 0.11$	Lap = 8.9, HAL = 6.9, $p = 0.58$	Complication: lap = 19%, HAL = 21%, $p = 0.68$
Jadlowiec et al. [23]	2005–2011	All diverticular: lap = 133, HAL = 291, open = 37	Lap = 180, HAL = 191.2, open = 204.4, $p = 0.0001$	Lap- > HAL = 8.5%, lap → open = 3.0%, HAL → open = 2.4%, $p = 0.02$	Lap = 4.45, HAL = 4.99, open = 6.52, $p < 0.0001$	Not calculated
Midura et al. [24]	2010–2014	All pathology: lap = 71, HAL = 57, lap-assist = 63	Lap = 165, HAL = 172.8, lap-assist = 132, $p < 0.001$	(only counted patients who were performed successfully)	Lap = 3.6, HAL = 4.1, lap-assist = 4.0, $p = 0.009$	Lap = 2.8%, HAL = 5.3%, lap-assist 3.2%, $p = 0.25$

Finally, there was no difference in complication occurrences between the two groups [15]. For this reason, in our patients who have the highest likelihood of conversion (obesity and complicated diverticulitis), we choose to start with a hand-assisted approach.

Conclusions

Laparoscopic or hand-assisted laparoscopic left/sigmoid colectomy is the preferred approach for patients with benign indications such as diverticulitis. Even diverticular disease complicated by abscess, phlegmon, or fistula should not preclude an attempt at a laparoscopic approach. In our practice, patients with repeated bouts of uncomplicated diverticulitis will undergo a straight laparoscopic approach, whereas patients with complicated disease or morbid obesity will undergo a planned hand-assisted procedure. Hand-assisted laparoscopy has a decreased conversion rate (in comparison to laparoscopic procedures) and facilitates increased adoption of minimally invasive colectomy in patients with complex diverticulitis and obesity or a combination of both.

References

1. Lacy AM, Garcia-Valdecasas JC, Delgado S, Castells A, Taura P, Pique JM, et al. Laparoscopy-assisted colectomy versus open colectomy for treatment of non-metastatic colon cancer: a randomised trial. Lancet. 2002;359(9325):2224–9.
2. Clinical Outcomes of Surgical Therapy Study G, Nelson H, Sargent DJ, Wieand HS, Fleshman J, Anvari M, et al. A comparison of laparoscopically assisted and open colectomy for colon cancer. N Engl J Med. 2004;350(20):2050–9.
3. Leung KL, Kwok SP, Lam SC, Lee JF, Yiu RY, Ng SS, et al. Laparoscopic resection of recto-sigmoid carcinoma: prospective randomised trial. Lancet. 2004;363(9416):1187–92.
4. Veldkamp R, Kuhry E, Hop WC, Jeekel J, Kazemier G, Bonjer HJ, et al. Laparoscopic surgery versus open surgery for colon cancer: short-term outcomes of a randomised trial. Lancet Oncol. 2005;6(7):477–84.
5. Schwenk W, Haase O, Neudecker J, Muller JM. Short term benefits for laparoscopic colorectal resection. Cochrane Database Syst Rev. 2005;(3):CD003145.
6. Klarenbeek BR, Veenhof AA, Bergamaschi R, van der Peet DL, van den Broek WT, de Lange ES, et al. Laparoscopic sigmoid resection for diverticulitis decreases major morbidity rates: a randomized control trial: short-term results of the Sigma Trial. Ann Surg. 2009;249(1):39–44.
7. Senagore AJ, Duepree HJ, Delaney CP, Dissanaike S, Brady KM, Fazio VW. Cost structure of laparoscopic and open sigmoid colectomy for diverticular disease: similarities and differences. Dis Colon Rectum. 2002;45(4):485–90.
8. Dwivedi A, Chahin F, Agrawal S, Chau WY, Tootla A, Tootla F, et al. Laparoscopic colectomy vs. open colectomy for sigmoid diverticular disease. Dis Colon Rectum. 2002;45(10):1309–14; discussion 14–5
9. Gervaz P, Inan I, Perneger T, Schiffer E, Morel P. A prospective, randomized, single-blind comparison of laparoscopic versus open sigmoid colectomy for diverticulitis. Ann Surg. 2010;252(1):3–8.

10. Raue W, Paolucci V, Asperger W, Albrecht R, Buchler MW, Schwenk W, et al. Laparoscopic sigmoid resection for diverticular disease has no advantages over open approach: midterm results of a randomized controlled trial. Langenbeck's Arch Surg. 2011;396(7):973–80.
11. Thaler K, Baig MK, Berho M, Weiss EG, Nogueras JJ, Arnaud JP, et al. Determinants of recurrence after sigmoid resection for uncomplicated diverticulitis. Dis Colon Rectum. 2003;46(3):385–8.
12. Benn PL, Wolff BG, Ilstrup DM. Level of anastomosis and recurrent colonic diverticulitis. Am J Surg. 1986;151(2):269–71.
13. Tocchi A, Mazzoni G, Fornasari V, Miccini M, Daddi G, Tagliacozzo S. Preservation of the inferior mesenteric artery in colorectal resection for complicated diverticular disease. Am J Surg. 2001;182(2):162–7.
14. Lehmann RK, Brounts LR, Johnson EK, Rizzo JA, Steele SR. Does sacrifice of the inferior mesenteric artery or superior rectal artery affect anastomotic leak following sigmoidectomy for diverticulitis? A retrospective review. Am J Surg. 2011;201(5):623–7.
15. Moloo H, Haggar F, Coyle D, Hutton B, Duhaime S, Mamazza J, et al. Hand-assisted laparoscopic surgery versus conventional laparoscopy for colorectal surgery. Cochrane Database Syst Rev. 2010;(10):CD006585.
16. Le TH, Gathright JB Jr. Reconstitution of intestinal continuity after extended left colectomy. Dis Colon Rectum. 1993;36(2):197–8.
17. Bartus CM, Lipof T, Sarwar CM, Vignati PV, Johnson KH, Sardella WV, et al. Colovesical fistula: not a contraindication to elective laparoscopic colectomy. Dis Colon Rectum. 2005;48(2):233–6.
18. Hand-assisted laparoscopic surgery vs standard laparoscopic surgery for colorectal disease: a prospective randomized trial. HALS Study Group. Surg Endosc. 2000;14(10):896–901.
19. Marcello PW, Fleshman JW, Milsom JW, Read TE, Arnell TD, Birnbaum EH, et al. Hand-assisted laparoscopic vs. laparoscopic colorectal surgery: a multicenter, prospective, randomized trial. Dis Colon Rectum. 2008;51(6):818–26; discussion 26–8
20. Targarona EM, Gracia E, Garriga J, Martinez-Bru C, Cortes M, Boluda R, et al. Prospective randomized trial comparing conventional laparoscopic colectomy with hand-assisted laparoscopic colectomy: applicability, immediate clinical outcome, inflammatory response, and cost. Surg Endosc. 2002;16(2):234–9.
21. Tuech JJ, Pessaux P, Rouge C, Regenet N, Bergamaschi R, Arnaud JP. Laparoscopic vs open colectomy for sigmoid diverticulitis: a prospective comparative study in the elderly. Surg Endosc. 2000;14(11):1031–3.
22. Anderson J, Luchtefeld M, Dujovny N, Hoedema R, Kim D, Butcher J. A comparison of laparoscopic, hand-assist and open sigmoid resection in the treatment of diverticular disease. Am J Surg. 2007;193(3):400–3.. discussion 3
23. Jadlowiec CC, Mannion EM, Thielman MJ, Bartus CM, Johnson KH, Sardella WV, et al. Evolution of technique in performance of minimally invasive colectomies. Dis Colon Rectum. 2014;57(9):1090–7.
24. Midura EF, Hanseman DJ, Davis BR, Johnson BL, Kuethe JW, Rafferty JF, et al. Laparoscopic sigmoid colectomy: Are all laparoscopic techniques created equal? Surg Endosc. 2016;30(8):3567–72.
25. Sonoda T. Hand-assisted laparoscopic total abdominal colectomy. In: Milsom J, Bohm N, Nakajima K, editors. Laparoscopic colorectal surgery. 2nd ed. New York: Springer Science + Business Media; 2006.
26. Leroy J, Henri M, Rubino F, Marescaux J. Sigmoidectomy. In: Milsom J, Bohm N, Nakajima K, editors. Laparoscopic colorectal surgery. 2nd ed. New York: Springer Science + Business Media; 2006.

Master Program Colorectal Pathway: Laparoscopic Splenic Flexure Release (Tips and Tricks)

4

Antonio Caycedo-Marulanda and John H. Marks

Introduction and Rationale

Splenic flexure release otherwise known as the mobilization splenic flexure is an essential skill for all general and colorectal surgeons who perform colonic resections. The fundamental benefit of mobilizing the splenic flexure is the construction of a tension-free anastomosis following left colectomy, sigmoid colectomy, anterior resection, low anterior resection, as well as total mesorectal resection resections (TME) with coloanal anastomosis. Additionally, SFR is routinely performed during total and subtotal colectomies.

The extra colonic length provided by SFR allows for the descending colon to reach down into the deep pelvis for restoration of bowel continuity. While SFR may be performed selectively by some, most surgeons routinely perform SFR for all left-sided colectomy to ensure an adequately perfused anastomosis without tension [1–3]. Distance from the anal verge plays a significant role as a risk factor for anastomotic leak in colorectal anastomoses, with tumors located 6 cm or less from the anal verge being at the highest risk [4]. It is possible that when creating these low colorectal or coloanal anastomoses, blood supply relies on the different connecting arcades, which may or may not be present, thus increasing the risk of leak secondary to ischemia [5].

A. Caycedo-Marulanda
Health Sciences North, Department of General Surgery, Division of Colorectal Surgery, Northern Ontario School of Medicine, Sudbury, ON, Canada

J. H. Marks (✉)
Lankenau Medical Center, Department of Colon and Rectal Surgery, Wynnewood, PA, USA
e-mail: marksj@mlhs.org

P. Sylla et al. (eds.), *The SAGES Manual of Colorectal Surgery*,
https://doi.org/10.1007/978-3-030-24812-3_4

Indications and Contraindications

Indications include resections involving the left side such as left colectomy, sigmoid colectomy, anterior resection, low anterior resection, ultralow anterior resection (with coloanal anastomosis), and total abdominal colectomy. As a general principle, colorectal anastomosis following sigmoid resection for diverticulitis or colon cancer should be performed to the rectum itself and not to the rectosigmoid, which usually requires additional colon length for reach and hence SFR. Studies have shown that the relapse rate is much higher for diverticulitis if the rectosigmoid and distal sigmoid colon are left in place [6]. In addition, anastomotic integrity relies on meticulous dissection, adequate blood supply, and lack of tension [1]; the last two are optimized by performing SFR. When the decision to perform SFR is left to the end rather than the start of the operation, it is usually fraught with more technical difficulties and usually results from poor preoperative planning.

In the current era, there is an increased interest in sphincter preservation and restoration of bowel continuity [7]. Low and ultralow rectal cancer surgery has become more prevalent, and newer approaches have been introduced, including the use of robotic platforms and those for transanal total mesorectal excision (taTME) [8–10]. In these cases, splenic flexure release is mandatory if reconstruction is to take place.

It is our opinion that SFR should be performed systematically and at the beginning of the case, particularly during sigmoid resection for diverticulitis, before any difficulties are encountered during pelvic dissection. SFR is also strongly recommended during TME with planned sphincter preservation for rectal cancer [11]. The specific SFR approach used is based on the surgeon's preference and patient's anatomy. There are no absolute contraindications to performing SFR. It should be noted, however, that in patients who have had previous gastric or left upper quadrant surgery as well as pancreatitis, the dissection might be more difficult.

Principles and Quality Benchmarks

The goal of this step in the operation is to return the left colon to its original embryologic state. The surgeon should be mindful of the fact that embryologically the hindgut and distal midgut are midline structures. Originally, the bowel is extra-abdominal and undergoes counter-clockwise rotation to be sealed to the lateral attachments along the line of Toldt (Fig. 4.1a–e). By fully releasing the mesentery of the distal and transverse colon, the left colon is returned to its embryologic midline state (Fig. 4.2). This is essential to allow for a tension-free anastomosis of the descending colon to the rectum. It is helpful for the surgeon to picture this as separating the pages in a book, such that the mesentery leaf is freed from the next page, which is the retroperitoneum.

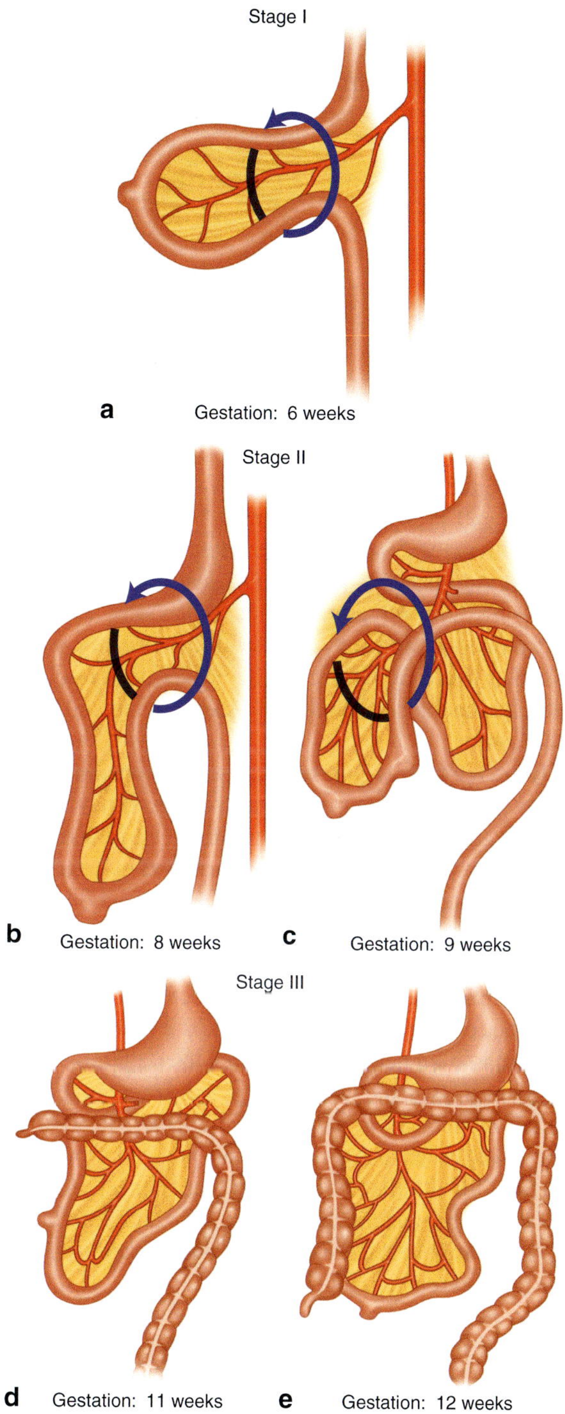

Fig. 4.1 (**a**–**e**) Embryonic bowel rotation. The embryologic bowel is extra-abdominal and undergoes counter-clockwise rotation to be sealed to the lateral attachments along the line of Toldt

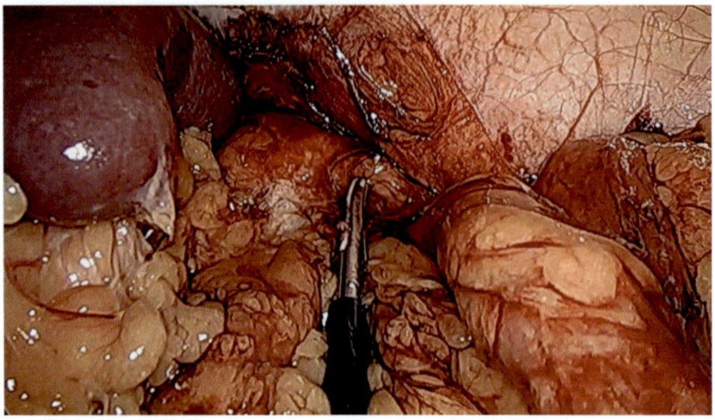

Fig. 4.2 Full splenic flexure release. The release of the mesentery of the distal transverse colon and the descending colon returns the left colon to its embryologic midline state

Perioperative Planning, Patient Workup, and Optimization

Patients undergoing SFR as part left-sided resection will undergo standard workup, staging, and preoperative planning based on the actual diagnosis. Almost invariably, patients will undergo computed tomography scanning (CT) as part of their workup. Additionally, a barium or gastrografin enema can be very helpful in demonstrating the configuration of the descending colon, the level and extent of diverticular disease, and may help with the decision-making related to extent of the resection that may be needed. However, it is rarely the case that any imaging is obtained for the sole reason of assessing the suitability of the splenic flexure for mobilization.

There is a lack of standardization of preoperative assessment of the blood supply of the splenic flexure, which has proven to have significant variability. Different recognizable patterns have been identified in a recent radiologic study, in which preoperative blood supply was determined by using CT angiography and CT colonography with 3-D reconstructions. In this publication, 39.7% of the blood supply was identified to originate from the left colic artery (LCA), 17.8% from the left branch of the middle colic artery, 9.9% from the LCA and the left branch of the middle colic artery, 4.2% from the accessory left colic artery, 2.6% from the LCA and the accessory left colic artery, and 25.8% from the marginal artery [12]. These newly classified patterns differ from the traditional belief that 85–89% of the blood supply of the splenic flexure originates from the left colic artery and 11–15% from the left branch of the middle colic artery [13]. That being said, we know that the descending colon and splenic flexure are well supplied by vascular arcades originating from the middle colic vessels that connect with blood supply that comes from the inferior mesenteric artery (Fig. 4.3), and it is extremely rare that ligation of the IMA proximal to the left colic results in frank ischemia in the left colon when the proximal mesentery is uninjured.

Technology to assess the blood supply of the large bowel preoperatively is available [14]. There is no evidence, however, to indicate that patients have a decrease in the rate of complications secondary to ischemia when they undergo preoperative assessment of the blood supply compared with those patients who do not, and this

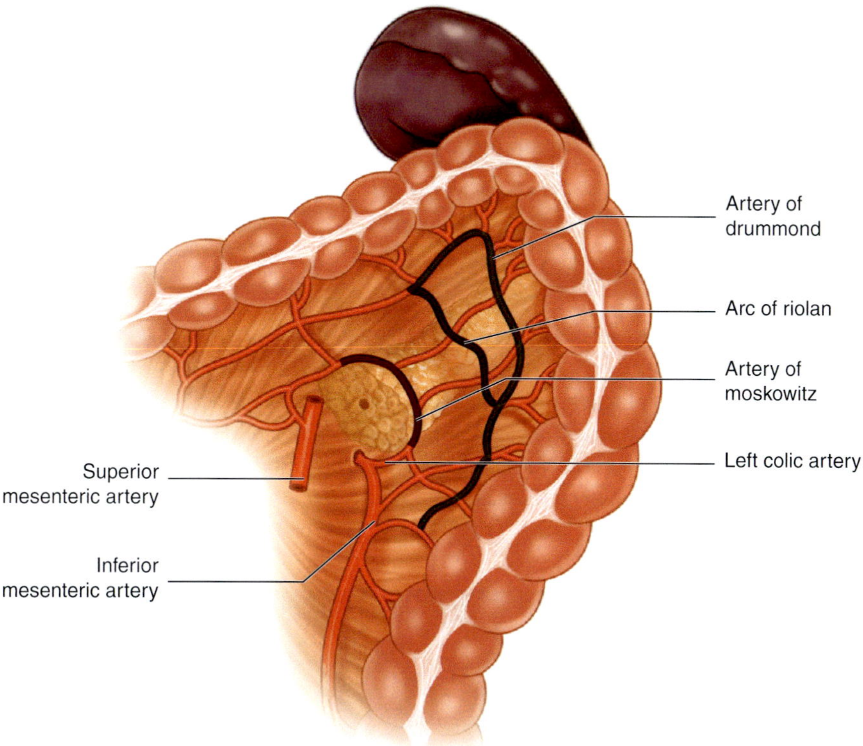

Fig. 4.3 Vascular arcades connecting the middle colic vessels to the blood supply of the IMA

does not play a role in routine preoperative planning for patients [15]. Please refer to Chap. 29 on best practices to assess the integrity and perfusion of left-sided anastomoses.

Operative Setup

The operative setup would be the same as for left-sided and pelvic procedures and/ or total abdominal colectomy. The optimal trocar position includes a 10–12 mm camera port through or near the umbilicus, a second 10–12 mm port in the right lower quadrant (main port for the left-sided dissection), a 5 mm port in the lower aspect of the right upper quadrant, close to the umbilicus, and a second 5 mm port on the contralateral side. The assistant should ideally stand either between the legs or on the right side of the patient with the primary surgeon standing on the right side during the SFR. The surgical table could either be on mild or full reverse Trendelenburg position. This is optional and depends on the surgeon's preference. In our practice, the patient remains in Trendelenburg position throughout the SFR.

Operative Technique: Surgical Steps

The operative approaches for release of the splenic flexure are well established and should be performed in a standardized fashion. There are three options available to the surgeon including the supramesocolic, the inframesocolic, and the lateral to medial approach.

Supramesocolic Approach

The patient is placed in a reverse Trendelenburg roughly five degrees, maximal right side down. The camera is trans- or supraumbilical; the left hand is used to grasp the gastrocolic ligament close to the stomach. Gravity allows for downward traction of the transverse colon, putting the gastrocolic ligament on stretch (Fig. 4.4). The right hand coming from the right lower quadrant is utilized to identify first and then incise the perforating veins between the gastroepiploic veins on the greater curvature and the transverse colon (Fig. 4.5). Once this space is entered, the lesser sac is

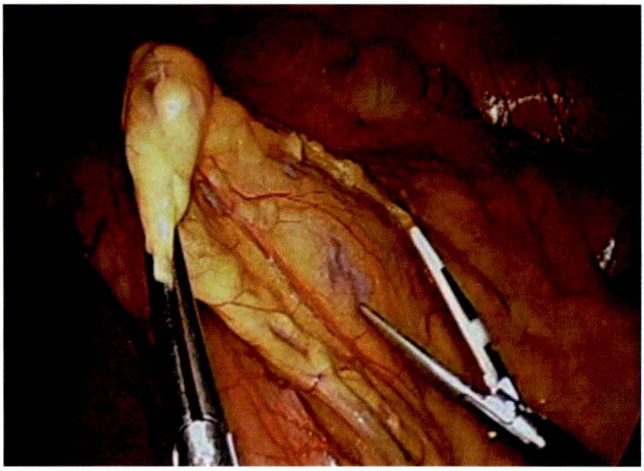

Fig. 4.4 Gastrocolic ligament on stretch. The camera is trans or supraumbilical, the left hand is used to grasp the gastrocolic ligament close to the stomach. Gravity allows for downward traction of the transverse colon, putting the gastrocolic ligament on stretch

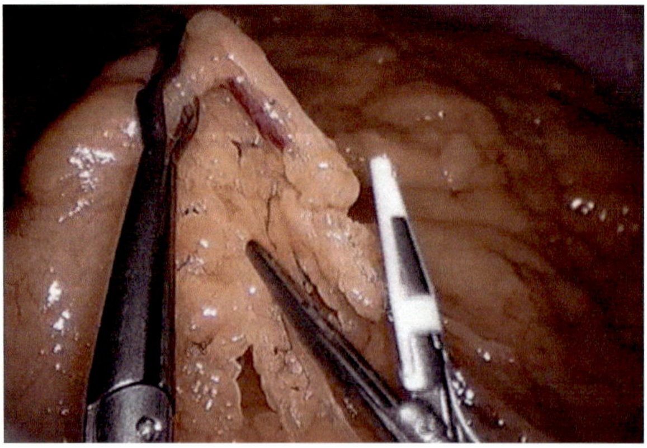

Fig. 4.5 Gastroepiploic vein. The right hand coming from the right lower quadrant is utilized to identify first and then incise the perforating veins between the gastroepiploic veins on the greater curvature and the transverse colon

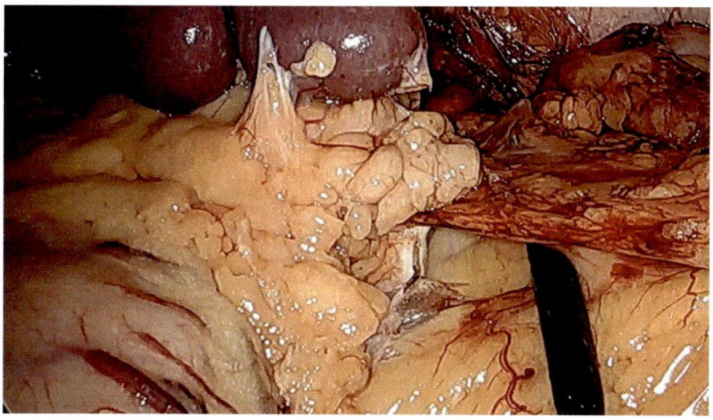

Fig. 4.6 The attachments of the retroperitoneum and the mesentery of the descending colon should be identified and pushed apart along an avascular plane. This can be developed bluntly and does not require any sharp dissection

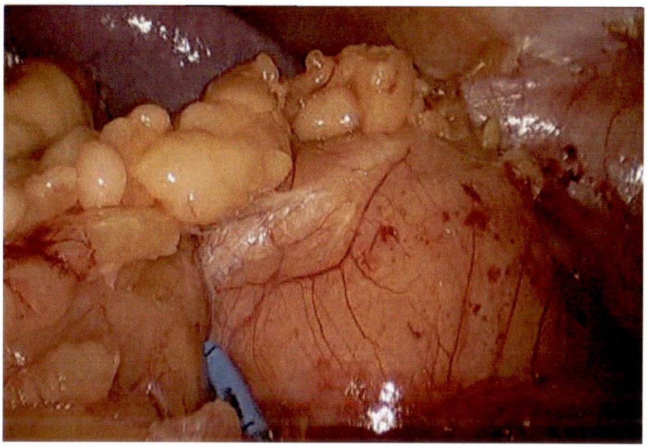

Fig. 4.7 Color and texture difference between Gerota's fascia and the colon mesentery

immediately visualized and incised in a central to lateral fashion from roughly the mid-transverse colon out to the splenic flexure through the gastrocolic ligament. The surgeon must be careful while performing this aspect of the operation to avoid going too deep and inadvertently injuring the mesentery of the transverse colon. This is a critical point as injury to the mesentery of the transverse colon will put at risk the blood supply to the descending colon, which is necessary for the anastomosis. The dissection should be carried out laterally as far as can easily be accomplished. The dissection should then be carried out toward the upper 10 cm of the line of Toldt along the proximal descending colon. The attachments of the retroperitoneum and the mesentery of the descending colon should be identified and pushed apart along an avascular plane. This can be developed bluntly and does not require any sharp dissection (Fig. 4.6). By paying strict attention here, the surgeon can notice the difference in color and texture of the fat of the colonic mesentery, deep to Gerota's fascia and retroperitoneal fat (Fig. 4.7). Once this is mobilized, the hands are switched so that the traction of the transverse colon is brought down to the left hip by the right hand, and the energy source is coming from the left hand, bringing the thermal spread and/or scissors away from the transverse colon and a wayward diverticulum. The attachments of the greater omentum to the spleen must be carefully divided. Care must be taken not to put undue traction on the colon or the

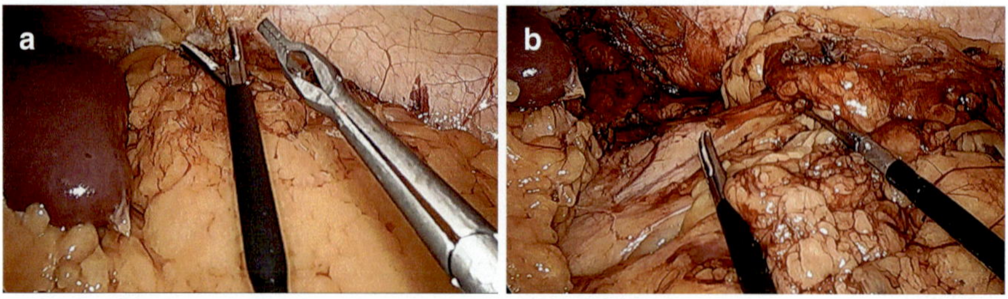

Fig. 4.8 (**a**, **b**) Left-right hand switch. Hands are switched so that the traction of the transverse colon is brought down to the left hip by the right hand and the energy source is coming from the left hand, bringing the thermal spread and or scissors away from the transverse colon and a wayward diverticulum

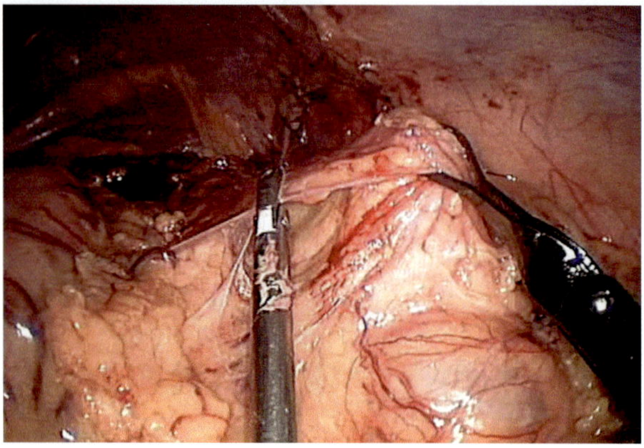

Fig. 4.9 Inferior border of the pancreas. Identifying the mesentery and incising it approximately a centimeter to the inferior border of the pancreas, the transverse colonic mesentery can be liberated from its attachment to the retroperitoneum and along Gerota's fascia

greater omentum. The greater omentum may be attached to the splenic capsule as this will potentially be an area where capsular tearing of the spleen can occur. It is always a good idea at this point of the operation to gently pull medially on the greater omentum while watching the spleen for movement, to gauge the adherence and possible danger of this manipulation. For lower anastomoses, where a coloanal or low rectal anastomosis is necessary, the mesentery must be released from the inferior border of the pancreas. By identifying the mesentery and incising it approximately 1 cm distal to the inferior border of the pancreas, the transverse colonic mesentery can be liberated from its attachment to the retroperitoneum and along Gerota's fascia. If all these steps are completed as described above, splenic flexure release will be complete (Figs. 4.8a, b and 4.9).

Inframesocolic Approach

The patient is positioned in steep Trendelenburg with maximal right side down, and the small bowel is fully retracted to the right side of the abdomen. An incision is made 1.5 cm above the insertion of the inferior mesenteric vein (IMV) into the splenic vein. By dissecting here in an avascular fashion, one will enter into the lesser sac anterior to the pancreas. Care must be taken not to be too superficial and enter into the mesentery of the transverse colon. Interruption of the blood supply here can put at risk the blood supply to the descending colon which is essential for a well-vascularized anastomosis to the rectum. However, when dissection is carried along this avascular plane, this greatly facilitates takedown of the transverse colonic mesentery from its attachments to the retroperitoneum and full mobilization of the mesentery of the transverse colon. This dissection is extended cephalad and laterally, remaining superficial to Gerota's fascia. During this dissection, it is imperative to distinguish the difference in consistency and discoloration of the fatty tissue and the inferior edge of the pancreas in order to stay on the anterior aspect of this latter organ. As the dissection progresses, the descending colon is visualized from the medial aspect. At this point, the lateral attachments are mobilized and the greater omentum is taken off the transverse colon. In this fashion, the colon is entirely mobilized. A considerable challenge of this approach is that, if the surgeon is not careful, she/he can end up posterior to the pancreas and risk injuring it as well as the splenic vein. While highly reliable and reproducible as a technique, this is the approach with the highest potential for complications. It is particularly challenging with obese patients. When learning this technique, it is advised that the surgeon have a low threshold to merge this with the other approaches until the surgeon is very familiar and comfortable with this anatomy and the outlined danger areas. However, with careful manipulation, this approach allows for mobilization of the colon without repositioning the patient.

Lateral to Medial Approach

This is the most commonly used SFR approach, and the one that most open surgeons are comfortable with. An incision is made along the line of Toldt and extended toward the splenic flexure. One must be mindful as one marches up the line of Toldt, not to inadvertently extend behind the kidney. As the surgeon gets close to the splenic flexure, the surgeon remembers that she/he needs to direct the dissection medially and not extend it cephalad. Cephalad extension will direct the surgeon posterior and lateral to the spleen and up to the diaphragm. That being said, by staying slightly medial and scoring the superficial layer of the omentum, it is easier to liberate the rest of the greater omentum off the transverse colon by applying a combination of blunt and sharp dissection. This facilitates full mobilization of the flexure, especially in situations when the omentum and the mesentery are prominent and fatty. From a minimally invasive standpoint, be it laparoscopic or robotic, the challenge with this approach is the energy source being used for dissection (e.g., an ultrasonic, bipolar, or monopolar energy). Lateral spread in this fashion invites the possibility of injury to the colon or an unrecognized diverticulum of the descending colon, distal transverse colon, or splenic flexure. Therefore the surgeon must be mindful at all times to protect the colon so as not to inadvertently injure it during mobilization. Again, if a lower anastomosis is necessary, further dissection may be necessary, including the mesentery of the transverse colon. This can be accomplished in a lateral to medial fashion. Care must be taken to avoid injury of the mesentery or any major nearby vascular structures.

Pros and Cons

In general terms, there are no specific contraindications for the procedure. However, the surgeon must bear in mind that critical structures are very closely related in the splenic flexure area (left kidney, left renal vein, splenic vein, superior mesenteric vessels, portal veins, pancreas). Any injury to those organs or entering into the wrong plane can have serious consequences. There are situations in which the procedure can become very challenging from a technical standpoint as in redo surgery, procedures in morbidly obese patients or in patients with prior pancreatitis or major surgery in left upper quadrant.

Pitfalls and Troubleshooting

Laparoscopic splenic flexure mobilization has traditionally been considered difficult and time-consuming. While some surgeons have advocated using the same standardized approach to SFT in every case, as practicing surgeons it is essential to be knowledgeable in all the different techniques so that difficult anatomy can be addressed safely and an alternative approach can be selected when appropriate [16]. This aspect of the procedure requires a thorough understanding of the anatomy of the neighboring structures in order to avoid injuries. As in any other laparoscopic interventions, the recognition of unsafe scenarios or lack of progress should prompt the surgeon to consider other strategies or conversion to an open approach.

Complications that can occur during SFR include injury to the mesentery of the transverse or descending colon, which can affect perfusion of the left conduit. Once the IMA is transected, colorectal and coloanal anastomoses are entirely dependent on the blood supply from the middle colic artery and accessory vascular arcades, including the marginal artery of Drummond, the arterial arc of Riolan, and the artery of Moskowitz [5] (Fig. 4.3).

Any injury to the marginal vessel that supplies the colon can render the anastomosis ischemic. Aside from dissecting into the wrong plane and inadvertently dividing the mesocolic vessels of the proximal colon, careless handling of the mesentery can be costly and result in devascularization of the proximal colon [17]. The intraoperative use of fluorescence imaging to assess perfusion can be helpful in gauging adequate blood supply for the left colon before and after constructing the anastomosis [11, 18]. If more proximal colon needs to be mobilized to achieve a well-vascularized anastomosis, the colon attachments should be released fully from the inferior border of the pancreas.

Other complications of SFR include splenic injury. The spleen is often not clearly visualized, and no effort should be made to routinely see it. Regardless of the surgeon's ability to see the spleen, it must be made certain that undue mobilization or traction do not occur. The most common mechanism whereby the spleen is injured during splenic mobilization involves excessive pulling on the descending or transverse colon when the greater omentum is attached to the splenic capsule. The result is avulsion of capsule and subsequent bleeding. When this occurs, generally the best approach is to pack the area and wait for hemostasis rather than resort to more aggressive strategies. That being said, clearly the best way to treat a splenic injury is to avoid it in the first place [19].

Other areas of risk involve injury to the pancreas, particularly in the area of the splenic hilum and the pancreatic tail. While mobilizing the splenic flexure, one must be certain to be anterior to the tail of the pancreas and away from the splenic hilum. It is not difficult when fully mobilizing the mesentery of the distal transverse colon and the proximal descending colon to delve too deep into the retroperitoneum and inadvertently dissect posterior to the pancreatic tail. This, in turn, takes the surgeon into the splenic hilum [19].

Lastly, a potential complication, which is unique to the inframesocolic approach, includes carrying the dissection at the IMV to posterior and coming underneath the inferior border of the pancreas. The real problem here is that if this is continued, one can enter the splenic vein, which could result in major bleeding. By recognizing this possibility, the surgeon should be able to avoid this issue entirely.

The inframesocolic approach is more difficult to adopt from a technical standpoint. It is the preferred approach during robotic dissection, when changes in table positioning are much more restricted. It is our recommendation that surgeons become facile with all three approaches. But while learning each technique, the surgeon should be aware of the limitations and risks of each approach and have a low threshold to convert to another approach or to an open approach.

Another area of difficulty that can be encountered is when the greater omentum is so prominent that it either entirely obscures the flexure and/or is densely fused with the mesentery (Fig. 4.10). This needs to be carefully released to obtain adequate length that can be carried out for a safe colorectal anastomosis.

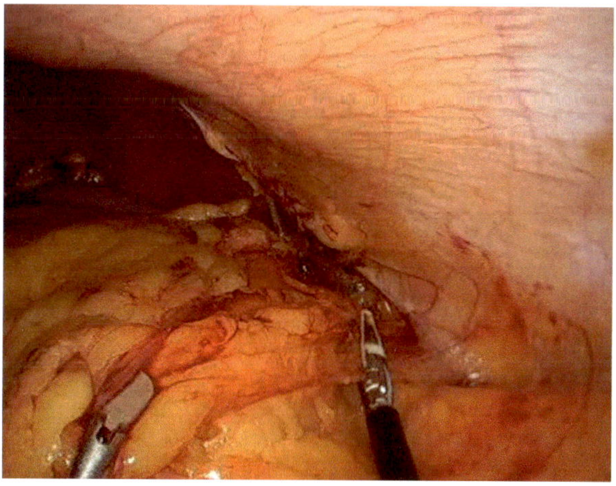

Fig. 4.10 Greater omentum covering the splenic flexure

Outcomes

Literature comparing different approaches for SFR is scarce. Perhaps the most significant publication is from Benseler and colleagues. This retrospective study compared the use of the three different approaches on 303 patients that underwent laparoscopic surgery for rectal cancer at a single center over a 12-year period. The authors identified a significantly higher rate of intraoperative complications ($p = 0.038$), including dissecting in the wrong plane, organ injury, and bleeding, for those patients that had SFR using the lateral approach. Postoperative morbidity was also higher on the same group, secondary to increased wound infection ($p = 0.001$) [20]. We cannot provide any rational explanation for these results nor would we allow this to factor into our decision-making for how to best approach this operative step.

Conclusions

Splenic flexure release is an integral part of the procedure for a multitude of colon surgeries. The general and colorectal surgeon must be entirely comfortable with the different approaches in order to carry this out in a routine fashion. In most cases, the splenic flexure can be released by using one of the above-described techniques. However, on occasion, a combination of approaches is required. We recommend that each surgeon develop their preferred technique which they use routinely but also become facile with the other approaches as these will be helpful at times, and it is best to be knowledgeable before trying a technique in a difficult situation.

We advocate the routine release of the splenic flexure for a safe anastomosis. It is the authors' opinion that consideration to releasing the splenic flexure be given early on during the procedure in a proactive fashion, rather than reserving it for when it is necessary in order to achieve adequate length for the anastomosis. Delaying the decision to complete splenic flexure takedown until the end of an otherwise difficult operation can complicate the procedure even further. Routine release using a standardized approach will result in better outcome for patients with colorectal disease.

References

1. Goulder F. Bowel anastomoses: the theory, the practice and the evidence base. WJGS. 2012;4(9):208–6.
2. Chand M, Miskovic D, Parvaiz AC. Is splenic flexure mobilization necessary in laparoscopic anterior resection? Dis Colon Rectum. 2012;55(11):1195–7.
3. Brennan DJ, Moynagh M, Brannigan AE, Gleeson F, Rowland M, O'Connell RP. Routine mobilization of the splenic flexure is not necessary during anterior resection for rectal cancer. Dis Colon Rectum. 2007;50(3):302–7.
4. Tortorelli A, Alfieri S, Sanchez A, Rosa F, Papa V, Di Miceli D, et al. Anastomotic leakage after anterior resection for rectal cancer with mesorectal excision: incidence, risk factors, and management. Am J Surg. 2015;81(1):41–7.

5. Toh JWT, Matthews R, Kim SH. Arc of Riolan-preserving splenic flexure takedown during anterior resection. Dis Colon Rectum. 2018;61(3):411–4.
6. Jurowich CF, Germer CT. Elective surgery for sigmoid diverticulitis – indications, techniques, and results. Visc Med. 2015;31(2):112–6.
7. Rullier E, Denost Q, Vendrely V, Rullier A, Laurent C. Low rectal cancer. Dis Colon Rectum. 2013;56(5):560–7.
8. Marks JH, Myers EA, Zeger EL, Denittis AS, Gummadi M, Marks GJ. Long-term outcomes by a transanal approach to total mesorectal excision for rectal cancer. Surg Endosc. 2017;31(12):5248–57.
9. Marks JH, Salem JF. From TATA to NOTES: how taTME fits into the evolutionary surgical tree. Tech Coloproctol. 2016;20(8):513–5.
10. Marks JH, Montenegro GA, Salem JF, Shields MV, Marks GJ. Transanal TATA/TME: a case-matched study of taTME versus laparoscopic TME surgery for rectal cancer. Tech Coloproctol. 2016;20(7):467–73.
11. Caycedo-Marulanda A, Ma G, Jiang HY. Transanal total mesorectal excision (taTME) in a single-surgeon setting: refinements of the technique during the learning phase. Tech Coloproctol. 2018;22(6):433–43.
12. Fukuoka A, Sasaki T, Tsukikawa S, Miyajima N, Ostubo T. Evaluating distribution of the left branch of the middle colic artery and the left colic artery by CT angiography and colonography to classify blood supply to the splenic flexure. Asian J Endosc Surg. 2016;10(2):148–53.
13. Sakorafas GH, Zouros E, Peros G. Applied vascular anatomy of the colon and rectum: clinical implications for the surgical oncologist. Surg Oncol. 2006;15(4):243–55.
14. Kawamoto A, Inoue Y, Okigami M, Yasuda H, Okugawa Y, Hiro J, et al. Preoperative assessment of vascular anatomy by multidetector computed tomography before laparoscopic colectomy for transverse colon cancer: report of a case. Int Surg. 2015;100(2):208–12.
15. McDermott S, Deipolyi A, Walker T, Ganguli S, Wicky S, Oklu R. The role of preoperative angiogram in colon interposition surgery. Diagn Interv Radiol. 2012;18(3):314–8.
16. Takeru M, Takeshi I, Kenro H, Daisuke T, Yutaka S, Yasuo S, et al. A three-step method for laparoscopic mobilization of the splenic flexure. Ann Surg Oncol. 2015;22(s335):1–1.
17. Garcia-Granero A, Sánchez-Guillén L, Carreño O, Sancho Muriel J, Alvarez Sarrado E, Fletcher Sanfeliu D, et al. Importance of the Moskowitz artery in the laparoscopic medial approach to splenic flexure mobilization: a cadaveric study. Tech Coloproctol. 2017;21(7):567–72.
18. Blanco-Colino R, Espin-Basany E. Intraoperative use of ICG fluorescence imaging to reduce the risk of anastomotic leakage in colorectal surgery: a systematic review and meta-analysis. Tech Coloproctol. 2017;22(1):15–23.
19. Merchea A, Dozois EJ, Wang JK, Larson DW. Anatomic mechanisms for splenic injury during colorectal surgery. Clin Anat. 2011;25(2):212–7.
20. Benseler V, Hornung M, Iesalnieks I, Breitenbuch von P, Glockzin G, Schlitt HJ, et al. Different approaches for complete mobilization of the splenic flexure during laparoscopic rectal cancer resection. Int J Color Dis. 2012;27(11):1521–9.

Bibliography

Atallah S, Albert M, Monson JRT. Critical concepts and important anatomic landmarks encountered during transanal total mesorectal excision (taTME): toward the mastery of a new operation for rectal cancer surgery. Tech Coloproctol. 2016;20(7):483–94.

Deijen CL, Tsai A, Koedam TWA, Veltcamp Helbach M, Sietses C, Lacy AM, et al. Clinical outcomes and case volume effect of transanal total mesorectal excision for rectal cancer: a systematic review. Tech Coloproctol. 2016;20(12):811–24.

Koedam TWA, van Ramshorst GH, Deijen CL, Elfrink AKE, Meijerink WJHJ, Bonjer HJ, et al. Transanal total mesorectal excision (TaTME) for rectal cancer: effects on patient-reported quality of life and functional outcome. Tech Coloproctol. 2017;21(1):25–33.

Lee L, De Lacy B, Gomez Ruiz M, Liberman AS, Albert MR, Monson JRT, et al. A multicenter matched comparison of transanal and robotic total mesorectal excision for mid and low-rectal adenocarcinoma. Ann Surg. 2018; https://doi.org/10.1097/SLA.0000000000002862. [Epub ahead of print]

Pasam RT, Trejo DE, Murray A, Lee-Kong S, Feingold D, Kiran RP. PTU-223 Conversion to open surgery from laparoscopy: to 'try and fail' or 'not try at all'? Gut. 2015;64(Suppl 1):A161.1–A161.

Sylla P, Rattner DW, Delgado S, Lacy AM. NOTES transanal rectal cancer resection using transanal endoscopic microsurgery and laparoscopic assistance. Surg Endosc. 2010;24(5):1205–10.

Wong-Chong N, Caycedo-Marulanda A. Transanal total mesorectal excision with retroileal colorectal anastomosis: combining old and new techniques. Color Dis. 2018;20(7):642–3.

Masters Program Colorectal Pathway: Laparoscopic Left Colon Resection for Complex Inflammatory Bowel Disease

5

Anuradha R. Bhama and Conor P. Delaney

Introduction and Rationale

Crohn's disease can be a challenging disease process for surgeons to treat. Patients often present with obstruction, an abscess, or fistula, frequently with septic complications of their disease [1]. When possible, these are initially treated nonoperatively with image-guided drainage procedures and antibiotics in order to stabilize the patient and clear the sepsis. This then allows for time to hold immunosuppressive medications and optimize nutritional parameters to allow for an elective resection. Less frequently, nonoperative preparation and preoperative optimization may not be possible, and the patient will require a more emergent operative procedure. This is usually related to intestinal obstruction or perforation of a previously contained abscess.

This chapter will focus on the specific considerations regarding fistula and abscess necessary in patients with CD. Fistulas can occur between the small bowel and colon with any adjacent structure including the bladder, the vagina, other gastrointestinal sites, or, more rarely, the skin (Figs. 5.1a, b and 5.2). In situations involving a fistula between the left colon and the small intestine, it is necessary to determine the segment of the diseased intestine that is the origin of the fistula, as the diseased segment is the portion of the bowel that should be resected. If the small intestine is diseased, then frequently only the small intestine requires resection, provided the sigmoid colon is free of disease and the fistulous opening is small and amenable to primary repair, as described below (Figs. 5.3, 5.4, 5.5, and 5.6a–c). Regardless, a laparoscopic approach can usually be utilized safely to perform a

A. R. Bhama
Department of Surgery, Division of Colorectal Surgery, Rush University Medical Center, Chicago, IL, USA

C. P. Delaney (✉)
Digestive Disease and Surgery Institute, Cleveland Clinic, Cleveland, OH, USA
e-mail: delanec@ccf.org

P. Sylla et al. (eds.), *The SAGES Manual of Colorectal Surgery*,
https://doi.org/10.1007/978-3-030-24812-3_5

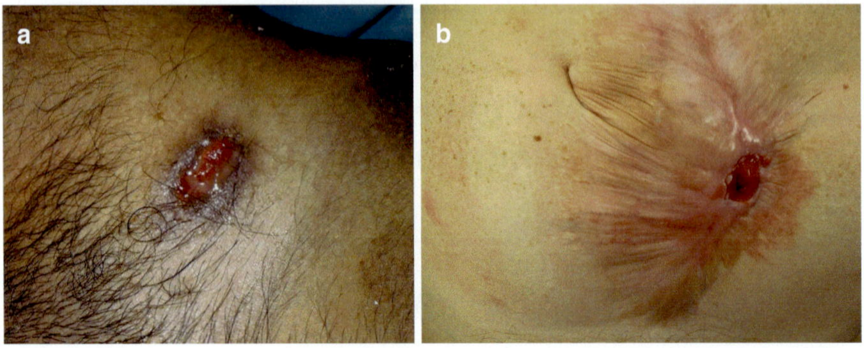

Fig. 5.1 (**a**, **b**) Examples of colocutaneous fistula in patients with inflammatory bowel disease

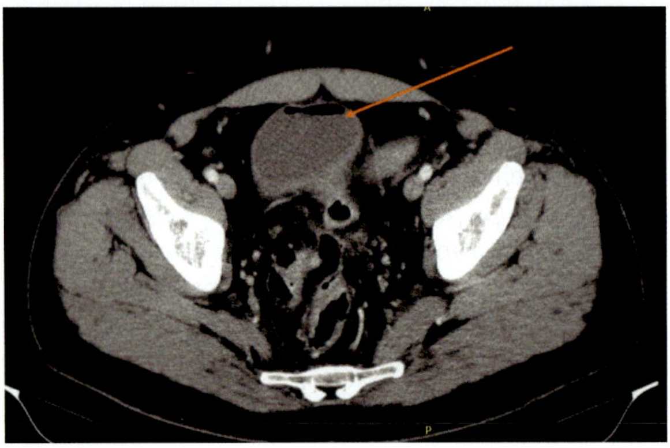

Fig. 5.2 CT scan of patient with colovesical fistula. Note air in the bladder

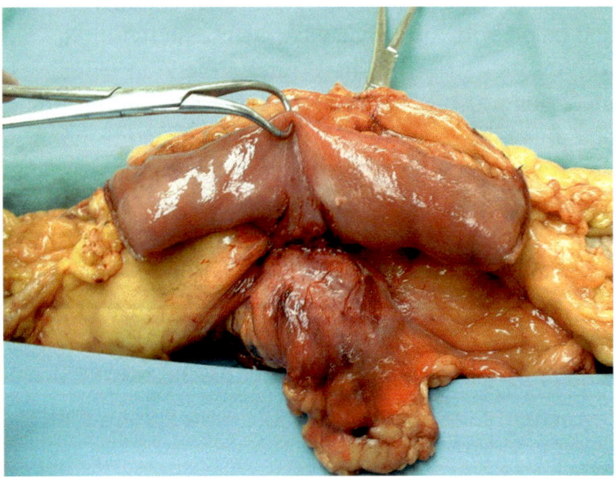

Fig. 5.3 Fistula between healthy small bowel and diseased segment of colon

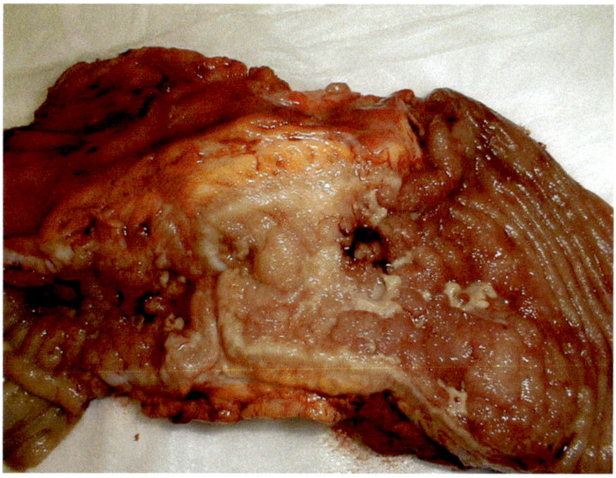

Fig. 5.4 Luminal view of enteric fistula in setting of active inflammatory Crohn's disease

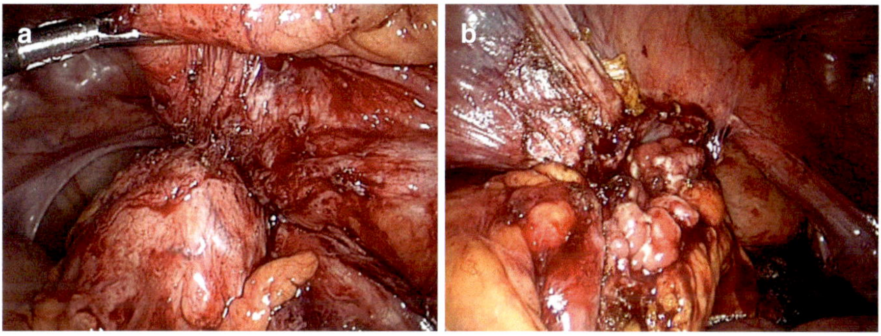

Fig. 5.5 (**a**, **b**) Laparoscopic views of fistulizing Crohn's disease

left-sided colon resection in most situations [2, 3]. Some patients with chronic complex diverticular disease may present with fistulas and abscesses that require similar management [4].

Indications and Contraindications

A laparoscopic approach is indicated in almost all patients. Inability to tolerate pneumoperitoneum and steep Trendelenburg position because of medical comorbidity or massive obesity are rare in this population. The primary contraindication is a prior history of multiple surgeries with obliterative adhesions. Anatomical considerations that may complicate laparoscopy include large hernias, dense adhesions from prior surgery, or enterocutaneous fistulas that require resection of the abdominal wall. Patients who are hemodynamically unstable generally cannot tolerate laparoscopy, as the positioning is typically more exaggerated, the operative times may be longer, and the pneumoperitoneum causes a decrease in cardiac preload. Patients

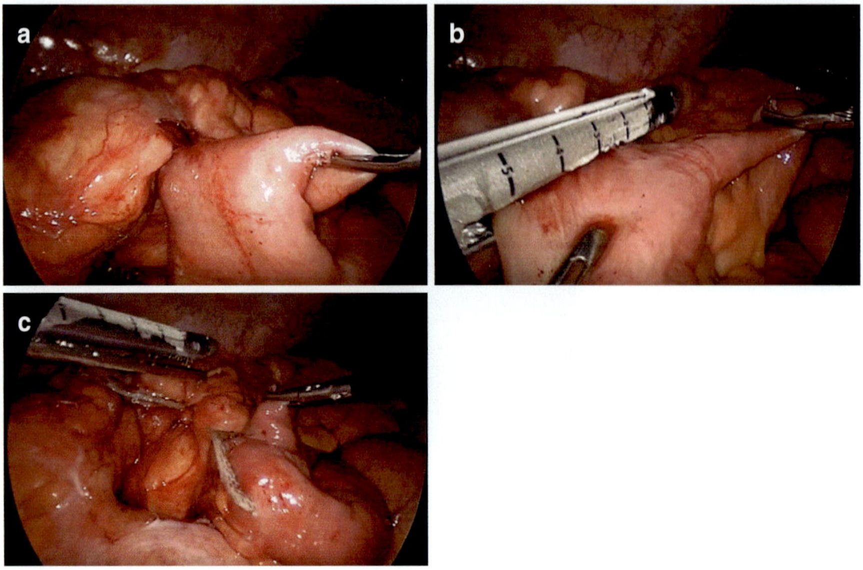

Fig. 5.6 (**a–c**) Crohn's ileosigmoid fistula. After confirming that the sigmoid is not primarily involved with active inflammatory Crohn's disease, the endoscopic stapler is used to transect across the fistula followed by resection of the disease terminal ileum and preservation of the sigmoid colon. (All: Courtesy of Daniel Popowich, MD)

must be able to tolerate the physiologic changes associated with laparoscopy in order to undergo this approach. This includes patients with severe pulmonary disease as well. In the vast majority of cases, however, laparoscopy can be attempted and if the patient does not tolerate a trial at positioning, or adhesions are too severe, conversion to an open procedure may be indicated. Other contraindications include lack of surgeon experience or lack of appropriate equipment.

There are some situations in which a large fistula is present that may require assistance from other subspecialty surgeons, such as a low bladder fistula or rare ureteric fistula. In such cases, it is necessary to coordinate preoperative planning with the assisting surgeons. Especially for the sigmoid colon, if it is possible to do the majority of the procedure laparoscopically and a portion of the procedure through a small Pfannenstiel incision, many of the benefits of laparoscopy may be provided to the patient by minimizing the size of the definitive incision. Careful preoperative planning in a team-based approach and clear communication with the operating room staff is necessary in these situations.

Segmental colon resection in the setting of CD remains somewhat controversial [5–10]. Although a full discussion of this topic is outside the confines of this chapter, a total colectomy is usually indicated for CD-related dysplasia or pancolitis, considering ileorectal anastomosis for those with rectal sparing and good continence [11]. Segmental colectomy, with or without a temporary diverting ileostomy, can be considered for those with short segment disease in whom the rectum, anus, and proximal colon appear salvageable.

Principles and Quality Benchmarks

The first principle of treating IBD associated with fistula and abscess is to ensure that the source of sepsis has been controlled, and the patient has been stabilized hemodynamically. These patients rarely present acutely. When possible, treatment with antibiotics and utilization of radiologic drainage as a bridge to surgery is advocated to clear sepsis and allow the patient to recover from systemic sepsis and allow for preoperative optimization. Nutritional optimization may need to be considered as well, and we primarily base assessment on weight loss, using prealbumin in those otherwise suspected to be malnourished. Patients are frequently evaluated by dieticians on the multidisciplinary team. If patients can tolerate enteral diets, they are educated on dietary choices and supplements that optimize their protein and calorie needs. If patients cannot tolerate oral intake, they are evaluated and followed carefully by members of a multidisciplinary nutritional support team to manage enteral or total parenteral nutrition. Ideally patients will demonstrate weight gain or stabilization of weight loss and normal serum markers of nutrition including albumin and prealbumin. There are instances where the disease severity is so great that surgical resection is necessary prior to improvement in nutritional status. For that reason, we generally are more concerned about getting 7–10 days of adequate nutrition, rather than waiting for laboratory values to normalize.

When proceeding with the operation, it is important to remember to evaluate the entire bowel for active disease, even if the indication for operation is colonic disease. The extent of disease is not always accurately identified preoperatively. Typically, preoperative evaluation includes colonoscopy and one or more means of small bowel assessment, such as CT or MR enterography. If no recent endoscopic assessment is available, preoperative colonoscopy should be performed to assess for the extent of colitis or proctitis and for any underlying malignancy, as it allows more accurate surgical planning and a better discussion with the patient. If patients are very symptomatic and/or preoperative colonoscopy cannot be completed, this can be performed intraoperatively. Even so, it is important to visually inspect the entire intestine for active disease and in our practice, we generally exteriorize and "run" or sequentially palpate the entire small intestine. At a minimum this can be done laparoscopically with a hand-over-hand technique of running the small bowel, with care taken to avoid injuring the bowel, although generally the small bowel can be exteriorized and palpated when a specimen is being removed.

When performing a resection for CD, it is important to preserve as much bowel as possible, though this is less directly relevant for colonic disease. Surgical margins should be grossly negative for active disease for 2 cm, as defined by the normal appearing bowel with absence of mesenteric inflammation. It is not necessary to have frozen section assessment of surgical margins. An anastomosis should not be created if there is active purulence in proximity to the anastomosis, such as a large pelvic abscess with resultant thickening and secondary inflammation of the distal rectum. A proximal diverting loop ileostomy should be considered if there are concerns about the quality of the remaining intestine for anastomosis, patient nutrition, or immunosuppression.

Preoperative Planning, Patient Workup, and Optimization

Except in the relatively rare situations of bleeding or acute perforation, preoperative optimization is essential for patients with IBD. Abscesses that can be drained are dealt with using image-guided techniques, including retroperitoneal abscesses, unless small. Smaller abscesses and some intramesenteric abscesses may be best left undrained and treated with antibiotics. Holding any immunosuppressive agents, such as biologic agents, is also recommended. Steroids are tapered if possible but can rarely be stopped in patients with these types of symptoms. There are no set guidelines for the duration of time of biologic agents to be held, though we generally wait 6–8 weeks prior to proceeding with an operation. The nutritional status of the patient should be assessed to determine the safety of proceeding with an operation and the likelihood of successful healing postoperatively. Evaluation of serum levels of albumin, prealbumin, and transferrin is useful. In patients who are malnourished, preoperative supplemental nutrition may be necessary. This can be done orally with high-protein supplements but may require enteral or parenteral nutrition, particularly in those who are chronically partially obstructed with their disease, or who have high-output or symptomatic fistulas which preclude intestinal feeding. Postoperative supplemental enteral or parenteral nutrition is generally unnecessary. Many patients are also routinely seen by our enterostomal team and given a temporary mark for a stoma. In cases requiring intraoperative decision-making, both left and right-sided marks are placed, taking care to be away from old scars and skinfolds.

Once surgery is scheduled, standard enhanced recovery protocols are applied [12]. Patients should be encouraged to stop smoking and limit alcohol intake, as these have been shown to have improved postoperative outcomes when done for greater than 4 weeks prior to operation. Patient education and setting clear postoperative expectations are paramount in preparation for surgery. This discussion includes expected goals regarding pain control, postoperative diet advancement, patient participation in recovery, and discharge criteria and planning.

In preparation for the operation, all patients who are not obstructed should undergo mechanical bowel preparation. Bowel preparation is commonly utilized as it provides several benefits in the laparoscopic setting. The decompressed bowel after mechanical bowel preparation allows for easier manipulation and specimen extraction. Particularly important is that the addition of oral neomycin and metronidazole with the mechanical bowel appears to be associated with a significant decrease in rate of postoperative surgical site infection.

Preoperative diet remains controversial, as patients traditionally fast from midnight the night prior to surgery. In our practice, consistent with anesthesia guidelines, patients are allowed to continue to consume clear liquids up until 2 hours prior to surgery. Some enhanced recovery protocols also provide patients with carbohydrate loading fluids to drink the morning of surgery. Patients with chronic obstructive disease who will not tolerate a bowel preparation are kept on a liquid diet for 48 hours and given two bottles of magnesium citrate, a milder preparation that is usually tolerated reasonably well. For more details on preoperative preparations, please refer to the chapters on enhanced recovery protocols in colorectal surgery (Chaps. 7 and 8).

Standard venous thromboembolism prophylaxis and preoperative intravenous antibiotics should be administered in accordance with SCIP (Surgical Care Improvement Project) guidelines [12]. This has been shown to minimize the risk of surgical site infection. Enhanced recovery programs also call for antinausea prophylaxis to be administered [12]. Currently, alvimopan is not indicated for laparoscopic surgery, as it has not been clearly shown to improve postoperative outcomes; however, we will give a single dose to patients at high risk of conversion, and this will continue postoperatively if the patient is converted to open surgery. For more details on enhanced recovery recommendations, please refer to the chapter on enhanced recovery protocols in colorectal surgery (Chaps. 7 and 8).

Operative Setup

Patients are placed in a modified lithotomy position, ensuring that the legs and arms are positioned appropriately to avoid nerve injury. The patient's arms should both be tucked by their sides, with the use of sleds if needed for larger patients. In order to overcome the steep Trendelenburg positioning, a bean bag may be placed underneath the patient, the chest may be taped to the table, or anti-sliding padding can be used. The lithotomy position is important so access to the anus is maintained.

Operative Technique: Surgical Steps

The basics steps of laparoscopic colectomy for CD follow similar principles to those described in the chapters on laparoscopic left and sigmoid colectomy for benign (Chap. 3) and malignant disease (Chap. 17). In cases of abscess and fistula with inflammatory bowel disease, and similar to some complex diverticular disease, there are several operative steps that are helpful.

Laparoscopic Access

Many of these cases are re-operative in nature. Even so, we start with a sub-umbilical cutdown to insert a Hasson balloon port. This commonly is quite straightforward. If there are adhesions or concerns of adherent intestine, a lateral 5 mm visual port is inserted, away from the area of the pathology. This guides placement of a second port which allows adhesiolysis and insertion of additional ports as required.

Definition of Anatomy and Pathology and Abscess Management

The procedure starts with a review of the area of pathology. Multiple small bowel loops may be involved and there may be extensive adhesions. The operation then starts with lysis of adhesions, separating each loop individually off the phlegmon.

In these cases, the entire small bowel will be examined extracorporeally, but if there are areas of particular concern, they are marked with a laparoscopic 3-0 polyglycolic acid suture. Loops of small bowel that contain fistulas are controlled by an endoloop suture, to minimize intraabdominal leakage and contamination. Generally, each adherent loop of bowel is separated so that they can be removed through a small incision for resection or examination.

Once the small bowel loops have been separated, the colon can be evaluated. The decision of whether the mesentery or bowel is mobilized first really depends on what step will facilitate dissection of the diseased segment most safely and effectively. Oftentimes, the best strategy is to start by mobilizing the bowel proximal to the pathology in order to define the correct anatomical planes. This will help identify anatomic landmarks and guide the dissection safely toward the diseased segments and associated phlegmons, abscess cavities, and/or fistulas. This dissection will lead next to taking down colovesical, colovaginal fistulas, or even left lower quadrant cutaneous fistulas. These are transected with a combination of sharp dissection with scissors and blunt dissection using a Maryland or bowel grasper. For those who like energy devices for dissection, these are particularly unsuitable in fistula and abscess cases, as the tissues are often so thickened that the energy devices cannot be closed effectively. When a pericolonic abscess cavity is unroofed, a suction device is immediately positioned into the cavity to aspirate out all pus before it contaminates the abdomen. The goal at this stage is simply to control and minimize spillage of purulence. The use of monopolar cautery should be minimized in order to avoid inadvertent burn injury to the bowel. Sponges can be very helpful to achieve hemostasis as well as to provide effective bowel retraction. Frequently ovaries, fallopian tubes, or the appendix may be adherent to the inflammatory phlegmon or abscess and must be carefully separated. If the appendix is involved, it is removed as per routine. Once the pathology and anatomy have been fully defined, the entire small bowel should be examined for disease, as described above.

Another important consideration is identification of the ureter. Frequently the ureter may be more medial than expected due to distorted anatomy from the inflammatory process. Consider ureteral stents, although these are generally not required except for cases with a psoas abscess, prior pelvic surgery, or some colovaginal fistulae with a phlegmon involving the pelvic sidewall.

Mobilization and Division of Mesentery

For the left colon, a low ligation of the inferior mesenteric vessels is adequate unless there is dysplasia or a concern for cancer. Our preferred approach in cancer is a medial to lateral approach to the mesentery. This frequently also works well in cases with inflammatory disease. Usually the easiest first step is to grasp the rectosigmoid mesentery and elevate it from the retroperitoneum and incise with scissors or cautery parallel to the inferior mesenteric vessels over the sacral promontory. This allows CO_2 to distend the presacral space, and the mesentery is mobilized as per routine. If there is too much tethering on the mesentery because of a vesical fistula, this is taken down first. The left colic vessels may need to be divided to achieve adequate length for tension-free colorectal anastomosis.

In cases where the abscess is medial, however, a medial approach is fraught with difficulty, and there is frequently too much inflammation to visualize any plane. Rather than transecting the mesentery blindly, we will switch to a lateral to medial approach. The planes there are often more manageable, even allowing mobilization as far medial as the ureter and presacral space. If that is not the case, move proximally on the descending colon, and a plane can usually be found. The last option is a high medial approach, coming between the duodenojejunal flexure and the inferior mesenteric vein, which generally allows entry to a clean anatomical plane.

If there is any doubt about an anatomical plane, stay inside the mesenteric fascia. While this causes a little more bleeding, it is much safer. It is important not to dissect blindly, particularly with an energy device, as these can so effectively stop bleeding that one may stray outside the correct plane and cause injury to surrounding urinary, vascular, or nerve structures.

Many of these abscesses and fistulas involve the left pelvic sidewall. In these cases, one must carefully combine blunt and sharp dissection techniques, and frequently switch from medial to lateral views, to progress gradually to completely dissect the mesentery off the abscess wall or pelvic sidewall. The goal is to have adequately mobilized the left colon, so that the diseased segment can be removed, with an adequate margin of normal tissue and adequate length for a tension-free anastomosis. Splenic flexure mobilization is almost routinely required in these cases but division of the inferior mesenteric vein again at the tail of the pancreas is rarely required. Please refer to specific laparoscopic techniques in Chap. 4 on laparoscopic splenic flexure release.

Colon Transection

Proximal colonic division is generally extracorporeal. The distal transection margin is critical and may be complex. The most frequent consideration is whether one is distal to the inflammation. Our goal is always to mobilize enough rectum and mesorectum so that we reach visibly and palpably normal tissue. Sometimes a loop of sigmoid is stuck in the pelvis, and this must be completely mobilized. Sometimes the upper rectal wall is thickened because of an adjacent abscess, and we generally mobilize more distally, sometimes below the peritoneal reflection until normal bowel can be identified. If the rectum does not look healthy enough for an anastomosis, it is transected as a Hartmann's stump and an end colostomy is brought out, which may subsequently be closed depending on a variety of factors such as pathology, patient status, etc. Indeed, the quality of the distal rectum is usually a predominant determinant of whether an anastomosis will be performed, or a Hartmann's stump left for safety. Additional considerations for anastomosis include the extent and severity of any residual proctitis in the rectal stump. For details on steps to take during Hartman's procedures, please refer to the chapter on Key steps to facilitate minimally invasive Hartmann's reversal (Chap. 20).

Specimen Extraction

In simple cases requiring a sigmoid or left colon resection, a left lower quadrant muscle splitting incision is made. This is technically straightforward with a low complication rate. If a diverting stoma is required, the specimen is removed through that opening, if necessary making a "key-hole" incision to enlarge the opening.

For patients with an enterocolic fistula that required dissection of tethered small bowel loops from an abscess or phlegmon, or with concurrent ileocolic and left colon disease, a short periumbilical midline incision is used. A wound protector is critical to prevent contamination by the abscess or fistula. This permits sequential exteriorization of the entire length of the small bowel, which can be examined, resected, or repaired as appropriate.

Anastomosis

Small bowel anastomoses are performed most frequently using a stapled side-side functional end-end approach. Left-sided anastomoses are stapled transanally. We use a 28 mm circular stapler to minimize anal stretching and to facilitate reaching the apex of the rectal stump. Sizers are not usually required for these cases, although they are sometimes used to gently stretch the rectum. In rare cases, a hand-sewn colorectal anastomosis may be performed, and this can be performed through a short Pfannenstiel incision.

Fistula Repair

The enteric and colon sides of fistulas are generally both resected as segmental resections (Fig. 5.3). In the setting of Crohn's disease, it is necessary to first evaluate both for active inflammation. If the tissues are actively inflamed, then a fistula repair is not advisable, and formal resection should be carried out (Figs. 5.4 and 5.5a, b). If there is no surrounding inflammation, a tiny fistula in small bowel may be managed with a wedge resection and hand-sewn closure of the enterotomy. While some surgeons advocate selective use of stapling across fistulas when only one of the bowel segments is involved with Crohn's disease, we do not routinely staple across fistula tracts, as we feel this is by definition abnormal tissue and at higher risk for recurrence. We tend to reserve this for patients with multiple prior Crohn's resections and less residual small bowel (Fig. 5.6a–c). For more discussions on laparoscopic management of complex Crohn's ileocolic disease, please refer to the chapter on advanced laparoscopic right colectomy techniques (Chap. 16).

Small colovesical fistulas are tested by distending the bladder with very dilute methylene blue. If there is no leak, they are not sutured. Larger fistulas are repaired with laparoscopic suturing. An omental pedicle graft should be placed next to the bladder, and a drain should be placed and monitored in case of a urine leak. A contrast study is done at 48 hours for small fistulas. Larger (sutured) fistulas are imaged at 2 weeks by cystography before removing the Foley catheter. Vaginal fistulas are left open unless they are large in which case they are sutured with absorbable sutures. An omental pedicle graft is placed over the defect when possible.

Other Steps

A segment of omentum is brought down as an omental pedicle graft between any remaining wall of a fistula or abscess cavity if reach permits. Drains are placed into residual contained abscess cavities, although not if the abscess cavity has not been mostly excised. Surgical wounds are closed in a standard fashion, and a wound protector is used in all cases. Vacuum-assisted (VAC) dressings are not used. In rare cases of extreme purulence or wound contamination, the wound is partially closed and a betadine wick is inserted and removed on POD3 for delayed primary closure. If there is a colocutaneous fistula that requires excision of the abdominal wall and skin (Fig. 5.1a, b), these defects are typically managed with wet to dry dressing changes, which can be switched to negative pressure dressing changes once healthy granulation tissue is visible. The utilization of laparoscopy helps reduce the rates of surgical site infection when compared to open operations. Standard enhanced recovery protocols and intraoperative surgical site infection measures are implemented.

Pitfalls and Troubleshooting

The level of difficulty can range from straightforward to highly complex depending on the degree of severity of the inflammation. The learning curve in general for laparoscopic left colectomy is upward of 50 cases and may not necessarily include the challenges specific to safely managing penetrating CD [13]. Common challenges include the ability to separate the colon from adjacent structures, identifying and protecting the left ureter, managing the difficult Crohn's mesentery, and closure of the fistula on the organ remaining in situ (typically bladder or vagina). When separating the colon from adjacent structures, if standard techniques are not successful, some surgeons favor conversion to hand-assist to optimize blunt dissection while minimizing the size of the incision to maintain the benefits of a laparoscopic approach.

Identifying the ureter can be difficult in the setting of severe inflammation. Keep in mind that the ureter may be more medial than normal. Ureteral stents may be placed preoperatively or intraoperatively if necessary [14]. We tend to favor selective intraoperative placement since a previous study we performed showed that this made surgery faster and was just as manageable for urology [14]. Typically, ureteral stents may help identify but not prevent ureteral injuries, and their presence should not supplant safe dissection and knowledge of the anatomy.

The mesentery in CD can be challenging as it is frequently thickened, friable, woody, and tends to bleed easily. Even when taking segments of mesentery with small vascular branches, blood loss can be quite significant. When using an energy device, it may be necessary to take the mesentery in layers and cauterize/seal the vessel in multiple locations prior to ligation. Endoloop® (Ethicon, Somerville, NJ, USA) and endoscopic clip appliers may be helpful when taking named vessels and should be available.

The predominant overarching theme in completing these cases laparoscopically should be safety. Safe and quality surgical technique should not be compromised for the sole purpose of completing the case in a minimally invasive fashion. Specifically, in cases where there is difficulty in managing a bleeding mesentery or a question of integrity of bowel, bladder, or vaginal repair; conversion is indicated. Conversion is also indicated for several technical reasons such as inability to establish or maintain pneumoperitoneum, inability to maintain adequate visualization, or inability to clear gross fecal contamination.

Outcomes

While no specific studies evaluate left-sided colectomy specifically, several studies have shown that segmental colectomy for CD can be performed safely [6, 7, 11, 15]. The review article by Lightner and colleagues examined the results of six studies looking at colectomy in Crohn's disease with a follow-up ranging from 5 to 14 years [11]. However, they conclude that 50–65% of patients will have recurrent disease involving the colon requiring additional immunosuppression. Furthermore, up to 57% will require additional operation, and 5–35% will have a permanent stoma due to medically refractory disease (Table 5.1).

A meta-analysis by Tekkis and colleagues included six studies comparing segmental resection vs subtotal/total colectomy with ileorectal anastomosis. A total of 488 patients with CD were included (223 ileorectal anastomosis patients and 265 segmental colectomy patients). The time to recurrence was longer in patients who had total colectomy with ileorectal anastomosis by 4.4 years (95% CI 3.1–5.8, $P < 0.001$), but there was no difference in the incidence of postoperative complications (OR = 1.4, 95% CI 0.16–12.74) or the need for a permanent stoma between the

Table 5.1 Recurrence rates after segment resection for Crohn's colitis

Author	Year published	Number of patients	Percent recurrence	Average length of follow-up (years)
Longo [8]	1988	21	62	5
Prabhakar[a]	1997	49	49	14
Makowiec [9]	1998	141	63	10
Andersson [5]	2002	31	39	13
Martel[b]	2002	4	65	8.7
Fichera [10]	2005	55	61	5.1

Modified with permission of Oxford University Press from Lightner [11]
[a]Prabhakar et al. [24]
[b]Martel et al. [25]

two groups (OR = 2.75, 95% CI 0.78–9.71) demonstrating that both segmental colectomy and total abdominal colectomy with ileorectal anastomosis were safe and effective treatment options for colonic CD, even though patients who underwent segmental colectomy exhibited earlier recurrence than those in the ileorectal anastomosis group. Their recommendation was that for patients with medically refractory CD, a segmental resection may be preferred in the setting of segmental colitis and absence of perianal disease since the disease recurs regardless of the operative approach. Total proctocolectomy with an end ileostomy remains the preferred approach in the setting of colonic dysplasia.

Regarding the use of minimally invasive surgery in CD, the benefits of laparoscopy for ileocolonic resections have been well-established even in the setting of abscess, fistula, and recurrent disease [2, 16–18]. The feasibility of laparoscopy for complex fistulizing disease has been described with similar outcomes to that of nonfistulizing disease [19–21]. In the prospective study by Goyer and colleagues, postoperative outcomes between patients with CD undergoing laparoscopic ileocolic resection for uncomplicated disease were compared with those undergoing laparoscopic ileocolic resection for complicated or recurrent disease [21]. A total of 124 consecutive patients were analyzed over a 9-year period. The indications for laparoscopic ileocolic resection within the cohort of complex CD included fistula (43%), abscess (30%), and recurrent disease after prior ileocolic resection (27%). Although complex disease was significantly associated with increased average operative time (214 ± 13 vs 191 ± 53 minutes, $P < 0.05$), increased conversion rate to open procedure (37% vs 14%, $P < 0.01$), and increased use of a temporary stoma (39% vs 9%, $P < 0.001$), the overall postoperative morbidity was similar between both groups (17% vs 17%, P = not significant(NS)), including major surgical postoperative complications (7% vs 6%, P = NS). The average hospital stay was also not statistically different between both groups (8 vs 7 days, P = NS) [21]. This prospective study of consecutive patients suggests that laparoscopy in complex CD is safe and feasible.

With regards to minimally invasive approach to colectomy in patients with CD, despite a paucity of contemporary studies on this topic, older studies have demonstrated laparoscopy to be safe and feasible when performed at centers of expertise. A single institutional experience was described by Holubar and colleagues identifying a total of 92 patients with CD undergoing minimal invasive colectomy from 1997 to 2008 [22]. Procedures included 43 total colectomies, 17 subtotal colectomies, and 32 segmental colectomies. Overall, straight laparoscopy was used in 57% of cases and 43% were hand-assisted with no significant difference in operative times between lap- and hand-assisted groups. The rate of conversion to open laparotomy was 16%, and only small bowel disease predicted conversion (OR 7 (1.6–35)). Conversion was not associated with increased length of hospital stay or postoperative complications. Overall postoperative length of stay was 5 (4–7) days with a 34% rate of early postoperative complications. Only perianal disease predicted complications after multivariate analysis (OR 2.6 (1.0–6.6)).

A case-matched study by da Luz Moreira and colleagues analyzing Crohn's patients undergoing laparoscopic vs open colectomy showed that although median operative times were significantly longer in the laparoscopic cohort (240 vs 150 min,

P <0.01), postoperative complications were similar and the laparoscopic group had shorter median length of stay (5 vs 6 days, *P* = 0.07) and median time to first bowel movement (3 vs 4 days, *P* = 0.4) [23].

Conclusions

Laparoscopy is feasible and safe in patients with abscess or fistula due to inflammatory bowel disease. It is important to thoroughly evaluate the patient and optimize preoperative parameters through management of medications, nutrition, and utilization of enhanced recovery pathways. It is important to recognize patient-specific contraindications and surgeon-specific limitations in attempting to approach these operations laparoscopically. Several unique considerations need to be observed in order to perform a safe operation, and conversion should be considered whenever safety or quality is in question.

References

1. Fleshman J, Peters W. The Management of Crohn's colitis. In: Cameron J, Cameron A, editors. Current surgical therapy. 12th ed. Philadelphia: Elsevier; 2017.
2. Duepree H, Senagore A, Delaney C, Brady K, Fazio V. Advantages of laparoscopic resection for ileocecal Crohn's disease. Dis Colon Rectum. 2002;45(5):605–10.
3. Delaney C, Lawrence J, Keller D, Champagne B, Senagore A. Operative techniques in laparoscopic colorectal surgery. Philadelphia: Lippincott, Wiliiams, & Wilkins; 2014.
4. Bosio R, Delaney C. Surgical treatment of diverticulitis and its complications. In: Fazio V, Church J, Delaney C, Kiran P, editors. Current therapy in colon and rectal surgery. Philadelphia: Elsevier; 2017.
5. Andersson P, Olaison G, Hallböök O, Sjödahl R. Segmental resection or subtotal colectomy in Crohn's colitis? Dis Colon Rectum. 2002;45(1):47–53.
6. Angriman I, Pirozzolo G, R B CF, Castoro C, Scarpa M. A systematic review of segmental vs subtotal colectomy and subtotal colectomy vs total proctocolectomy for colonic Crohn's disease. Color Dis. 2017;19(8):279–87.
7. Sanfey H, Bayless T, Cameron J. Crohn's disease of the colon. Is there a role for limited resection? Am J Surg. 1984;147(1):38–42.
8. Longo W, Ballantyne G, Cahow C. Treatment of Crohn's colitis. Segmental or total colectomy? Arch Surg. 1988;123(5):588–90.
9. Makowiec F, Paczulla D, Schmidtke C, Starlinger M. Long-term follow-up after resectional surgery in patients with Crohn's disease involving the colon. Z Gastroenterol. 1998;36(8):619–24.
10. Fichera A, McCormack R, Rubin M, Hurst R, Michelassi F. Long-term outcome of surgically treated Crohn's colitis: a prospective study. Dis Colon Rectum. 2005;48(5):963–9.
11. Lightner A. Segmental resection versus total proctocolectomy for Crohn's colitis: what is the best operation in the setting of medically refractory disease or dysplasia? Inflamm Bowel Dis. 2018;24(3):532–8.
12. Delaney C, Bosio R. Chapter 7: Optimizing outcomes with enhanced recovery. In: Steele S, Hull T, Read T, Saclarides T, Senagore A, Whitlow C, et al., editors. The ASCRS textbook of colon and rectal surgery. 3rd ed. New York: Springer International Publishing; 2017.
13. Toledano Trincado M, Sánchez Gonzalez J, Blanco Antona F, Martín Esteban M, Colao García L, Cuevas Gonzalez J, et al. How to reduce the laparoscopic colorectal learning curve. JSLS. 2014;18(3):e2014.00321.

14. Pokala N, Delaney C. A randomized controlled trial comparing simultaneous intra-operative vs sequential prophylactic ureteric catheter insertion in re-operative and complicated colorectal surgery. Int J Color Dis. 2007;22(6):683–7.
15. Tekkis P, Purkayastha S, Lanitis S, Athanasiou T, Heriot A, Orchard T, et al. A comparison of segmental vs subtotal/total colectomy for colonic Crohn's disease: a meta-analysis. Color Dis. 2006;8(2):82–90.
16. Favuzza J, Delaney C. Laparoscopic ileocecectomy small bowel resection and strictureplasty for Crohn's disease. In: Nguyen N, Scott-Conner C, editors. The SAGES manual. 2nd ed. New York: Springer International Publishing; 2012.
17. Heimann T, Swaminathan S, Greenstein A, Greenstein A, Khaitov S, Steinhagen R, et al. Can laparoscopic surgery prevent incisional hernia in patients with Crohn's disease: a comparison study of 750 patients undergoing open and laparoscopic bowel resection. Surg Endosc. 2017;31(12):5201–8.
18. Nguyen S, Teitelbaum E, Sabnis A, Bonaccorso A, Tabrizian P, Salky B. Laparoscopic resection for Crohn's disease: an experience with 335 cases. Surg Endosc. 2009;23(10):2380–4.
19. Pokala N, Delaney C, Brady K, Senagore A. Elective laparoscopic surgery for benign internal enteric fistulas: a review of 43 cases. Surg Endosc. 2005;19(2):222–5.
20. Wen Y, Althans A, Brady J, Dosokey E, Choi D, Nishtala M, et al. Evaluating surgical management and outcomes of colovaginal fistulas. Am J Surg. 2017;213(3):553–7.
21. Goyer P, Alves A, Bretagnol F, Bouhnik Y, Valleur P, Panis Y. Impact of complex Crohn's disease on the outcome of laparoscopic ileocecal resection: a comparative clinical study in 124 patients. Dis Colon Rectum. 2009;52(2):205–10.
22. Holubar S, Dozois E, Privitera A, Pemberton J, Cima R, Larson D. Minimally invasive colectomy for Crohn's colitis: a single institution experience. Inflamm Bowel Disease. 2010;16(11):1940–6.
23. da Luz Moreira A, Stocchi L, Remzi F, Geisler D, Hammel J, Fazio V. Laparoscopic surgery for patients with Crohn's colitis: a case-matched study. J Gastrointest Surg. 2007;11(11):1529–33.
24. Prabhakar LP, Laramee C, Nelson H, Dozois RR. Avoiding a stoma – role for segmental or abdominal colectomy in Crohn's colitis. Dis Colon Rectum. 1997;40(1):71–8.
25. Martel P, Betton PO, Gallot D, Malafosse M. Crohn's colitis: experience with segmental resections; results in a series of 84 patients. J Am Coll Surg. 2002;194(4):448–53.

Part II

Preoperative Considerations

6 Laparoscopy Versus Open Colorectal Surgery: How Strong Is the Evidence?

Katerina Wells and James Fleshman

Introduction and Rationale

The original concept of laparoscopic colectomy was to minimize the surface impact on the abdominal wall, while the same extent of resection was being performed on the colon, as might be accomplished through an open large incision. Since that concept was proposed and started in 1991 with the first case report of a laparoscopic right colectomy, the ability of laparoscopic surgeons has increased to the point that almost all operations on the entire gastrointestinal tract can be accomplished laparoscopically. It is remarkable that laparoscopic technique and instrumentation have not changed much from the initial explosion of long straight instruments inserted through the abdominal wall access ports which mirrored most of the instruments used in open operations. Laparoscopy is considered standard of care for most general surgical procedures, and the same can be said for colorectal operations, even though some surgeons lag behind in adoption of the approach. The evidence is mature and fills the surgical literature with solid evidence that laparoscopic techniques can be utilized for almost all routine and even some advanced colorectal procedures.

Levels of Evidence and Data Quality

As we consider recent publications on outcomes from laparoscopic operations, we should only accept Level 1 or 2 evidence to make our decisions and adhere to the principles of evidence-based practice. The early reports of laparoscopic techniques and outcomes were in the form of case reports or small, single-institution, retrospective

K. Wells · J. Fleshman (✉)
Baylor University Medical Center, Department of Surgery, Texas A & M Health Science Center, Dallas, TX, USA
e-mail: Katerina.wells@bswhealth.org; James.fleshman@bswhealth.org

P. Sylla et al. (eds.), *The SAGES Manual of Colorectal Surgery*,
https://doi.org/10.1007/978 3 030-24812-3_6

reviews of consecutive patient series with, at best, a case-matched retrospective historical control group of patients treated with open technique. This barely qualified as Level 4 evidence on the literature quality scale, where randomized controlled trials (RCTs) are considered Level 2 and systematic meta-analysis of data from similar-design, RCTs is considered Level 1 evidence (e.g., Cochrane Database Systematic Reviews) [1, 2]. In the early days of laparoscopic general surgery, very few randomized controlled trials for comparison of outcomes between minimally invasive and open procedures were performed. Fortunately, comparison of large retrospective series with historic outcomes measures was able to detect a rise in complication rates (e.g., bile duct injury during cholecystectomy). Efforts were redirected to make the minimally invasive approach as safe as the open approach while maintaining the benefits of minimally invasive access to abdominal organs (e.g., development of the critical view of the portal structures and cystic duct in cholecystectomy). Meta-analysis of these retrospective series reviews, without case matching or propensity score-controlled adjustment, does not improve the quality of the data because the biases of selection and partial follow-up persist. Combining data simply increases the number of subjects to make a comparison statistically significant.

Fortunately, colorectal surgeons have learned that RCTs will answer specific questions without controversy in most circumstances. The area of laparoscopic resection for colorectal cancer has been the most studied [3–13]. The complexity of designing an RCT is based on selecting a homogeneous population with as few confounding factors as possible and applying a consistent approach to the disease and patient to achieve predetermined primary and secondary outcomes. Randomization can remove almost all selection bias from the process, and prospectively collected data are usually more complete and less likely to be manipulated. Colon and rectal cancers have been the focus of most RCTs in colorectal surgery and continue to populate the literature. As mentioned above, the meta-analysis of the combined data from RCTs can provide the clearest answer to a major question like cancer treatment. It is important to try to standardize the confounding factors in each trial to make the combined analysis meaningful. For example, the definition of the rectum or the segments of the colon used in the study will make a difference in the ability to draw a conclusion. Dr. Lars Pahlmann took the data from the early RCTs studying laparoscopic colectomy for cancer to provide a meta-analysis of combined trials and confirmed equivalence of laparoscopic and open approaches to colon cancer [14]. It is hoped that combined data analysis of the recently published rectal cancer trials will give us the same confidence in the use of laparoscopy in patients with rectal cancer.

Reviews of large administrative databases (e.g., National Inpatient Sample [15] and Premier Prospective Database [16] and California Cross Section Database [17]) provide adequate numbers of patients to result in statistical significance for even small differences in outcomes across a wide spectrum of patients, hospitals, and surgeons. It is important to remember that these large databases are usually reservoirs of data from hospitals and insurance companies that utilize relatively untrained personnel to enter the data at the patient interface. The data are collected with limited filters, other than the fact that the patient had a procedure or a disease process based on codes. Some databases are able to include severity of illness information and enhance comparison of patients based on comorbidities and other individual features of the patient. The integration of disease codes, procedure codes, and billing codes can sometimes be faulty and give a false sense of security and accuracy based on large numbers alone.

The best technique for managing retrospective data is achieved by educated, specifically trained, data abstractors and entry personnel focused on a set of definitions, rules, and criteria for specific conditions and outcomes. The National Surgical Quality Improvement Project (NSQIP) [18], the Society of Thoracic Surgery (STS) database, and the National Cancer Database (NCDB) at the American College of Surgeons are examples of trustworthy databases that can give a reliable answer even within the limitations of retrospective data. The quality of the data needs to be considered when evaluating outcomes of different techniques. Each database has its own limitations based on the comprehensiveness of the data collected, which is constrained by time, resources, and storage capacity. Fortunately, the newest data collection effort in colorectal surgery is supported by the NCDB with prospective rectal cancer-specific data collection through the National Accreditation Program in Rectal Cancer (NAPRC) managed by the American College of Surgeons. These data elements were collaboratively defined by consensus within the multidisciplinary OSTRiCh (Optimizing Surgical Treatment of Rectal Cancer) Consortium during the design phase of the NAPRC. As the NAPRC functions, data points will be changed to answer new questions relevant to clinical practice.

If laparoscopic colorectal surgery is to be considered as standard of care over open surgery, we need contemporary data and reports from the literature to confirm ongoing safety and quality of outcomes from the laparoscopic approach. A search of the surgical literature back to 2006 yielded a large number of reports (134) comparing open and laparoscopic colorectal surgery. A selection process that focused on resection of the colon and rectum and comparison of the 2 approaches yielded 25 articles that deserve discussion. Comparison of different aspects of the procedure and a range of outcomes have been reported in the past decade in large database reviews, systematic meta-analysis, randomized controlled trials, and prospective non-randomized series. The bottom line reflects the ability of laparoscopic colorectal surgery to achieve excellent outcomes and improve on some of the aspects of recovery over the open approach.

Outcomes

The benefit of laparoscopy is most realized in the short-term outcomes of length of stay and postoperative pain. These are uniformly superior to the open technique. Mortality after a laparoscopic colorectal procedure has been reported to be less than after an open resection (0.52% vs 1.24%) (relative risk = 0.69) (0.4% vs 2.0%) [15, 19–28]. Length of stay is always shorter by multiple days for laparoscopic resections compared to open [6, 15–28]. Complications over a broad spectrum of definitions are always fewer for laparoscopic procedures [16, 19–28]. Laparoscopy acts in conjunction with protocols for enhanced recovery after surgery to improve outcomes after colectomy [6, 23].

The cost of laparoscopic procedures to the system, while higher in the operating room, has been shown to be lower overall, due to reduced complications and length of stay [15, 16]. Cost comparisons warrant further investigation as the application of technologic advances including robotic-assisted surgery increases in colorectal surgery. Cancer outcomes after laparoscopic surgery have been shown to be the same as for open operation including survival, recurrence, lymph node harvest, and ability to resect locally advanced, emergently operated, obstructed tumors from all sections of the colon and the rectum and in elderly and high-risk patients [4–6, 15, 20, 22, 24–30]. Several rectal cancer trials have developed the concept of the composite pathologic assessment as an immediate oncologic outcome. Long-term outcomes of 3- or 5-year overall survival, disease-free survival, and local recurrence are considered non-inferior and therefore acceptable as a preferred standard owing to its short-term benefits.

Hand-assisted laparoscopic techniques have been shown to provide equivalent outcomes to open and straight laparoscopic colorectal resections with a lower conversion rate and shortened learning curve [19, 31, 32]. Sexual and bladder function may be impacted by laparoscopic techniques used in low rectal resection; otherwise, quality of life is similar to open results [3, 5]. Conversion from laparoscopic to open operation has been shown to impact outcomes adversely [3, 32, 33]. Conversion is associated with longer length of stay, higher rates of readmission, and higher rates of postoperative complications. Studies have reported negative oncologic outcomes following conversion; however, when adjusting for other factors, perioperative outcomes and pathologic features are more predictive of oncologic endpoints such that conversion may be a proxy for more biologically aggressive disease or a more susceptible patient [34].

Laparoscopy for the management of benign disease including inflammatory bowel disease and diverticulitis is well studied and is extensively covered in several subsequent chapters. In the two available randomized controlled trials that consider laparoscopic over open ileocolic resection for Crohn's disease, despite a longer operative time with laparoscopy, laparoscopy was found to be feasible, safe, and with low conversion rate provided procedures were performed with proper patient selection and by experienced surgeons. There is strong evidence that laparoscopic sigmoid resection offers the benefit of reduction in major complications and shorter hospital stay over open resection [35–37]. There are no randomized data for laparoscopic treatment of small intestinal obstruction [2].

See Table 6.1.

Table 6.1 Summary of best quality evidence for laparoscopic colorectal surgery

Study	Type	N	Indications	Endpoint	Conclusion
COST (2007) Fleshman et al. [7]	RCT non-inferiority	872	Colon cancer Stage I–III	Time to recurrence	"Laparoscopic colectomy for curable colon cancer is not inferior to open surgery based on long-term oncologic endpoints"
COLOR (2005) Veldkamp et al.[a]	RCT non-inferiority 7% margin	1248	Colon cancer Stage I–IV	3-yr DFS	"…the difference in disease-free survival between groups was small and, we believe, clinically acceptable, justifying the implementation of laparoscopic surgery into daily practice" "Laparoscopic surgery [has]…similar rates of disease-free survival, overall survival and recurrences as open surgery at 10-year follow-up"
CLASICC[b,c] (2005, 2012)	RCT	794	Colon and rectal cancer Stage I–IV	Multiple OS, DFS, LR	"…impaired short-term outcomes after laparoscopic-assisted anterior resection for cancer of the rectum do not yet justify its routine use" "Long-term results…support the use of laparoscopic surgery for both colonic and rectal cancer"
ALCCaS (2018) McCombie et al. [5]	RCT	601	Colon cancer Stage I–III	5-year OS, DFS, freedom from recurrence	"… laparoscopic colorectal resection was not inferior to open colorectal resection in direct measures of survival and recurrence"
COREAN (2014) Jeong et al. [4]	RCT non-inferiority 15% margin	340	Rectal cancer Stage II–III	3-year DFS	"…laparoscopic resection for locally advanced rectal cancer after preoperative chemoradiotherapy provides similar outcomes for disease-free survival as open resection, thus justifying its use"
COLOR II (2015) [13]	RCT non-inferiority 5% margin	1044	Rectal cancer Stage I–III	3-year LR	"…laparoscopic surgery is as safe and effective as open surgery in patients with rectal cancers without invasion of adjacent tissues"
Z6051 (2015, 2018) Fleshman et al. [8, 9]	RCT non-inferiority 6% margin	486	Rectal cancer Stage I–III	Composite pathology 2-year DFS, recurrence	"Laparoscopic assisted resection of rectal cancer was not found to be significantly different to OPEN resection of rectal cancer based on the outcomes of DFS and recurrence"

(continued)

Table 6.1 (continued)

Study	Type	N	Indications	Endpoint	Conclusion
AlaCaRT (2018) Stevenson et al. [11]	RCT non-inferiority 8% margin	475	Rectal cancer (0–15 cm) Stage I–IV	Composite pathology 2-year LR, DFS	"Laparoscopic surgery for rectal cancer did not differ significantly from open surgery in effects on 2-year recurrence or DFS and OS"
Maartense et al. (2006)[d]	RCT	60	Ileocolic Crohn's disease	3-month QoL	"QoL …was not different for laparoscopic-assisted compared with the open ileocolic resection, morbidity, hospital stay, and costs were significantly lower"
Milsom et al. (2001) [35] Stocchi et al. (2008)[e]	RCT	60	Ileocolic Crohn's disease	Recurrence Postoperative complications	"Laparoscopic ileocolectomy is at least comparable to open ileocolectomy…"
Sigma trial Klarenbeek et al. [f] (2009)	RCT	104	Diverticulitis	Mortality Postoperative complications	"Laparoscopic surgery was associated with a 15.4% reduction in major complication rates, less pain, improved quality of life, and shorter hospitalization at the cost of a longer operating time"
Gervaz et al. (2010, 2011)[g,h]	RCT	113	Diverticulitis	Postoperative pain Duration of ileus duration of LOS	"Laparoscopic sigmoid resection is associated with a 30% reduction in duration of postoperative ileus and hospital stay"

DFS disease-free survival, *OS* overall survival, *LR* local recurrence, *RCT* randomized controlled trial, *QoL* quality of life, *LOS* length of hospital stay
[a]Veldkamp et al. [38]
[b]Guillou et al. [39]
[c]Green et al. [40]
[d]Maartense et al. [41]
[e]Stocchi et al. [42]
[f]Klarenbeek et al. [37]
[g]Gervaz et al. [36]
[h]Gervaz et al. [43]

Conclusion

In summary, there is high-quality evidence the supports laparoscopic treatment of most colorectal diseases. Outcomes are generally equivalent if not better than open operation in almost all parameters. Laparoscopy for both benign and malignant colorectal diseases should be considered whenever possible, and surgeons should now consider laparoscopy as standard of care. As technological advances in the field of minimally invasive surgery continue to evolve, surgeons must continue to validate the safety and feasibility of these newer technologies with high-quality evidence.

References

1. Dasari BV, McKay D, Gardiner K. Laparoscopic versus open surgery for small bowel Crohn's disease. Cochrane Database Syst Rev. 2011;19(1):CD006956.
2. Cirocchi R, Abraha I, Farinella E, Montedori A, Sciannameo F. Laparoscopic versus open surgery in small bowel obstruction. Cochrane Database Syst Rev. 2010;17(2):CD007511.
3. Jayne DG, Brown JM, Thorpe H, Walker J, Quirke P, Guillou PJ. Bladder and sexual function following resection for rectal cancer in a randomized clinical trial of laparoscopic versus open technique. Br J Surg. 2005;92(9):1124–32.
4. Jeong SY, Park JW, Nam BH, Kim S, Kang SB, Lim SB, et al. Open versus laparoscopic surgery for mid-rectal or low-rectal cancer after neoadjuvant chemoradiotherapy (COREAN trial): survival outcomes of an open-label, non-inferiority, randomized controlled trial. Lancet Oncol. 2014;15(7):767–74.
5. McCombie AM, Frizelle F, Bagshaw PF, Frampton CM, Hewett PJ, McMurrick PJ, et al. The ALCCaS trial: a randomized controlled trial comparing quality of life following laparoscopic versus open colectomy for colon cancer. Dis Colon Rectum. 2018;61(10):1156–62.
6. King PM, Blazeby JM, Ewings FPJ, Longman RJ, Kendrick AH, et al. Randomized clinical trial comparing laparoscopic and open surgery for colorectal cancer within an enhanced recovery programme. Br J Surg. 2006;93(3):300–8.
7. Fleshman J, Sargent DJ, Green E, Anvari M, Stryker SJ, Beart RW Jr, et al. Laparoscopic colectomy for cancer is not inferior to open surgery based on 5-year data from the COST Study Group trial. Ann Surg. 2007;246(4):655–62; discussion 662–664
8. Fleshman J, Branda M, Sargent DJ, Boller AM, George V, Abbas M, et al. Effect of laparoscopic-assisted resection vs open resection of stage II or III rectal cancer on pathologic outcomes: the ACOSOG Z6051 randomized clinical trial. JAMA. 2015;314(13):1346–55.
9. Fleshman J, Branda ME, Sargent DJ, Boller AM, George VV, Abbas MA, et al. Disease-free survival and local recurrence for laparoscopic resection compared to open resection of stage II to III rectal cancer: follow-up results of the ACOSOG Z6051 randomized controlled trial. Ann Surg. 2019;269(4):589–95.
10. Stevenson AR, Solomon MJ, Lumley JW, Hewett P, Clouston AD, Gebski VJ, et al. Effect of laparoscopic-assisted resection vs open resection on pathological outcomes in rectal cancer: the ALACaRT Randomized Clinical Trial. JAMA. 2015;314(13):1356–63.
11. Stevenson ARL, Solomon MJ, Brown CSB, Lumley JW, Hewett P, Clouston AD, et al. Disease-free survival and local recurrence after laparoscopic-assisted resection or open resection for rectal cancer: the Australasian Laparoscopic Cancer of the Rectum Randomized Clinical Trial. Ann Surg. 2019;269(4):596–602.
12. COLOR Study Group. COLOR: a rancomized clinical trial comparing laparoscopic and open resection for colon cancer. Dig Surg. 2000;17(6):617–22.
13. COLOR II Study Group, Buunen M, Bonjer HJ, Hop WC, Haglind E, Kurlberg G, et al. COLOR II. A randomized clinical trial comparing laparoscopic and open surgery for rectal cancer. Dan Med Bull. 2009;56(2):89–91.
14. Bonjer HJ, Brown J, Delgado S, Kuhrij E, Haglind E, Pahlmann L. Laparoscopically assisted vs open colectomy for colon cancer: a meta-analysis. Arch Surg. 2007;142(3):298–303.
15. Lee MTG, Chiu CC, Wang CC, Chang CN, Lee SH, Lee M, et al. Trends and outcomes of surgical treatment for colorectal cancer between 2004 and 2012 – an analysis using national inpatient database. Sci Rep. 2017;7(1):2006.

16. Keller DS, Delaney CP, Hashemi HEM. A national evaluation of clinical and economic outcomes in open versus laparoscopic colorectal surgery. Surg Endosc. 2016;30(10):4220–8.
17. Patel SS, Patel MS, Mahanti S, Ortega A, Ault GT, Kaiser AM, et al. Laparoscopic versus open colon resections in California: a cross-sectional analysis. Am Surg. 2012;78(10):1063–5.
18. Ballian N, Weisensel N, Rajamanickam V, Foley EF, Heise CP, Harms BA, et al. Comparable postoperative morbidity and mortality after laparoscopic and open emergent restorative colectomy: outcomes from the ACS NSQIP. World J Surg. 2012;36(10):2488–96.
19. Zhang X, Wu Q, Gu C, Hu T, Bi L, Wang Z. Hand-assisted laparoscopic surgery versus conventional open surgery in intraoperative and postoperative outcomes for colorectal cancer. An updated systematic review and meta-analysis. Medicine. 2017;96:33(e7794).
20. Cirocchi R, Campanile FC, Di Saverio S, Popivanov G, Carlini L, Pironi D, et al. Laparoscopic versus open colectomy for obstructing right colon cancer: a systematic review and meta-analysis. J Visc Surg. 2017;154:387–99.
21. Malczak P, Mizera M, Torbica G, Witowski J, Major P, Pisarska M, et al. Is the laparoscopic approach for rectal cancer superior to open surgery? A systematic review and meta-analysis on short-term surgical outcomes. Wideochir Inne Tech Maloinwazyine. 2018;13(2):129–40.
22. Nagasue Y, Akiyoshi T, Ueno M, Fukunaga Y, Nagayama S, Fujimoto Y, et al. Laparoscopic versus open multivisceral resection for primary colorectal cancer: comparison of perioperative outcomes. J Gastrointest Surg. 2013;17(7):1299–305.
23. Zhuang CL, Huang DD, Chen FF, Zhou CJ, Zheng BS, Chen BC, et al. Laparoscopic versus open colorectal surgery within enhanced recovery after surgery programs: a systematic review and meta-analysis of randomized controlled trials. Surg Endosc. 2015;9(8):2091–100.
24. Yamaguchi S, Tashiro J, Araki R, Okuda J, Hanai T, Otsuka K, et al. Laparoscopic versus open resection for transverse and descending colon cancer: short-term and long-term outcomes of a multicenter retrospective study of 1830 patients. Asian J Endosc Surg. 2017;10(3):268–75.
25. Yamamoto S, Hinoi T, Niitsu H, Okajima M, Ide Y, Murata K, et al. Influence of previous abdominal surgery on surgical outcomes between laparoscopic and open surgery in elderly patients with colorectal cancer: subanalysis of a large multicenter study in Japan. J Gastroenterol. 2017;52(6):695–704.
26. Zeng WG, Zhou ZX, Hou HR, Liang JW, Zhou HT, Wang Z, et al. Outcome of laparoscopic versus open resection for rectal cancer in elderly patients. J Surg Res. 2015;193(2):613–8.
27. Hida K, Hasegawa S, Kinjo Y, Yoshimura K, Inomata M, Ito M, et al. Open versus laparoscopic resection of primary tumor for incurable stage IV colorectal cancer: a large multicenter consecutive patients cohort study. Ann Surg. 2012;255(5):929–34.
28. Hemandas AK, Abdelrahman T, Flashman KG, Skull AJ, Senapati A, O'Leary DP, et al. Laparoscopic colorectal surgery produces better outcomes for high risk cancer patients compared to open surgery. Ann Surg. 2010;252(1):84–9.
29. Athanasiou CD, Robinson J, Yiasemidou M, Lockwood S, Markides GA. Laparoscopic vs open approach for transverse colon cancer. A systematic review and meta-analysis of short and long term outcomes. Int J Surg. 2017;41:78–85.
30. Han SA, Lee WY, Park CM, Yun SH, Chun HK. Comparison of immunologic outcomes of laparoscopic vs open approaches in clinical stage III colorectal cancer. Int J Color Dis. 2010;25(5):631–8.
31. Duraes L, Schroeder DA, Dietz DW. Modified pfannenstiel open approach as an alternative to laparoscopic total proctocolectomy and IPAA: comparison of short- and long-term outcomes and quality of life. Dis Colon Rectum. 2018;61(5):573–8.
32. Ozturk E, Kiran RP, Remzi F, Geisler D, Fazio V. Hand-assisted laparoscopic surgery may be a useful tool for surgeons early in the learning curve performing total abdominal colectomy. Color Dis. 2010;12(3):199–205.
33. Masoomi H, Moghadamyeghaneh A, Mills S, Carmichael JC, Pigazzi A, Stamos MJ. Risk factors for conversion of laparoscopic colorectal surgery to open surgery: does conversion worsen outcome? World J Surg. 2015;39(5):1240–7.
34. Leijssen LGJ, Dinaux AM, Kunitake H, Bordeianou LG, Berger DL. Is there a drawback of converting a laparoscopic colectomy in Colon Cancer? J Surg Res. 2018;232:595–604.

35. Milsom JW, Hammerhofer KA, Böhm B, Marcello P, Elson P, Fazio VW. Prospective, randomized trial comparing laparoscopic vs. conventional surgery for refractory ileocolic Crohn's disease. Dis Colon and Rectum. 2001;44(1):1–8. Discussion 8–9
36. Gervaz P, Inan I, Perneger T, Schiffer E, Morel P. A prospective, randomized, single-blind comparison of laparoscopic versus open sigmoid colectomy for diverticulitis. Ann Surg. 2010;252(1):3–8.
37. Klarenbeek BR, Veenhof AA, Bergamaschi R, van der Peet DL, van den Broek WT, de Lange ES. Laparoscopic sigmoid resection for diverticulitis decreases major morbidity rates: a randomized control trial. Ann Surg. 2009;249(1):39–44.
38. Veldkamp R, Kuhry E, Hop WC, Jeekel J, Kazemier G, Bonjer HJ, et al. Laparoscopic surgery versus open surgery for colon cancer: short-term outcomes of a randomised trial. Lancet Oncol. 2005;6(7):477–84.
39. Guillou PJ, Quirke P, Thorpe H, Walker J, Jayne DG, Smith AM, et al. Short-term endpoints of conventional versus laparoscopic-assisted surgery in patients with colorectal cancer (MRC CLASICC trial): multicentre, randomised controlled trial. Lancet. 2005;365(9472):1718–26.
40. Green BL, Marshall HC, Collinson F, Quirke P, Guillou P, Jayne DG, et al. Long-term follow-up of the Medical Research Council CLASICC trial of conventional versus laparoscopically assisted resection in colorectal cancer. Br J Surg. 2013;100(1):75–82.
41. Maartense S, Dunker MS, Slors JF, Cuesta MA, Pierik EG, Gouma DJ, et al. Laparoscopic-assisted versus open ileocolic resection for Crohn's disease: a randomized trial. Ann Surg. 2006;243(2):143–9; discussion 150–3
42. Stocchi L, Milsom JW, Fazio VW. Long-term outcomes of laparoscopic versus open ileocolic resection for Crohn's disease: follow-up of a prospective randomized trial. Surgery. 2008;144(4):622–7; discussion 627–8
43. Gervaz P, Mugnier-Konrad B, Morel P, Huber O, Inan I. Laparoscopic versus open sigmoid resection for diverticulitis: long-term results of a prospective, randomized trial. Surg Endosc. 2011;25(10):3373–8.

Debunking Enhanced Recovery Protocols in Colorectal Surgery: Minimal Requirements for Maximum Benefit

7

Deborah S. Keller and Lawrence Lee

Introduction and Rationale

Despite significant improvements in perioperative care and surgical technique, major surgery is still associated with significant morbidity that can delay recovery and increase healthcare costs [1]. In the late 1990s, Henrik Kehlet proposed that to understand postoperative morbidity, it is necessary to understand the components of the surgical stress response [2]. They addressed the multiple components in a multimodal rehabilitation or "fast-track" pathway, designed to achieve early recovery for patients undergoing major surgery [3, 4]. These protocols eliminate outdated perioperative care principles, implement evidence-based innovations to expedite recovery, and reduce physiological stress and postoperative organ dysfunction by optimizing perioperative care and recovery. While originally used in open surgery, the same principles apply, and results are amplified in combination with minimally invasive surgery. The key tenets focus on patient education, multimodal opioid-sparing analgesia, reduction of surgical stress via fluid management, minimal invasive surgery, optimizing nutrition, and stressing early ambulation, diet, and defined discharge criteria. Traditional perioperative care principles such as immobilization, nasogastric tubes, and fasting were eliminated, and innovations such as carbohydrate-loading liquids before surgery, regional anesthetic techniques, maintenance of normal temperature during surgery, optimal treatment of postoperative pain and prophylaxis, and minimally invasive laparoscopic surgical techniques were implemented. The replacement of these traditional approaches in surgical care with evidence-based practices has demonstrated that surgical recovery can be accelerated

D. S. Keller (✉)
Division of Colorectal Surgery, Department of Surgery, New York Presbyterian Hospital-Columbia University Medical Center, New York, NY, USA

L. Lee
Department of Surgery, McGill University Health Centre, Montreal, QC, Canada
e-mail: Larry.lee@mcgill.ca

P. Sylla et al. (eds.), *The SAGES Manual of Colorectal Surgery*,
https://doi.org/10.1007/978-3-030-24812-3_7

and convalescence decreased [5]. Since their introduction, volumes of work have established that these pathways can reduce the stress response, postoperative morbidity, length of hospital stay, and overall costs. Enhanced recovery was initiated in colorectal surgery, and the largest body of literature is still based in the colorectal field; however, the concept and benefits rapidly spread to a variety of surgical specialties [6].

With the undisputed improvement in clinical and financial outcomes using enhanced recovery protocols and need to improve surgical quality and value, this is a topic relevant to all surgeons who perform colorectal procedures. As enhanced recovery evolves, there are several important points for providers to keep in mind. First, the term "enhanced recovery after surgery" is a misnomer, as the order sets cover the entire patient surgical experience, and the preoperative, intraoperative, and postoperative periods need to be incorporated for best success. In addition, simply having a protocol is also not enough to reap the benefits of enhanced recovery; experience and better organization of care are necessary for success [7]. Finally, the implementation process involves the entire multidisciplinary team; all staff members that care for the surgical patient should be educated in the protocols and supportive. In this chapter, we debunk common assumptions around ERPs and use a simple approach to help put an ERP into practice using minimal requirements for maximal benefit in colorectal surgery.

Reviewing the Evidence: The Clinical Case for ERP

The benefits of ERPs are becoming unquestionably clear based on a growing body of literature. Multiple randomized trials have demonstrated the clinical benefits of ERPs. The most recent systematic review and meta-analysis included 25 randomized trials comparing ERP versus conventional care in patients undergoing colorectal surgery. In this meta-analysis, there were significant reductions in length of stay and perioperative morbidity in favor of ERP, without differences in readmissions or mortalities (Table 7.1) [8]. These overall effects remained significant regardless of open versus laparoscopic approach or by indication for surgery (colorectal cancer, rectal cancer, or benign disease). A similar meta-analysis in patients undergoing major non-colorectal

Table 7.1 Results from a meta-analysis of 25 randomized trials comparing ERP and conventional care in patients undergoing colorectal surgery

Outcome	Number of comparisons included	Effect
Length of stay	24	Mean difference: −2.62 days (95% CI −3.22, −2.02)
Perioperative morbidity	19	Risk ratio: 0.66 (95% CI 0.54, 0.80)
Mortality	22	Risk ratio: 1.79 (95% CI 0.81, 3.95)
Readmissions	19	Risk ratio: 1.10 (95% CI 0.81, 1.50)
Surgical site infections	17	Risk ratio: 0.75 (95% CI 0.52, 1.07)

Table 7.2 Results of a meta-analysis comparing ERP and conventional care in patients undergoing major non-colorectal abdominal surgery (randomized trials only)

Outcome	Number of comparisons included	Effect
Length of stay	11	Mean difference: −2.6 days (95% CI −3.5, −1.7)
Perioperative morbidity	12	Risk ratio: 0.68 (95% CI 0.43, 1.10)
Readmissions	7	Risk ratio: 1.60 (95% CI 0.87, 2.96)

abdominal surgery also demonstrated a significant decrease in length of stay without a difference in readmissions, although the effect on complications was not statistically significant (Table 7.2) [9]. Analysis of return of GI function has reported significant reductions in time to first flatus and time to first bowel movement for both upper GI and colorectal procedures [10]. Nonetheless, the effect sizes for these three important outcomes are remarkably similar between colorectal and non-colorectal abdominal surgery, suggesting the robustness of ERP principles. The generalizability of ERPs is especially important, as the initial effort and resource investments and expertise development for a colorectal ERP can then be applied for other procedures and specialties. With this evidence, methods to develop, implement, and measure outcomes with ERP are key for surgeons performing colorectal surgery.

Solicit Institutional Support

Institutional support from hospital administrators is a necessary step for success, as for senior level buy-in sets the tone for the culture change with ERP implementation, and demonstrates to all staff that the institution supports dedicating the time and resources that are required to implement and maintain these pathways. Institutional support for ERP is necessary to identify where support can be offered, such as in the provision of an ERP facilitator, purchasing decisions, reallocation of staff and support services, education sessions in relation to ERPs, and the development of strategies to improve multidisciplinary buy-in and participation [11]. A recent study of SAGES members reported the single most important roadblock to successful ERP implementation was the lack of support from the hospital administration [12]. Thus, the visible top-down support of the institution and administration is key to drive the awareness and implementation of an ERP. As you put an ERP into practice, the next step after reviewing the evidence and building a clinical case is to present this evidence to the institutional administration to ensure high-level support of the initiative.

Defining Leaders and Creation of the Multidisciplinary Team

With support of the administration, the next step is to build the multidisciplinary team. A successful ERP requires active collaboration and participation from the entire healthcare provider team, to ensure that all involved stakeholders feel accountable for the implementation and maintenance processes [13]. It is essential to define leaders and assemble a multidisciplinary team, identifying champions from all involved specialties that will take the lead in organizing, implementing, and maintaining their specialty's respective roles in the ERP. The team begins with defining a local clinical champion, who recognizes its benefits. This individual then forms a working group of similar-minded individuals from all involved parties into a steering committee, which should be able to effectively disseminate the clinical and economic benefits of the ERP approach to their colleagues, implement, and monitor changes. This steering committee should consist of representatives from the involved specialties, as well as allied health professionals that are essential for patient care. This multidisciplinary team is recommended to include surgeons, anesthesiologists, internists, nursing representatives from the preoperative center, postanesthesia care unit, surgical ward, physiotherapists, pharmacists, and nutritionists that meet on a regular schedule. Each of these individuals represents an essential component in the patient's perioperative journey. The role of the surgeon and anesthesiologist is obvious; however other specialties and team members should also be recruited. For example, much of the preoperative testing and evaluation can be streamlined to minimize patient burden and resource utilization. In this regard, the inclusion of a representative of the medical specialty in charge of preoperative center is crucial. Operating room, perioperative care, and ward nursing representation are also critical, to ensure education, acceptance, and compliance with the ERP items during surgery and the patient's stay in the postanesthesia recovery unit and inpatient floor. Similarly, allied health professionals that provide much of the care processes in the perioperative period should also be included. Pharmacists are an essential team member for agreement with medications included in the pathways and ease of future clinical trials. Nutrition, physical therapy, and wound ostomy care nurses are invaluable for input on managing high-risk and frail patients during the prehabilitation and postoperative periods. In most hospital systems, trainees are actively involved in patient care and may actually have the primary role of putting in orders and patient education. Thus, surgical resident involvement for ownership and buy-in of the care practices by the house staff is critical. For centers with the means or desire to publish, a librarian who can provide detailed literature searches on the best available evidence can also facilitate the dissemination process and pathway design. Once protocols have been developed and approved, the Information Technologies department can help streamline the implementation and audit processes, by integrating the pathways into the electronic medical record with automated order sets, back-end databases, and personalized queries on outcomes metrics. Finally, a dedicated ERP facilitator is one of the essential elements commonly overlooked. The facilitator is paramount for successful ERP implementation and subsequent audit processes [14, 15]. The ERP facilitator is mostly a nurse, nurse practitioner, or physician assistant (most common in the United States). Their responsibilities include reviewing the literature and evidence-based guidelines; shepherding the pathways through the approval process; maintaining momentum; creating patient education material; coordinating education sessions, meetings, and launch; and, finally, conducting postlaunch feedback and audit [15]. In cases where there is a dedicated colorectal unit, the facilitator could also be the nurse manager of the dedicated unit, helping to assure training and compliance with postoperative care principles. The ERP coordinator is a vital member of the team who is responsible for overseeing each of these key steps and coordinating among specialties.

Reviewing Current Data

Once the team is created, it is important to provide clear goals for your ERP. The first step in this process is to review specific institutional practice patterns and outcomes. Determine what the current outcome and process measure data are at your institution. Process measures cover what the institution does to maintain or improve care; these measures typically reflect generally accepted recommendations for clinical practice. Examples include use of bowel prep, blood sugar control before surgery, and the delivery of timely prophylactic antibiotics to reduce surgical site infection. Outcome measures reflect the impact of interventions on the patient's care and include metrics such as hospital length of stay, readmissions, and common complications. From these data, develop a specific needs assessment for change and initial goals for the ERP, such as reducing the rate of surgical site infections, reducing length of stay, or reducing opioid use. Provide the group with your institution's current processes and outcomes, as well as the same metrics for other hospitals and national benchmarks to emphasize the need and help prove the need for the change. These are basics of patient improvement, financial benefits, and clinical outcomes, to give the team a sense of urgency and need to implement a protocol. Without these data, there may be resistance to change from healthcare providers that do not see any advantages of the ERP approach over their current practice or fear the process change will be cumbersome and expensive [12].

Creating an Education Program

With the current state of your institution and ERP goals defined, the next step involves education of these providers on current best practices and evidence-based recommendations and their potential improvements in clinical and financial outcomes. It is imperative to provide education for all staff at the appropriate levels, as well as to create a sense of urgency to drive change initiatives. This approach has been shown to be effective in a business setting, as well as in healthcare [11, 13]. Literature on the basic principles and successful outcomes of ERP can be sent for the team to review as pre-learning, prior to meeting in person. Suggested landmark background papers are seen in Box 7.1. Next, targeted education specific to each team member's contribution is essential for the team to understand their role and essential contribution to the overall success of an ERP. Ideas for education include presenting the initiative at grand rounds for each department involved and trainees, staff meetings, designated education sessions, and ward "huddles" or sign-out sessions and creating handouts for the staff with the protocol and their main role highlighted. For the nursing and allied health staff, assure presentations occur at multiple periods to include staff that work on evening or weekend shifts. With education, acceptance of the culture change will come, followed by willing participation and then finally excitement for the new standard and identification of ERP champions. It is especially important to educate the primary caretakers, including nursing and other allied health professionals in the preoperative clinic, postanesthesia care unit, and postoperative surgical ward, as ERPs may require significant departures from long-standing practices. Specific changes like removing patient-controlled analgesia (PCAs) after surgery and removing the practice of preoperative fasting starting at midnight the night before surgery require changes across multiple providers, preoperative clinic, admitting office, pre-anesthesia clinic and anesthesiologists, and postoperative and ward nursing. These changes can be facilitated with the support of the champions, who can effectively set goals, disseminate the evidence and benefits underlying the proposed changes, and support the implementation [1].

Box 7.1 Suggested Reading for Surgeons to Review Evidence for Enhanced Recovery

1. King PM, Blazeby JM, Ewings P, et al. The influence of an enhanced recovery programme on clinical outcomes, costs and quality of life after surgery for colorectal cancer. Colorectal Dis. 2006;8:506–13.
2. Kehlet H, Wilmore DW. Evidence-based surgical care and the evolution of fast-track surgery. Ann Surg. 2008;248:189–98.
3. Vlug MS, Wind J, Hollmann MW, Ubbink DT, Cense HA, Engel AF, Gerhards MF, van Wagensveld BA, van der Zaag ES, van Geloven AA, Sprangers MA, Cuesta MA, Bemelman WA, LAFA study group. Laparoscopy in combination with fast track multimodal management is the best perioperative strategy in patients undergoing colonic surgery: a randomized clinical trial (LAFA-study). Ann Surg. 2011;254:868–75.
4. Smart NJ, White P, Allison AS, Ockrim JB, Kennedy RH, Francis NK. Deviation and failure of enhanced recovery after surgery following laparoscopic colorectal surgery: early prediction model. Colorectal Dis. 2012;14:e727–34.
5. Aarts MA, Okrainec A, Glicksman A, Pearsall E, Victor JC, McLeod RS. Adoption of enhanced recovery after surgery (ERAS) strategies for colorectal surgery at academic teaching hospitals and impact on total length of hospital stay. Surg Endosc. 2012;26:442–50.
6. Lawrence JK, Keller DS, Samia H, et al. Discharge within 24 to 72 hours of colorectal surgery is associated with low readmission rates when using enhanced recovery pathways. J Am Coll Surg. 2013;216:390–4.
7. Keller DS, Bankwitz B, Woconish D, et al. Predicting who will fail early discharge after laparoscopic colorectal surgery with an established enhanced recovery pathway. Surg Endosc. 2014;28:74–9.
8. Lee L, Mata J, Augustin B, Ghitulescu GA, Boutros M, Charlebois P, Stein B, Liberman AS, Fried GM, Morin N, Carli F, Latimer E, Feldman LS. Cost-effectiveness of enhanced recovery versus conventional

perioperative management for colorectal surgery. Ann Surg. 2015; 262(6):1026–33.
9. Stone AB, Grant MC, Pio Roda C, et al. Implementation costs of an enhanced recovery after surgery program in the United States: a financial model and sensitivity analysis based on experiences at a Quaternary Academic Medical Center. J Am Coll Surg. 2016;222:219–25.
10. Keller DS, Delaney CP, Senagore AJ, Feldman LS, SAGES SMART Task Force. Uptake of enhanced recovery practices by SAGES members: a survey. Surg Endosc. 2017;31(9):3519–26. https://doi.org/10.1007/s00464-016-5378-8.
11. Carmichael JC, Keller DS, Baldini G, Bordeianou L, Weiss E, Lee L, Boutros M, McClane J, Steele SR, Feldman LS. Clinical practice guideline for enhanced recovery after colon and rectal surgery from the American Society of Colon and Rectal Surgeons (ASCRS) and Society of American Gastrointestinal and Endoscopic Surgeons (SAGES). Surg Endosc. 2017;9.
12. Jurt J, Slieker J, Frauche P, Addor V, Solà J, Demartines N, Hübner M. Enhanced recovery after surgery: can we rely on the key factors or do we need the bel ensemble? World J Surg. 2017;41(10):2464–70. https://doi.org/10.1007/s00268-017-4054-z.
13. Berian JR, Ban KA, Liu JB, Ko CY, Feldman LS, Thacker JK. Adherence to enhanced recovery protocols in NSQIP and association with colectomy outcomes. Ann Surg. 2017.
14. Stone AB, Yuan CT, Rosen MA, Grant MC, Benishek LE, Hanahan E, Lubomski LH, Ko C, Wick EC. Barriers to and facilitators of implementing enhanced recovery pathways using an implementation framework: a systematic review. JAMA Surg. 2018;03.

Overcoming Barriers Through Culture Change

ERPs may represent a significant culture change – departures from long-standing clinical practices – and there may be initial resistance to change, especially if awareness of the benefits of the ERP is poor [14]. Resistance to change has been identified as one of the major barriers to ERP implementation, yet it is one that can be slowly broken down through enhanced multidisciplinary collaboration and communication, as well as support from hospital administration [16, 17]. Other potential barriers that are often encountered include lack of manpower, knowledge, hospital resources, buy-in, poor communication among team members, and patient factors [12]. There may also be specialty-specific barriers and concerns. From the nursing point of view, a potential lack of manpower and time is often viewed as potential barriers to ERP implementation, as nurses may be resistant to interventions that increased their workload and thus compound staffing shortages [16]. However, studies have reported decreased or unchanged nursing workload as a result of pathway implementation [18]. Surgeons often cite personal preferences, feeling little room for improvement from their current outcomes, lack of time to learn new methods, inconsistency with covering teams and partners, and comfort with long-standing practices as barriers to implementation [12]. Anesthesiologists were concerned about the surgeons' willingness to cede control of perioperative elements traditionally under their control. One common theme across specialties is that they often saw other specialties as potential barriers, such as surgeon concerns about ward nursing not adopting many of the perioperative interventions. Many of these potential barriers can be overcome through improved organizational culture, communication, and education on everyone's role in reaching the common goal of improved patient recovery. Another common barrier to adoption is the perceived additional costs and resources that these pathways require [16]. A review of the economic data (described in more detail below) will show that there are important cost savings associated with these pathways, and any initial resource investments can be recovered by the clinical and economic benefits [19, 20]. With the common barriers and obstacles to success identified, the steering committee can proactively develop action plans to overcome them and adjust the plans during regular meetings to address new issues that arise.

Overcoming Barriers by Building the Business Case for Enhanced Value with ERPs

One of the oft-stated barriers to ERP adoption is the perception that significant time, money, and resources are required. While certainly some investments in time and healthcare resources are necessary, especially when it comes to a dedicated ERP facilitator, these overall costs are often more than recovered based from the overall cost savings associated with ERPs. It is also important to frame the benefits of ERP through the "value" perspective. Value in healthcare is defined as the outcomes achieved per dollar spent [21]. Value is always defined around the customer, which is the surgical patient. Value depends on results, and it is important to realize that cost reduction without regard to the outcomes achieved is dangerous and self-defeating, leading to false "savings" and potentially ineffective care and poor outcomes. Conversely, when value improves, patients, payers, providers, and suppliers all benefit, and the economic sustainability of the healthcare system increases [21]. Improving the quality and cost-effectiveness of healthcare requires that we decrease or eliminate care that provides no benefit or offer interventions that provide good value for their cost [22]. ERPs eliminate surgical practices that are outdated, have no evidence-based benefit, and may be harmful – such as perioperative starvation and prolonged postoperative bedrest – and replace them with multiple evidence-based interventions within a single perioperative strategy that may reduce waste and variability and improve outcomes. There is a cost to set up an ERP, with much of the expense to cover salary of the ERP coordinator. However, these costs can be spread across a large number of patients, especially as ERP principles can be easily applied across different procedure groups, thus resulting in a negligible per patient cost. In addition, even including all input and maintenance costs, there is an overall cost

Table 7.3 Breakdown of McGill University Health Centre Surgical Recovery (SuRe) workgroup program costs over a 1-year period

Full-time ERP nurse coordinator (yearly salary)	81,225
Opportunity costs of ERP steering group (1 hr./meeting × 26 meetings)	14,320
Nurse specialists and managers, nutritionist, physiotherapist, librarian, clinical leaders from surgery, and anesthesia ($550 per meeting)	
Patient education material (operating costs of work performed by a medical informatics center)	13,225
Total	108,770

Used with permission of Wolters Kluwer Health from Lee et al. [20]

benefit for the savings resulting from the accelerated recovery and use of resources during the hospital stay; these saving are furthered by the reduction of postdischarge healthcare resources, complications, and readmissions with ERP. Several studies have proven this overall cost benefit. In a cost-effectiveness analysis comparing ERP with conventional care in colorectal surgery, Lee and colleagues found the yearly cost of the ERP was $108,770 (2103 CAD); this cost was spread across multiple patients and specialties managed by ERPs, resulting in a mean overall cost of the multidisciplinary program to approximately $153 (2013 CAD) per patient [20] (Table 7.3). The authors found no shift in the burden of care to the outpatient setting, either resulting an overall significantly lower societal costs (productivity losses and caregiver burden) or total cost savings with ERP of $2985 ($373–$5753) per patient [20]. The available economic data generally support the cost-effectiveness of ERP, with lower total and direct costs [23–29]. At one institution, there was a per patient reduction of $7129 in direct costs, corresponding to a cost savings of $777,061 in the 6-month study period the ERP group [26]. The cost-effectiveness was generalizable to all patient populations, with the cost benefit for ERP expected to generate cost savings in at least 85% of unadjusted and 82% of adjusted cost samples [27]. Another study estimated that the implementation of ERP across an entire provincial hospital network in Alberta, Canada, reported that an upfront investment of $528,459 CAN over 2 years was required [30]. The "break-even point" – where the cost savings would be greater than the implementation costs – was estimated at 93 to 236 cancer resections or 38 to 80 noncancer resections. Based on these data, it was further estimated that every $1 invested would result in $3.8 (range 2.4–5.1) in return [31]. Data from an academic US center reported similar results (Table 7.4) [19]. All of these studies support the notion of higher value care with ERP, with provision of better outcomes at the same cost, identical outcomes at the same cost, or better outcomes at lower costs.

Developing the Protocols

After reviewing the evidence, current outcome, and process measure data and developing the multidisciplinary team, the next step is writing the detailed care plans. In the ERP development, it is necessary to consider the preoperative, intraoperative, and postoperative periods, and then drill down on the distinct elements you want to cover in each time frame. The specific elements included will depend on the

Table 7.4 Implementation costs at an American quaternary academic medical center

	Annual no. of ERAS cases		
Costs	100	250	500
Implementation costs, $	10,000	10,000	10,000
Site visits/training course	0	73,700	135,839
Surgeon/anesthesia/nursing leadership time	0	25,000	50,000
Capita expenses, equipment, $			
Annual costs, $			
Personnel			
Project manager	100,875	100,875	126,094
Acute pain nurse	0	56,950	113,900
Preoperative support	0	28,475	56,950
Materials			
Education materials	2000	5000	10,000
Carbohydrate drinks/nutritional supplements	5000	12,500	25,000
Disposable materials related to fluid therapy monitor or other ERAS equipment	0	12,500	25,000
Total first-year costs, $	117,875	325,00	552,783
Annual maintenance costs, $	107,875	216,300	356,944
Cost per patient, year 1, $	1179	1300	1106
Cost per patient, nonyear 1, $	1079	865	714

Used with permission of Elsevier from Stone et al. [19]

PREOPERATIVE	INTRAOPERATIVE	POSTOPERATIVE
	Education	
Incentive spirometry	Antibiotic prophylaxis	Diet
Exercise	Multimodal analgesia	Ambulation
Smoking Cessation	PONV prophylaxis	Multimodal analgesia
Nutrition	Goal directed fluid therapy	PONV treatment
Carbohydrate loading	Anesthetic management	IV Fluid management
Premedication	MIS approach	Bowel motility
Bowel prep	Glycemic control	Tubes/Drains
Bowel motility agent	Temperature control	Daily Care Plan
Multimodal analgesia	Neuromuscular blockade	Defined Discharge Criteria
Glycemic control	NG Tube and Drains	Scheduled Follow Up
	Audit Processes and Outcomes	

Fig. 7.1 Enhanced recovery protocol template. (Used with permission of the Society of American Gastrointestinal and Endoscopic Surgeons (SAGES) from SAGES SMART Program. Available online at: http://www.sages.org/smart-enhanced-recovery-program)

individual institution and the ERP goals, but there are essential elements to cover in all protocols. Samples and guidelines can be found on the SAGES SMART Enhanced Recovery Program site [32]. A general template is seen in Fig. 7.1. In the preoperative period, patient education and setting expectations should be the

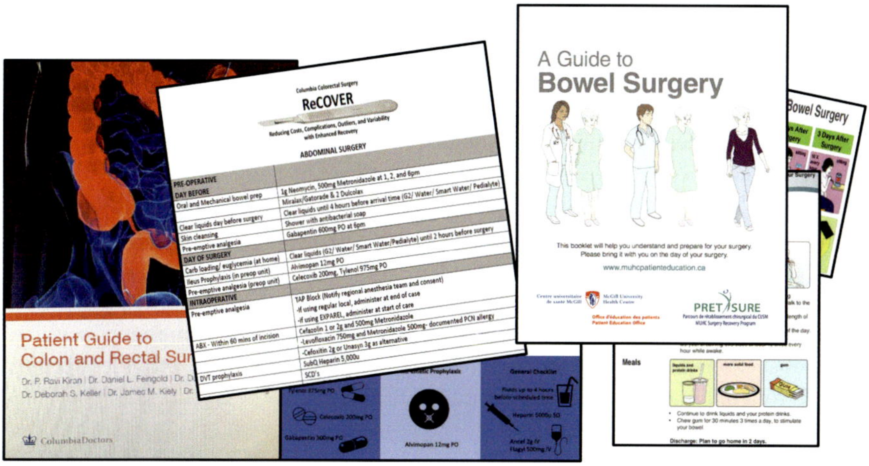

Fig. 7.2 Enhanced recovery protocol educational material

cornerstone of every ERP [33]. Preoperative education is essential; the need for more education and counseling has been identified as a barrier to ERP success [34]. Thus, information should be repeated at different points in time and via different means – words, pictures, electronic media, or mobile health apps – to increase patient engagement in their recovery process (Fig. 7.2) [15, 33, 35]. The bowel preparation should be detailed; the current standard of care is mechanical and oral antibiotics to reduce surgical site infection [36, 37]. There may also be a role for a prehabilitation program prior to surgery, with nutrition, regular exercise, smoking cessation, and anxiety/stress management facilitate return to baseline functional status; this is especially important in colorectal cancer and frail patients [38–40]. Other tenets for the preoperative period are fluid and carbohydrate loading, clear liquids until 2 hours before surgery, and preemptive pain and ileus management [6]. During the intraoperative period, attention should focus on multimodal pain management, minimally invasive approaches instead of large incisions when feasible, goal-directed fluid therapy, and avoidance of unnecessary drains and tubes. Postoperatively, important elements include early ambulation; early removal of catheters, drains, and tubes; early resumption of diet and cessation of supplemental intravenous fluids, and multimodal opioid-sparing pain management. Patients should also have a scheduled follow-up visit before discharge to reduce anxiety during the transition of care from hospital to home.

Measuring and Further Improving Outcomes

Audit of processes and outcomes is a common theme across all periods. The designated coordinator can document compliance with the protocol overall and individual ERP elements and evaluate the process and outcome variables for key metrics.

Programs such as the American College of Surgeons National Surgical Quality Improvement Program (NSQIP) are a useful tool to help with quality improvement after ERP implementation. NSQIP produces risk-adjusted reports tracking institutional outcomes and can compare outcomes to both your historical and national rates. The Enhanced Recovery in NSQIP (ERIN) program has ERP-specific variables that can be collected within the NSQIP and can be a useful tool for audit [41]. The ERAS Society has also developed an interactive audit tool specifically to measure and track care processes and outcomes for ERPs [42]. For institutions without access to NSQIP or the ability to use the ERAS Society tool, the most simple option is to create your own report using a spreadsheet, such as Microsoft Excel, where customized audit reports can be easily created showing overall compliance with the individual elements of a protocol, trends over time, and even provider-specific reports for continuous quality improvement (Fig. 7.3).

After the initial implementation, effective integration with existing clinical systems, such as creating standardized electronic order sets, and using audit and feedback to report to hospital stakeholders have been identified as technical enablers to success [17]. It is important to set a regular schedule to audit the outcomes, such as every month initially and then every quarter, and transition the results back to the unit champions and stakeholders. Audit of outcomes regularly allows for refinement, celebrating accomplishments, and continued administrative and departmental support. With the audit results, the team can revise the protocol, education documents, and any other aspect of the program to meet changing needs and goals. Auditing can also help identify outliers and patients who fail to meet expectations on an ERP to maximize identification of defects in and improve on further pathway implementation and success [1, 43, 44]. To date, there are no standardized frameworks to guide data

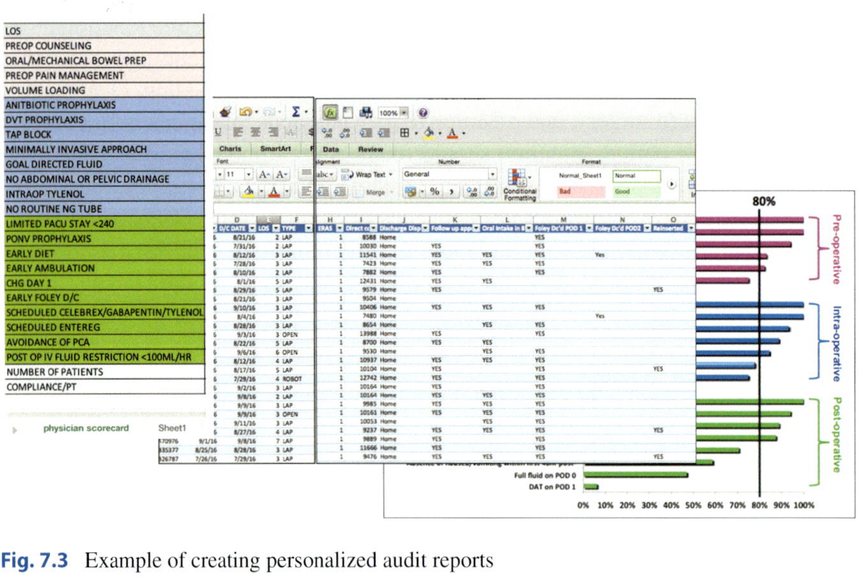

Fig. 7.3 Example of creating personalized audit reports

collection or audit or to assess the effectiveness of implementation, but an international expert consensus is underway to maximize outcomes [14].

The impact of ERP compliance on postoperative outcomes has been studied; showing increasing compliance independently improves outcomes, with fewer complications and shorter primary hospital length of stay [45]. The association of compliance with improved clinical outcomes was shown specifically in major colorectal cancer surgery, indicating a dose-response relationship [46]. Thus, continued quality improvement should target increasing compliance with all elements of the ERP. While compliance improves outcomes, ERPs are not an all-or-none phenomenon. Non-compliance occurs mostly in the postoperative period and may be due to lack of education, logistical issues, or medical necessity [47]. Patients will still experience benefits in clinical and functional improvement following parts of the pathways as the team strives for complete implementation to maximize the benefits [48].

Conclusions

Enhanced recovery protocols are proven to improve the clinical and financial outcomes in colorectal surgery. Development of ERPs is commonly thought of as a complicated, expensive, and labor-intensive practice, and while there is a large volume of literature on outcomes, there is little written on the actual implementation science of ERPs at the institutional level. In this chapter, we moved through the stepwise development, methods to successfully translate the ERP into clinical practice and auditing results using the minimal requirements for maximal benefit. This framework can assist all surgeons practicing colorectal surgery in the process of defining their goals; obtaining institutional support; creating their multidisciplinary team, business case, and specific protocols; overcoming the cultural change when rolling out the protocols; and auditing results for ongoing quality improvement. It is important to remember that ERPs are a process and to have patience with the results and acceptance of the process. With time and perseverance, barriers and enablers will be identified, and ERP will prove to be incorporated as everyday practice with ongoing benefits.

References

1. Keller DS, Bankwitz B, Woconish D, Champagne BJ, Reynolds HL Jr, Stein SL, et al. Predicting who will fail early discharge after laparoscopic colorectal surgery with an established enhanced recovery pathway. Surg Endosc. 2014;28:74–9.
2. Kehlet H. Multimodal approach to control postoperative pathophysiology and rehabilitation. Br J Anaesth. 1997;78:606–17.
3. Kehlet H, Wilmore DW. Multimodal strategies to improve surgical outcome. Am J Surg. 2002;183:630–41.
4. Wilmore DW, Kehlet H. Management of patients in fast track surgery. BMJ. 2001;322:473–6.

5. Kehlet H, Wilmore DW. Evidence-based surgical care and the evolution of fast-track surgery. Ann Surg. 2008;248:189–98.
6. Ljungqvist O, Scott M, Fearon KC. Enhanced recovery after surgery: a review. JAMA Surg. 2017;152(3):292–8.
7. Maessen J, Dejong CH, Hausel J, Nygren J, Lassen K, Andersen J, et al. A protocol is not enough to implement an enhanced recovery programme for colorectal resection. Br J Surg. 2007;94:224–31.
8. Greer NL, Gunnar WP, Dahm P, Lee AE, MacDonald R, Shaukat A, et al. Enhanced recovery protocols for adults undergoing colorectal surgery: a systematic review and meta-analysis. Dis Colon Rectum. 2018;61:1108–18.
9. Visioni A, Shah R, Gabriel E, Attwood K, Kukar M, Nurkin S. Enhanced recovery after surgery for noncolorectal surgery?: a systematic review and meta-analysis of major abdominal surgery. Ann Surg. 2018;267:57–65.
10. Lau CS, Chamberlain RS. Enhanced recovery after surgery programs improve patient outcomes and recovery: a meta-analysis. World J Surg. 2017;41:899–913.
11. Hogan C, Barry M, Burke M, Joyce P. Healthcare professionals' experiences of the implementation of integrated care pathways. Int J Health Care Qual Assur. 2011;24:334–47.
12. Keller DS, Delaney CP, Senagore AJ, Feldman LS, Task Force SAGESSMART. Uptake of enhanced recovery practices by SAGES members: a survey. Surg Endosc. 2017;31(9):3519–26.
13. McLeod RS, Aarts MA, Chung F, Eskicioglu C, Forbes SS, Conn LG, et al. Development of an enhanced recovery after surgery guideline and implementation strategy based on the knowledge-to-action cycle. Ann Surg. 2015;262:1016–25.
14. Francis NK, Walker T, Carter F Hübner M, Balfour A, Jakobsen DH, et al. Consensus on training and implementation of enhanced recovery after surgery: a Delphi Study. World J Surg. 2018;42:1919–28.
15. Brady KM, Keller DS, Delaney CP. Successful implementation of an enhanced recovery pathway: the nurse's role. AORN J. 2015;102:469–81.
16. Pearsall EA, Meghji Z, Pitzul KB, Aarts MA, McKenzie M, McLeod RS, et al. A qualitative study to understand the barriers and enablers in implementing an enhanced recovery after surgery program. Ann Surg. 2015;261:92–6.
17. Gotlib Conn L, McKenzie M, Pearsall EA, McLeod RS. Successful implementation of an enhanced recovery after surgery programme for elective colorectal surgery: a process evaluation of champions' experiences. Implement Sci. 2015;10:99.
18. Hübner M, Addor V, Slieker J, Griesser AC, Lécureux E, Blanc C, et al. The impact of an enhanced recovery pathway on nursing workload: a retrospective cohort study. Int J Surg. 2015;24:45–50.
19. Stone AB, Grant MC, Pio Roda C, Hobson D, Pawlik T, Wu CL, et al. Implementation costs of an enhanced recovery after surgery program in the United States: a financial model and sensitivity analysis based on experiences at a Quaternary Academic Medical Center. J Am Coll Surg. 2016;222:219–25.
20. Lee L, Mata J, Ghitulescu GA, Boutros M, Charlebois P, Stein B, et al. Cost-effectiveness of enhanced recovery versus conventional perioperative management for colorectal surgery. Ann Surg. 2015;262:1026–33.
21. Porter ME. What is value in health care. N Engl J Med. 2010;363:2477–81.
22. Owens DK, Qaseem A, Chou R, Shekelle P, Clinical GCOTACOP. High-value, cost-conscious health care: concepts for clinicians to evaluate the benefits, harms, and costs of medical interventions. Ann Intern Med. 2011;154:174–80.
23. Lemanu DP, Singh PP, Stowers MD, Hill AG. A systematic review to assess cost effectiveness of enhanced recovery after surgery programmes in colorectal surgery. Color Dis. 2014;16:338–46.
24. Lee L, Li C, Landry T, Latimer E, Carli F, Fried GM, et al. A systematic review of economic evaluations of enhanced recovery pathways for colorectal surgery. Ann Surg. 2014;259:670–6.
25. Jung AD, Dhar VK, Hoehn RS, Atkinson SJ, Johnson BL, Rice T, et al. Enhanced recovery after colorectal surgery: can we afford not to use it. J Am Coll Surg. 2018;226:586–93.

26. Thiele RH, Rea KM, Turrentine FE, Friel CM, Hassinger TE, McMurry TL, et al. Standardization of care: impact of an enhanced recovery protocol on length of stay, complications, and direct costs after colorectal surgery. J Am Coll Surg. 2015;220:430–43.
27. Miller TE, Thacker JK, White WD, Mantyh C, Migaly J, Jin J, et al. Reduced length of hospital stay in colorectal surgery after implementation of an enhanced recovery protocol. Anesth Analg. 2014;118:1052–61.
28. Ren L, Zhu D, Wei Y, Pan X, Liang L, Xu J, et al. Enhanced Recovery After Surgery (ERAS) program attenuates stress and accelerates recovery in patients after radical resection for colorectal cancer: a prospective randomized controlled trial. World J Surg. 2012;36:407–14.
29. Roulin D, Donadini A, Gander S, Griesser AC, Blanc C, Hübner M, et al. Cost-effectiveness of the implementation of an enhanced recovery protocol for colorectal surgery. Br J Surg. 2013;100:1108–14.
30. Nelson G, Kiyang LN, Chuck A, Thanh NX, Gramlich LM. Cost impact analysis of Enhanced Recovery After Surgery program implementation in Alberta colon cancer patients. Curr Oncol. 2016;23:e221–7.
31. Thanh NX, Chuck AW, Wasylak T, Lawrence J, Faris P, Ljungqvist O, et al. An economic evaluation of the Enhanced Recovery After Surgery (ERAS) multisite implementation program for colorectal surgery in Alberta. Can J Surg. 2016;59:415–21.
32. SAGES SMART Enhanced Recovery Program. https://www.sages.org/smart-enhanced-recovery-program/.
33. Sjöstedt L, Hellström R, Stomberg MW. Patients' need for information prior to colonic surgery. Gastroenterol Nurs. 2011;34:390–7.
34. Alawadi ZM, Leal I, Phatak UR, Flores-Gonzalez JR, Holihan JL, Karanjawala BE, et al. Facilitators and barriers of implementing enhanced recovery in colorectal surgery at a safety net hospital: a provider and patient perspective. Surgery. 2016;159:700–12.
35. Keller DS, Chand M. Increasing patient engagement to move enhanced recovery forward. Ann Laparosc Endosc Surg. 2017;2:155.
36. Kiran RP, Murray AC, Chiuzan C, Estrada D, Forde K. Combined preoperative mechanical bowel preparation with oral antibiotics significantly reduces surgical site infection, anastomotic leak, and ileus after colorectal surgery. Ann Surg. 2015;262:416–25; discussion 423
37. Klinger AL, Green H, Monlezun DJ, Beck D, Kann B, Vargas HD, et al. The role of Bowel preparation in colorectal surgery: results of the 2012-2015 ACS-NSQIP Data. Ann Surg. 2019;269(4):671–7.
38. Gillis C, Li C, Lee L, Awasthi R, Augustin B, Gamsa A, et al. Prehabilitation versus rehabilitation: a randomized control trial in patients undergoing colorectal resection for cancer. Anesthesiology. 2014;121:937–47.
39. Carli F, Zavorsky GS. Optimizing functional exercise capacity in the elderly surgical population. Curr Opin Clin Nutr Metab Care. 2005;8:23–32.
40. Barberan-Garcia A, Ubré M, Roca J, Lacy AM, Burgos F, Risco R, et al. Personalised prehabilitation in high-risk patients undergoing elective major abdominal surgery: a Randomized Blinded Controlled Trial. Ann Surg. 2018;267:50–6
41. Berian JR, Ban KA, Liu JB, Sullivan CL, Ko CY, Thacker JKM, et al. Association of an enhanced recovery pilot with length of stay in the National Surgical Quality Improvement Program. JAMA Surg. 2018;153:358–65.
42. ERAS Society. Interactive Audit. https://www.encare.net/healthcare-professionals/products-and-services/eras-interactive-audit-system-eias.
43. Grant MC, Galante DJ, Hobson DB, Lavezza A, Friedman M, Wu CL, et al. Optimizing an enhanced recovery pathway program: development of a postimplementation audit strategy. Jt Comm J Qual Patient Saf. 2017;43:524–33.
44. Keller DS, Stulberg JJ, Lawrence JK, Delaney CP. Process control to measure process improvement in colorectal surgery: modifications to an established enhanced recovery pathway. Dis Colon Rectum. 2014;57:194–200.
45. ERAS Compliance Group. The impact of enhanced recovery protocol compliance on elective colorectal cancer resection: results from an International Registry. Ann Surg. 2015;261:1153–9.

46. Gustafsson UO, Hausel J, Thorell A, Ljungqvist O, Soop M, Nygren J. Adherence to the enhanced recovery after surgery protocol and outcomes after colorectal cancer surgery. Arch Surg. 2011;146:571–7.
47. Roulin D, Muradbegovic M, Addor V, Blanc C, Demartines N, Hübner M. Enhanced recovery after elective colorectal surgery – reasons for non-compliance with the protocol. Dig Surg. 2017;34:220–6.
48. Martin D, Roulin D, Addor V, Blanc C, Demartines N, Hübner M. Enhanced recovery implementation in colorectal surgery-temporary or persistent improvement. Langenbeck's Arch Surg. 2016;401:1163–9.

Bowel Preparation in Colorectal Surgery: Impact on SSIs and Enhanced Recovery Protocols

8

Traci L. Hedrick and Stefan D. Holubar

Introduction and Rationale

There are few topics more widely debated in the gastrointestinal surgical literature than the use of mechanical bowel preparation (MBP) for colorectal surgery. Some of the controversy arises from differences in practice patterns between the United States and Europe. However, much of the discrepancy arises from methodological differences between studies with regard to bowel preparation recipes including the osmolarity of the cathartic and the presence or absence of oral antibiotics (OAs). The variations in study methodology (specifically with regard to the omission of OAs) have led to misinterpretation of the data and changes in practice. As a result, practice patterns vary widely (Fig. 8.1) [1–3]. In this chapter, we will review the evolution of the MBP including the most up-to-date literature specifically with regard to the role of MBP in the prevention of surgical site infection (SSI) and use within an enhanced recovery protocol (ERP).

Efficacy of Mechanical Bowel Preparation (MBP) in Colorectal Surgery

The efficacy of the MBP combined with OAs for elective intestinal surgery was first demonstrated in the 1970s when the Nichols-Condon bowel preparation (typically a clear liquid diet for 24 hours followed by neomycin and erythromycin in addition to vigorous mechanical cleansing) was described [4–6]. This demonstrated a

T. L. Hedrick (✉)
University of Virginia Health System, Department of Surgery, Charlottesville, VA, USA
e-mail: Th8q@virginia.edu

S. D. Holubar
Department of Colon and Rectal Surgery, Cleveland Clinic Foundation, Cleveland, OH, USA
e-mail: holubas@ccf.org

P. Sylla et al. (eds.), *The SAGES Manual of Colorectal Surgery*,
https://doi.org/10.1007/978-3-030-24812-3_8

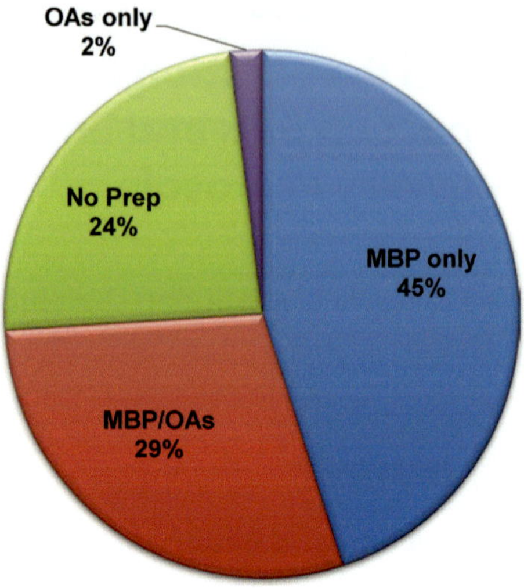

Fig. 8.1 Graphic representation of practice patterns throughout the United States with regard to mechanical bowel preparation demonstrating that 24% of surgeons omit a mechanical bowel prep, 29% use MBP with oral antibiotics, and 45% use MBP in the absence of oral antibiotics. (Data from Refs. [1–3])

reduction in SSI following colorectal surgery from 43% to 9%. Following this sentinel publication, the Nichols-Condon bowel preparation became the gold standard for the following two decades with widespread, global use and adoption of this "aggressive" cathartic prep, which was often poorly tolerated by patients [7, 8]. However, the modern use of the MBP has been called into question due to a number of secular trends in surgery including patient satisfaction/tolerance, concern of overall renal failure with hyperosmotic preparations, the development of broader spectrum parenteral (IV) antibiotics, and finally the advent of enhanced recovery programs (ERPs). As a result, there has been a proliferation of research into the efficacy of the MBP (with or without OAs), which continues to this day (Fig. 8.2).

With the development of parenteral third-generation cephalosporins and other parenteral antibiotics, many of the MBP trials conducted in the early 2000s *omitted* OAs based on the assumption that IV antibiotics would mitigate the need for OAs [9, 10]. This was in stark contrast to the initial trials conducted during the 1970s. It subsequently became evident that a MBP *in the absence of* OAs results in liquid, bacteria-laden stool that is more likely to contaminate the operative field than formed stool in the unprepped colon [11, 12]. Due to the omission of OAs in a majority of these studies, clinical trials and meta-analyses from the early 2000s failed to demonstrate efficacy in SSI or anastomotic leak prevention with MBP [9, 10, 13–15]. In fact, the 2005 Cochrane meta-analysis suggested that, compared to no prep at all, MBP alone may result in a higher rate of anastomotic leakage and surgical site infection [14]. Thus, the omission of the MBP became standard practice and one of the primary tenets of the early ERP movement [16]. Many ERP protocols to this day still recommend omission of mechanical bowel preparations altogether. Please refer to the chapters on ERPs in colorectal surgery for more details regarding specific protocols (Chaps. 7 and 8).

In a Cochrane Collaboration meta-analysis published in 2009, Nelson and coauthors demonstrated the importance of OAs in the presence of prophylactic IV

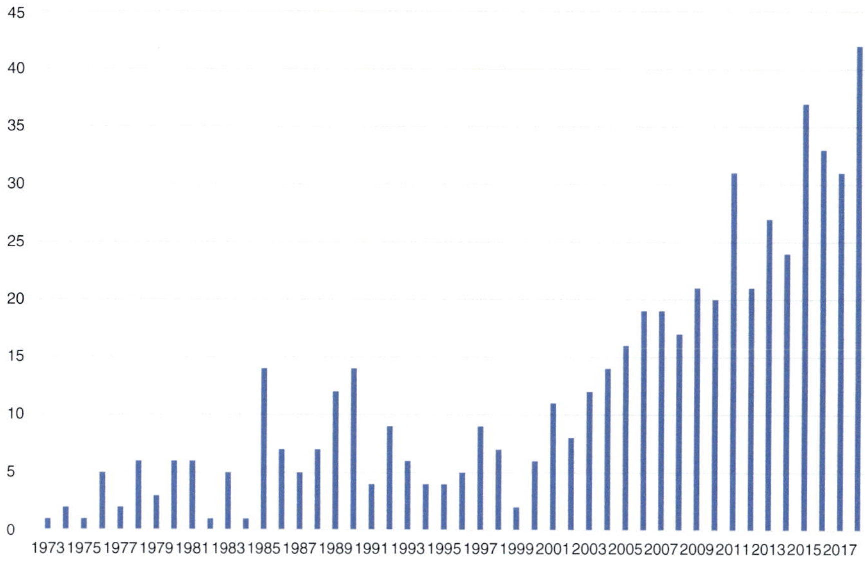

Fig. 8.2 Graphic representation of the number of published manuscripts within PubMed per year on the use of mechanical preparation prior to surgery

antibiotics and a MBP. Their review of 182 RCTs found that OAs administered in the presence of a MBP in addition to IV antibiotics for prophylaxis were associated with a 75% reduction in the rate of SSI [17]. This subsequently led to the publication of several studies evaluating the efficacy of OA combined with the MBP. Multiple large risk-adjusted national database studies including the National Surgical Quality Improvement Program (NSQIP) and the Michigan Surgical Quality Collaborative-Colectomy Best Practices Project demonstrated significant reduction in infectious morbidity (SSI and anastomotic leak) associated with the use of a MBP *when combined* with oral antibiotics [1, 18–25]. Furthermore, the addition of OAs does not seem to increase the risk of *Clostridium difficile* infection and may, in fact, reduce the risk through the prevention of SSI and subsequent need for broad-spectrum antibiotics [26]. The recommendation for the use of a MBP in the presence of OAs is now supported by multiple meta-analyses [27].

Taken together, these data demonstrate that a MBP alone in the absence of OAs cannot be recommended. However, based on several prospective randomized controlled trials (RCTs) and databases studies totaling over 100,000 patients, a combination of a MBP and nonabsorbable OAs is associated with the lowest rate of infectious morbidity following elective colorectal surgery. This distinction in the use of MBP *with and without* OAs is critical when interpreting available literature to optimize surgical outcomes [1, 2, 20, 28].

There are emerging data suggesting that OAs may be beneficial at reducing SSI in elective colorectal surgery *in the absence of MBP*, at least relative to regimens without OAs [29, 30]. Several recent large NSQIP studies have examined the role of OA prep without MBP. Atkinson and coauthors [31] conducted a study of just over

6000 patients, demonstrating that OA alone, without MBP, was associated with a reduction in SSI rates from 13.7% to 9.7% ($p = 0.01$). Klinger and coauthors [23] examined roughly 30,000 colectomy patients within NSQIP and found that while a combined MBP with OAs was superior, OA alone was favorable to omission of MBP in terms of SSIs. A significant limitation of this study was that only 6% (1374) of the cohort received OA alone, suggesting significant selection bias.

Finally, Garfinkle and coauthors [30] in a similar study with over 40,000 colectomies found that OA alone and combined OA + MBP resulted in an equivalently low rate of SSI, leak, and ileus, suggesting that the combined prep offered no advantage over OAs alone. These studies have been included in a recent networked meta-analysis whose findings were that overall combined MBP + OAs produced the lowest rate of infectious complications with OAs alone as the next best option for obtaining the lowest rate of SSIs [21]. There are no RCTs examining OAs alone compared to other strategies. Therefore, whether or not isolated OAs in the absence of a mechanical preparation is truly effective in reducing infectious morbidity remains to be seen.

To assess current practice regarding current bowel prep use, the authors conducted a Twitter® poll, of mostly academic surgeons, from around the globe. This included 141 votes from a variety of different countries and showed that a combined MBP and OA prep is now the most commonly used preparation (59%), while 21% of surgeons omit use of any MBP. A similar contemporaneous poll regarding sigmoid colectomies showed similar results with the addition that some surgeons prescribe enemas for left-sided procedures (Fig. 8.3).

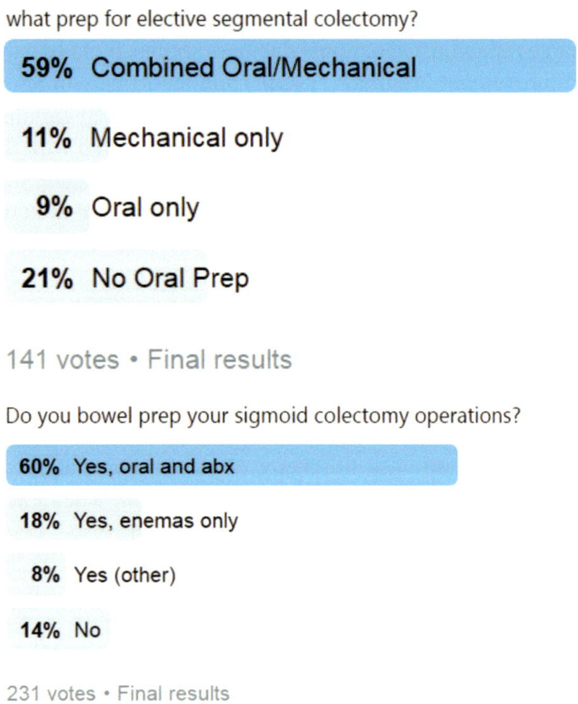

Fig. 8.3 Results of recent Twitter (Twitter Inc., San Francisco, CA, USA) poll on the use of bowel preparations by academic surgeons

Bowel Preparations and Laparoscopic Colorectal Surgery

Aside from the salutary effect of MBPs on SSIs, the MBP offers a practical and technical benefit specific to intestinal surgery through decompression of the bowel. This allows for easier manipulation of the colon, particularly with laparoscopy. In addition, a mechanical preparation is obviously preferable should an intraoperative colonoscopy become necessary (e.g., unable to locate the lesion intraoperatively) which could force the decision to abandon surgery or perform an extended resection with hopes of resecting the lesion. Thus, many colorectal surgeons who perform mostly laparoscopic surgery, including the authors of this chapter and their respective partners, prefer a combined preparation for these reasons.

Types of Mechanical Bowel Preparations

One common misconception held by many perioperative care providers is that all MBPs cause dehydration, electrolyte imbalance, and detrimental physiologic effects. Although many of the early hyperosmotic phosphate-based solutions did lead to dehydration, the isosmotic solutions in most current MBP regimens are better tolerated. Table 8.1 describes the clinical characteristics of various MBP regimens.

In contrast to isosmotic preparations, hyperosmotic preparations such as magnesium citrate and sodium phosphate draw water into the intestine through an osmotic

Table 8.1 Various mechanical bowel preparations and their properties

Name	Properties
Polyethylene glycol (PEG, GoLYTELY® [Braintree Laboratories, Braintree, MA, USA], Colyte® [Pendopharm, Montreal, Canada])	Safe, large volume, poor taste
Sulfate-free PEG (NuLytely® [Braintree Laboratories, Braintree, MA, USA], TriLyte® [Schwarz Pharma, Milwaukee, WI, USA])	Safe, large volume, better taste
Low-volume PEG and bisacodyl (HalfLytely® [Braintree Laboratories, Braintree, MA, USA])	Safe, lower volume (2 L)
Low-volume sulfate solution (SUPREP® [Braintree Laboratories, Braintree, MA, USA])	Low volume, risk of electrolyte abnormalities and renal dysfunction
Ascorbic acid lavage (MoviPrep® [Salix Pharmaceuticals, Bridgewater, NJ, USA])	Safe, better taste, caution in patients with G6PD deficiency
Sodium phosphate Liquid form Visicol® tablets (Salix Pharmaceuticals, Bridgewater, NJ, USA) OsmoPrep® tablets (Salix Pharmaceuticals, Bridgewater, NJ, USA)	Low volume, electrolyte and fluid shifts, caution in cardiac/liver/renal dysfunction; elderly/dehydrated, those taking angiotensin-converting enzyme inhibitors or angiotensin receptor blockers
Magnesium citrate as adjunct to PEG	Lower volume, caution in renal dysfunction

effect. As a result, hyperosmotic preparations can be administered in smaller volumes resulting in higher patient satisfaction. However, as opposed to the safer isosmotic solutions, the hyperosmotic solutions can be associated with significant fluid and electrolyte shifts and renal damage [32–34]. Hence, hyperosmotic bowel preparation solutions are not generally recommended prior to colorectal surgery.

Polyethylene glycol (PEG), an osmotically balanced electrolyte lavage solution, is the most commonly used agent for MBP in elective colorectal surgery. It is standardly administered in a 4 liter preparation that many patients dislike due to volume and taste. The major advantage is that the high-molecular weight, nonabsorbable polymer passes directly through the GI tract without net absorption or secretion. Fluid and electrolyte shifts are thereby generally avoided. Up to 17% of patients will experience adverse effects such as nausea and vomiting with PEG [9]. Standard full-volume PEG preparations include GoLYTELY® (Braintree Laboratories, Braintree MA, USA), Colyte® (Pendopharm, Montreal, Canada), NuLytely® (Braintree Laboratories, Braintree, MA, USA), and TriLyte® (Schwarz Pharma, Milwaukee, WI, USA). Low-volume PEG preparations (HalfLytely® [Braintree Laboratories, Braintree, MA, USA], MoviPrep® [Salix Pharmaceuticals, Bridgewater, NJ, USA], MiraLax® [Bayer, Whippany, NJ, USA], and BiPeglyte® [Pendopharm, Montreal, Canada]) have been developed in combination with other cathartic agents to make the solution more palatable. There is a paucity of literature evaluating the efficacy of these low-volume preparations specific to colorectal surgery. However, the low-volume solutions have been demonstrated to result in similar preparation for colonoscopy procedures.

Bowel Preparations and Enhanced Recovery Protocols (ERPs)

To date, limited research has focused on the intersection between the mechanical bowel preparation and enhanced recovery. Even ERP guidelines from Europe and North America are contradictory, with the ERAS society advocating for omission of the MBP, while the aforementioned ASER guideline recommended routine combined MBP + OA prep [35].

The most recent guideline on ERP for colon and rectal surgery was a joint ASCRS/SAGES publication. That guideline stated that MBP + OA is the preferred preparation and is associated with reduced complication rates (grade of recommendation 2B, weak recommendation based on moderate quality evidence) [36]. In addition to that resource, readers are referred to the SAGES SMART Enhanced Recovery Program (https://www.sages.org/smart-enhanced-recovery-program/). The position that SAGES has taken is that bowel preparations should be used selectively, but their recommendations are congruent with the above recommendations. Specifically, they recommend inclusion of oral antibiotics if a mechanical bowel preparation is used, as this combination has been shown to decrease infections when used. However, a definitive recommendation was not made for rectal surgery as it was felt more data are required (https://www.sages.org/enhanced-recovery/bowel-preparation/).

In addition to the bowel preparation itself, one must consider how the preparation affects oral carbohydrate loading. Hendry and coauthors [37] demonstrated the feasibility of oral carbohydrate loading with MBP in patients undergoing elective left colon and rectal resections with no adverse events. Subsequently, numerous successful ERPs have been published incorporating use of an isosmotic MBP with oral antibiotics. Thiele and colleagues demonstrated that MBP with oral antibiotics could successfully be incorporated into an ERP, demonstrating a 2.2 day reduction in length of stay and a reduction in overall complications by 48.8% (p <0.0001) [38]. Likewise, Keenan and colleagues [39] demonstrated a further reduction in infectious morbidity and length of stay following the addition of a SSI prevention bundle that included, among various other things, the routine use of a MBP to their existing successful ER program. These results demonstrate that use of a PEG-based MBP in the presence of oral antibiotics is not detrimental to an ER program. Finally, MBP + OA has been endorsed not only by ASCRS and SAGES but also by the American Society for Enhanced Recovery (ASER) and Perioperative Quality Initiative (POQI) to prevent infectious complications following elective colorectal surgery in the setting of an ERP [40].

A sample MBP that can be utilized within an ERP is demonstrated in Box 8.1. Prophylactic antiemetics may attenuate the postoperative nausea and vomiting associated with the emetogenic nature of the large-volume preparations and high-dose metronidazole and the prokinetic effects of the high-dose erythromycin. Finally, patients should be encouraged to drink electrolyte-rich fluids throughout their preparation up until 2 hours before surgery.

Box 8.1 Sample bowel preparation in enhanced recovery protocol

- Clears starting at 6 am in the morning the day before surgery.
- 4 liters of GoLYTELY® (Braintree Laboratories, Braintree, MA, USA) starting at 5:00 PM.
- Erythromycin (1 g administered orally at 1:00 pm, 2:00 pm, and 10:00 PM)[a], [b].
- Neomycin (1 g administered orally at 1:00 pm, 2:00 pm, and 10:00 PM).
- Clear liquids can be consumed ad libitum until 2 hours prior to surgery.
- A 20 oz Gatorade® (PepsiCo, Chicago, IL, USA) is consumed 2 hours prior to surgery.

[a]May substitute 1 g of metronidazole for the erythromycin

[b]Alternative dose/timing 2 g of the antibiotics given at 6 pm and 10 pm

Conclusion

An isosmotic MBP in combination with OAs is associated with the lowest attainable rates of infectious morbidity following elective colorectal surgery. The use of these preparations can be effectively utilized within an enhanced recovery protocol without untoward effects on the recovery process. Preparation use may be optimized by addition of simple measures such as use of palatable lower volume solutions, prophylactic antiemetics, and electrolyte-rich drinks.

References

1. Morris MS, Graham LA, Chu DI, Cannon JA, Hawn MT. Oral antibiotic bowel preparation significantly reduces surgical site infection rates and readmission rates in elective colorectal surgery. Ann Surg. 2015;261(6):1034–40.
2. Kiran RP, Murray AC, Chiuzan C, Estrada D, Forde K. Combined preoperative mechanical bowel preparation with oral antibiotics significantly reduces surgical site infection, anastomotic leak, and ileus after colorectal surgery. Ann Surg. 2015;262(3):416–25; discussion 23–5
3. Scarborough JE, Mantyh CR, Sun Z, Migaly J. Combined mechanical and oral antibiotic bowel preparation reduces incisional surgical site infection and anastomotic leak rates after elective colorectal resection: an analysis of colectomy-targeted ACS NSQIP. Ann Surg. 2015;262(2):331–7.
4. Bartlett JG, Condon RE, Gorbach SL, Clarke JS, Nichols RL, Ochi S. Veterans Administration Cooperative Study on Bowel Preparation for Elective Colorectal Operations: impact of oral antibiotic regimen on colonic flora, wound irrigation cultures and bacteriology of septic complications. Ann Surg. 1978;188(2):249–54.
5. Nichols RL, Condon RE, DiSanto AR. Preoperative bowel preparation. Erythromycin base serum and fecal levels following oral administration. Arch Surg. 1977;112(12):1493–6.
6. Nichols RL, Condon RE, Gorbach SL, Nyhus LM. Efficacy of preoperative antimicrobial preparation of the bowel. Ann Surg. 1972;176(2):227–32.
7. Nichols RL, Broido P, Condon RE, Gorbach SL, Nyhus LM. Effect of preoperative neomycin-erythromycin intestinal preparation on the incidence of infectious complications following colon surgery. Ann Surg. 1973;178(4):453–62.
8. Clarke JS, Condon RE, Bartlett JG, Gorbach SL, Nichols RL, Ochi S. Preoperative oral antibiotics reduce septic complications of colon operations: results of prospective, randomized, double-blind clinical study. Ann Surg. 1977;186(3):251–9.
9. Dahabreh IJ, Steele DW, Shah N, Trikalinos TA. Oral mechanical bowel preparation for colorectal surgery: systematic review and meta-analysis. Dis Colon Rectum. 2015;58(7):698–707.
10. Guenaga KF, Matos D, Wille-Jorgensen P. Mechanical bowel preparation for elective colorectal surgery. Cochrane Database Syst Rev. 2011;(9):CD001544.
11. Mahajna A, Krausz M, Rosin D, Shabtai M, Hershko D, Ayalon A, et al. Bowel preparation is associated with spillage of bowel contents in colorectal surgery. Dis Colon Rectum. 2005;48(8):1626–31.
12. Anjum N, Ren J, Wang G, Li G, Wu X, Dong H, et al. A randomized control trial of preoperative oral antibiotics as adjunct therapy to systemic antibiotics for preventing surgical site infection in clean contaminated, contaminated, and dirty type of colorectal surgeries. Dis Colon Rectum. 2017;60(12):1291–8.
13. Guenaga KK, Matos D, Wille-Jorgensen P. Mechanical bowel preparation for elective colorectal surgery. Cochrane Database Syst Rev. 2009;(1):CD001544.
14. Guenaga KF, Matos D, Castro AA, Atallah AN, Wille-Jorgensen P. Mechanical bowel preparation for elective colorectal surgery. Cochrane Database Syst Rev. 2005;(1):CD001544.
15. Guenaga KF, Matos D, Castro AA, Atallah AN, Wille-Jorgensen P. Mechanical bowel preparation for elective colorectal surgery. Cochrane Database Syst Rev. 2003;(2):CD001544.
16. Gustafsson UO, Scott MJ, Schwenk W, Demartines N, Roulin D, Francis N, et al. Guidelines for perioperative care in elective colonic surgery: Enhanced Recovery After Surgery (ERAS(R)) Society recommendations. Clin Nutr. 2012;31(6):783–800.
17. Nelson RL, Glenny AM, Song F. Antimicrobial prophylaxis for colorectal surgery. Cochrane Database Syst Rev. 2009;(1):CD001181.
18. Englesbe MJ, Brooks L, Kubus J, Luchtefeld M, Lynch J, Senagore A, et al. A statewide assessment of surgical site infection following colectomy: the role of oral antibiotics. Ann Surg. 2010;252(3):514–9; discussion 9–20
19. Kim EK, Sheetz KH, Bonn J, DeRoo S, Lee C, Stein I, et al. A statewide colectomy experience: the role of full bowel preparation in preventing surgical site infection. Ann Surg. 2014;259(2):310–4.

20. Moghadamyeghaneh Z, Hanna MH, Carmichael JC, Mills SD, Pigazzi A, Nguyen NT, et al. Nationwide analysis of outcomes of bowel preparation in colon surgery. J Am Coll Surg. 2015;220(5):912–20.
21. Toh JWT, Phan K, Ctercteko G, Pathma-Nathan N, El-Khoury T, Richardson A, et al. The role of mechanical bowel preparation and oral antibiotics for left-sided laparoscopic and open elective restorative colorectal surgery with and without faecal diversion. Int J Color Dis. 2018;33(12):1781–91.
22. Kaslow SR, Gani F, Alshaikh HN, Canner JK. Clinical outcomes following mechanical plus oral antibiotic bowel preparation versus oral antibiotics alone in patients undergoing colorectal surgery. BJS Open. 2018;2(4):238–45.
23. Klinger AL, Green H, Monlezun DJ, Beck D, Kann B, Vargas HD, et al. The role of bowel preparation in colorectal surgery: results of the 2012-2015 ACS-NSQIP Data. Ann Surg. 2019;269(4):671–7.
24. Koller SE, Bauer KW, Egleston BL, Smith R, Philp MM, Ross HM, et al. Comparative effectiveness and risks of bowel preparation before elective colorectal surgery. Ann Surg. 2018;267(4):734–42.
25. Dolejs SC, Guzman MJ, Fajardo AD, Robb BW, Holcomb BK, Zarzaur BL, et al. Bowel preparation is associated with reduced morbidity in elderly patients undergoing elective colectomy. J Gastrointest Surg. 2017;21(2):372–9.
26. Al-Mazrou AM, Hyde LZ, Suradkar K, Kiran RP. Effect of inclusion of oral antibiotics with mechanical bowel preparation on the risk of Clostridium Difficile infection after colectomy. J Gastrointest Surg. 2018;22(11):1968–75.
27. McSorley ST, Steele CW, McMahon AJ. Meta-analysis of oral antibiotics, in combination with preoperative intravenous antibiotics and mechanical bowel preparation the day before surgery, compared with intravenous antibiotics and mechanical bowel preparation alone to reduce surgical-site infections in elective colorectal surgery. BJS Open. 2018;2(4):185–94.
28. European Society of Coloproctology collaborating g. Association of mechanical bowel preparation with oral antibiotics and anastomotic leak following left sided colorectal resection: an international, multi-centre, prospective audit. Color Dis. 2018;20(Suppl 6):15–32.
29. Atkinson SJ, Swenson BR, Hanseman DJ, Midura EF, Davis BR, Rafferty JF, et al. In the absence of a mechanical bowel prep, does the addition of pre-operative oral antibiotics to parental antibiotics decrease the incidence of surgical site infection after elective segmental colectomy? Surg Infect. 2015;16(6):728–32.
30. Garfinkle R, Abou-Khalil J, Morin N, Ghitulescu G, Vasilevsky CA, Gordon P, et al. Is there a role for oral antibiotic preparation alone before colorectal surgery? ACS-NSQIP analysis by coarsened exact matching. Dis Colon Rectum. 2017;60(7):729–37.
31. Atkinson SJ, Swenson BR, Hanseman DJ, Midura EF, Davis BR, Rafferty JF, et al. In the absence of a mechanical bowel prep, does the addition of pre-operative oral antibiotics to parental antibiotics decrease the incidence of surgical site infection after elective segmental colectomy? Surg Infect. 2015;16(6):728–32.
32. Holte K, Nielsen KG, Madsen JL, Kehlet H. Physiologic effects of bowel preparation. Dis Colon Rectum. 2004;47(8):1397–402.
33. Ackland GL, Harrington J, Downie P, Holding JW, Singh-Ranger D, Griva K, et al. Dehydration induced by bowel preparation in older adults does not result in cognitive dysfunction. Anesth Analg. 2008;106(3):924–9, table of contents
34. Ackland GL, Singh-Ranger D, Fox S, McClaskey B, Down JF, Farrar D, et al. Assessment of preoperative fluid depletion using bioimpedance analysis. Br J Anaesth. 2004;92(1):134–6.
35. Slim K, Kartheuser A. Mechanical bowel preparation before colorectal surgery in enhanced recovery programs: discrepancy between the American and European Guidelines. Dis Colon Rectum. 2018;61(2):e13–e4.
36. Carmichael JC, Keller DS, Baldini G, Bordeianou L, Weiss E, Lee L, Boutros M, McClane J, Feldman LS, Steele SR. Clinical practice guidelines for enhanced recovery after colon and rectal surgery from the American Society of Colon and Rectal Surgeons and Society of American Gastrointestinal and Endoscopic Surgeons. Dis Colon Rectum. 2017;60(8):761–84.

37. Hendry PO, Balfour A, Potter MA, Mander BJ, Bartolo DC, Anderson DN, et al. Preoperative conditioning with oral carbohydrate loading and oral nutritional supplements can be combined with mechanical bowel preparation prior to elective colorectal resection. Colorectal Dis. 2008;10(9):907–10.
38. Thiele RH, Rea KM, Turrentine FE, Friel CM, Hassinger TE, McMurry TL, et al. Standardization of care: impact of an enhanced recovery protocol on length of stay, complications, and direct costs after colorectal surgery. J Am Coll Surg. 2015;220(4):430–43.
39. Keenan JE, Speicher PJ, Nussbaum DP, Adam MA, Miller TE, Mantyh CR, et al. Improving outcomes in colorectal surgery by sequential implementation of multiple standardized care programs. J Am Coll Surg. 2015;221(2):404–14 e1.
40. Holubar SD, Hedrick T, Gupta R, Kellum J, Hamilton M, Gan TJ, et al. American Society for Enhanced Recovery (ASER) and Perioperative Quality Initiative (POQI) joint consensus statement on prevention of postoperative infection within an enhanced recovery pathway for elective colorectal surgery. Perioper Med (Lond). 2017;6:4.

Checklist for Patients and OR Team in Preparation for Laparoscopic Colorectal Surgery

9

Samuel Eisenstein and Alexis L. Grucela

Introduction and Rationale

Preoperative preparation for laparoscopic colon and rectal surgery should include careful evaluation and planning on the part of the surgeon. Knowledge of comorbidities dictates need for further preoperative testing or intervention in order to prevent complications within the perioperative period. Furthermore, prior pelvic radiation or pelvic surgery plays an important role in operative planning. Preoperative mechanical bowel preparation (MBP), judicious use of antibiotics, and prophylaxis for venous thromboembolic events (VTE) are essential aspects of perioperative patient care. Once a patient is deemed appropriate and ready for surgery, the surgeon must carefully plan their approach and know what instruments are required to achieve the desired outcome.

The checklist for the surgeon and OR team can be conceptualized in two phases:

1. Preoperative (outpatient) preparation and prevention.
2. Preoperative preparation in the operating room.

S. Eisenstein
University of California San Diego Health Systems, Department of Surgery, Division of Colon and Rectal Surgery, La Jolla, CA, USA
e-mail: seisenstein@ucsd.edu

A. L. Grucela (✉)
New York University Langone Health, New York University, Department of Surgery, Division of Colon and Rectal Surgery, New York, NY, USA

P. Sylla et al. (eds.), *The SAGES Manual of Colorectal Surgery*,
https://doi.org/10.1007/978-3-030-24812-3_9

Preoperative Planning, Patient Workup, and Optimization

Preoperative Risk Assessment

A systems-based approach to the preoperative assessment is essential with particular emphasis on cardiac and pulmonary risk factors. There are clinical risk factors based on patients' comorbidities which are used to assess perioperative risk of morbidity and mortality. The American Society of Anesthesiologists physical status classification is used to assess general risk (Table 9.1) [1]. American Society of Anesthesiologists class III or higher should prompt preoperative risk assessment by internist or medical subspecialist (i.e., cardiologist, pulmonologist). This provides dialogue between the surgeon and consultant and determines if further preoperative diagnostics or interventions are necessary prior to surgery. Box 9.1 lists patient

Table 9.1 American Society of Anesthesiologists physical status classification

ASA PS classification	Definition	Examples, including, but not limited to:
ASA I	A normal healthy patient	Healthy, non-smoking, no or minimal alcohol use
ASA II	A patient with mild systemic disease	Mild diseases only without substantive functional limitations. Examples include (but not limited to) current smoker, social alcohol drinker, pregnancy, obesity (30< BMI <40), well-controlled DM/HTN, mild lung disease
ASA III	A patient with severe systemic disease	Substantive functional limitations: one or more moderate to severe diseases. Examples include (but not limited to) poorly controlled DM or HTN, COPD, morbid obesity (BMI ≥40), active hepatitis, alcohol dependence or abuse, implanted pacemaker, moderate reduction of ejection fraction, ESRD undergoing regularly scheduled dialysis, premature infant PCA <60 weeks, history (>3 months) of MI, CVA, TIA, or CAD/stents.
ASA IV	A patient with severe systemic disease that is a constant threat to life	Examples include (but not limited to) recent (<3 months) MI, CVA, TIA, or CAD/stents, ongoing cardiac ischemia or severe valve dysfunction, severe reduction of ejection fraction, sepsis, DIC, ARD, or ESRD not undergoing regularly scheduled dialysis
ASA V	A moribund patient who is not expected to survive without the operation	Examples include (but not limited to) ruptured abdominal/thoracic aneurysm, massive trauma, intracranial bleed with mass effect, ischemic bowel in the face of significant cardiac pathology or multiple organ/system dysfunction
ASA VI	A declared brain-dead patient whose organs are being removed for donor purposes	

DM diabetes melitus, *HTN* hypertension, *ESRD* end-stage renal disease, *MI* myocardial infarction, *TIA* transient ischemic attack, *CVA* cerebrovascular accident, *DIC* disseminated intravascular coagulation, *CAD* coronary artery disease

Used with permission of the American Society of Anesthesiologists [1]

Box 9.1 Patient Factors Associated with Perioperative Complications

Patient factors

- Age
- Smoking
- Dyspnea at rest or on exertion
- Poor functional status
- Cerebrovascular accident
- Disseminated cancer
- Preoperative open wound
- Immunosuppression
- Preoperative weight loss >10%
- Preoperative anemia or need for >4 units of PRBC within 72 hours of surgery
- Body mass index (BMI)
- Preoperative leukocytosis

characteristics shown to be independent risk factors associated with perioperative complications in patients undergoing surgery.

Extremes of body mass index (BMI) (<20 kg/m^2 or >35 kg/m^2) are associated with significant risk of 30-day mortality, and BMI >35 kg/m^2 is associated with increase in 30-day morbidity (urinary tract infection, wound infection, sepsis, VTE) [2, 3]. These patients should undergo nutrition counseling at first preoperative visit in order to optimize weight and nutritional status before surgery. A conversation between the operating surgeon and the morbidly obese patient should occur communicating the increased risk of morbidity and mortality incurred based on the patient's BMI. An anesthesia preoperative assessment is also recommended for these patients, as factors such as challenging airways can exist.

The goal of preoperative cardiac risk assessment is to identify those who have recently experienced myocardial infarction (MI) and those at high risk of perioperative MI in order to prevent perioperative cardiac complications. Recent MI requiring percutaneous coronary intervention presents a challenge due to the requirement of dual antiplatelet therapy (aspirin and clopidogrel) in the post intervention period [4, 5]. Bare-metal stents require antiplatelet therapy for a minimum of 4–6 weeks post procedure and drug-eluting stents a minimum 1 year post procedure before stopping for elective surgery [4, 5]. In the setting of malignancy or acute ulcerative colitis, one may not have the ability to concede to these time restraints. Therefore, the risk of perioperative MI versus postoperative bleeding on antiplatelet therapy must be carefully weighed, and a discussion between cardiologist, surgeon, and patient is of utmost importance in such circumstances. Some institutions have their own policies on this and continue at least aspirin throughout the operation on patients with cardiac stents.

The Revised Cardiac Risk Index (RCRI) [6] and Gupta score [7] are two clinical indices commonly used to assess patients at high risk for experiencing perioperative cardiac events. Patients with scores predicting higher risk may need more extensive diagnostic investigation and possible intervention prior to elective surgery. For

Box 9.2 Revised Cardiac Risk Index (RCRI)

- Revised Cardiac Risk Index (RCRI): independent risk factors associated with increased incidence of perioperative cardiac events in patients undergoing non-cardiac surgery

1. High-risk surgery
2. Ischemic heart disease
3. History of congestive heart failure
4. History of cerebrovascular disease
5. Insulin therapy for diabetes
6. Preoperative serum creatinine >2.0 mg/dL

Box 9.3 Gupta Score

- *Gupta score:* independent risk factors associated with greater potential to identify increased risk of perioperative cardiac event compared with RCRI
  - ASA class
  - Dependent functional status
  - Age
  - Abnormal creatinine (>1.5 mg/dL)
  - Type of surgery

Table 9.2 Recommend time for discontinuation of anticoagulation prior to surgery

Drugs	Mechanism of action	Hold time
Heparin	Promote antithrombin	6–12 hours
Low molecular weight heparin	Factor Xa inhibitor	12–24 hours
Warfarin	Vitamin K antagonist	5 days
Argatroban	Direct thrombin inhibitors	3–9 hours
Bivalirudin	Direct thrombin inhibitors	1.5–3 hours
Dabigatran	Direct thrombin inhibitors	24–96 hours (more if patient has renal impairment)
Rivaroxaban	Factor Xa inhibitor	24–48 hours
Apixaban	Factor Xa inhibitor	24–48 hours
Edoxaban	Factor Xa inhibitor	48 hours
Aspirin	Cyclooxygenase inhibitor	Unnecessary (7–10 days for reversal of effect)
Clopidogrel	Platelet P2Y12 receptor inhibitor	5 days
Prasugrel	Platelet P2Y12 receptor inhibitor	5 days
Ticagrelor	Platelet P2Y12 receptor inhibitor	5 days
Ticlopidine	Platelet P2Y12 receptor inhibitor	5 days

example, in the RCRI (Box 9.2) for each risk factor, a patient is given a score of 1, and for those with a total score of ≥2, further testing may be of clinical utility. Patients with low scores do not need further testing. The Gupta score (Box 9.3) is scoring index that is also used to identify high-risk patients for perioperative cardiac complications [7]. This scoring index is reported to be more accurate than RCRI; however, it is more difficult to calculate and, therefore, less frequently used. Patients with cardiac risk factors may be on a variety of anticoagulants. Standard recommendations for holding anticoagulants are included in Table 9.2.

Special Considerations

Immune Suppression

Patients undergoing colon and rectal surgery may suffer from baseline immunosuppression for a variety of reasons. Patients with inflammatory bowel disease (IBD) are often taking a variety of medications including biologic agents, steroids, and thiopurines which impair their immune response, cancer patients may have been exposed to chemotherapy, transplant patients may require long-term immune suppression, and the malnourished may have baseline immune dysfunction. When possible, it is advantageous to stop immune suppression and allow it to wash out of the system; however, this is not often an option as stopping these medications could cause the patients to deteriorate and opens up other potential risks.

There is a significant body of literature demonstrating that steroids significantly increase the risk of septic complications during colon and rectal surgery [8–12]. This effect appears to be dose related, and it does seem clear that patients taking less than 20 mg of prednisone daily are at a lower risk of complications than those on more than 20 mg daily. These patients are still, however, at an increased risk of complications compared to those who are entirely off of steroids [12]. The use of perioperative stress-dose steroids has also fallen out of favor. Perioperative adrenal insufficiency is an extremely rare condition, and there is a greater risk of steroid-related complications [13]. Patients have been assessed for mild symptoms such as orthostasis in the perioperative period, and there is no difference based on whether they received a stress dose of steroids at the time of surgery [14]. The current recommendation is for the patient to take their standard steroid dose on the day of surgery and then begin a taper in the postoperative period. Stress-dose steroids should only be administered in the setting of symptomatic adrenal insufficiency. There is also excellent evidence showing that thiopurines do not appear to increase the risk of postoperative complications in patients with IBD [15].

There is much greater controversy surrounding the effect that biologics have on perioperative outcomes in IBD surgery. There have been several papers showing an increase in perioperative infection rate [16–18] and several and many others showing no increased rate of infection [19–22]. There are valid arguments on both sides as to whether biologic agents should be stopped or washed out of the system prior to surgery, but the full argument is well beyond the scope of this chapter. Likely biologic agents are markers for severity of disease, and patients who have failed

Table 9.3 Half-life and washout time of biologic treatments for IBD

Medication	Half-life (d)	Washout (d)
Infliximab	8–9.5	40–47.5
Adalimumab	14	70
Certolizumab	14	70
Golimumab	9–15	45–75
Vedolizumab	25	125
Natalizumab	10–11	40–45
Ustekinumab	15(IV) 45.6 (SQ)	75 (IV) 228 (SQ)
Tofacitinib	0.13	3

Half-lives and washout times for biologic therapies for IBD listed in days (*IV* intravenous, *SQ* subcutaneous)

multiple biologics likely have the most severe disease. This needs to be taken into consideration when planning surgery, and these patients should be treated as though they have more severe illness than they may exhibit. A common approach to patients on biologics is to wait until they are at the nadir of their dose, usually around the time they are about to receive their next dose, delay that dose, perform their surgery, and restart medication if medically necessary several weeks after surgery. It should be remembered that these patients still have active therapy in their system, and the only true way to ensure there is no drug present is to allow for a full washout which is equivalent to five half-lives of the medication (Table 9.3).

Ideally, chemotherapy should be allowed to wash out of the patient's system prior to undergoing elective colorectal procedures. Chemotherapy can impair wound healing, cause myelosuppression, impair immune responses, and lead to a variety of other different issues which can increase the risk of postoperative complications. When feasible, it is best to wait at least 6 weeks after any dose of chemotherapy to allow for washout. This is particularly true of bevacizumab, a monoclonal antibody against vascular endothelial growth factor (VEGF), which impairs angiogenesis. These patients are at a significant risk of postoperative bleeding. Waiting for surgery is not always feasible, and in the acute setting, patients undergoing chemotherapy sometimes require urgent surgical intervention. When this occurs, it is always important to take the chemotherapy into consideration when planning the type of surgery and consider smaller, more temporizing procedures knowing that significant intervention may lead to significant complication.

Smokers

Smoking is a well-documented risk factor for complications after colon and rectal surgery. Smoking has shown to contribute to increased risk of VTE, wound infection, anastomotic dehiscence, and hernia formation [23–25]. The effects of smoking on the airway are also extensive. Carbon monoxide has deleterious effects on the cardiovascular system and can persist for several hours after inhalation. Airway sensitivity is increased, and these effects last 2–10 days after inhalation. Mucus secretion is also altered, and these effects can last for many weeks [26]. Smoking cessation should be instituted at least 4 weeks prior to surgery, and it has been shown that there is increasing benefit for every week beyond 4 that the patient is able to stop smoking [23]. However, for those who have quit smoking for less than 4 weeks, the alteration of mucus secretion may lead to greater risk of respiratory complications from general anesthesia, and ideally it is best to wait until mucus secretion and cilliation returns to its normal state [26].

One should consider canceling elective surgery in patients who are actively smoking, and any patient who actively smokes and presents for surgery should be counseled on smoking cessation techniques. The surgeon should seek help from the patient's primary care physician as they will often have a greater depth of experience in assisting the patients to adequate cessation. Several aides have also been used in promoting smoking cessation. These include varenicline, bupropion, and nicotine replacement. In a randomized controlled trial, varenicline demonstrated a 3.6-fold increase in smoking cessation compared to placebo, while bupropion and nicotine replacement demonstrated a two-fold increase [27].

These techniques for smoking cessation are often not effective, and so many surgeons will test their patient's blood, urine, or saliva for nicotine or the by-product of nicotine metabolism cotinine. Nicotine will only stay positive on a blood test for several days after consumption, whereas cotinine may remain positive for several weeks and is therefore a better test of long-term cessation than nicotine testing alone. It should be noted that patients taking nicotine replacement will also test positive for nicotine and cotinine, and so this should be taken into consideration when counseling patients on their optimal cessation technique.

Malnutrition

It is also critical to ensure your patient's nutritional status is optimized prior to undergoing major abdominal surgery. Nutrition can be measured in many different ways, whether its body mass index (BMI), weight loss, or hypoalbuminemia. It is important to take all of these into consideration when evaluating a patient for surgery, but the single best test is likely hypoalbuminemia, which has been shown to be the best predictor of most surgical complications as well as length of stay and overall complication rates when compared to weight loss and BMI in patients with colorectal cancer [28]. Malnutrition has been shown to increase the risk of almost every potential complication, from a variety of infectious and septic conditions, to VTE and DVT, to anesthesia-related complications, as poor nutrition impairs every major organ system, leaving patients open to postoperative dysfunction.

Improving upon patient nutrition prior to surgical intervention is necessary to minimize the risk of complications. Patients who are at risk for malnutrition should be assessed prior to surgery with an albumin and prealbumin levels. It should be remembered that albumin is a better marker of chronic nutrition with a half-life of 20–22 days, while prealbumin has a half-life of 2–4 days and is a better gauge of the direction a patient's nutrition is trending. If a patient is determined to be malnourished, then intervention should be considered. Intervention should be chosen based on the factors which led to the patient's malnutrition as well as the acuity of the problem and the timing of surgical intervention. Generally those who are in a catabolic condition should take in between 1.5 and 1.8 g of protein per Kg of body weight per day [29]. Vitamin D supplementation can also help increase muscle mass and should also be considered [29].

Standard dietary supplementation with high-quality protein supplements (>30 g protein/serving) can be helpful, particularly if there is only mild malnutrition. Total parenteral nutrition (TPN) should be considered in patients who are unable to take enteral nutrition. These patients are at higher risk of line-related complications, but this risk is trivial in comparison with those complications that the patient may encounter due to their malnutrition. Enteral nutrition (EN) consists of elemental or semi-elemental feeds delivered to the gut which recently has been shown to be the preferred approach when possible. These data have been borne out in the IBD community where historically patients underwent prolonged usage of TPN for malabsorption and short gut. While studies have shown both TPN and EN are effective at decreasing the risk of surgical complications compared to standard dietary intervention, EN has been shown to be superior to TPN with a number needed to treat of 2 to prevent surgical complications [30]. One downside of EN, however, is that the enteral feeds tend to be foul tasting and difficult to ingest, requiring prolonged placement of a nasogastric tube for up to 4 weeks prior to surgery. TPN tends to be easier to administer, and thus, when given the options, patients will often prefer TPN.

Preoperative immunonutrition is also a useful adjunct in colon and rectal surgery. It is well documented that surgery leads to a state of relative immune suppression in the perioperative period. Immunonutrition usually consists of supplements taken for a week prior to surgery consisting of some combination of arginine, glutamine, branched-chain amino acids, omega-3 fatty acids, and nucleotides. These are designed to target mucosal barrier function, cellular defense, and local and systemic inflammation [31]. A large meta-analysis of immunonutrition showed that while it does not improve mortality, it does decrease the risk of overall complication and infectious complications and shortened hospital stay. The caveat to these data is that when substratified to industry-sponsored vs nonsponsored trials, only the industry sponsored trials demonstrated these benefits [32].

Obesity

Obesity has been shown to increase the risk of almost every type of surgical complication in the colon and rectal surgery patient [33]. Having a plan in place for mitigating the risks of obesity is critical in ensuring optimal patient outcomes. The extremely obese should not be considered for elective surgery without undergoing some manner of weight loss program. This may ultimately include the consideration of bariatric surgery prior to elective colorectal procedures in an attempt to optimize the patient. There are also newer endoluminal approaches to weight loss which carry a lower risk of complications while still achieving modest improvements in both weight loss and correcting the various comorbidities associated with obesity [34]. Morbidly obese patients who can delay their colorectal procedure should be referred to a surgical weight loss team to undergo evaluation.

Many patients will not be able to undergo this long course of evaluation and treatment prior to their surgical intervention. A very low calorie liquid diet has been shown to decrease fat and in particular visceral fat in the preoperative period [35,

36]. By decreasing visceral fat, specifically a surgeon can gain length and reach of bowel. This diet can be particularly helpful in procedures such as low anterior resections and ileal pouch-anal anastomosis where bowel length is crucial. Very low calorie liquid diets usually have the patient consume nutritional shakes that make up less than 800 kcal/day for 1–4 weeks. The amount of fat loss correlates to the time the patient consumes this diet, and it should be done under the direction of a medical or surgical weight loss specialist to ensure that the patients are consuming the appropriate macronutrients.

For those patients who must undergo surgery prior to weight loss, it is important to understand the risks obesity imparts upon the colon and rectal surgery patient. Hernia rates and wound complications are significantly increased in these patients. A minimally invasive approach and off-midline extraction may be helpful in minimizing these wound complications [33, 37]. Surgical site infections are also increased in this population [33]. This may mean that an otherwise uneventful case may still benefit from anastomotic diversion in an attempt to minimize the risk of a leak. These patients may also benefit from drains in their subcutaneous tissues to minimize the risk of infected fat necrosis. Obese patients are also at an increased risk of respiratory and cardiovascular complications from anesthesia [33]. Therefore, it is helpful to include the anesthesia team in your surgical planning and consider prolonged postoperative monitoring for adverse events.

Renal Impairment

Chronic dialysis has been demonstrated to increase the risk of major complications from elective colorectal procedures by at least 2.5-fold and mortality by seven-fold [38]. These patients are particularly difficult to manage postoperatively especially with regard to managing their fluid balance. If these patients present with sepsis, it can be quite difficult to ensure that they maintain the appropriate intravascular volume to support their circulatory system without putting the patient into pulmonary edema. These patients are at a significantly increased risk of both bleeding and VTE [38]. And because of this, it is crucial to carefully manage any postoperative anticoagulation. Patients on dialysis should be managed in conjunction with a nephrologist who should see the patient prior to surgery to ensure that they are optimized. Dialysis should be optimally timed for surgery. It has been shown that an interval of less than 7 hours between dialysis and surgery can lead to postoperative hypotension due to the depleted intravascular state with which these patients undergo surgery [39]. Therefore, it is likely best to dialyze a patient the day prior to surgery to ensure they are undergoing their procedure at euvolemia.

Chronic kidney disease (CKD) not on dialysis also imparts an increased risk of perioperative complications. CKD patients undergoing colorectal resections were more likely to develop cardiovascular complications postoperatively and have a greater than two-fold risk of 30-day mortality [40]. These patients have the potential to be more dysregulated than the dialysis patients depending on their degree of renal impairment. Uremia can lead to a pro-inflammatory state which can lead to an increased risk of atherosclerotic complications as well as infections and bleeding problems. These patients are also often malnourished and volume overloaded, their electrolytes are unbalanced, and they have relative immune suppression. These patients are also often anemic and may benefit from preoperative erythropoietin. When possible their renal function should be optimized as much as possible, and electrolytes should be checked immediately prior to surgery and frequently throughout their procedures.

Preoperative Stoma Marking

Preoperative stoma marking should be arranged for all patients undergoing colon and rectal surgery who may require a stoma at the time of their procedure. A frank conversation about the risks of colostomy or ileostomy is absolutely necessary before attempting bowel surgery. Patients should be aware of the likelihood of this outcome prior to undergoing surgery.

The surgeon may elect to perform their own marking, taking into consideration where the patient's belt line may fall and then evaluating the abdominal contours. The patient should be evaluated in a variety of positions including sitting and supine. Creases, folds, and surgical scars should be avoided as they are a common site of leakage. Stoma marking should occur medial to the lateral border of the rectus abdominis muscle which can be easily palpated by having the patient sit up part way from the supine position, putting this muscle on tension. Oftentimes, it is necessary to mark multiple locations, either bilaterally or in the upper and lower abdomen depending on the patient's habitus and the potential for different types of stomas which could be created at the time of surgery.

It is often much more beneficial for the patient to be marked by an enterostomal therapist (EST) or a wound, ostomy, and continence nurse (WOCN). These specialists not only mark the patient prior to surgery, but they help educate the patient on what life with a stoma may be like. They introduce the patients to the equipment and help them gain a familiarity. Oftentimes these nurses will see the patients in the hospital and continue their education prior to and post discharge. For more details on stomas, please refer to Chap. 36 on optimizing stoma function and quality of life.

Preoperative Patient Education

Patient education is a critical part of the enhanced recovery process and of managing expectations of what they will experience during their postop period/hospital stay and at home. Patient education materials should be distributed including the preoperative plan and preparation and what to expect. See Fig. 9.1 for an example. These materials have been demonstrated to help assuage patient's fears of the unknown and have been demonstrated to decrease length of hospital stay [41].

Current enhanced recovery and surgical site infection (SSI) prevention protocol bundles may include aspects to improve return of bowel function, improved length of stay, and decrease wound infection rates. These are often institution-specific but

Patient Education

NYU Langone
MEDICAL CENTER

COLORECTAL SURGERY

HOW TO PREPARE FOR YOUR OPERATION

HOW TO PREPARE FOR YOUR OPERATION

You are scheduled to have colorectal surgery soon. There are 2 very important things you need to do to get ready for this surgery:

IMPORTANT

✓ **Bowel preparation**
✓ **TWO (2) special showers with CHG soap**
- We will give you a special antibacterial soap to use called Chlorhexidine Gluconate (CHG) 4% antiseptic solution (ex. Hibiclens.)

Here are step-by-step instructions on how to do the bowel preparation ("bowel prep") and special showers:

- Two (2) days before surgery, go to your pharmacy and:
  - ✓ Buy *Boost* (or *Boost Diabetic* if you have diabetes)
  - ✓ Fill the prescriptions needed for bowel prep:
    - NuLYTELY
    - 2 different antibiotics
      - metronidazole (Flagyl)
      - Neomycin sulfate.

THE DAY BEFORE SURGERY

Bowel Prep Instructions

✓ Drink only clear liquids throughout the day:
water, gelatin desserts, juice (no pulp), popsicles, clear broth (no vegetables or noodles), sports drinks, or tea and coffee without milk.
✓ 1:00 p.m.: take 1 metronidazole pill and 2 Neomycin pills.
✓ 2:00 p.m.: take 1 metronidazole pill and 2 Neomycin pills.

1

Created: 01/2016

Fig. 9.1 NYU Langone Medical Center colon pathway. (Used with permission. Copyright © NYU Langone Health)

Bowel Prep Instruction (continued)

- 3:00 p.m.: start drinking the NuLYTELY.
  - ✓ Drink a large glass (about 8 oz.) every 10 minutes. It is best to drink the whole glass very fast, rather than sipping small amounts for a longer time. *Keep drinking until the gallon is gone.*
  - Feeling bloated and/or nauseated is common after the first few glasses. This is temporary and will get better once bowel movements begin.
- ✓ 11:00 p.m.: take 1 metronidazole pill and 2 Neomycin pills.
- ✓ 11:00 p.m.: drink the *Boost* or *Boost Diabetic*.

IMPORTANT

Drink plenty of clear liquids (sports drinks are best) the evening before surgery to keep from getting dehydrated. **Do not eat or drink anything after Midnight (12:00 a.m.).**

Shower Instructions

- ✓ Take the first of your 2 showers the night before surgery.
- ✓ Wash and rinse your hair first using your regular shampoo.
- ✓ Wet your skin in the shower and then turn the water off.
- ✓ Using the CHG soap, gently lather your whole body from the chin down. You may use a washcloth.
- ✓ Wash your whole body but pay special attention to your neck, chest, belly, and groin, including groin creases. Please include belly folds, belly button and under the breasts.
- ✓ **AVOID** getting the soap in your eyes, ears, mouth or nose.
- ✓ Let the lather remain in contact with your skin for at least 15-20 seconds. Rinse well.
- ✓ **DO NOT** rewash with regular soap.
- ✓ After your shower, pat yourself dry with a clean, freshly washed towel.
- ✓ **DO NOT** apply lotions, perfumes, hair products or makeup.
- ✓ **DO NOT** shave yourself in the surgical area. This can increase the chance of infection.

2

Created: 01/2016

HOW TO PREPARE FOR YOUR OPERATION

Fig. 9.1 (continued)

THE DAY OF YOUR SURGERY

✓ Take the second of the 2 showers with the CHG soap in the morning before leaving home. (See above instructions.)
✓ Arrive at the pre-operative area at your scheduled time.

The following information will help you understand your hospital stay and what you can expect as you recover from surgery. These guidelines will help you recover as quickly as possible, as well as reduce the risks of some potential complications.

- When you wake from surgery you will likely have an IV tube. This IV is connected to a pain pump that you can control to help manage your pain after surgery. (The nurses will show you how to use it).
- Because the medications used to make you sleep during surgery will temporarily keep you from urinating on your own, you will also have a catheter (a thin, flexible tube) to drain urine from your bladder.

✓ When you are fully awake, start your breathing exercises. The nurses will show you how to do these exercises.

✓ If recommended by your doctor and only with help from a nurse, you should try to get out of bed in your hospital room and sit in a chair. Take short walks if you can, also only if recommended by your doctor.

- You may drink liquids but only if you feel up to it.

AFTER SURGERY: DAYS 1 & 2, and DAY 3 THROUGH DISCHARGE

Days 1 & 2

- The bladder drain will likely be removed on the first day.

✓ Keep doing your breathing exercises.
✓ Get out of bed and take short walks in the hallways at least 5 times today, if your doctor advises.
✓ Use your pain medication (either the pain pump or pain pills) to stay comfortable.

- You will be on a liquid diet at first, and then advanced to solid food if you continue to do well with the liquids. Eat or drink only what you feel you are able to without feeling discomfort.

2

Created: 01/2016

HOW TO PREPARE FOR YOUR OPERATION

Fig. 9.1 (continued)

Day 3 Through Discharge Day

- If you have been doing well, continue with your breathing exercises, short walks in the halls and controlling your pain. We are just waiting for your system to wake up before we send you home. We know your system is awake if you pass gas or have a bowel movement. This typically happens sometime between Day 2 and Day 4 but remember: everyone is different and these are only guidelines.

4

Created: 01/2016

HOW TO PREPARE FOR YOUR OPERATION

Fig. 9.1 (continued)

may include mechanical and antibiotic bowel preparation, carbohydrate loading/drinks, chlorhexidine shower, or wipes. For more specific recommendations, please refer to the chapters on enhanced recovery protocols (Chap. 7) in colorectal surgery and on bowel preparation (Chap. 8) in colorectal surgery.

Operative Setup, Pitfalls, and Troubleshooting

Local, Regional, and Epidural Anesthesia

Multimodal analgesia is an important part of postoperative recovery after laparoscopic colon and rectal surgery as minimizing the use of narcotics aids in intestinal recovery. Patients should be evaluated prior to surgery for any effective adjunct to their postoperative pain control which may help minimize the postoperative use of narcotics and thus facilitate a quicker return of bowel function.

Transversus abdominis plane (TAP) blocks are a mainstay of perioperative abdominal anesthesia. Local anesthetic is injected into the neurovascular plane between the transversus abdominis and the internal oblique. This effectively blocks T7-L1 innervation to the abdominal wall for up to the first 24 hours after surgery, depending on the type of local anesthetic used. This can be done during laparoscopic surgery under direct visualization, or it can be done preoperatively using ultrasound guidance by the surgeon or anesthesiologist. Studies comparing TAP block to local wound infiltration have demonstrated similar visual analog scale (VAS) pain scores during the first 24 hours, but they have also demonstrated a significant decrease in narcotic use during that same time period [42, 43], demonstrating that this can be a useful adjunct in aiding return of bowel function to expedite postoperative recovery.

There is extensive evidence that thoracic epidural anesthesia (TEA) decreases postoperative pain and narcotic use, expediting the recovery of bowel function in open surgery. The evidence for TEA usage in laparoscopic surgery is less conclusive. Several studies have examined the impact of epidural anesthesia on postoperative outcomes from laparoscopic colectomy and proctectomy. Most have shown that TEA leads to longer hospital stay, increased costs, and no decrease in postoperative ileus [44–46]. Pain score improvement versus conventional postoperative narcotic analgesia varies but generally is not better [44–46]. These studies do have several problems, however, as there is some heterogeneity as to which patients receive epidural narcotics as opposed to just local anesthetic as well as including a diverse group of surgeries. Many of the studies are also retrospective, and therefore the TEA patients tend to be the ones with more risk factors for postoperative complications. Patients being considered for laparoscopic procedures who have a high risk of conversion based on preoperative factors to open should be considered for TEA as this can be removed in the early postoperative period if the surgery stays minimally invasive.

Intravenous lidocaine infusions have been used as an adjunct both during anesthesia and postoperatively in the recovery and on the floor. Preliminary results of multiple studies have shown less postoperative pain, less narcotic use with earlier return of bowel function, and no adverse events [47, 48]. Patients need to be monitored, which can result in resistance in adaptation; however, cardiac complications such as arrhythmias and other adverse effects are rare. With a sound, data-driven protocol and team education, this can be easily employed.

Another option for patients undergoing laparoscopic colorectal surgery is adjunct spinal analgesia. This is a single preoperative injection of a combination of morphine and long-acting local anesthetic into the L3-L4 space. Although not studied extensively, this modality has been shown in limited studies to provide as much as 3 days of postoperative analgesia, generally decreasing narcotic requirements and pain scores, without affecting other postoperative outcome [49].

Prevention of Venous Thromboembolism

Venous thromboembolic events (VTE), which include deep vein thrombosis (DVT) and pulmonary embolism (PE), remain the most preventable cause of perioperative morbidity and mortality in hospitalized patients. Over 250,000 patients are diagnosed with DVT, and 50,000 patients are diagnosed with PE each year [50]. A quarter of patients with PE present with sudden death [51]. Colorectal surgical patients are at a four- to fivefold higher risk of PE relative to other general surgery patients. Rectal surgery places patients at higher risk of VTE due to extensive pelvic dissection, prolonged placement of patient in Trendelenburg position, and prolonged operative time. In addition, obesity, malignancy, and inflammatory bowel disease [52, 53] have a greater risk of VTE.

Current CHEST and SAGES guidelines for VTE prophylaxis for laparoscopic surgery stratify surgical patients into four categories of risk based on the Caprini Score (Table 9.4) [54–56]: very low (no risk factors), low (one to two points), moderate (three to four points), and high (five points and greater). Patients at moderate

Table 9.4 Caprini Score

One point	Two points	Three points	Four points
Age 41–60 years Swollen legs (current) Varicose veins BMI >25 Minor surgery Sepsis (within last month) Serious lung disease Oral contraceptives Pregnancy or postpartum <1 month History of stillborn infant, recurrent spontaneous abortion, premature birth Acute myocardial infarction History of inflammatory bowel disease History of prior major surgery (<1 month) Abnormal pulmonary function	Age 61–74 years Arthroscopic surgery Malignancy Laparoscopic surgery (>45 minutes) Patients confined to bed rest (>72 hours) Immobilizing plaster Cast (>1 month) Central venous access Major surgery (>45 minutes)	Age >75 years History of DVT/PE Factor V Leiden Elevated homocysteine Heparin-induced thrombocytopenia Elevated anticardiolipin Lupus anticoagulant Prothrombin 202110A Family history of thrombosis	Stroke (<1 month) Elective lower extremity arthroplasty Hip, pelvis, or leg fracture (<1 month) Acute spinal cord injury (<1 month) Multiple trauma (<1 month)

risk and greater require chemical and mechanical VTE prophylaxis. Chemical prophylaxis entails 5000 U of unfractionated heparin administered subcutaneously three times daily. Mechanical VTE prophylaxis entails use of graduated compression boots placed prior to anesthesia induction, and after induction, 5000 U of unfractionated heparin is administered subcutaneously.

Parenteral Antibiotics

The benefit of perioperative prophylactic parenteral antibiotic use has been well established. Current Surgical Care Improvement Project (SCIP) guidelines and SSI protocol bundles require administration of parenteral antibiotics within 1 hour of incision (preferably within 30 minutes) [57, 58]. Multiple antibiotic regimens (Box 9.4) are suitable for elective colorectal surgery. These regimens should be tailored to accommodate institutional variations of species sensitivities. All antibiotics should be re-dosed per protocols based on antibiotics and case length. Parenteral antibiotics may be continued postoperatively, but are generally not, and should be discontinued within 24 hours of operative end time.

Box 9.4 Antibiotic Prophylaxis for Elective Colon and Rectal Surgery

- Ampicillin-sulbactam
- Cefoxitin, cefotetan (second-generation cephalosporin with aerobic and anaerobic activity)
- Cefazolin plus metronidazole
- Ceftriaxone plus metronidazole (institutions with increased resistance to second-generation cephalosporins)
- Cefuroxime plus metronidazole
- Ertapenem
- Alternatives for patients with beta-lactam allergy:
  - Clindamycin or vancomycin plus aminoglycoside, aztreonam, or fluoroquinolone
  - Metronidazole plus aminoglycoside or fluoroquinolone
  - (Metronidazole should not be combined with aztreonam as this will have no aerobic gram-positive coverage)

Positioning

Careful patient positioning is critical to ensure that the surgeon and assistant have access to the anatomy and that dexterity is not limited by patient habitus. Careful positioning is also important in preventing pressure-related injuries during the procedure.

Lithotomy or split leg position should generally be used for patients undergoing pelvic procedures. This should be performed with the anus just past the lower break of the table. This is important because access to the anus is often part of critical steps during the procedure such as the placement of an EEA stapler or in performing flexible endoscopy. Lithotomy should be undertaken with padded Allen stirrups. The legs should be placed carefully, the pressure points should be padded, and the weight should be placed on the patient's heel and off of their calf to help prevent peroneal nerve injury or compartment syndrome. During the procedure, when the anus is not being accessed, it is often helpful to bring the legs down so the thighs are parallel to the floor. This will help prevent instrument limitation by the legs.

Both of the arms should be tucked during laparoscopic surgery. While this does limit the anesthesiologist's access to the arms, and their vascular access, it facilitates surgeon positioning and access during the case, especially for pelvic dissections. It is important to discuss this with the anesthesiologist prior to positioning so they have all access planned, which is required for the case. Pressure points, such as the elbows, and the hypothenar aspect of the hand should be carefully padded to prevent pressure injury prior to tucking.

Patients should be affixed to the bed in multiple points to prevent any slippage during surgery. Pelvic surgery often requires steep Trendelenburg positioning, and this may cause the patient's anus to slip above the bed break. Similarly in a total colectomy or flexure mobilization, the patient may go through extremes in positioning from Trendelenburg to reverse Trendelenburg and steep lateral positioning. In patients undergoing surgery in a supine position, it is helpful to place a strap across the thighs as well and the chest, taking care to avoid the patient's neck. In lithotomy position, the stirrups will serve as one point of fixation, and a chest strap should act as a second. We also recommend the use of fixation pads such as the Pink Pad™ (Xodus Medical, New Kensington, PA, USA). These devices are pads consisting of a high-friction foam which prevents patient slippage during extreme positioning.

Urinary Catheterization and Ureteral Stenting

Generally urinary catheters are placed preoperatively and removed within 12–24 hours of surgery. Catheters allow for decompression of the bladder, thus avoiding injury on trocar placement and allowing access/visualization in the pelvis. Catheters can often be avoided in brief procedures by having the patient void their bladder contents just prior to surgery.

In the setting of laparoscopic surgery, the surgeon is not afforded the opportunity to appreciate the ureters by palpation. Stents have not been shown to decrease rates of injury [59]. However, the use of preoperatively placed ureteral stents allows for the early identification and repair of ureteral injury [60, 61]. Stents are of particular benefit in the setting of prior pelvic surgery, inflammation, locally advanced cancers, or prior pelvic radiation. Any such circumstances can make pelvic dissection more difficult. Historically lighted stents have only been useful in the thinnest of patients as thick tissue has made it difficult to appreciate the luminescence. A newer technique which is more cost-effective which allows for better

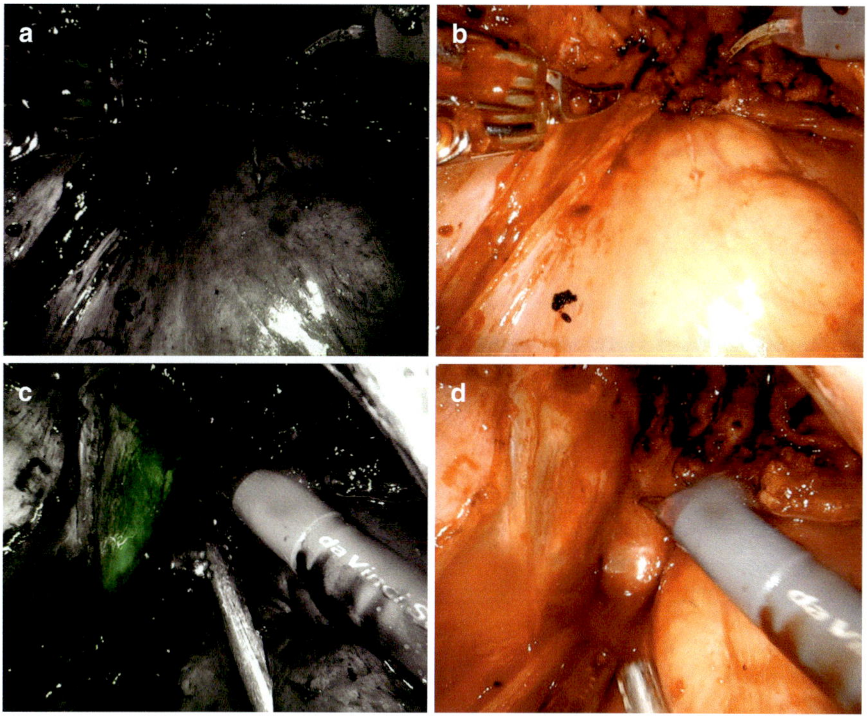

Fig. 9.2 (**a**–**d**) Ureteral stent with ICG

visualization is injecting indocyanine green (ICG), which fluoresces under infrared light (Fig. 9.2a–d). There are little data to date to demonstrate the efficacy of these technologies, however.

OR Setup and Equipment

Each team member has a specific role and responsibility in setting up the operating room and ensuring necessary equipment is available and functioning properly. The duties specific to the circulating nurse, scrub person, surgeon/surgery team, and anesthesiologist both prior to and after the patient enters the OR and after prepping and draping is outlined comprehensively in Fig. 9.3 [62].

Surgical Time-Out

The surgical time-out should consist of a verbal checklist of all the abovementioned factors to ensure they are all properly performed prior to incision. The WHO also has a checklist which is incorporated in many institution's time-out procedures (Fig. 9.4) [63].

MIS Safety Checklist

1. Pre-Patient Entry

A. Circulating Nurse Duties

Parameter	*Actions*
Surgeon Preference Card	☐ Reviewed
OR Table Position	☐ Correct orientation and weight capacity
	☐ Bean bag mattress (if indicated)
	☐ Table accessories (eg spreader bars/leg supports/foot board as indicated)
	☐ Positioned for fluoroscopy if indicated
Power sources	☐ Connected and linked to all devices
CO2 insufflator	☐ Check CO2 volume, pressure and flow
	☐ Backup cylinder and accessories (wrench and key) in place Filter for CO2 unit or tubing
Video monitors	☐ Position per procedure
	☐ Test pattern present
Suction/irrigation	☐ Cannister set
	☐ Irrigation and pressure bag available
Alarms	☐ Turned on and audible
Video documentation	☐ Recording media available and operational (DVD, print, etc.)

B. Scrub Person Duties

Parameter	*Actions*
Reusable instruments	☐ Check movement handles and jaws, all screws present
	☐ Check sealing caps
	☐ Instrument vents closed
	☐ Check cautery insulation
Veress needle	☐ Check plunger/spring action
	☐ Flush needle and stopcock Saline solution available
Hasson cannula	☐ Check valves, plunger, and seals
Trocars/Ports	☐ Check appropriate size/type
	☐ Close stopcocks
Laparoscope	☐ Size and type per preference
	☐ Check lens clarity
	☐ Anti-fog solution or warmed saline for lens cleaning

2. After Patient Entry

Parameter	*Actions*
Patient position	☐ Secured to OR table, safety strap on
	☐ Pressure sites padded
	☐ Arms out or tucked per procedure
Sequential compression device	☐ On and connected to device
Electrosurgical unit	☐ Ground pad applied
Foot controls	☐ Positioned for surgeon access
Power sources (camera, insufflator, light source, monitors, cautery, ultrasonics, bipolar)	☐ Turned on (on standby)
Miscellaneous	☐ Foley catheter (if indicated)
	☐ Naso- or orogastric tube (bougies if indicated)
Antibiotics	☐ Given as indicated

3. After Prep and Drape

Parameter	*Actions*
Electrosurgical unit	☐ Cautery cords connected to unit
Monopolar cautery	☐ Tip protected
Ultrasonic or bipolar device	☐ Connected to unit ☐ Activation test performed
Line connections	☐ Camera cord
	☐ Light source (on standby)
	☐ CO2 tubing (connected and flushed)
	☐ Suction/irrigation (suction turned on)
	☐ Smoke evacuation filter connected
Local anesthetic	☐ Syringe labeled and filled with anesthetic of choice needle connected
Fluoroscopy case	☐ Mix and dilute contrast appropriately and label
	☐ Clear tubing, syringe, catheter of air bubbles, label syringes

SAGES This checklist has been developed by SAGES and AORN to aid operating room personnel in the preparation of equipment and other duties unique to laparoscopic surgery cases. It should not supplant the surgical time out or other hospital-specific patient safety protocols. AORN

Fig. 9.3 SAGES/AORN MIS safety checklist. (Used with permission of the Society of American Gastrointestinal and Endoscopic Surgeons from: https://www.sages.org/wp-content/uploads/SAGES_AORN_MIS_Checklist.pdf)

Surgical Safety Checklist

World Health Organization | Patient Safety — A World Alliance for Safer Health Care

Before induction of anaesthesia → **Before skin incision** → **Before patient leaves operating room**

Before induction of anaesthesia

(with at least nurse and anaesthetist)

Has the patient confirmed his/her identity, site, procedure, and consent?
- ☐ Yes

Is the site marked?
- ☐ Yes
- ☐ Not applicable

Is the anaesthesia machine and medication check complete?
- ☐ Yes

Is the pulse oximeter on the patient and functioning?
- ☐ Yes

Does the patient have a:

Known allergy?
- ☐ No
- ☐ Yes

Difficult airway or aspiration risk?
- ☐ No
- ☐ Yes, and equipment/assistance available

Risk of >500ml blood loss (7ml/kg in children)?
- ☐ No
- ☐ Yes, and two IVs/central access and fluids planned

Before skin incision

(with nurse, anaesthetist and surgeon)

- ☐ **Confirm all team members have introduced themselves by name and role.**
- ☐ **Confirm the patient's name, procedure, and where the incision will be made.**

Has antibiotic prophylaxis been given within the last 60 minutes?
- ☐ Yes
- ☐ Not applicable

Anticipated Critical Events

To Surgeon:
- ☐ What are the critical or non-routine steps?
- ☐ How long will the case take?
- ☐ What is the anticipated blood loss?

To Anaesthetist:
- ☐ Are there any patient-specific concerns?

To Nursing Team:
- ☐ Has sterility (including indicator results) been confirmed?
- ☐ Are there equipment issues or any concerns?

Is essential imaging displayed?
- ☐ Yes
- ☐ Not applicable

Before patient leaves operating room

(with nurse, anaesthetist and surgeon)

Nurse Verbally Confirms:
- ☐ The name of the procedure
- ☐ Completion of instrument, sponge and needle counts
- ☐ Specimen labelling (read specimen labels aloud, including patient name)
- ☐ Whether there are any equipment problems to be addressed

To Surgeon, Anaesthetist and Nurse:
- ☐ What are the key concerns for recovery and management of this patient?

This checklist is not intended to be comprehensive. Additions and modifications to fit local practice are encouraged. Revised 1 / 2009 © WHO, 2009

Fig. 9.4 World Health Organization surgical safety checklist. (Used with permission of the World Health Organization: whqlibdoc.who.int/publications/2009/9789241598590_eng_Checklist.pdf)

Conclusion

Each team member plays a critical role in preoperative preparation for laparoscopic colorectal surgery. Careful preoperative prevention and planning along with patient education and preoperative preparation in the operating room result in successful laparoscopic colon and rectal surgery.

References

1. American Society of Anesthesiologists. Schaumburg. Available from: https://www.asahq.org/standards-and-guidelines/asa-physical-status-classification-system.
2. Smith RK, Broach R, Traci H, Mahmoud NN, Paulson EC. Impact of BMI on postoperative outcomes in patients undergoing proctectomy for rectal cancer: A National Surgical Quality Improvement Program analysis. Dis Colon Rectum. 2014;57:687–93.
3. van Vugt JLA, Cakir H, Kornmann VNN, Doodeman HJ, Stoot JH, Boerma D, et al. The new body mass index as a predictor of postoperative complications in elective colorectal cancer surgery. Clin Nut. 2015;34(4):700–40.
4. Odonkor PN, Grigore AM. Patients with ischemic heart disease. Med Clin N Am. 2013;97:1033–50.
5. Fleisher LA, Bechman JA, Brown KA, Calkins H, Chaikof E, Fleischmann KE, et al. ACC/AHA 2007 guidelines on perioperative cardiovascular evaluation and care for noncardiac surgery: executive summary. JACC. 2007;50:1707–32.
6. Lee TH, Marcantonio ER, Mangione CM, Thomas EJ, Polanczyk CA, Cook EF, et al. Circulation. 1999;100:1043–9.
7. Gupta S, Gupta H, Sundaram A, Kaushik M, Fang X, Miller WJ, et al. Development and validation of a risk calculator for prediction of cardiac risk after surgery. Circulation. 2011;124:381–7.
8. Markel TA, Lou DC, Pfefferkorn M, Scherer LR 3rd, West K, Rouse T, et al. Steroids and poor nutrition are associated with infectious wound complications in children undergoing first stage procedures for ulcerative colitis. Surgery. 2008;144:540–5.
9. Fleshner P, Ippoliti A, Dubinsky M, Ognibene S, Vasiliauskas E, Chelly M, et al. A prospective multivariate analysis of clinical factors associated with pouchitis after ileal pouch-anal anastomosis. Clin Gastroenterol Hepatol. 2007;5:952–8.
10. Lim M, Sagar P, Abdulgader A, Thekkinkattil D, Burke D. The impact of preoperative immunomodulation on pouch-related septic complications after ileal pouch-anal anastomosis. Dis Colon Rectum. 2007;50:943–51.
11. Lake JP, Firoozmand E, Kang JC, Vassiliu P, Chan LS, Vukasin P, et al. Effect of high-dose steroids on anastomotic complications after proctocolectomy with ileal pouch anal anastomosis. J Gastrointest Surg. 2004;8:547–51.
12. Ziv Y, Church JM, Fazio VW, King TM, Lavery IC. Effect of systemic steroids on ileal pouch-anal anastomosis in patients with ulcerative colitis. Dis Colon Rectum. 1996;39:504–8.
13. Kelly KN, Domajnko B. Perioperative stress-dose steroids. Clin Colon and Rectal Surg. 2013;26:163–7.
14. Zaghiyan K, Melmed GY, Berel D, Ovsepyan G, Murrell Z, Fleshner P. A prospective, randomized, noninferiority trial of steroid dosing after major colorectal surgery. Ann Surg. 2014;259:32–7.
15. Mahadevan U, Loftus EV Jr, Tremaine WJ, Pemberton JH, Harmsen WS, Schleck CD, et al. Azathioprine or 6-mercaptopurine before colectomy for ulcerative colitis is not associated with increased postoperative complications. Inflamm Bowel Dis. 2002;8:311–6.

16. Huang W, Tang Y, Nong L, Sun Y. Risk factors for postoperative intra-abdominal septic complications after surgery in Crohn's disease: a meta-analysis of observational studies. J Crohns Colitis. 2015;9:293–301.
17. Selvaggi F, Pellino G, Canonico S, Sciaudone G. Effect of preoperative biologic drugs on complications and function after restorative proctocolectomy with primary ileal pouch formation: systematic review and meta-analysis. Inflamm Bowel Dis. 2015;21(1):79–92.
18. Mor IJ, Vogel JD, da Luz Moreira A, Shen B, Hammel J, Remzi FH. Infliximab in ulcerative colitis is associated with an increased risk of postoperative complications after restorative proctocolectomy. Dis Colon Rectum. 2008;51:1202–10.
19. Coquet-Reinier B, Berdah SV, Grimaud JC, Birnbaum D, Cougard PA, Barthet M, et al. Preoperative infliximab treatment and postoperative complications after laparoscopic restorative proctocolectomy with ileal pouch-anal anastomosis: a case-matched study. Surg Endosc. 2010;24:1866–71.
20. Narula N, Charleton D, Marshall JK. Meta-analysis: peri-operative anti-TNFα treatment and post-operative complications in patients with inflammatory bowel disease. Aliment Pharmacol Ther. 2013;37:1057–64.
21. Nørgård BM, Nielsen J, Qvist N, Gradel KO, de Muckadell OB, Kjeldsen J. Pre-operative use of anti-TNF-α agents and the risk of post-operative complications in patients with ulcerative colitis – a nationwide cohort study. Aliment Pharmacol Ther. 2012;35:1301–9.
22. Lau C, Dubinsky M, Melmed G, Vasiliauskas E, Berel D, McGovern D, et al. The impact of preoperative serum anti-TNFα therapy levels on early postoperative outcomes in inflammatory bowel disease surgery. Ann Surg. 2015;261:487–96.
23. Hawn MT, Houston TK, Campagna EJ, Graham LA, Singh J, Bishop M, et al. The attributable risk of smoking on surgical complications. Ann Surg. 2011;254:914–20.
24. Sorensen LT. Wound healing and infection in surgery: the pathophysiological impact of smoking, smoking cessation, and nicotine replacement therapy: a systematic review. Ann Surg. 2012;255:1069–79.
25. Sorensen LT. Wound healing and infection in surgery. The clinical impact of smoking and smoking cessation: a systematic review and meta-analysis. Arch Surg. 2012;147:373–83.
26. Lumb AB. Pre-operative respiratory optimisation: an expert review. Anaesthesia. 2019;74 Suppl 1:43–8.
27. Anthenelli RM, Benowitz NL, West R, St Aubin L, McRae T, Lawrence D, et al. Neuropsychiatric safety and efficacy of varenicline, bupropion, and nicotine patch in smokers with and without psychiatric disorders (EAGLES): a double-blind, randomised, placebo-controlled clinical trial. Lancet. 2016;387:2507–20.
28. Hu WH, Cajas-Monson L, Eisenstein S, Parry L, Cosman B, Ramamoorthy S. Preoperative malnutrition assessments as predictors of postoperative mortality and morbidity in colorectal cancer: an analysis of ACS-NSQIP. Nutr J. 2015;14:91.
29. van Rooijen S, Carli F, Dalton S, Thomas G, Bojesen R, Le Guen M, et al. Multimodal prehabilitation in colorectal cancer patients to improve functional capacity and reduce postoperative complications: the first international randomized controlled trial for multimodal prehabilitation. BMC Cancer. 2019;19:98.
30. Brennan GT, Ha I, Hogan C, Nguyen E, Jamal MM, Bechtold ML, et al. Does preoperative enteral or parenteral nutrition reduce postoperative complications in Crohn's disease patients: a meta-analysis. Eur J Gastroenterol Hepatol. 2018;30:997–1002.
31. Calder PC. Immunonutrition. BMJ. 2003;327:117–8.
32. Probst P, Ohmann S, Klaiber U, Hüttner FJ, Billeter AT, Ulrich A, et al. Meta-analysis of immunonutrition in major abdominal surgery. Br J Surg. 2017;104:1594–608.
33. Wahl TS, Patel FC, Goss LE, Chu DI, Grams J, Morris MS. The obese colorectal surgery patient: surgical site infection and outcomes. Dis Colon Rectum. 2018;61:938–45.
34. Hill C, Khashab MA, Kalloo AN, Kumbhari V. Endoluminal weight loss and metabolic therapies: current and future techniques. Ann N Y Acad Sci. 2018;1411:36–52.
35. Faria SL, Faria OP, de Almeida Cardeal M, Ito MK. Effects of a very low calorie diet in the preoperative stage of bariatric surgery: a randomized trial. Surg Obes Relat Dis. 2015;11:230–7.

36. Yolsuriyanwong K, Thanavachirasin K, Sasso K, Zuro L, Bartfield J, Marcotte E, et al. Effectiveness, compliance, and acceptability of preoperative weight loss with a liquid very low-calorie diet before bariatric surgery in real practice. Obes Surg. 2019;29:54–60.
37. Aquina CT, Rickles AS, Probst CP, Kelly KN, Deeb AP, Monson JR, et al. Visceral obesity, not elevated BMI, is strongly associated with incisional hernia after colorectal surgery. Dis Colon Rectum. 2015;58:220–7.
38. Sirany AM, Chow CJ, Kunitake H, Madoff RD, Rothenberger DA, Kwaan MR. Colorectal surgery outcomes in chronic dialysis patients: an American College of Surgeons National Surgical Quality Improvement Program Study. Dis Colon Rectum. 2016;59:662–9.
39. Deng J, Lenart J, Applegate RL. General anesthesia soon after dialysis may increase postoperative hypotension – a pilot study. Heart Lung Vessel. 2014;6:52–9.
40. Currie A, Malietzis G, Askari A, Nachiappan S, Swift P, Jenkins JT, et al. Impact of chronic kidney disease on postoperative outcome following colorectal cancer surgery. Color Dis. 2014;16:879–85.
41. Cavallaro PM, Milch H, Savitt L, Hodin RA, Rattner DW, Berger DL, et al. Addition of a scripted pre-operative patient education module to an existing ERAS pathway further reduces length of stay. Am J Surg. 2018;216(4):652–7.
42. Park JS, Choi GS, Kwak KH, Jung H, Jeon Y, Park S, et al. Effect of local wound infiltration and transversus abdominis plane block on morphine use after laparoscopic colectomy: a nonrandomized, single-blind prospective study. J Surg Res. 2015;195:61–6.
43. Abdallah FW, Chan VW, Brull R. Transversus abdominis plane block: a systematic review. Reg Anesth Pain Med. 2012;37:193–209.
44. Courtot L, Le Roy B, Memeo R, Voron T, de Angelis N, Tabchouri N, et al. Risk factors for postoperative ileus following elective laparoscopic right colectomy: a retrospective multicentric study. Int J Color Dis. 2018;33:1373–82.
45. Halabi WJ, Kang CY, Nguyen VQ, Carmichael JC, Mills S, Stamos MJ, et al. Epidural analgesia in laparoscopic colorectal surgery: a nationwide analysis of use and outcomes. JAMA Surg. 2014;149:130–6.
46. Borzellino G, Francis NK, Chapuis O, Krastinova E, Dyevre V, Genna M. Role of epidural analgesia within an ERAS program after laparoscopic colorectal surgery: a review and meta-analysis of randomised controlled studies. Surg Res Pract. 2016;2016:7543684.
47. Ventham NT, Kennedy ED, Brady RR, Paterson HM, Speake D, Foo I, et al. Efficacy of intravenous lidocaine for postoperative analgesia following laparoscopic surgery: a meta-analysis. World J Surg. 2015;39:2220–34.
48. Herroeder S, Pecher S, Schönherr ME, Kaulitz G, Hahnenkamp K, Friess H, et al. Systemic lidocaine shortens length of hospital stay after colorectal surgery: a double-blinded, randomized, placebo-controlled trial. Ann Surg. 2007;246:192–200.
49. Day AR, Smith RV, Scott MJ, Fawcett WJ, Rockall TA. Randomized clinical trial investigating the stress response from two different methods of analgesia after laparoscopic colorectal surgery. Br J Surg. 2015;102:1473–9.
50. McNally MP, Burns CJ. Venous thromboembolic disease in colorectal patients. Clin Colon Rectal Surg. 2009;22:34–40.
51. Bergqvist D. Venous thromboembolism: a review of risk and prevention in colorectal surgery patients. Dis Colon Rectum. 2006;49:1620–8.
52. Buchberg B, Masoomi H, Lusby K, Choi J, Barleben A, Magno C, et al. Incidence and risk factors of venous thromboembolism in colorectal surgery. Arch Surg. 2011;146:739–43.
53. Gross ME, Vogler SA, Mone MC, Sheng X, Sklow B. Postoperative venous thromboembolism prophylaxis in IBD: a National Surgical Quality Improvement Program analysis. Dis Colon Rectum. 2014;57:482–9.
54. Bahl V, Hu HM, Henke P, Wakefield TW, Campbell DA Jr, Caprini JA. A validation study of retrospective venous thromboembolism risk scoring method. Ann Surg. 2010;251:344–50.
55. Pollak AW, McBane RD. Succinct review of the new VTE prevention and management guidelines. Mayo Clinic Proc. 2014;89:394–408.

56. Richardson WS, Hamad GG, Stefanidis D. VTE prophylaxis for laparoscopic surgery guidelines: an update [Internet] 2017. Available from: https://www.sages.org/publications/guidelines/guidelines-for-deep-venous-thrombosis-prophylaxis-during-laparoscopic-surgery/.
57. National Guideline Clearinghouse. Rockville. Available from: http://www.guideline.gov/content.aspx?id=39533.
58. Bratzler DW, Dellinger EP, Olsen KM, Perl TM, Auwaerter PG, Bolon MK, et al. Clinical practice guidelines for antimicrobial prophylaxis in surgery. Am J Health Syst Pharm. 2013;70:195–283.
59. Leff EI, Groff W, Rubin RJ, Eisenstat TE, Salvati EP. Use of ureteral catheters in colonic and rectal surgery. Dis Colon Rectum. 1982;25:457–60.
60. Nam YS, Wexner SD. Clinical value of prophylactic ureteral stent indwelling during laparoscopic colorectal surgery. J Korean Med Sci. 2002;17:633–5.
61. Tsukinaka S, Wexner SD, DaSilva G. Prophylactic ureteric catheters in laparoscopic colorectal surgery. Tech Coloproctol. 2008;12:45–50.
62. MIS Safety Checklist [Internet]. Available from: https://www.sages.org/wp-content/uploads/SAGES_AORN_MIS_Checklist.pdf.
63. Surgical Safety Checklist [Internet]. Available from: whqlibdoc.who.int/publications/2009/9789241598590_eng_Checklist.pdf.

Essentials on Troubleshooting During Laparoscopic Colorectal Surgery

10

Alexander T. Hawkins and Craig H. Olson

Introduction

Laparoscopic surgery involves a complex interplay between the surgeon, technology, and the patient. For a case to go well and the patient to have a successful outcome, all aspects of the procedure must be carefully coordinated. However, this is not always the case, and the laparoscopic surgeon needs to have the knowledge and skills to correct things when an operation is deviating from the intended plan. This chapter presents a number of potential issues with laparoscopic surgery – including port placement, equipment, patient physiology, exposure, and inadvertent injury – as well as methods to rescue successful surgery.

Preoperative Preparation

Troubleshooting should begin even before the patient enters the operating room. It is important to engage in early discussion with the anesthesia team, circulating nurse, and scrub technician prior to the procedure. Items for discussion include patient positioning as well as the need to change positions, e.g., flipping prone for an abdominal perineal resection. For robotic surgery, thought must be given to where the robot will dock, along with where the assistants will stand. The appropriate table needs to be in the room, along with any other positioning equipment such as a footboard, beanbag, or straps. The proper case carts, equipment, supplies, and instruments should be in the rooms and checked to make sure they are operational. This particularly applies to

A. T. Hawkins
Vanderbilt University Medical Center, Department of General Surgery, Nashville, TN, USA
e-mail: Alex.hawkins@vumc.org

C. H. Olson (✉)
Clements University Hospital, University of Texas Southwestern, Dallas, TX, USA
e-mail: Craig.olson@utsouthwestern.edu

P. Sylla et al. (eds.), *The SAGES Manual of Colorectal Surgery*,
https://doi.org/10.1007/978-3-030-24812-3_10

the laparoscopic tower and its gas supply. Energy devices, such as the electrosurgical unit, should be inspected. Connections should be checked, settings confirmed and integrity of protective sheets on bipolar/monopolar devices closely inspected. If fluoroscopy is needed, the table must be radiolucent, and proper shielding equipment should be available for all members of the team.

Once the patient enters the room and is placed under general anesthesia, a Foley catheter and orogastric tube should be placed. Prior to any incision, a hard stop time-out should be conducted to confirm the patient's identity, procedure, medication administration, and any anticipated difficulties [1, 2].

Laparoscopic Access

Choice of Entry Technique

The establishment of pneumoperitoneum and initial port placement is one of the most critical parts of a laparoscopic procedure. Three main options exist for laparoscopic entry: an open (Hasson), closed (Veress), and optical port technique. The bulk of data that exists focuses on comparing the first two techniques. A recent meta-analysis concluded that there is insufficient evidence to recommend one laparoscopic entry technique over another. An open-entry technique is associated with a reduction in failed entry when compared to a closed-entry technique, with no evidence of a difference in the incidence of visceral or vascular injury. An advantage of direct trocar entry over Veress needle entry was noted for failed entry and vascular injury. They found that the evidence was generally of very low quality with small numbers of participants in most studies and that the findings should be interpreted with caution [3]. Further retrospective reviews suggest a trend toward reduction of the risk of major complications with either open access techniques or an optical port technique [4]. In terms of injury patterns for closed or Veress technique, 38 selected articles including 696,502 laparoscopic procedure cumulatively reported 1575 injuries (0.23%), 126 (8%) of which involving blood vessels or hollow viscera (0.018% of all laparoscopies). Of the 98 vascular injuries, 8 (8.1%) were injuries to major retroperitoneal vessels. There were 34 other reported retroperitoneal injuries, but the authors were not specific as to which vessel was injured. Of the 28 injuries to hollow viscera, 17 were considered major injuries, i.e., 60.7% (0.0024% of the total cases assessed) [5]. In the absence of definitive data to recommend one technique over another, surgeons are encouraged to employ whichever entry technique they are most comfortable with.

Special Considerations

For patients who have undergone previous abdominal surgery, either MIS or open, laparoscopic entry is still possible but requires some additional planning. Attempts should be made to establish access at a site remove from previous surgery and suspected adhesions. No one technique has demonstrated superiority in reoperative access. Basic principles include avoiding previous scars, a low threshold to modify the approach technique if initial attempts fail, and close inspection of the area once pneumoperitoneum is gained [6].

Laparoscopic entry in the obese patient can be significantly more difficult given the amount of subcutaneous tissues and the subsequent increase in distance between skin and fascia. To begin, larger Veress needles or Hasson trocars are necessary. Anatomically, obesity modifies the relationship of the umbilicus to the aortic bifurcation. Utilizing computed tomography, Hurd and colleagues demonstrated that the umbilicus migrates caudally in relation to the aortic bifurcation as the BMI increases [7]. Because of this, recommendations are for a 90° angle of insertion of the Veress needle. In terms of technique, Pasic and colleagues retrospectively analyzed outcomes in separate cohorts of obese and nonobese patients, focusing on multiple-entry approaches. The only group that demonstrated a significantly higher failure rate for obese patients was the open approach. Ultimately, the authors recommended using the Veress needle in the left upper quadrant for obese patients [8]. Despite these conclusions, we advocate whatever approach the surgeons feel most comfortable using while acknowledging the challenges that the obese patient poses.

Pitfalls and Troubleshooting

Complicated Peritoneal Entry

For the closed or Veress approach for abdominal access, inability to establish pneumoperitoneum will be noted by low pressure and high flow on the insufflator. Initial attempts may be tried at the same position, but if multiple attempts are unsuccessful, another site should be used. Palmer's point, at two fingerbreadths below the costal margin in the left midaxillary line, is usually a safe position unless previous surgery has taken place in the left upper quadrant (Fig. 10.1). If multiple attempts are unsuccessful, another entry technique should be used. If bile, enteric contents, or blood returns at placement of the Veress needle, the needle should be left in place, and alternative access gained immediately. The alternative access may be laparoscopic if it is safe to do so. If the bleeding is significant or if hypotension is noted, open laparotomy is required.

Regardless of the technique chosen for entry, the first step following port placement should be a visual inspection of the abdomen for injury. This can include the obvious, such as bleeding or enteric contents or the subtle, such as a retroperitoneal hematoma or hollow viscus injury. Any failed entry site should be inspected to assess for any associated injury. Hollow viscus injury may be repaired with oversewing as appropriate. Small bleeding can be controlled with an energy device. Larger bleeding may require vascular repair, and early consultation from a vascular surgeon is recommended. Bladder injury may require closure in layers and use of a Foley catheter for decompression for an extended period postoperatively. Urology consultation is recommended.

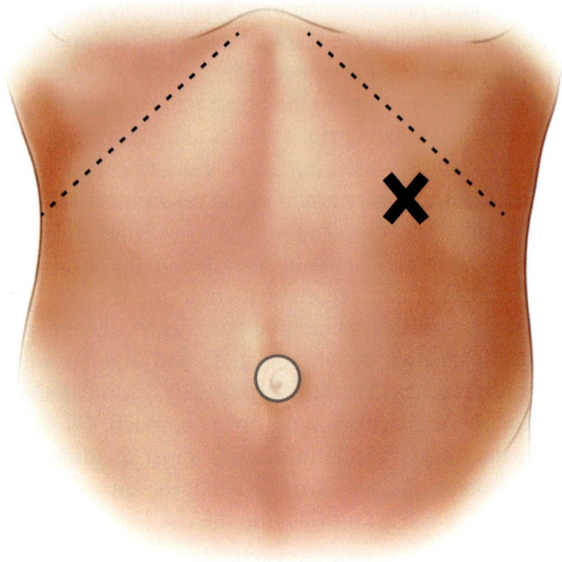

Fig. 10.1 Palmer's point: two fingerbreadths below the left costal margin in the midaxillary line

Laparoscopic entry can cause injury to vessels of the abdominal wall. Access sites are carefully chosen to avoid major vessels. Abdominal wall bleeding may not be immediately apparent until after the port is removed because the port may tamponade muscular or subcutaneous bleeding. In addition to visually inspecting the access site upon its creation, all laparoscopic port sites should also be observed during and following port removal. Bleeding points can usually be identified and managed with electrocautery or sutures as necessary. If bleeding persists, a Foley catheter may be inserted, inflated, and pulled back against the abdominal wall to tamponade the site. U-stitches can then be placed into the abdominal wall under direct laparoscopic visualization using a suture passer with absorbable braided suture. With uncontrolled bleeding, the skin incision may need to be enlarged to control the bleeding. Both proximal and distal to the injured portion of the vessel must be sutured.

Equipment Issues

Once pneumoperitoneum has been established and ports are placed, there are a few potential issues that can take place with any laparoscopy equipment. Major issues include low pressure, high pressure, problems with lighting, and problems with the picture. Troubleshooting tips are summarized in Table 10.1. A couple of issues will be highlighted here in the text.

Low pressure can be due to several etiologies. First, check that the CO_2 tank is full and that all lines and stopcocks are open or closed as appropriate. Next, check to make sure the ports are not leaking. If a port leaks during surgery, it can be due to the fascial defect being too large or excessive port angulation. Leaks can also be decreased with additional sutures or the placement of a towel clamp to cinch the

Table 10.1 Troubleshooting guide

Problem	Cause	Solution
Poor insufflation/loss of pneumoperitoneum	CO_2 tank empty	Change tank
	Accessory port stopcock(s) not properly adjusted	Inspect all accessory ports. Open or close stopcock(s) as needed
	Leak in sealing cap or stopcock	Change cap or cannula
	Excessive suctioning	Allow time to reinsufflate
	Loose connection of insufflator tubing at source or at port	Tighten connections
	Hasson stay sutures loose	Replace or secure sutures
	Tubing disconnection from insufflator	Connect tubing
	Flow rate set too low	Adjust flow rate
Excessive pressure required for insufflation (initial or subsequent)	Veress needle or cannula tip not in free peritoneal cavity	Reinsert needle or cannula
	Occlusion of tubing (kinking, table joints, etc.)	Inspect full length of tubing. Replace with proper size as necessary
	Port stopcock turned off	Fully open stopcock
	Patient is "light"	Give more muscle relaxant
	Cannula tip not in peritoneal space	Advance cannula under visual control
Inadequate lighting (partial/complete loss)	Loose connection at source or scope	Adjust connector
	Light is on "manual-minimum"	Go to "automatic"
	Bulb is burned out	Replace bulb
	Fiber optics are damaged	Replace light cable
	Automatic iris adjusting to bright reflection from instrument	Reposition instruments or switch to "manual"
	Monitor brightness turned down	Readjust setting
	Room brightness floods monitors	Dim room lights
Lighting too bright	Light is on "manual-maximum"	Go to "automatic"
	"Boost" on light source is activated	Deactivate "boost"
	Monitor brightness turned up	Readjust setting

(continued)

Table 10.1 (continued)

Problem	Cause	Solution
No picture on monitor(s)	Camera control or other components (printer, light source, monitor) not "on"	Make sure all power sources are plugged in and turned on
	Cable connector between camera control unit and/or monitors not attached properly	Cable should run from "video out" on camera control unit to "video in" on primary monitor. Use compatible cables for camera unit and light source
	Cable between monitors not connected	Cable should run from "video out" on primary monitor to "video in" on secondary monitor
	Input select button on monitor doesn't match "video in" choice	Assure matching selections
Poor picture quality		
Fogging/haze	Condensation on lens from cold scope entering warm abdomen	Gently wipe lens on viscera; use antifog solution or warm water
	Condensation on scope eyepiece, camera lens, coupler lens	Detach camera from scope (or camera from coupler), and inspect and clean lens as needed
Flickering electrical interference	Moisture in camera cable connecting plug	Use suction or compressed air to dry out moisture (don't use cotton tip applicators on multipronged plug)
	Poor cable shielding	Move electrosurgical unit to different circuit or away from video equipment
	Insecure connection of video cable between monitors	Reattach video cable at each monitor
Blurring, distortion	Incorrect focus	Adjust camera focus ring
	Cracked lens, internal moisture	Inspect scope/camera, and replace if needed
	Too grainy	Adjust enhancement and/or grain settings for units with this option

Adapted with the permission of the Society of American Gastrointestinal and Endoscopic Surgeons. From: SAGES Laparoscopy Troubleshooting Guide https://www.sages.org/wp-content/uploads/troubleshootingchart.pd

tissue closed around the trocar. Petrolatum-coated gauze may also be used to reduce the flow of any air leak. If available, balloon-tipped trocars can be used to eliminate a leak.

High pressure can result from several factors. Begin by inspecting insufflation tubing and stopcocks and that the insufflator is set on the correct pressure. High pressure can also be a result of the patient being inadequately paralyzed. Discussion with anesthesia regarding redosing of muscle relaxant is appropriate.

Investigation of poor lighting begins with tracing the light cord back to the light source and ensuring an appropriate connection. The light source itself should be checked and make sure the bulb is lit. The laparoscope should be cleaned to remove any material that may block the light. Finally, consider replacing the light cord as the fiber-optic cables can crack over time.

Troubleshooting an inadequate picture on the monitor involves a number of steps. As with the above issues, first start by tracing the camera cord and ensuring all cables are plugged in to the appropriate sites. The camera connection with the laparoscope should be examined and made sure it is tight. The laparoscope should be cleaned of any debris. If these measures fail, first replace the camera and then the laparoscopic tower.

Should any of these measures fail to fix the problem, the local representative of the laparoscopic equipment should be contacted for assistance.

Physiologic Issues

Laparoscopic surgery utilizes gas (usually CO_2) to insufflate the abdominal cavity to supernormal intra-abdominal pressures. The elevated intra-abdominal pressure, along with patient positioning and carbon dioxide absorption, can cause changes in physiology, especially in the respiratory and cardiovascular system. In most instances, the body can adapt to these changes without significant issues. But in certain scenarios, physiologic changes may become life threatening.

Nodal rhythm, sinus bradycardia, and asystole can all result from stretching of the peritoneum. Such effects usually take place at the beginning of insufflation because of the rapid stretching of the peritoneum. Should any arrhythmias be noted, immediate communication between the anesthesia and surgery team should take place. The abdomen should be desufflated as quickly as possible, and pharmacologic correction of the arrhythmia should be initiated.

The most frequently used gas for insufflation is CO_2. It is colorless, nontoxic, and nonflammable and has the greatest margin of safety in the event of a venous embolus as it is highly soluble. As it is readily absorbed from the peritoneum, it can cause an increase in $PaCO_2$. This has direct, as well as indirect (by raising catecholamine levels), effects on the cardiovascular system. Tachycardia, increased cardiac contractility, and reduction in diastolic filling can result in decreased myocardial oxygen supply to demand ratio and greater risk of myocardial ischemia. Constant monitoring of the ECG rhythm strip for signs of ischemia is essential. Any evidence of ischemia should be communicated, and the abdomen should be desufflated promptly.

If CO_2 is insufflated directly into a blood vessel or if gas is drawn into an open vessel by the Venturi effect, venous gas embolism can occur. This is a rare but potentially fatal occurrence. The physiologic effects of carbon dioxide are less than that with air because of the greater blood solubility. The clinical signs of a venous gas embolus begin with an abrupt decrease in the end-tidal CO_2 levels and are accompanied by hypotension and desaturation. A "mill wheel" murmur may be auscultated on physical exam. A transesophageal echocardiogram is usually required to evaluate the embolism. Treatment includes rapid deflation of the abdomen placement of the patient in the left lateral Trendelenburg position and resuscitation. If severe, the gas can be aspirated with a central line.

Optimizing Laparoscopic Exposure

OR Table Positioning

Obtaining proper exposure is one of the key elements to successful completion of any surgical procedure. As opposed to open surgery, where retractors can be easily placed, laparoscopic surgery presents more of a challenge. Gravity remains the greatest retractor available to the laparoscopic surgeon, and its use requires safe manipulation of the operating table to achieve exposure of the intended operative field. Mobilization of the splenic flexure can be aided by placing the patient in reverse Trendelenburg; rectal surgery is aided by placing the patient in Trendelenburg. Additional exposure can be provided by rotating the operative bed to the right or the left. Beyond gravity, additional ports and intraperitoneal retractors can be helpful as well. Position changes and additional retractors all introduce new complexities to the operation and provide opportunities for complications. Appropriate foreknowledge of these pitfalls can help to avoid them.

Trendelenburg exposure, or placement of the patient in the supine position, with the feet elevated above the head with the bed placed at an incline relative to the floor, is essential in pelvic laparoscopy (Fig. 10.2a, b). This position allows the intestine and peritoneal organs to fall upward toward the chest, providing a clear view of the pelvis. This introduces many challenges, both operative and anesthetic. From a very basic point of view, the patient must be securely placed on the operating table. Patient movement on the operative table can lead to surgical injuries, positioning injuries including neuropathies, and, in the extreme case, trauma from an unexpected fall. Physiologic risks of the Trendelenburg position include lower extremity compartment syndromes, increase in intraocular pressure, decrease in cerebral oxygenation, and a reduction in pulmonary compliance.

Nerve injury is the most common injury associated with the Trendelenburg position. In one series, brachial plexus injuries were seen in 6.6% of patients undergoing robotic urologic surgery [9]. Factors that contributed to neuropathies included arm positioning (patients with their arms tucked at the sides had half the rate of neuropathic injury compared to those with their arms extended) as well as length of operation. There are also reports of brachial plexus injuries resulting from the use of shoulder braces as well as wristlets intended to prevent the patient from sliding cephalad [10]. For this reason, it is recommended that the patient be secured to the bed with cross-chest straps, with arms at the side and thumbs pointing upward (Fig. 10.3). Other commercially available Trendelenburg positioning systems accomplish this through the use of a viscoelastic foam pad combined with a cross-chest hook and loop fastener.

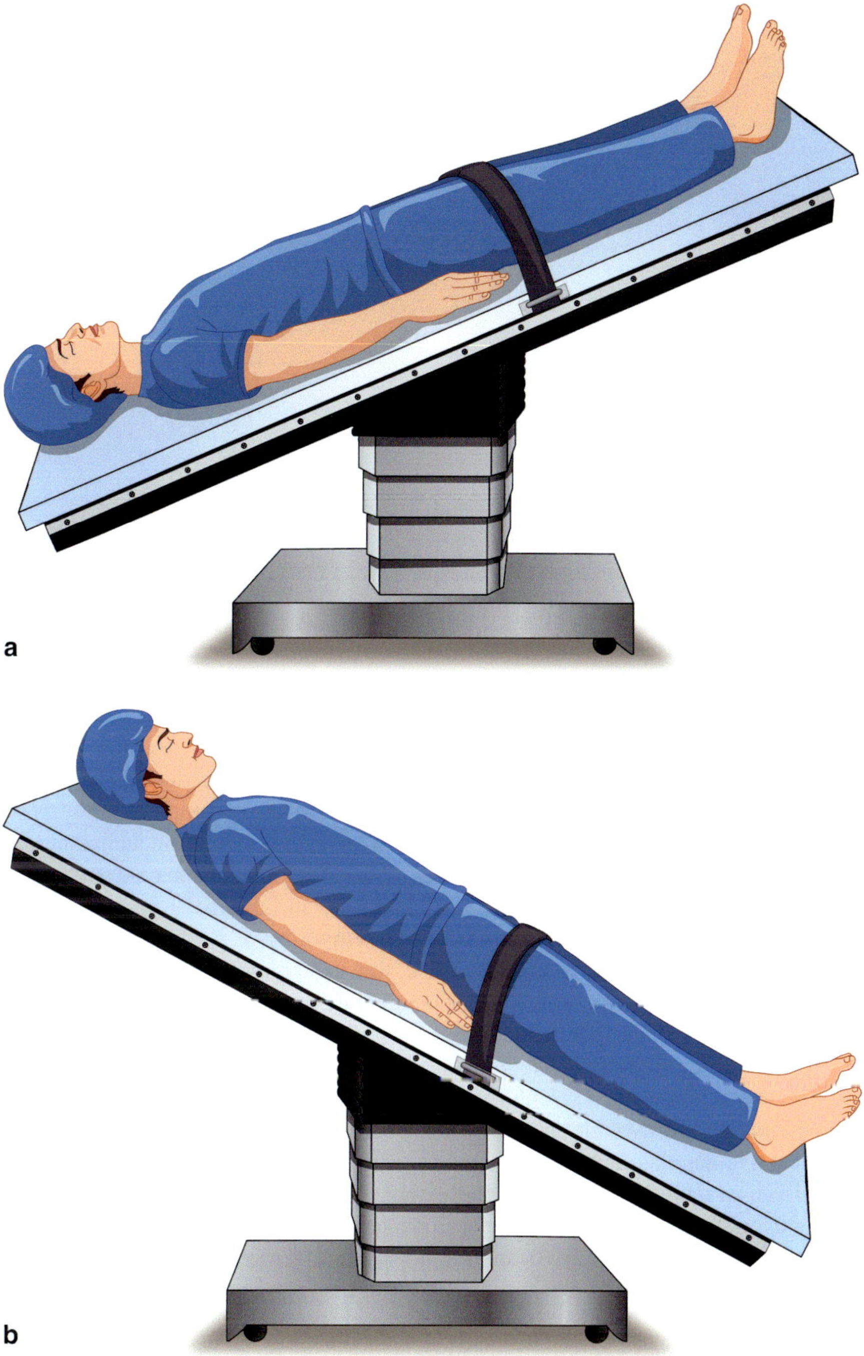

Fig. 10.2 (**a**, **b**) **a** Represents Trendelenburg positioning, while **b** represents reverse Trendelenburg

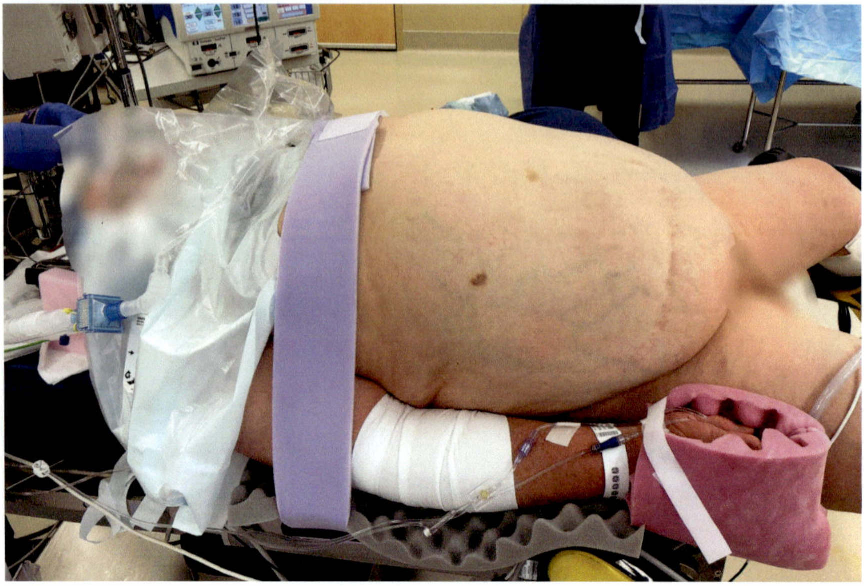

Fig. 10.3 The patient is positioned on a nonslip pad with arms tucked at side and fingers up to reduce risk of brachial plexus injury during Trendelenburg positioning

Physiologic changes associated with the Trendelenburg position can also create challenges. Most frequently, problems with oxygenation can be seen given the reduction in pulmonary compliance. This is best addressed by reducing the degree of Trendelenburg if possible. Other strategies include insuring complete paralysis of the patient, increasing peak airway pressure, and negative ventilation techniques. It is good practice to reevaluate the need for extreme angles during the case and lessen the degree of Trendelenburg if necessary. Increases in intraocular pressure occur and can lead to optic nerve injury resulting in temporary or permanent blindness. Patients with glaucoma are at increased risk; this can be mitigated through the use of appropriate ophthalmic medications and reducing the degree and length of Trendelenburg as much as possible [11]. Lower extremity compartment syndromes leading to fasciotomies and rhabdomyolysis have been reported as well and have been reviewed in the past [12]. Guidance provided by the authors suggests the risk can be mitigated by avoiding pressure on the calves in the lithotomy stirrup, avoiding excessive angulation of the hips and avoiding raising the legs as much as possible. Even an increase in intracranial pressure with a resultant decrease in cerebral oxygenation occurs with Trendelenburg positioning; however, the clinical significance remains uncertain [13]. As an overarching theme, minimizing the degree and length of Trendelenburg as much as possible will help to avoid these complications. In long cases, it may be advisable to intermittently return the patient to the supine position for a few minutes prior to reassuming the Trendelenburg position and continuing the operation.

Reverse Trendelenburg positioning has utility in colorectal surgery. In this position, the viscera fall into the pelvis, and exposure of the transverse colon and associated hepatic and splenic flexures improves. Reverse Trendelenburg is associated with fewer physiologic complications as opposed to the Trendelenburg position; however, the opportunity for patient motion on the table and associated nerve injury remains. Therefore, having the patient securely and appropriately attached to the bed and appropriately placed in lithotomy stirrups remains vital (Fig. 10.2a, b).

Left and right tilt can be applied to the bed in either the Trendelenburg or reverse Trendelenburg positions to increase exposure of the left or right colon, respectively. There are minimal physiologic changes that occur with bed tilt, but increased table motion increases the chance for patient motion and possible nerve injury or patient fall from the operative table.

Assistant Ports and Retraction

Placement of additional laparoscopic port sites can allow for improved retraction via the use of a surgical assist. The bowel can be manipulated with atraumatic graspers, laparoscopic fans, or even the placement of intraperitoneal surgical sponges (Figs. 10.4 and 10.5a–c). Additionally, intracorporeally placed retractors or sutures can be used in some instances. For example, a suture can be used to retract the uterus cephalad, and stay sutures can be used to assist in suturing on the bowel [14]. External retractors can also be helpful: the uterus can be retracted cephalad with the aid of a uterine manipulator, and the rectum can be moved through the use of sizers

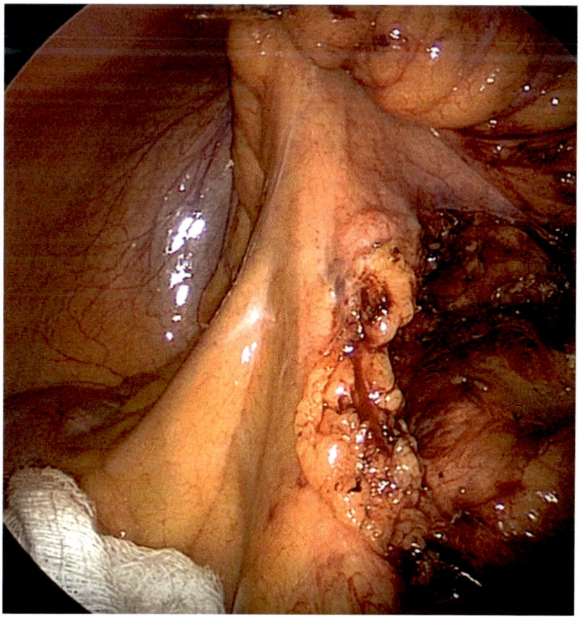

Fig. 10.4 During medial to lateral dissection of the inferior mesenteric artery (IMA), exposure is achieved with bowel retractors. An intra-abdominal sponge is used to retract the small bowel at the base of the mesentery to prevent inadvertent thermal injury. (Courtesy of Patricia Sylla, MD)

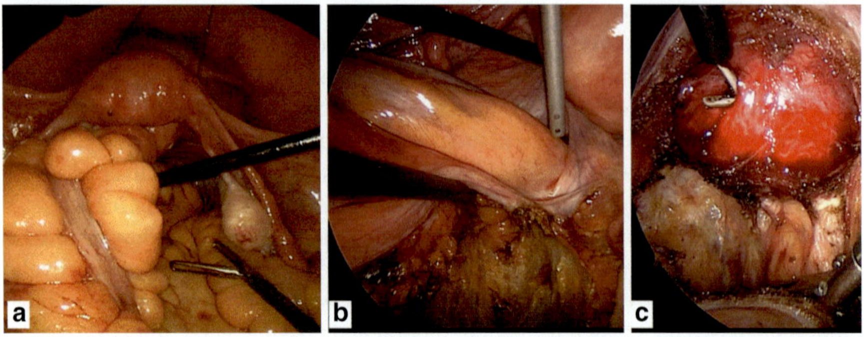

Fig. 10.5 (**a**–**c**) Three different techniques to retract the uterus, cul-de-sac, and vagina during low anterior resection. (**a**) A suture is placed laparoscopically through the uterus using a Keith needle, and the uterus is suspended superiorly. (**b**) Multiple retractors are used to retract the uterus and cul-de-sac superiorly in order to expose the anterior rectal wall. (**c**) A sizer is inserted transvaginally and used to retract the vaginal anteriorly and facilitate exposure of the rectovaginal plane. (All: Courtesy of Patricia Sylla, MD)

(Fig. 10.5a–c). Magnetic retractors that work through the abdominal wall have also been developed and have demonstrated clinical utility [15]. All these techniques introduce additional complexity to an operation, and close attention must be paid to the location of assistant's instruments, and in the case of intraperitoneal retractors/assists, these are removed at the completion of the operation.

Laparoscopic Visualization

Poor visualization can hamper the safe completion of laparoscopic procedures. Ideally, a clear view of the operative field should be present at all times. Fogging is a common problem which can be remedied by using pre-warmed laparoscopic lenses, warm air insufflation, and moving the insufflator away from the camera port. Fogging from smoke production during use of cautery or energy devices also occurs and can be improved by use of suction irrigation, venting a laparoscopic port, and use of a smoke evacuation device. Specialized laparoscopes with built-in heaters to warm the lens are available; also, the use of conductive lubrication on cautery instruments can greatly reduce the amount of smoke produced. Other impediments to visualization include dirty lenses from passing the scope through soiled ports. Here, cleaning the port regularly can help, as well as upsizing the port to allow for easier introduction of the lens. The suction irrigator can also be used to clean the lens by blowing clear fluid across it and then using the suction to remove remaining water vapor.

Control of Surgical Bleeding

Bleeding is a common operative problem and can be the cause of conversion to an open procedure. Increasing operative experience decreases the number of significant bleeding complications as well as the need to convert the case to address bleeding [16]. As always, prevention is better than reaction, and appropriate exposure of the operative field can reduce the incidence of bleeding and facilitate control. The first response should generally be control of the bleeding as quickly as possible using an instrument already present in the abdomen. This could be either a grasper or an energy device. Modern laparoendoscopic energy devices use endothermal bipolar vessel sealing or ultrasonic energy to coagulate tissue. Both can close vessels up to 7 mm in diameter; however, endothermal bipolar vessel sealing devices have significantly less heat production, decreasing possible thermal injury to nearby structures. A small randomized controlled trial showed a significant reduction in blood loss and operative times with the use of endothermal bipolar devices [17]. The choice of particular device is largely dependent on individual surgeon's preference and experience.

In the event bleeding cannot be controlled with an energy device, other options are available. Larger vessels with significant calcification may not be adequately sealed with coagulation alone. It is important to note that bipolar devices will malfunction when in proximity to a foreign body such as metal. Bleeding through staple lines must be controlled with alternative measures. Laparoscopic clips or endoloops are more effective means of control. Clips are available in either the traditional metal style or locking plastic clips. Endoloops are very effective to control bleeding from a major colonic vessel such as the ileocolic, inferior mesenteric, or middle colic pedicle. Slow bleeding through a staple line can also be managed with monopolar cautery, suture ligature, or application of a laparoscopic hemostatic agent.

Splenic Bleeding

Bleeding from the spleen can be difficult to control and lead to conversion to open and even splenectomy, which has long-term immunologic consequences. Rates of splenic injury vary from 0.5 to 1% for laparoscopic colorectal resections. For minor splenic bleeding, the best initial route is application of a surgical hemostatic agent and tamponade. If this proves ineffective, monopolar cautery or argon beam coagulation can be attempted; however, these can worsen the area of injury and lead to more severe bleeding. Devascularization of the inferior pole of the spleen has also been reported as a salvage technique and may prove effective [18]. Should splenectomy be required, the patient should receive the appropriate vaccinations prior to hospital discharge.

Organ Injury

Organ injuries that occur during laparoscopic colorectal resection should ideally be identified and repaired at the time of the procedure. Commonly injured organs include the small bowel and ureter, and special precautions can be taken to help avoid these complications. Other organs at risk include the spleen, pancreas, liver, bladder, and vagina. As with many aspects of surgery, most repairs can be accomplished laparoscopically; however, a low threshold for conversion to an open is appropriate. Knowledge of the anatomy and proper exposure are the first line of defense. Please see Chap. 31 on strategies to minimize conversion in laparoscopic colorectal surgery for more technical details.

Small Bowel Injury

Serosal tears affect the outer muscular layer of the intestine while leaving the inner muscular layer and mucosa intact. Small serosal tears likely require no repair. Larger tears benefit from closure with Lembert sutures. This can be accomplished laparoscopically in the traditional interrupted fashion or as a running suture. Absorbable sutures should be used, and unidirectional sutures can be employed as well. Repair should occur in a transverse fashion to avoid stenosis of the bowel lumen. Full thickness injuries of the intestine mandate repair. These are repaired most effectively with a running suture, and the use of unidirectional suture greatly facilitates laparoscopic closure and has been shown to be safe (Fig. 10.6) [19]. Again, repair should occur along the transverse axis of the bowel. Thermal injuries to the intestine are more difficult to identify [20]. Signs of thermal injury can be subtle, and surgeons should have a high index of suspicion if energy was used in close proximity to the bowel. Thermal injury can appear as a whitish discoloration, or in severe cases, the tissues may appear bruised or charred and have a contracted appearance. Often, these injuries may be missed altogether. If an area of injury is identified, it should be debrided and repaired as a full thickness injury.

Ureteral Injury

Injuries to the ureter occur in up to 1% of all laparoscopic colorectal operations and are one of the most commonly litigated areas in colorectal surgery [21]. Repair of ureter injuries should involve the consult of a urologic surgeon and ideally be identified and performed at the time of surgery. Delay in identification of ureteral injuries leads to increased risk of loss of kidney function and further complications [21].

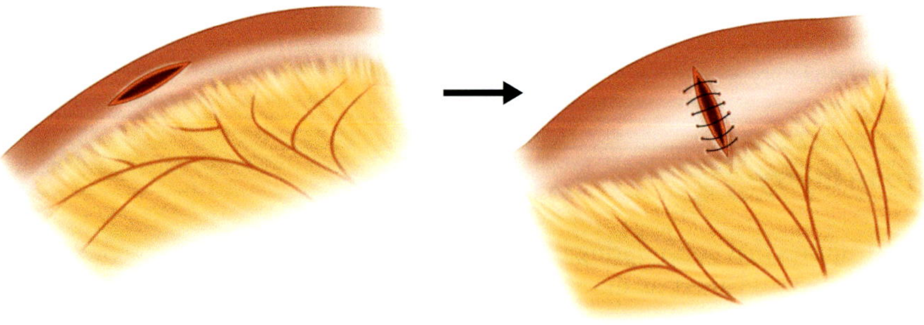

Fig. 10.6 Bowel repair. Repair of bowel injuries is performed transversely to avoid structuring of the intestine

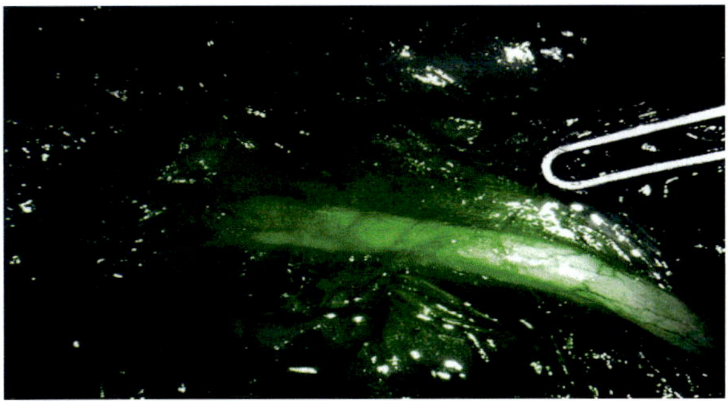

Fig. 10.7 Indocyanine green dye can be injected through ureteral stents to aid in ureteral visualization. (Courtesy of Jeffrey Gahan, MD, UT Southwestern Medical Center)

Prevention of ureter injuries is guided primarily by knowledge of the pelvic anatomy, proper exposure, and review of preoperative imaging. Ureteral stents can also play an important role. Stents are unlikely to prevent injuries but may aid intraoperative recognition of ureteral injuries, facilitating early repair. A 2018 analysis of NSQIP data demonstrated a protective effect of ureteral stents in high-risk cases [22]. Newer technologies such as lighted stents and immunofluorescence can aid further in intraoperative identification of the ureters, saving operative time and possibly reducing injury rates (Fig. 10.7) [23, 24]. Complications of ureteral stent placements occur approximately 2% of cases and include acute renal injury, obstruction and hydronephrosis, urinary tract infection, and ureteral perforation [25]. For this reason, many employ a selective stenting policy based on preoperative index of suspicion for a difficult case.

Trocar Site Closure

Hernias at port sites occur, and the question of which port sites to close remains controversial to this day. Generally, 5 mm port sites have a low risk of hernia, and closure is unnecessary. Consideration to closure should be given if the port has fallen out and been replaced several times during the operation, inadvertently creating a larger fascial defect. Hernias at 8 mm ports have been reported; however, common practice remains to not close the fascia at these defects as large series show these hernias are rare [26]. 10 12 mm ports have reported rates of hernia around 1%, making some authors recommend fascial closure of port site [27]. Risks of closure include vessel injury and bleeding, as well as increased postoperative pain. Port site closure can be accomplished with a laparoscopic suture passer or one of the several commercially available devices.

Conclusion

Laparoscopic colorectal surgery is a challenging endeavor that requires greater cognitive involvement and training when compared to traditional open surgery. Constant vigilance and anticipation and knowledge of potential problems can lead to improved intraoperative management and patient outcomes.

References

1. Gillespie BM, Chaboyer W, Thalib L, John M, Fairweather N, Slater K. Effect of using a safety checklist on patient complications after surgery: a systematic review and meta-analysis. Anesthesiology. 2014;120(6):1380–9.
2. Haynes AB, Weiser TG, Berry WR, Lipsitz SR, Breizat AH, Dellinger EP, et al. A surgical safety checklist to reduce morbidity and mortality in a global population. N Engl J Med. 2009;360(5):491–9.
3. Ahmad G, Gent D, Henderson D, O'Flynn H, Phillips K, Watson A. Laparoscopic entry techniques. Cochrane Database Syst Rev. 2015;(8):CD006583.
4. Merlin TL, Hiller JE, Maddern GJ, Jamieson GG, Brown AR, Kolbe A. Systematic review of the safety and effectiveness of methods used to establish pneumoperitoneum in laparoscopic surgery. Br J Surg. 2003;90(6):668–79.
5. Azevedo JL, Azevedo OC, Miyahira SA, Miguel GP, Becker OM Jr, Hypólito OH, et al. Injuries caused by Veress needle insertion for creation of pneumoperitoneum: a systematic literature review. Surg Endosc. 2009;23(7):1428–32.
6. Arnell TD. Minimally invasive reoperation following laparotomy. Clin Colon Rectal Surg. 2006;19(4):223–7.
7. Hurd WW, Bude RO, DeLancey JO, Pearl ML. The relationship of the umbilicus to the aortic bifurcation: implications for laparoscopic technique. Obstet Gynecol. 1992;80(1):48–51.
8. Pasic R, Levine RL, Wolf WM Jr. Laparoscopy in morbidly obese patients. J Am Assoc Gynecol Laparosc. 1999;6(3):307–12.
9. Mills JT, Burris MB, Warburton DJ, Conaway MR, Schenkman NS, Krupski TL. Positioning injuries associated with robotic assisted urological surgery. J Urol. 2013;190(2):580–4.
10. Shveiky D, Aseff JN, Iglesia CB. Brachial plexus injury after laparoscopic and robotic surgery. J Minim Invasive Gynecol. 2010;17(4):414–20.
11. Lee M, Dallas R, Daniel C, Cotter F. Intraoperative management of increased intraocular pressure in a patient with glaucoma undergoing robotic prostatectomy in the trendelenburg position. A A Case Rep. 2016;6(2):19–21.
12. Rao MM, Jayne D. Lower limb compartment syndrome following laparoscopic colorectal surgery: a review. Color Dis. 2011;13(5):494–9.
13. Robba C, Cardim D, Donnelly J, Bertuccio A, Bacigaluppi S, Bragazzi N, et al. Effects of pneumoperitoneum and Trendelenburg position on intracranial pressure assessed using different non-invasive methods. Br J Anaesth. 2016;117(6):783–91.
14. Choo SH, Jung W, Jeong U, Jeong BC, Han DH. Initial experiences of a novel self-retaining intracorporeal retractor device for urologic laparoendoscopic single-site surgery. J Endourol. 2014;28(4):404–9.
15. Rivas H, Robles I, Riquelme F, Vivanco M, Jiménez J, Marinkovic B, et al. Magnetic surgery: results from first prospective clinical trial in 50 patients. Ann Surg. 2018;267(1):88–93.
16. Kambakamba P, Dindo D, Nocito A, Clavien PA, Seifert B, Schäfer M, et al. Intraoperative adverse events during laparoscopic colorectal resection–better laparoscopic treatment but unchanged incidence. Lessons learnt from a Swiss multi-institutional analysis of 3,928 patients. Langenbeck's Arch Surg. 2014;399(3):297–305.
17. Campagnacci R, de Sanctis A, Baldarelli M, Rimini M, Lezoche G, Guerrieri M. Electrothermal bipolar vessel sealing device vs. ultrasonic coagulating shears in laparoscopic colectomies: a comparative study. Surg Endosc. 2007;21(9):1526–31.
18. Larkin JO, Carroll PA, McCormick PH, Mehigan BJ. Control of splenic bleeding during splenic flexure mobilisation by devascularisation of the inferior pole of the spleen. Tech Coloproctol. 2012;16(6):459–61.
19. Lee SW, Kawai M, Tashiro K, Nomura E, Tokuhara T, Kawashima S, et al. Laparoscopic gastrointestinal anastomoses using knotless barbed absorbable sutures are safe and reproducible: a single-center experience with 242 patients. Jpn J Clin Oncol. 2016;46(4):329–35.
20. Cassaro S. Delayed manifestations of laparoscopic bowel injury. Am Surg. 2015;81(5):478–82.

21. Marcelissen TA, Den Hollander PP, Tuytten TR, Sosef MN. Incidence of iatrogenic ireteral injury during open and laparoscopic colorectal surgery: a single center experience and review of the literature. Surg Laparosc Endosc Percutan Tech. 2016;26(6):513–5.
22. Coakley KM, Kasten KR, Sims SM, Prasad T, Heniford BT, Davis BR. Prophylactic ureteral catheters for colectomy: a National Surgical Quality Improvement Program-Based analysis. Dis Colon Rectum. 2018;61(1):84–8.
23. Al-Taher M, van den Bos J, Schols RM, Bouvy ND, Stassen LP. Fluorescence ureteral visualization in human laparoscopic colorectal surgery using methylene blue. J Laparoendosc Adv Surg Tech A. 2016;26(11):870–5.
24. Chahin F, Dwivedi AJ, Paramesh A, Chau W, Agrawal S, Chahin C, et al. The implications of lighted ureteral stenting in laparoscopic colectomy. JSLS. 2002;6(1):49–52.
25. Pathak RA, Taylor AS, Alford S, Broderick GA, Igel TC, Petrou SP, et al. Urologic-induced complications of prophylactic ureteral localization stent placement for colorectal surgery cases. J Laparoendosc Adv Surg Tech A. 2015;25(12):966–70.
26. Harr JN, Juo YY, Luka S, Agarwal S, Brody F, Obias V, et al. Incisional and port-site hernias following robotic colorectal surgery. Surg Endosc. 2016;30(8):3505–10.
27. Moran DC, Kavanagh DO, Sahebally S, Neary PC. Incidence of early symptomatic port-site hernia: a case series from a department where laparoscopy is the preferred surgical approach. Ir J Med Sci. 2012;181(4):463–6.

Principles of Complete Mesocolic Excision for Colon Cancer

11

Ian M. Paquette and Fergal Fleming

Introduction and Rationale

Since the initial description by Heald of total mesorectal excision (TME) [1–3], there has been a steady interest in the relationship between the quality of a rectal cancer resection and oncologic outcomes. The fact that a well-executed TME as judged by the quality of the mesorectal specimen is clearly associated with better oncologic outcomes has led to some authors to postulate that similar principles should be applied to colon cancer. The current point of controversy is the role for complete mesocolic excision (CME) in colon cancer surgery [4]. The effort to standardize colon cancer surgery has brought forth many new and often contradicting definitions. CME, "high-tie," "D3" resection, and others are often incorrectly used interchangeably in the literature. To be able to understand the literature on this topic, we must first understand the meaning of the various definitions which have been proposed. We will then examine the impact of these techniques on survival after colon cancer surgery and the evolving role of minimally invasive surgery in these techniques.

Definitions

Many reports in the literature use the terms CME and central vascular ligation (CLV) interchangeably. There are three components to CME. The first component involves sharp dissection between the parietal fascia and mesenteric plane and

I. M. Paquette (✉)
University of Cincinnati College of Medicine, Cincinnati, OH, USA
e-mail: ian.paquette@uc.edu

F. Fleming
Department of Colorectal Surgery, University of Rochester Medical Center, Rochester, NY, USA

P. Sylla et al. (eds.), *The SAGES Manual of Colorectal Surgery*,
https://doi.org/10.1007/978-3-030-24812-3_11

removal of the mesenteric tissue within a complete envelope of fascia and peritoneum [5]. The second component is the central vascular tie at the most proximal extent of the feeding blood vessel, and the final component is removal of an adequate length of bowel either side of the tumor to remove potentially involved lymph nodes in a longitudinal direction [6]. Where the confusion often arises is in the extent of lymphadenectomy that is done. CME requires proximal vascular ligation at the origin of the feeding vessels but does not require dissection of the root vessels (e.g., superior mesenteric artery or vein). The definitions of extent of lymph node dissection described in the following sections are based on the guidelines of the Japanese Society of Cancer of the Colon and Rectum (JSCCR) [7, 8] It is important to note that most of the literature reported below describes a CME dissection with a standard high ligation of the feeding vessel and does not include an extended lymphadenectomy.

D3

The Japanese classification references levels as D1–D3, as highlighted in Fig. 11.1. D1 lymph node resection represents transection of the mesenteric vessels at the level of the marginal vessel; D2 is a more traditional resection of the main feeding vessel to a given colonic segment at its origin. D2 dissection is equivalent to transection of the ileocolic artery at its origin off the superior mesenteric artery (SMA) or ligation of the inferior mesenteric artery at the takeoff of the left colic artery. A D3 dissection for a right-sided tumor includes lymph nodes along the anterior aspect of the superior mesenteric vein (SMV) and SMA (central lymph nodes) and for a left-sided tumor includes lymph nodes around the inferior mesenteric artery at the origin off the aorta [7].

Central Venous Ligation (CVL)

The group from Erlangen, Germany, has proposed nodal dissection even more extended than the D3 standard proposed by the Japanese, noted as central vascular ligation [7]. This description is pertinent to a right colectomy. Dissection in the plane of Toldt's fascia between the mesocolic fascia and the retroperitoneum is performed with sharp dissection. Surgery involves a Kocher maneuver and takedown of the mesenteric attachments to the duodenum and uncinate process of the pancreas with complete dissection around the superior mesenteric vein and superior mesenteric artery. For tumors of the cecum and proximal ascending colon, the right branches of the middle colic artery and middle colic vein are ligated centrally. For tumors located more distally in the ascending colon, hepatic flexure or proximal transverse colon (proximal to the left branch of middle colic artery) lymph node removal is taken down to origin of the middle colic and ileocolic artery with these arteries divided centrally. For tumor in the distal transverse colon, lymph nodes in the gastrocolic ligament are included in the resection, as are gastroepiploic vessels,

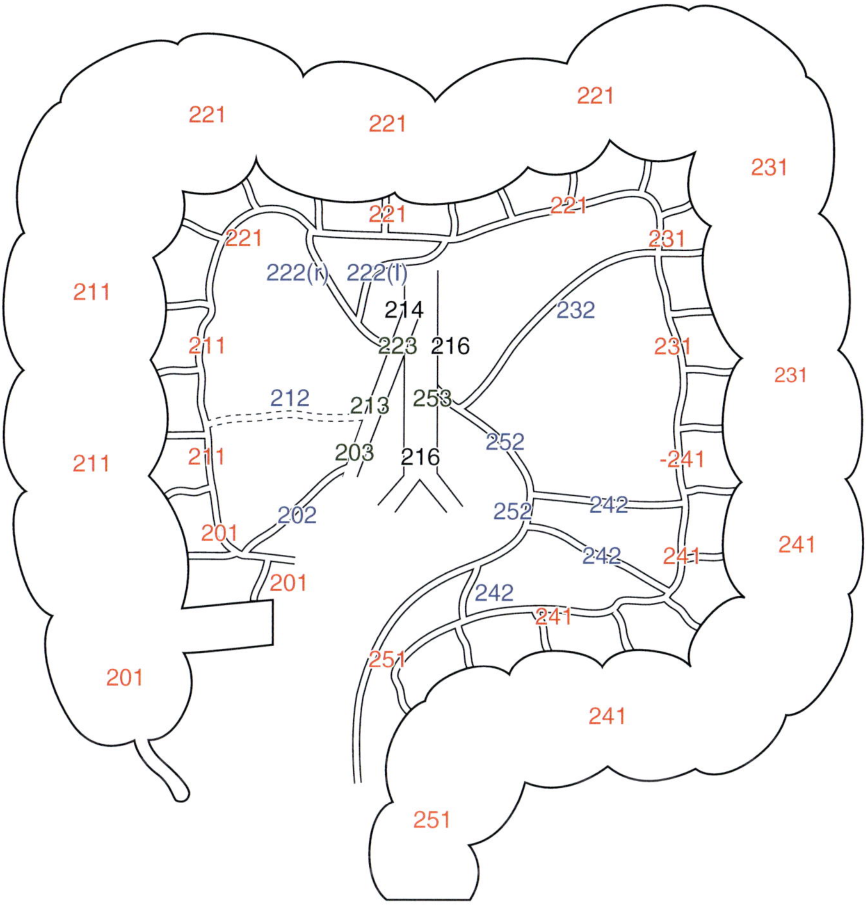

Fig. 11.1 Mesocolic lymph node stations according to the Japanese Society for Cancer of the Colon and Rectum. D1–D4 defined by colors: D1 red, D2 blue, D3 green, and D4 black. Right colic artery (dotted). (Used with permission of Wolters Kluwer from Bertelsen et al. [41])

and their branches to the stomach are divided for a length of approximately 10 cm either side of the tumor. It is important to understand this definition, in contrast to the definition of D3, and they are often inappropriately discussed interchangeably in the literature.

Role for Minimally Invasive Surgery in CME

Laparoscopic colectomy is widely accepted as a preferred surgical technique for colon cancer [9]. CME was initially described as a massive open operation, albeit with good oncologic outcomes. The challenge for the surgeon is to use minimally invasive techniques to achieve the same oncologic outcomes while maintaining the benefits of MIS approach. Many reports continue to emerge describing the technical considerations for achieving a CME resection for colon cancer using laparoscopic or robotic surgery [10–15]. Most of these studies examine outcomes in resection of either the right colon or the transverse colon, as a proximal lymphadenectomy in a left colectomy is not technically difficult and is often performed [10]. Of these types of resection, transverse colectomy tends to be more technically difficult, with longer operative times due to increased technical complexity [16]. The technical complexity comes from dealing with the intricacies of the middle colic vessels, which are often shorter and have more varied branching patterns than often seen in other segments of the colon. A study by Spinoglio and coauthors of 202 robotic vs. 101 laparoscopic right colectomies with CME indicated a lower rate of conversion to open surgery (0% vs. 6.9%) in robotic vs. laparoscopic surgery ($p = 0.01$), with no difference in 5-year overall or disease-free survival [17]. A recent literature review comparing laparoscopic vs. open CME included 1 RCT and 11 non-randomized studies (4 from Europe and 7 from Asia) [14]. As expected, laparoscopic surgery offered faster return of gastrointestinal function and less complications. There were no differences in the quality of the resected specimen based on lymph node harvest and distance from tumor to the mesenteric transection. The laparoscopic approach offered better 3-year overall survival (OR 2.02, $p = 0.001$) and disease-free survival (PR 1.45, $p = 0.05$) [14]. These results suggest that a minimally invasive approach is at least feasible, but the survival results need to be interpreted with some caution as these studies were fraught with selection bias, and in many instances, laparoscopic resections were offered to lower-risk tumors. Although little has been published on the learning curve during CME, the few publications on this topic have demonstrated a long learning curve as demonstrated by longer operative time and time to achieve CME specimens of satisfactory quality [18, 19].

Please refer to Chap. 13 on laparoscopic right colectomy for malignant disease for details on operative setup and techniques of laparoscopic right colectomy with CME.

Perioperative Outcomes of CME

The extensive dissection close to or around the root of the major blood vessels in both CME and D3 lymphadenectomy has led to understandable concerns about possible morbidity compared to conventional colon cancer resection which does not mandate as an extensive dissection. Tables 11.1 and 11.2 summarize publications to date where either CME or D3 resections were compared to either a concurrent or historical control group who underwent conventional or "standard" colon cancer resection. Operative blood loss was reported on in three studies, with one study reporting a significantly higher blood loss in the CME group, with no difference noted in the other two studies [20–22] (Table 11.1). A recent pooled analysis by Alhassan and coauthors comparing [23] conventional colectomy and CME for colon cancer found a similar rate of pooled overall complications for conventional resection of 19.6% (95% CI:13.6–25.5) and 22.5% (95% CI:18.4–26.6) for CME

Table 11.1 Studies comparing conventional colectomy and CME or D3 lymphadenectomy with respect to operative and 30-day outcomes

Study	Study period	Country	Surgical approach	Number	OR time (mins)	Blood loss (ml)	Complication rate (%)	30-day mortality (%)
West	1999–	Denmark	Conventional	170	–	–	–	–
et al. [39]	2008		CME	93	–	–	–	–
Bertelson	2007–	Denmark	Conventional	93	–	270	20	7.
et al. [22]	2009		CME	105	–	250	22.6	6.
Galizia	2004–	Italy	Conventional	58	130*	200*	12.1	–
et al. [20]	2012		CME	45	178	280	13.3	–
Bertelson	2008–	Denmark	Conventional	1031	–	–	–	4
et al. [34]	2011		CME	364	–	–	–	5
Bertelson	2008–	Denmark	Conventional	1701	–	–	28.5	–
et al. [40]	2013		CME	529	–	–	30.6	–
Merkel	1978–	Germany	Conventional	429	–	–	17.2*	3.7
et al. [24]	2014		CME	1099	–	–	21.3	2.7
Olofsson	2007–	Sweden	Conventional	390	148	204	20.8	0.8
et al. [21]	2009		CME	1694	155	232	22.8	3.6*
Kotake	1985–	Japan	Conventional	3425	–	–	–	–
et al. [26]	1994		D3 resection	3425	–	–	–	–
Kotake	1995–	Japan	Conventional	463	–	–	–	–
et al. [27]	2004		D3 resection	463	–	–	–	–

*: $P < 0.05$

[20–22, 24, 25]. However, the sole paper to date to report on intraoperative complications did note a significantly higher rate of intraoperative organ injuries in patients undergoing CME resection (CME 9.1% vs. 3.6% conventional resection, $p < 0.001$), notably splenic and superior mesenteric vein injury [25]. These findings suggest that a surgeon should be careful in performing dissection close to the root of major feeding vessels, as there is a risk of injury to structures such as the duodenum, pancreas, and SMV.

Oncologic Outcomes of CME

Pathological Outcomes

All three studies that reported on distance from the tumor to the high ligation tie reported a significantly longer distance from tumor to tie in the CME group compared to conventional surgery (Table 11.2). Lymph node yield was significantly higher in all six studies for CME group. Kotake and coauthors reported [26, 27] on two patient cohorts where a D3 lymphadenectomy was compared to conventional resection and observed a significantly higher lymph node yield for the D3 cohort in both studies compared to conventional resection.

To better understand the potential impact of central lymphadenectomy for colon cancer, one must first understand the incidence of central nodal positivity when these resections are done. Some reports have upstaged up to 5% of patients from N0

Table 11.2 Studies comparing conventional colectomy and CME or D3 lymphadenectomy with respect to pathological and long-term survival

Study	Surgical approach	Large bowel specimen length (mean)	Distance from tumor to high tie (cm)	Lymph node yield (mean)	Overall survival (%)	Disease-specific survival (%)
West et al. [39]	Conventional CME	24.7 (median) 31.5	8.4 (median)* 10.5	18* 28	– –	– –
Bertelson et al. [22]	Conventional CME	– –	7.1* 9.6	24.5* 26.7	– –	– –
Galizia et al. [20]	Conventional CME	27.4 28.8	8.7* 10.6	15* 20	– –	87 3 years 95
Bertelson et al. [34]	Conventional CME	– –	– –	– –	69.8 (5 years) 74.5	73.4* 4 years 85.8
Bertelson et al. [40]	Conventional CME	– –	– –	20* 36	– –	– –
Merkel et al. [24]	Conventional CME	– –	– –	25* (median) 27	Stage III 53.1* (5 years) Stage III 69.7	Stage III 61.7* 5 years Stage III 80.9
Olofsson et al. [21]	Conventional CME	– –	– –	17.5* 19.2	78.5 (3 years) 79.4	69.4 73.8
Kotake et al. [26]	Conventional D3 resection	– –	– –	14.9* 21.8	No difference at 5 years	– –
Kotake et al. [27]	Conventional D3 resection	– –	– –	11.6* 18.1	90.6 (5 years) 91.9	– –

*: $P < 0.05$

to N3 disease. Review of the literature involving D3 vascular ligation indicates that the central nodal basin is positive approximately 1–8% of the time. Right-sided tumors are estimated to metastasize to central vasculature between 3 and 5% of the time [7, 28–32], while left-sided lesions metastasize to the root of the IMA between 1.7 and 8% of the time [29, 33]. The true incidence of central nodal positivity is largely unknown because most colon cancer resections are done at the D2 level. Positive nodes in the central location would really be the only clinical reason to undertake such an extensive central resection.

Long-Term Survival

Attempts to compare survival between conventional colectomy for colon cancer and CME or D3 lymphadenectomy are difficult due to multiple potential confounding factors. Few studies compare CME to high-quality D2 resection, and the concepts of CME and CVL are often used interchangeably. There is a paucity of studies which directly compare high-quality conventional colectomy (D2 lymphadenectomy) with either D3 lymphadenectomy or CVL with lymphadenectomy along the root vessels. Many of the studies use historical controls when less attention was paid to lymph node retrieval and pathological assessment. Only one study reported significantly higher survival for stage 3 patients in the CME group compared to conventional resection group [13] (Table 11.2). The other four studies did not demonstrate a difference in overall survival between conventional and CME resections. Disease-specific survival was higher in two of the four studies [13, 34] which reported this endpoint. Despite the CME groups and D3 lymphadenectomy cohorts all having a significantly longer distance from tumor to high tie and lymph node yields, this apparent improvement in pathological surrogates has not been associated with a consistent improvement in survival (Table 11.2). This raises the question of what is the incremental benefit of an "extended" lymphadenectomy with respect to oncologic outcomes. The following section highlights some studies where CME or D3 resections are compared to a more standardized approach involving D2 lymphadenectomy.

Hohenberger and coauthors reported their experience with over 2000 patients who underwent colon cancer resection over a 35-year period with the period 1978–1984 represented the baseline group prior to a policy change, and routine use of CME colon cancer surgery was practiced in the two latter time periods (2003–2009–1994 and 2010–2014) [13]. They found a significant decrease in overall locoregional recurrence for the latter time period (2003–2009) (3.6%) compared to the earliest time period (1978–1984) (6.5%). For cancer-related survival, a significant improvement over time was found, from 78.9 to 90.6% (hazard ratio 0.54, 95% CI 0.38–0.77, $p = 0.001$), though no significant improvement in overall survival was seen. The results must be viewed within the context that the study was comparing patients from an era when no patients received adjuvant chemotherapy compared to the latter period where nearly 80% of patients with stage III patients received chemotherapy and no data were available on the mesenteric dissection plane or adequacy of the nodal assessment from the earlier study periods.

Kawamura and coauthors wished to explore the impact of ligation level (intermediate or high ligation) on survival for colon cancer over a very long time period (1963–1999) [35]. High ligation was not associated with an improvement in survival, regardless of level of lymph node positivity (pericolic, intermediate, or central lymph node positivity), though the results must be viewed within the context that the number of patients with intermediate or central lymph node positivity was very small ($n = 53$).

Kotake and coauthors explored the association of extent of lymphadenectomy (D3 versus D2 lymphadenectomy) using a match propensity score design for patients with a pathological stage T3 or T4 cancer from the time period 1985–1994. There was a significant difference in OS between the matched groups, favoring the D3 lymphadenectomy group (HR 0.81; 95% CI:0.73–0.90,

$p = 0.0001$), though the findings may have been confounded by the fact that even after matching the D2 group had a significantly higher proportion of stage 3 patients [26]. The same group subsequently examined the association between level of lymphadenectomy for pathological T2 tumor who underwent D2 versus D3 resection and found no difference in overall survival between patients who underwent a D2 versus D3 resection [27].

Bokey and coauthors compared two consecutive periods of time (1971–1979 vs. 1980–1995). Patients in the latter time period were defined as having undergone a standardized surgery with sharp mesocolic dissection with transection of the relevant vessels "close to the origin" of the feeding vessel. Patients in the latter standardized surgery group had a significantly better 5-year disease-specific survival (76.5% vs. 66.4%), though as with all these studies who use historical controls, the lack of receipt of chemotherapy in the stage 3 patients in the early time period must be considered [36]. The potential impact of a surgical education program was examined by Storli and associates who compared the outcomes of a group of patients ($n = 89$) after a CME training program and compared the outcomes to patients treated in different hospitals where conventional colectomy was performed ($n = 105$). The CME cohort had a lower local recurrence, and 3-year survival was higher than seen in the group who underwent conventional colectomy [37]. These studies do suggest that a standardized approach to colon cancer resection are important, though the precise contributions of the various elements of CME (sharp dissection in the mesocolic plane, lymphadenectomy to the D3 levels, and "wide" bowel resection) require further study.

A recent systematic review by Alhassan and associates of 14 studies compared short- and long-term outcomes between conventional colectomy and CME for colon cancer. The authors concluded that the evidence base for CME was limited and did not reveal a clear benefit over conventional colectomy in accordance with a previous study [12, 38].

Conclusion

Current data support resection of the complete mesocolic envelope with a D2 lymphadenectomy for colon cancer. Metastasis to central lymph nodes is a relatively rare event (1–8% of patients), and it is unclear whether extended lymphadenectomy confers a survival benefit. Minimally invasive techniques to these resections are technically feasible but are associated with a long learning curve. The recent resurgence of interest in the operative approach in colon cancer is to be welcomed as it has refocused attention on the integral role of optimal surgical technique in the management of colon cancer. Future studies should involve a standardized definition of what constitutes a CME with a prospective comparison between CME and a D2 lymphadenectomy with sharp dissection in the mesocolic plane to determine the optimal surgical technique.

References

1. Heald R, Moran B, Pahlman L, Christensen HK. Optimising surgery for rectal cancer. Ugeskr Laeger. 2011;173:1044–7.
2. Heald RJ. A new approach to rectal cancer. Br J Hosp Med. 1979;22:277–81.
3. Heald RJ. The 'Holy Plane' of rectal surgery. J R Soc Med. 1988;81:503–8.
4. Paquette IM, Madoff RD, Sigurdson ER, Chang GJ. Impact of proximal vascular ligation on survival of patients with colon cancer. Ann Surg Oncol. 2018;25:38–45.
5. West NP, Hohenberger W, Weber K, Perrakis A, Finan PJ, Quirke P. Complete mesocolic excision with central vascular ligation produces an oncologically superior specimen compared with standard surgery for carcinoma of the colon. J Clin Oncol. 2010;28:272–8.
6. Sondenaa K, Quirke P, Hohenberger W, Sugihara K, Kobayashi H, Kessler H, et al. The rationale behind complete mesocolic excision (CME) and a central vascular ligation for colon cancer in open and laparoscopic surgery : proceedings of a consensus conference. Int J Color Dis. 2014;29:419–28.
7. Hohenberger W, Weber K, Matzel K, Papadopoulos T, Merkel S. Standardized surgery for colonic cancer: complete mesocolic excision and central ligation--technical notes and outcome. Colorectal Dis: Off J Assoc Coloproctol Great Br Ireland. 2009;11:354–64.. discussion 364–5
8. Watanabe T, Itabashi M, Shimada Y, Tanaka S, Ito Y, Ajioka Y, et al. Japanese Society for Cancer of the Colon and Rectum (JSCCR) guidelines 2010 for the treatment of colorectal cancer. Int J Clin Oncol. 2012;17:1–29.
9. Fleshman J, Sargent DJ, Green E, Anvari M, Stryker SJ, Beart RW Jr, et al. Laparoscopic colectomy for cancer is not inferior to open surgery based on 5-year data from the COST Study Group trial. Ann Surg. 2007;246:655–62.. discussion 662–4
10. Ozben V, de Muijnck C, Esen E, Aytac E, Baca B, Karahasanoglu T, et al. Is robotic complete mesocolic excision feasible for transverse colon cancer? J Laparoendosc Adv Surg Tech A. 2018; https://doi.org/10.1089/lap.2018.0239. [Epub ahead of print].
11. Ozben V, Aytac E, Atasoy D, Erenler Bayraktar I, Bayraktar O, Sapci I, et al. Totally robotic complete mesocolic excision for right-sided colon cancer. J Robot Surg. 2019 Feb;13(1):107–14.
12. Cengiz TB, Aytac E, Gorgun E. Robotic complete mesocolic excision with high vascular tie and intracorporeal side-to-side anastomosis with omental pedicle flap - a video vignette. Colorectal Dis: Off J Assoc Coloproctol Great Br Ireland. 2018;20:453–4.
13. Wang Y, Zhang C, Zhang D, Fu Z, Sun Y. Clinical outcome of laparoscopic complete mesocolic excision in the treatment of right colon cancer. World J Surg Oncol. 2017;15:174.
14. Negoi I, Hostiuc S, Negoi RI, Beuran M. Laparoscopic vs open complete mesocolic excision with central vascular ligation for colon cancer: a systematic review and meta-analysis. World J Gastrointest Oncol. 2017;9:475–91.
15. Miyo M, Takemasa I, Ishihara H, Hata T, Mizushima T, Ohno Y, et al. Long-term outcomes of single-site laparoscopic colectomy with complete mesocolic excision for colon cancer: comparison with conventional multiport laparoscopic colectomy using propensity score matching. Dis Colon Rectum. 2017;60:664–73.
16. Cao J, Ji Y, Peng X, Wu W, Cheng L, Zhou Y, Yang P. Efficacy evaluation of laparoscopic complete mesocolic excision for transverse colon cancer. Zhonghua wei chang wai ke za zhi = Chinese J Gastrointest Surg. 2017;20:545–9.
17. Spinoglio G, Bianchi PP, Marano A, Priora F, Lenti LM, Ravazzoni F, et al. Robotic versus laparoscopic right colectomy with complete mesocolic excision for the treatment of colon cancer: perioperative outcomes and 5-year survival in a consecutive series of 202 patients. Ann Surg Oncol. 2018 Nov;25(12):3580–6.
18. Melich G, Jeong DH, Hur H, Baik SH, Faria J, Kim NK, et al. Laparoscopic right hemicolectomy with complete mesocolic excision provides acceptable perioperative outcomes but is lengthy-analysis of learning curves for a novice minimally invasive surgeon. Can J Surg. 2014;57:331–6.

19. Munkedal DL, West NP, Iversen LH, Hagemann-Madsen R, Quirke P, Laurberg S. Implementation of complete mesocolic excision at a university hospital in Denmark: an audit of consecutive, prospectively collected colon cancer specimens. Eur J Surg Oncolol. 2014;40:1494–501.
20. Galizia G, Lieto E, De Vita F, Ferraraccio F, Zamboli A, Mabilia A, et al. Is complete mesocolic excision with central vascular ligation safe and effective in the surgical treatment of right-sided colon cancers? A prospective study. Int J Color Dis. 2014;29:89–97.
21. Olofsson F, Buchwald P, Elmstahl S, Syk I. No benefit of extended mesenteric resection with central vascular ligation in right-sided colon cancer. Color Dis. 2016;18:773–8.
22. Bertelsen CA, Bols B, Ingeholm P, Jansen JE, Neuenschwander AU, Vilandt J. Can the quality of colonic surgery be improved by standardization of surgical technique with complete mesocolic excision? Color Dis. 2011;13:1123–9.
23. Alhassan N, Yang M, Wong-Chong N, Liberman AS, Charlebois P, Stein B, et al. Comparison between conventional colectomy and complete mesocolic excision for colon cancer: a systematic review and pooled analysis : a review of CME versus conventional colectomies. Surg Endosc. 2019 Jan;33(1):8–18.
24. Merkel S, Weber K, Matzel KE, Agaimy A, Gohl J, Hohenberger W. Prognosis of patients with colonic carcinoma before, during and after implementation of complete mesocolic excision. Br J Surg. 2016;103:1220–9.
25. Bertelsen CA, Neuenschwander AU, Jansen JE, Kirkegaard-Klitbo A, Tenma JR, Wilhelmsen M, et al. Short-term outcomes after complete mesocolic excision compared with 'conventional' colonic cancer surgery. Br J Surg. 2016;103:581–9.
26. Kotake K, Mizuguchi T, Moritani K, Wada O, Ozawa H, Oki I, et al. Impact of D3 lymph node dissection on survival for patients with T3 and T4 colon cancer. Int J Color Dis. 2014;29:847–52.
27. Kotake K, Kobayashi H, Asano M, Ozawa H, Sugihara K. Influence of extent of lymph node dissection on survival for patients with pT2 colon cancer. Int J Color Dis. 2015;30:813–20.
28. Kanemitsu Y, Komori K, Kimura K, Kato T. D3 lymph node dissection in right hemicolectomy with a no-touch isolation technique in patients with colon cancer. Dis Colon Rectum. 2013;56:815–24.
29. Kanemitsu Y, Hirai T, Komori K, Kato T. Survival benefit of high ligation of the inferior mesenteric artery in sigmoid colon or rectal cancer surgery. Br J Surg. 2006;93:609–15.
30. Huh JW, Kim YJ, Kim HR. Distribution of lymph node metastases is an independent predictor of survival for sigmoid colon and rectal cancer. Ann Surg. 2012;255:70–8.
31. Hohenberger W, Merkel S, Weber K. Lymphadenectomy with tumors of the lower gastrointestinal tract. Der Chirurg; Zeitschrift fur alle Gebiete der operativen Medizen. 2007;78:217–25.
32. Hohenberger W, Lux P, Merkel S, Weber K. Lymph node dissection for carcinomas of the lower gastrointestinal tract. What is evidence-based? Der Chirurg; Zeitschrift fur alle Gebiete der operativen Medizen. 2011;82:1096–105.
33. Chin CC, Yeh CY, Tang R, Changchien CR, Huang WS, Wang JY. The oncologic benefit of high ligation of the inferior mesenteric artery in the surgical treatment of rectal or sigmoid colon cancer. Int J Color Dis. 2008;23:783–8.
34. Bertelsen CA, Neuenschwander AU, Jansen JE, Wilhelmsen M, Kirkegaard-Klitbo A, Tenma JR, et al. Disease-free survival after complete mesocolic excision compared with conventional colon cancer surgery: a retrospective, population-based study. Lancet Oncol. 2015;16:161–8.
35. Kawamura YJ, Umetani N, Sunami E, Watanabe T, Masaki T, Muto T. Effect of high ligation on the long-term result of patients with operable colon cancer, particularly those with limited nodal involvement. Eur J Surg. 2000;166:803–7.
36. Bokey EL, Chapuis PH, Dent OF, Mander BJ, Bissett IP, Newland RC. Surgical technique and survival in patients having a curative resection for colon cancer. Dis Colon Rectum. 2003;46:860–6.
37. Storli KE, Sondenaa K, Furnes B, Nesvik I, Gudlaugsson E, Bukholm I, et al. Short term results of complete (D3) vs. standard (D2) mesenteric excision in colon cancer shows improved

outcome of complete mesenteric excision in patients with TNM stages I-II. Tech Coloproctol. 2014;18:557–64.
38. Killeen S, Mannion M, Devaney A, Winter DC. Complete mesocolic resection and extended lymphadenectomy for colon cancer: a systematic review. Colorectal Dis: Off J Assoc Coloproctol Great Br Ireland. 2014;16:577–94.
39. West NP, Sutton KM, Ingeholm P, Hagemann-Madsen RH, Hohenberger W, Quirke P. Improving the quality of colon cancer surgery through a surgical education program. Dis Colon Rectum. 2010;53:1594–603.
40. Bertelsen CA. Complete mesocolic excision an assessment of feasibility and outcome. Dan Med J 2017;64.
41. Bertelsen CA, Kirkegaard-Klitbo A, Nielsen M, Leotta SM, Daisuke F, Gögenur I. Pattern of colon cancer lymph node metastases in patients undergoing central mesocolic lymph node excision: a systematic review. Dis Colon Rectum. 2016;59(12):1209–21.

Part III

Rights-Sided Resections

Unexpected Findings at Appendectomy 12

Emily Steinhagen and Garrett M. Nash

Introduction and Rationale

Laparoscopic appendectomy is one of the most frequently performed general surgery operations. With the widespread availability of cross-sectional imaging and improved expertise with ultrasound, the number of patients undergoing surgery for presumed appendicitis with a normal appendix has diminished. However, there are many entities that may be found during appendectomy that should prompt the surgeon to reevaluate their operative strategy prior to performing the planned appendectomy procedure.

Normal Appendix with Unexpected Other Source of Pathology

When laparoscopy is performed for a presumptive diagnosis of appendicitis and intraoperative findings suggest that the appendix is not the problem, a careful inspection of the abdomen to identify a source of inflammation or infection should be completed. Many entities may overlap with the clinical presentation of appendicitis and therefore should be systematically excluded (Box 12.1).

E. Steinhagen (✉)
University Hospitals Cleveland Medical Center, Case Western Reserve University, Cleveland, OH, USA
e-mail: emily.steinhagen@uhhospitals.org

G. M. Nash
Department of Surgery, Memorial Sloan Kettering Cancer Center, Weill Cornell Medical College, New York, NY, USA

P. Sylla et al. (eds.), *The SAGES Manual of Colorectal Surgery*,
https://doi.org/10.1007/978-3-030-24812-3_12

Box 12.1 Differential Diagnosis When the Appendix Is Normal

Inflamed Meckel's diverticulum
Cecal diverticulitis
Sigmoid diverticulitis
Epiploic appendagitis
Crohn's disease
Cecal cancer
Cholecystitis
Gynecologic pathology

- Tubo-ovarian abscess
- Pelvic inflammatory disease
- Ovarian torsion
- Ruptured ectopic pregnancy
- Ovarian cyst
- Hydrosalpinx
- Endometriosis

Inflamed Meckel's Diverticulum

Meckel's diverticulum is an embryologic remnant of the omphalomesenteric or vitelline duct found in approximately 2% of individuals; the vast majority is asymptomatic [1]. The most common presentations are bleeding and infection. Bleeding occurs most commonly in younger patients because of ectopic gastric mucosa and resulting acid secretion and ulceration. Like the appendix, it can get obstructed from inspissated bowel contents or enlarged lymphoid tissue. When this happens, it can become inflamed or infected in a phenomenon similar to appendicitis. Because of the location of the Meckel's, typically 40 cm from the ileocecal valve, clinical signs and symptoms may mimic appendicitis. Furthermore, on imaging when the appendix is small and non-visualized, an inflamed Meckel's in the right lower quadrant could feasibly be confused for an inflamed appendix. In addition, a Meckel's can perforate and cause free fluid or an abscess that is easily confused with that of a perforated appendicitis [2].

Potential etiologies of Meckel's diverticulitis may be because of torsion from the mesodiverticular band that attaches the tip of the diverticula to the mesentery or abdominal wall, ulceration in the presence of ectopic gastric mucosa leading to perforation, obstruction of the lumen typically from normal intestinal contents, and more rarely from seeds or bones that have been ingested.

When the appendix is found to be normal at exploration, a search for alternative sources is conducted, and the small bowel is run. When an inflamed Meckel's diverticulum is identified, it should be removed. A diverticulectomy is usually feasible given the typical anti-mesenteric position of the diverticulum as long as the base of the diverticulum is normal. This can be done with a technical approach similar to an appendectomy by utilizing a stapler, endo-loops, or suture ligating the stump. Care should be taken to avoid narrowing the small bowel lumen from which the diverticulum arose. In general, diverticulectomy can safely be performed with a laparoscopic approach. Routine exteriorization of the bowel for direct palpation is an option that may avoid laparotomy but is not, in general, required [3]. In some instances, small bowel resection may be necessary either due to the amount of inflammation and involvement of the associated small bowel or because of anatomic concerns. Diverticulectomy alone is sufficient for clearing all heterotopic tissue that may be present while also decreasing postoperative complications compared to segmental small bowel resection [4].

When diverticulectomy for inflamed Meckel's is performed, it may still be reasonable to perform a prophylactic appendectomy as it adds minimal morbidity to the procedure and has the potential to prevent later pathology. There is virtually no literature to guide this decision. However, whether to perform a prophylactic diverticulectomy in the setting of appendicitis is discussed in the literature. The rationale includes a small risk of becoming symptomatic and a very low risk of malignancy. The overall risk of symptoms from a Meckel's ranges from 4 to 16%, and an estimated morbidity from the procedure ranges from 0 to 6% [1]. It is impossible to make a strong management recommendation in the absence of evidence. However, a reasonable approach may be to remove a Meckel's with features that may represent a higher risk of becoming symptomatic, namely, those in male patients, those under age 50 years, diverticular length greater than 2 cm, and those with heterotopic tissue felt on palpation [5].

Cecal Diverticulitis

Cecal diverticulitis is a relatively rare problem that accounts for approximately 3% of all diverticulitis. Compared to appendicitis, it is also very rare (0.4–2.1% compared to ~7%). Given the association between the cecum and the appendix, diagnostic uncertainty based on clinical signs and symptoms as well as imaging findings is understandable. Up to 70% of patients diagnosed with this problem in the operating room had a preoperative diagnosis of appendicitis on imaging [6]. The classic presentation is a patient with right lower quadrant pain, tenderness on examination, and fever. Leukocytosis is common as is an inflammatory reaction in the right lower quadrant on imaging. Authors that attempt to differentiate suggest that the course of cecal diverticulitis may be more indolent than appendicitis, and the pain does not begin in the epigastrium [7]. Unlike left-sided diverticuli, cecal diverticuli tend to be true diverticuli consisting of all layers of the bowel wall though traditional false diverticuli may also occur. They are seen more frequently in men of Asian descent, and the true diverticuli are considered a congenital phenomenon.

When it is diagnosed preoperatively, cecal diverticulitis may be managed nonoperatively in the majority of cases similarly to left-sided diverticulitis. Surgical treatment of this entity includes right hemicolectomy, ileocecal resection, or simple diverticulectomy or inversion of the diverticulum [6, 8]. When diagnosed intraoperatively, recommendations are based on a grading system: Grade I describes a protruding, easily identifiable cecal diverticuli, grade II is an inflamed cecal mass, grade III is a localized abscess or fistula, and grade IV represents a free perforation [9]. In cases of grade I cecal diverticulitis, simple diverticulectomy and appendectomy are recommended. For grades II–IV, the suggested treatment is ileocecectomy or right hemicolectomy [10]. In practice, cecal diverticulitis may be impossible to distinguish from a mass intraoperatively, and in those cases, an oncologic right hemicolectomy is the prudent choice. In some clinical scenarios, it may be the most prudent option to simply terminate the procedure and treat the diverticulitis with antibiotics until the diverticulum can be definitively addressed in the elective setting.

Sigmoid Diverticulitis

A redundant sigmoid may lie in the midline, in the pelvis, or even in the right lower quadrant. Inflammation of the sigmoid colon may appear similar to appendicitis on clinical history, physical exam, and laboratory evaluations. On CT scan, inflammatory changes may appear in the right lower quadrant, and the appendix may also appear thickened or secondarily inflamed. In this situation, the appendiceal inflammation is due to proximity rather than inherent pathology. There is often a serositis on direct observation. In this situation, appendectomy is not indicated, but consideration for removal to prevent future complications can be considered. Treatment of complicated sigmoid diverticulitis is discussed in Chap. 28.

Epiploic Appendagitis

Inflammation of an epiploic appendage may partially mimic appendicitis clinically with acute onset right lower quadrant pain that is progressive. However, patients are usually afebrile and without leukocytosis, nausea, or vomiting. The right colon is the third most common site for appendagitis, following the sigmoid and descending colon. The etiology of epiploic appendagitis is torsion of the appendage causing venous occlusion that can result in ischemia, thrombosis, or infarction. It is benign and self-limited, requiring no specific treatment. Patients typically improve with oral anti-inflammatory medications over 4–7 days. Rarely, an inflamed epiploic appendage will become infected and develop into an abscess, cause a bowel obstruction, or act as a lead point for intussusception.

On imaging, it should be feasible to differentiate this entity from appendicitis; the patient should have a normal appendix, and on CT scan there is inflammatory infiltration of the fat around the offending epiploic appendage. There is a characteristic central lucency [11]. With ultrasound, an inflamed epiploic appendage will appear as an oval, non-compressible mass with no central flow on Doppler when the probe is placed over the point of maximal tenderness [12]. In cases of severe inflammation, it could appear that the inflammation is surrounding the appendix and can lead to diagnostic confusion.

Given the widespread use of imaging, this is a diagnosis that is typically not made in the operating room at this point. However, if imaging is not utilized or not available and it is found in the context of a normal appendix, the appendix should not be removed. There is no evidence whether it is necessary to remove the offending epiploic appendage once identified.

Crohn's Disease

On laparoscopy, features of Crohn's disease may be visualized including creeping fat, thickened mesentery, inflamed bowel, abscess, and strictures. When these are found, it must first be determined if there is a perforation. If there is a bowel perforation, an appropriate resection should be performed with or without a stoma depending on patient and surgeon factors. When there is no perforation and particularly when the diagnosis has not previously been made, no resection should be performed. The remainder of the bowel should be carefully examined to determine the extent of the disease. Areas of inflammation, mesenteric thickening, and creeping fat should be noted. Strictures are also a common finding and may or may not be associated with proximal bowel dilation depending on the severity. The position and distance between abnormal segments should be documented. Following the operation, a careful history should be taken with the new diagnosis in mind, and patients should be seen by a gastroenterologist to direct further workup and treatment.

While certainly it is possible for a patient with a new diagnosis of Crohn's disease to have appendicitis as well, it is somewhat rare to have two simultaneous problems. The commonly taught adage to remove the appendix if the base and cecum are normal and to leave it if they are not is a reasonable approach despite no specific evidence in either direction. The goal of this approach is to reduce diagnostic confusion in the future between a Crohn's flare and appendicitis. The appendix, however, should not be removed if the cecal inflammation involves the base of the appendix given the risk of postoperative stump leak. Given the availability of imaging, this is less important, but since the morbidity of the appendectomy is minimal, it is still appropriate.

Gynecologic Pathology

Many gynecologic and obstetric conditions may mimic the clinical signs and symptoms of appendicitis. Even on imaging, some entities may demonstrate right lower quadrant inflammatory changes. Therefore, if the appendix is normal on laparoscopy, the pelvis should be carefully evaluated. Diagnoses such as tubo-ovarian abscess, pelvic inflammatory disease, ovarian torsion, ruptured ectopic pregnancy, ovarian cyst, hydrosalpinx, or even severely symptomatic endometriosis may mimic appendicitis.

Whenever possible, the assistance of a gynecologist should be utilized in dealing with these entities. If that is not feasible, any infection or sepsis should be drained;

nonviable tissue should be removed with the goal of preserving both ovaries and fallopian tubes whenever possible.

Pelvic inflammatory disease (PID) is a usually polymicrobial infection of the upper part of the female reproductive system (uterus, fallopian tubes, ovaries). Symptoms include pain, fever, and vaginal discharge. The pain may be pelvic or lower abdominal. On exam, cervical motion tenderness and adnexal tenderness may be noted. There is typically mucopurulent cervicitis. The most frequently implicated organisms are *Neisseria gonorrhoeae* or *Chlamydia trachomatis*, but polymicrobial infection with a number of other bacteria is also common [13, 14]. The diagnosis is often made clinically and based on physical exam and therefore requires a high degree of suspicion. Tubo-ovarian abscess is a late complication of pelvic inflammatory disease. If the abscess ruptures, it can result in peritonitis and sepsis. The abscess is often visible on ultrasound or cross-sectional imaging such as CT scan but on the right side could appear similar to appendicitis if the inflammation is extensive and the appendix lays in the pelvis. On laparoscopy, there may be a confined abscess. In addition, inflammatory changes consistent with Fitz-Hugh-Curtis perihepatitis may be seen. PID is usually treated with antibiotics alone. When tubo-ovarian abscess requires surgery, operative therapy may include either drainage or salpingo-oophorectomy.

Ovarian torsion occurs when the ovary rotates on its vascular pedicle and the vessels are occluded. This leads to unilateral pain and is often associated with nausea and vomiting. It may be more common in the setting of ovarian masses or cysts. When suspected, the diagnosis can often be made with Doppler sonography that demonstrates a loss of blood flow to the affected ovary. When diagnosed preoperatively on imaging, a gynecologist should be consulted. When found incidentally in the operating room, the treatment for ovarian torsion is surgical detorsion and pexy; if the ovary is necrotic or nonviable, it should be removed.

Ectopic pregnancy occurs when the embryo implants outside of the uterine cavity. The fallopian tube is the most common site of implantation [15]. Common symptoms are abdominal/pelvic pain associated with vaginal bleeding in the setting of a positive pregnancy test. Nauseas and vomiting are less frequent. Most women present between 4 and 8 weeks after the last menstrual period [16]. On ultrasound, there is no evidence of intrauterine pregnancy. When diagnosed early, medical management with methotrexate and serial laboratory monitoring is often feasible. Ruptured ectopic pregnancy, however, is a surgical emergency because of the risks for severe bleeding and hemorrhagic shock. When possible, consultation to gynecology should be made prior to going to the operating room. In the operating room, the affected fallopian tube is incised, and the contents are removed; alternatively, salpingectomy may be required. The ovary should be preserved when possible.

Appendiceal Mass

The other occasional unexpected intraoperative finding during appendectomy is an appendiceal mass or mucocele (dilated mucin-filled appendix), which occurs in less than 2% of appendectomy specimens [17]. Recent database studies suggest that the

Box 12.2 Appendiceal Neoplasms
Epithelial neoplasms

- Adenocarcinoma (mucinous and non-mucinous)
- Low-grade mucinous appendiceal neoplasm (LMAN)
- Signet ring carcinoma
- Goblet cell carcinoma[1]

Non-epithelial neoplasms

- Carcinoid tumor
- Lymphoma
- Leiomyoma
- Leiomyosarcoma

incidence of appendiceal tumors may be increasing from 0.63 to 0.97 per 100,000 persons; however, this may be a consequence of more selective appendectomy or more thorough pathologic evaluation [18, 19]. While many appendiceal neoplasms are not identified until the pathologist is examining the specimen, when noted in the operating room, an appendiceal mass requires thoughtful treatment about how to proceed.

Appendiceal neoplasms may be broadly classified into epithelial and non-epithelial tumors (Box 12.2). Epithelial tumors include mucinous or non-mucinous adenocarcinoma, low-grade appendiceal mucinous neoplasm, and signet ring carcinomas. Non-epithelial neoplasms include carcinoid tumors, lymphomas, leiomyomas, and leiomyosarcomas. Goblet cell carcinoids are mixed epithelial and non-epithelial neoplasms but with an adenocarcinoma phenotype. An additional feature common to epithelial tumors is associated mucin in the peritoneal cavity. When there is large-volume mucinous ascites, the clinical syndrome is referred to as pseudomyxoma peritonei; however, this is rarely an unexpected finding. Nevertheless, smaller areas of mucinous peritoneal implants, which were not identified on imaging, may be seen during surgery and should be evaluated for if there is a suspicion for an appendiceal neoplasm at exploration.

It is not always feasible to confirm malignancy at the time of surgery, even if there is mucin present on the serosa of the appendix or on the nearby or remote peritoneal surfaces. However, it is important to note whether the mass is at the tip of the appendix or at the base. The remainder of the peritoneal cavity must also be carefully surveyed to look for mucin or nodular lesions on the peritoneum, mesentery, or other organs.

[1] Mixed epithelial and non-epithelial neoplasms but with an adenocarcinoma phenotype.

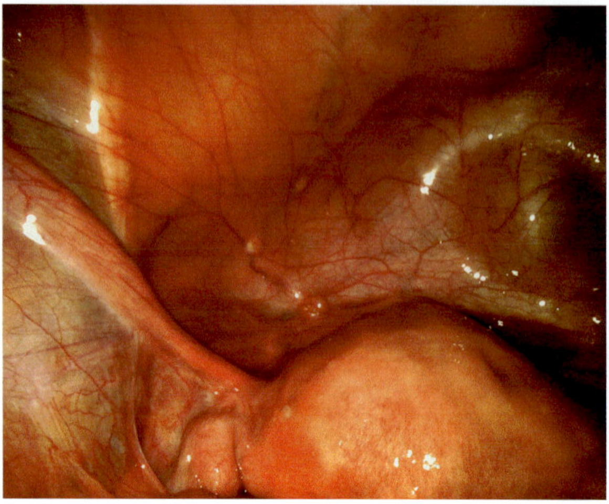

Fig. 12.1 Peritoneal implant

In general, the surgical approach to an unexpected appendiceal mass during a laparoscopy for presumed appendicitis should be as follows:

- Carefully inspect the pelvis, ovaries, both hemidiaphragms, liver, omentum, mesentery, and bowel serosa at the beginning of the operation accompanied by photo documentation and extensive sampling of suspicious or indeterminate peritoneal lesions in four quadrants (Fig. 12.1). These should be sent for permanent rather than frozen section as it may not be truly representative due to tumor heterogeneity. If it is not the practice of your hospital to routinely section the entire appendix, ensure that this is requested for this patient.
- When peritoneal disease is seen, avoid laparoscopic ports or incisions in the rectus muscle and keep in the midline if possible as incisional metastases may occur and are more difficult to manage off the midline.
- The goal of surgery in this setting is to address urgent symptoms/conditions related to the mass such as appendicitis or bowel obstruction. However, it is prudent to limit surgery to appendectomy and biopsy of peritoneal disease whenever possible as right colectomy, hysterectomy, or any organ resection may be unnecessary, in the setting of a benign mass, or may complicate future management, in the setting of malignancy [20].
- There is no absolute contraindication to laparoscopy for appendiceal tumors, and surgical approach should depend on surgeon experience. The tumor should not be directly grasped to avoid rupture.
- If the patient has not had completed cross-sectional imaging of abdomen and pelvis prior to surgery, this should be performed if malignancy is identified on final pathology. If preoperative ultrasound is suspicious for an appendiceal mass in the setting of appendicitis, obtaining cross-sectional imaging preoperatively may assist in decision-making.

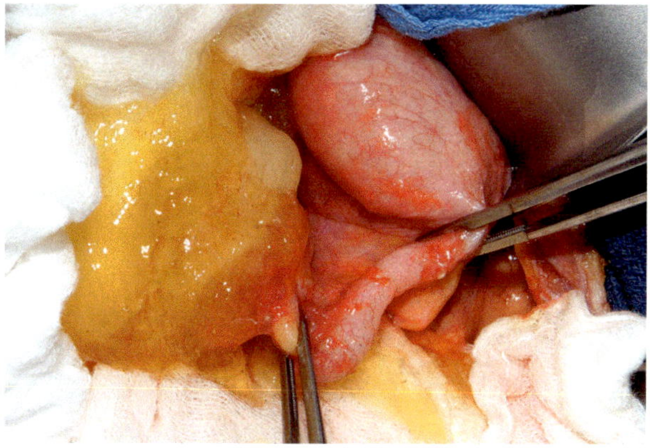

Fig. 12.2 Ruptured low-grade appendiceal mucinous neoplasm (LAMN) with peritoneal mucin

Appendiceal adenocarcinoma is a rare cancer with an estimated incidence of 2.6 per one million per year. These tumors are thought to arise from adenomas and are most commonly mucinous or intestinal type though some harbor a variety of elements. Mechanical rupture of these tumors does not necessarily lead to peritoneal metastases, and many will have established metastases prior to symptoms of rupture [21]. The typical pattern of metastasis is to the parietal and visceral peritoneum rather than along lymphatics, particularly in low-grade primary tumors [22]. However, the intestinal type is thought to progress along the adenoma to carcinoma sequence and is comparable to colon cancer, yet solid organ metastases are not common as initial site of metastatic disease [21]. Signet ring cell appendiceal adenocarcinoma is a particularly rare subset of mucinous adenocarcinoma. It is rarely confined at diagnosis and may infiltrate below mucosal surfaces. Unfortunately, the majority of appendiceal cancers may have spread at the time of diagnosis, though estimates vary greatly by series [17, 23–25]. Mucin may be found throughout the abdomen and easily visualized in more advanced cases (Fig. 12.2); in other situations, there may be small mucin deposits which are subtle and are only seen after meticulous inspection. For the low-grade lesions, right hemicolectomy typically does not play a role in staging as lymph node positivity rate may be as low as 5%; however, in higher-grade primary tumors, lymph nodes have been shown to be predictive of recurrence [22, 23]. As a result, given the uncertain nature of the disease at time of index surgery and the more extensive treatment that will likely be required particularly for many appendiceal cancers, right colectomy is best reserved for an elective operation after appropriate pathology review and patient counseling.

A low-grade appendiceal mucinous neoplasm (LAMN) is a well-differentiated tumor which grows slowly and tends to have a fibrotic, sometimes calcified appendiceal wall and is commonly described as a mucocele by radiologist; however, it is important to note that mucocele is not a pathologic diagnosis (Fig. 12.3). LAMNs may extrude mucin on the nearby serosal surfaces. When a mucinous lesion is suspected, it is important to avoid directly grasping it as it may rupture and increase the risk of subsequent recurrence within the peritoneal cavity if the mucin harbors neoplastic epithelium.

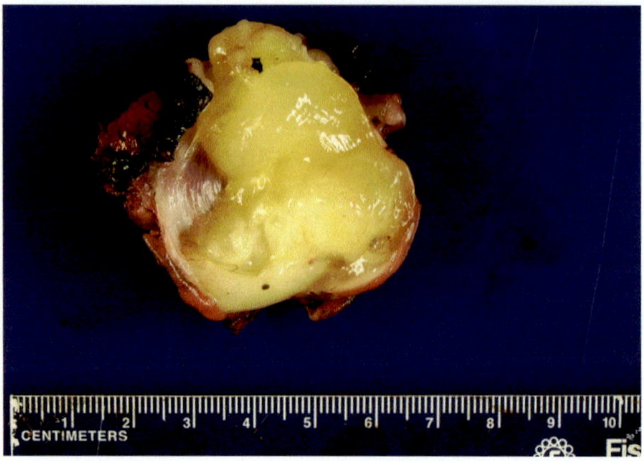

Fig. 12.3 Intact low-grade appendiceal mucinous neoplasm (LAMN) opened for pathologic examination

When LAMNs are confined to the mucosa of the appendix, as proven by complete sectioning of the appendix and careful examination of the peritoneum by imaging and during surgery, appendectomy with negative margins is curative, and no specific follow-up is necessary. However, when there is intramural or extra-appendiceal mucin present, further follow-up and, possibly, treatment are necessary. When the mucin is acellular and seen within the wall of the appendix or confined to the serosa of the appendix or periappendicular tissue, the entity is referred to as LAMN of uncertain malignant potential (UMP) and is associated with a 5% risk of subsequent recurrence. However, cellular mucin carries a higher risk of recurrence, and consideration of subsequent treatment at a specialty center should be given [26, 27]. Simple appendectomy is typically sufficient for diagnostic and therapeutic purpose for LAMN and LAMN/UMP. However, partial cecectomy or ileocecectomy is occasionally necessary to clear the margin for neoplastic tissue. Formal right colectomy is unnecessary as the initial treatment as most mucinous neoplasms seen on preoperative imaging do not harbor invasive cancer and are not at risk for lymph node metastases. Baseline serum tumor markers including CEA, CA-125, and CA19-9 may be useful for monitoring LAMN/UMP and can be drawn pre- and postoperatively if a LAMN is suspected. There are no formal guidelines for surveillance of LAMN/UMP; however, imaging and serum markers more frequently than once a year appear unnecessary given the low risk of recurrence and indolent course for those who recur.

While definitive management of appendiceal carcinoma may ultimately include right hemicolectomy and/or intraperitoneal chemotherapy (IPC), the most appropriate course of action upon recognizing this unexpected finding is to remove the appendix, biopsy suspected metastatic disease, and close without additional organ resection. Neither the surgeon nor the patient may be prepared for a more significant undertaking. If the next step in a patient's treatment involves systemic chemotherapy or cytoreductive surgery, a more extensive operation may delay initiation of that treatment. A right hemicolectomy alone does not provide any survival advantage over appendectomy alone in stage IV disease nor does it particularly help with

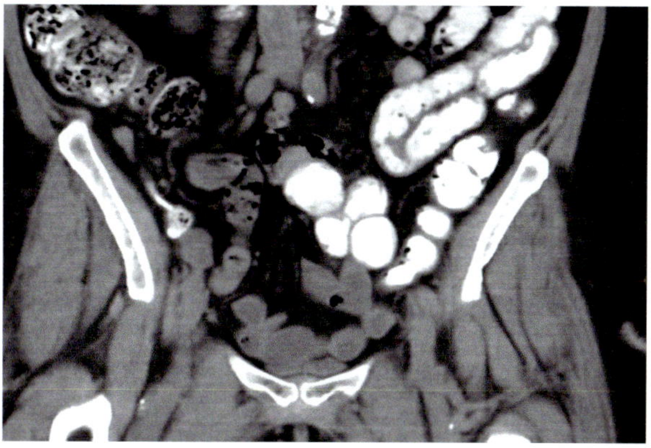

Fig. 12.4 Neoendocrine tumor (NET) on CT

staging in many cases [22, 28]. Furthermore, studies have suggested improved efficacy of IPC with a lower prior surgical score which is calculated based on extent of previous surgery [29]. Therefore, while it is certainly appropriate to remove the appendix and perform any other necessary biopsies, a more extensive right hemicolectomy is not warranted in most cases.

Carcinoid tumors, also known as neuroendocrine tumors (NET), of the appendix have an incidence of 0.15 per 100,000 per year (Fig. 12.4) [30, 31]. Approximately 75% occur at the tip of the appendix, 15% in the mid-appendix, and 10% at the base. Size is one of the critical features of staging for carcinoid tumor; fortunately the majority are less than 1 cm at the time of removal, and only 6% are more than 2 cm [32]. With increasing size, penetration of the appendiceal wall and infiltration of the mesoappendix become more likely. However, size is the most significant predictor of prognosis, rather than depth of invasion and lymphatic or perineural invasion. In a carcinoid <1 cm in size, lymph node metastases are rare. In tumors over 2 cm, the risk is approximately 20–30% [33]. Distant metastasis for appendiceal carcinoid is rare at diagnosis. In general, definitive management of non-metastatic appendiceal carcinoids >2 cm, those at the base or with positive margins, or those with adverse histologic features or radiologic evidence or locoregional nodal involvement is right hemicolectomy, though it is important to note that there are no data to address the benefit of this intervention. Nevertheless, pathologic diagnosis must be made; therefore, appendectomy alone is the first treatment. Once the diagnosis of appendiceal NET is made, workup including cross-sectional imaging should be performed. Octreotide scans and serum markers are unnecessary in the absence of symptoms consistent with metastatic disease, such as carcinoid syndrome. Staging right colectomy is recommended for tumors greater than 2 cm, and no specific follow-up is necessary for tumors less than 1.5 cm. The management of tumors between 1.5 and 2 cm after appendectomy remains controversial. The two largest series of appendiceal NET report no cases of lymph node metastases in patients with <2 cm tumors; however, there are only seven patients reported in case series with lymph node metastases and tumors <2 cm. [34–36] Though small bowel NET is associated with synchronous additional small bowel lesions, this has not been described in appendiceal NET.

Conclusions

When intraoperative findings do not match up to preoperative expectations, a thoughtful approach is required. The remainder of the abdomen must be examined if the appendix is normal to identify the etiology of the patients' symptoms. An abnormality that likely explains the clinical picture should be appropriately addressed; others such as epiploic appendicitis and some presentations of Crohn's disease do not require any intervention. The impulse to intervene because the operation is underway should be tempered by careful judgement about what might have been done differently if the correct diagnosis was apparent and the potential for harm. When a mass or mucin is encountered, the operation should be limited to appendectomy and biopsies to definitively stage the patient whenever possible. Patients will benefit from definitive pathology and preoperative planning if any further intervention is considered.

References

1. Sagar J, Kumar V, Shah DK. Meckel's diverticulum: a systematic review. J R Soc Med. 2006;99(10):501–5.
2. Levack MM, Fiedler AG, Kaafarani H, King DR. Perforation of a mesenteric Meckel's diverticulum. J Surg Case Rep. 2018;2018(6):rjy126.
3. Ezekian B, Leraas HJ, Englum BR, Gilmore BF, Reed C, Fitzgerald TN, et al. Outcomes of laparoscopic resection of Meckel's diverticulum are equivalent to open laparotomy. J Pediatr Surg. 2019;54(3):507–10.
4. Robinson JR, Correa H, Brinkman AS, Lovvorn HN. Optimizing surgical resection of the bleeding Meckel diverticulum in children. J Pediatr Surg. 2017;52(10):1610–5.
5. Park JJ, Wolff BG, Tollefson MK, Walsh EE, Larson DR. Meckel diverticulum: the Mayo Clinic experience with 1476 patients (1950-2002). Ann Surg. 2005;241(3):529–33.
6. Fang J-F, Chen R-J, Lin B-C, Hsu Y-B, Kao J-L, Chen M-F. Aggressive resection is indicated for cecal diverticulitis. Am J Surg. 2003;185(2):135–40.
7. Koshy RM, Abusabeib A, Al-Mudares S, Khairat M, Toro A, Di Carlo I. Intraoperative diagnosis of solitary cecal diverticulum not requiring surgery: is appendectomy indicated? World J Emerg Surg. 2016;11(1):1.
8. Connolly D, McGookin R, Gidwani A, Brown M. Inflamed solitary caecal diverticulum – it is not appendicitis, what should I do? Ann R Coll Surg Engl. 2006;88(7):672–4.
9. Cecal diverticulitis. In: Welch JP, Cohen JL, Sardella WV, Vignati PV, editors. Diverticular disease, management of the difficult surgical case. Baltimore: Williams and Watkins; 1998:428–441.
10. Hall J, Hammerich K, Roberts P. New paradigms in the management of diverticular disease. Curr Probl Surg. 2010;47(9):680–735.
11. Singh AK, Gervais DA, Hahn PF, Sagar P, Mueller PR, Novelline RA. Acute epiploic appendagitis and its mimics. Radiographics. 2005;25(6):1521–34.
12. Mollà E, Ripollés T, Martínez MJ, Morote V, Roselló-Sastre E. Primary epiploic appendagitis: US and CT findings. Eur Radiol. 1998;8(3):435–8.
13. Mitchell C, Prabhu M. Pelvic inflammatory Disease. Infect Dis Clin N Am. 2013;27(4):793–809.
14. Sharma H, Tal R, Clark N, Segars J. Microbiota and pelvic inflammatory disease. Semin Reprod Med. 2014;32(01):043–9.
15. Mausner Geffen E, Slywotzky C, Bennett G. Pitfalls and tips in the diagnosis of ectopic pregnancy. Abdom Radiol. 2017;42(5):1524–42.

16. Kirk E, Bottomley C, Bourne T. Diagnosing ectopic pregnancy and current concepts in the management of pregnancy of unknown location. Hum Reprod Update. 2014;20(2):250–61.
17. Benedix F, Reimer A, Gastinger I, Mroczkowski P, Lippert H, Kube R, et al. Primary appendiceal carcinoma – epidemiology, surgery and survival: results of a German multi-center study. Eur J Surg Oncol. 2010;36(8):763–71.
18. Whitfield CG, Amin SN, Garner JP. Surgical management of primary appendiceal malignancy. Color Dis. 2012;14(12):1507–11.
19. Overman MJ, Fournier K, Hu C-Y, Eng C, Taggart M, Royal R, et al. Improving the AJCC/TNM staging for adenocarcinomas of the appendix: the prognostic impact of histological grade. Ann Surg. 2013;257(6):1072–8.
20. Sugarbaker PH, Chang D. Results of treatment of 385 patients with peritoneal surface spread of appendiceal malignancy. Ann Surg Oncol. 1999;6(8):727–31.
21. Marmor S, Portschy PR, Tuttle TM, Virnig BA. The rise in appendiceal cancer incidence: 2000-2009. J Gastrointest Surg. 2015;19(4):743–50.
22. González-Moreno S, Sugarbaker PH. Right hemicolectomy does not confer a survival advantage in patients with mucinous carcinoma of the appendix and peritoneal seeding. Br J Surg. 2004;91(3):304–11.
23. Nash GM, Smith JD, Tang L, Weiser MR, Temple LK, O'Reilly E, et al. Lymph node metastasis predicts disease recurrence in a single-center experience of 70 stages 1–3 appendix cancers: a retrospective review. Ann Surg Oncol. 2015;22(11):3613–7.
24. Roy P, Chetty R. Goblet cell carcinoid tumors of the appendix: an overview. World J Gastrointest Oncol. 2010;2(6):251–8.
25. McGory ML, Maggard MA, Kang H, O'Connell JB, Ko CY. Malignancies of the appendix: beyond case series reports. Dis Colon Rectum. 2005;48(12):2264–71.
26. Yantiss RK, Shia J, Klimstra DS, Hahn HP, Odze RD, Misdraji J. Prognostic significance of localized extra-appendiceal mucin deposition in appendiceal mucinous neoplasms. Am J Surg Pathol. 2009;33(2):248–55.
27. Roxburgh CS, Fenig YM, Cercek A, Shia J, Rassam RM, Paty PB, et al. Outcomes of low-grade appendiceal mucinous neoplasms with remote acellular mucinous peritoneal deposits. Ann Surg Oncol. 2019;26(1):118–24.
28. Sugarbaker PH. When and when not to perform a right colon resection with mucinous appendiceal neoplasms. Ann Surg Oncol. 2017;24(3):729–32.
29. Paul BK, Ihemelandu C, Sugarbaker PH. Prior surgical score. Dis Colon Rectum. 2018;61(3):347–54.
30. Maggard MA, O'Connell JB, Ko CY. Updated population-based review of carcinoid tumors. Ann Surg. 2004;240(1):117–22.
31. Goede AC, Caplin ME, Winslet MC. Carcinoid tumour of the appendix. Br J Surg. 2003;90(11):1317–22.
32. Komminoth P, Arnold R, Capella C, Klimstra DS, Klöppel G, Solcia E, et al. Neuroendocrine neoplasms of the appendix. In: Bosman FT, Carneiro F, Hruban RH, Theise ND, editors. WHO classification of tumors of the digestive system (IARC WHO classification of tumours). 4th ed. Lyon: IARC Press; 2010.
33. Spanos CP, Kaiser AM. Appendiceal neoplasms. In: Steele SR, Hull TL, Read TE, Saclarides TJ, Senagore AJ, Whitlow CB, editors. The ASCRS textbook of colon and rectal surgery. 3rd ed. Cham: Springer International Publishing; 2016.
34. Moertel CG, Weiland LH, Nagorney DM, Dockerty MB. Carcinoid tumor of the appendix: treatment and prognosis. N Engl J Med. 1987;317(27):1699–701.
35. Roggo A, Wood WC, Ottinger LW. Carcinoid tumors of the appendix. Ann Surg. 1993;217(4):385–90.
36. Thirlby RC, Kasper CS, Jones RC. Metastatic carcinoid tumor of the appendix. Report of a case and review of the literature. Dis Colon Rectum. 1984;27(1):42–6.

Laparoscopic Right Colectomy for Malignant Disease

13

Hermann Kessler and Jeremy M. Lipman

Introduction and Rationale

Laparoscopic right hemicolectomy is oncologically effective for malignant disease and associated with improved patient outcomes when compared to open operations [1, 2]. This approach has therefore become an important tool in the arsenal of surgeons who perform right colon resections. Compared with an open approach, minimally invasive surgery has been associated with reduced length of hospital stay, faster return to work, earlier normalization of diet, decreased perioperative pain, improved cosmesis, lower incidence of incisional hernia, lower narcotic utilization, decreased transfusion requirement, and improved quality of life.

Laparoscopic right hemicolectomy was first described in the early 1990s following the success of laparoscopic cholecystectomy [3, 4]. The initial reports of the procedure utilized between four and six laparoscopic trocars to perform a lateral-to-medial mobilization and intracorporeal mesenteric ligation; however, the anastomosis was performed extracorporeally. The variation of a hand-assisted laparoscopic surgery (HALS) approach showed equivalent short- and long-term recovery and oncological outcomes when compared with traditional laparoscopic surgery, but longer operative times were reported for hand-assisted laparoscopic surgery [5]. Even for those surgeons who prefer straight laparoscopy for a right colectomy, the hand-assisted approach can be an excellent adjunct to prevent conversion to laparotomy.

H. Kessler (✉)
Cleveland Clinic, Department of Colorectal Surgery, Cleveland, OH, USA
e-mail: kessleh@ccf.org

J. M. Lipman
Cleveland Clinic, Lerner College of Medicine of Case Western Reserve University, Cleveland, OH, USA

P. Sylla et al. (eds.), *The SAGES Manual of Colorectal Surgery*,
https://doi.org/10.1007/978-3-030-24812-3_13

Over time, the laparoscopic dissection technique has evolved. The medial-to-lateral dissection gained acceptance and was increasingly favored based on shorter operative times, improved exposure, and equivalent oncologic outcomes when compared with a lateral-to-medial dissection [6, 7].

Adhering to the basic principles of oncologic resection, single-incision laparoscopic approaches have been employed. Single-incision right colectomy claimed improved cosmetic results, while it was shown to have equivalent operative times and blood loss when compared to traditional laparoscopic resection [8]. A large randomized controlled trial comparing single-incision and multi-port laparoscopy for colon resection suggested that the cosmetic result was only improved for those undergoing a truly single-incision resection [9]. The single-incision approach therefore remains a viable option for patients who desire the best possible cosmetic result.

The most recent evolution to minimally invasive right colectomy is robotic surgery. A randomized controlled trial comparing the robotic to traditional laparoscopic approach found similar oncologic results and short- and long-term outcomes. However, longer operative times and increased cost lead some to question its role for right-sided colon cancer [10]. The robot, however, offers opportunities for advanced minimally invasive techniques even for right colectomy, e.g., facilitating performance of an intracorporeal anastomosis (ICA). Data suggest that robotic right hemicolectomy with ICA may result in a shorter time to return of bowel function and decreased overall incision length, at the cost of higher expense and longer operative times [11]. For more details on techniques and results, please refer to the chapters on robotic right-sided colon resection (Chap. 15) and options for ileocolonic reconstruction (Chap. 14).

In the current chapter, the oncologic principles of a right hemicolectomy performed for malignancy will be reviewed, with emphasis on complete mesocolic excision (CME) and laparoscopic techniques.

Indications and Contraindications

Laparoscopic right hemicolectomy is an appropriate operation for the majority of right-sided colon malignancies [12]. Several well-designed, large, multinational, randomized controlled trials have shown mostly equivalent oncologic outcomes for laparoscopic and open approaches to right-sided colon cancers [13–16]. The non-inferiority of oncologic outcomes, coupled with decreased length of hospital stay, wound complication rates, blood loss, and time to return of work, have led most surgeons to view this as a safe and effective technique for managing right-sided colon cancers.

Care must be taken to assure that the laparoscopic operation accomplishes the same dissection as a laparotomy. Regardless of the pathology or the technical experience of the surgeon, an appropriate oncologic resection must be achieved in the end.

Careful patient selection is important to identify those who are appropriate for a laparoscopic resection. In particular, tumors invading the abdominal wall or other organs can pose significant technical challenges to a laparoscopic resection and may be better suited to a laparotomy. Likewise, perforated tumors with extensive adjacent inflammatory changes present a unique challenge in pursuit of an R0 resection. These patients carry a high risk for peritoneal recurrence and therefore warrant meticulous attention to assure a complete resection [17]. Perforated tumors may also result in sepsis, and the hemodynamic instability may be exacerbated with the creation of CO_2 pneumoperitoneum, possibly as a result of decreased venous return from gas compression of the inferior vena cava. Active communication with the anesthesiology team is essential in such cases.

Patients presenting with obstructing right-sided colon cancers may not be amenable to a laparoscopic resection due to poor visualization from dilated bowel if their ileocecal valve is incompetent. These patients are also at high risk for dehydration and benefit from fluid resuscitation prior to operation.

Principles and Quality Benchmarks

The key benchmarks are the oncologic outcomes of patients and the quality of the resection. The tumor must be resected to include at least 5 cm negative margins and the entire lymphovascular drainage system [18]. The arterial supply to the portion of colon containing the tumor should be excised at the takeoff of its feeding vessel.

The importance of total mesorectal excision has been well described for rectal cancer. Extrapolating from this, the concepts of complete mesocolic excision (CME) and central vascular ligation (CVL) have evolved in the treatment of right-sided colon malignancies. For tumors in the cecum and ascending colon, the ileocolic artery (and if present the right colic artery) should be divided at the takeoff from the superior mesenteric artery. While for these tumors the trunk of the middle colic artery does not need to be divided, the right branch of the middle colic artery should be ligated. The colon should be divided at the level of the middle colic artery [19, 20]. This will assure a complete lymphovascular en bloc excision which must achieve a minimum of 12 lymph nodes in the specimen, as the patient's survival may otherwise be negatively impacted [21]. For more details on this topic, please refer to Chap. 11 on principles of complete mesocolic excision (CME) for colon cancer.

Conversion to an open operation should never be viewed as a complication and should be undertaken whenever the safety or effectiveness of a laparoscopic resection is in doubt. As was noted above, the addition of a hand port may allow for preservation of the minimally invasive advantages while avoiding a conversion to full laparotomy. In a recent meta-analysis, a conversion rate of 2–13% was reported from comparable studies of laparoscopic right hemicolectomy [22]. Individual surgeons should be encouraged to follow their conversion rates and to be cognizant if higher than expected.

Preoperative Planning, Patient Work-Up, and Optimization

Preoperative planning for a laparoscopic right hemicolectomy for malignancy should begin with appropriate staging. This should include a CT scan of the chest, abdomen, and pelvis to ensure that no metastatic disease is present. Complete blood count (CBC), serum chemistry, and carcinoembryonic antigen (CEA) level are also recommended by the National Comprehensive Cancer Network (NCCN) as part of the initial cancer staging [23]. A complete colonoscopy is also recommended, as synchronous lesions are not infrequent and may change the operative plan.

Endoscopic tattooing of the lesion is useful in patients planned for laparoscopic right hemicolectomy. Misidentification of the segment of colon in which a lesion sits occurs around 20% of the time after colonoscopy [24]. As such, it is imperative to assure accurate localization of the involved colon segment prior to resection. Laparoscopic colectomy does not provide much tactile feedback about the colon, and visualization is limited to the serosa. Therefore, a colonoscope should be available in the operating room to permit on-table localization if needed.

A preoperative mechanical bowel preparation with antibiotics has been shown to reduce the incidence of anastomotic leak, surgical site infection, and ileus [25, 26]. Many combinations of antibiotics and mechanical preparation agents exist, though none have yet been reported superior to another. It does seem clear, however, that bowel preparation alone without antibiotics is not sufficient to achieve these improved outcomes [27]. For more details on this topic, please refer to Chaps. 7 and 8 on enhanced recovery protocols in colorectal surgery.

Operative Setup

The patient is placed under general anesthesia, ideally in an OR that is specially equipped for minimally invasive procedures. At least two monitors should be available, one on each side of the patient. A 10-mm laparoscopic camera with a 30-degree optical system is ideal. The patient may be positioned modified-lithotomy or split-leg to facilitate hepatic flexure mobilization from between the legs if needed. The anus needs to remain easily accessible in the event intraoperative endoscopy is required. The patient's abdomen is disinfected and draped.

Operative Technique: Surgical Steps, Medial-to-Lateral Approach

For an open access, a vertical 1.5-cm midline incision is made near the umbilicus, and the abdominal cavity is opened stepwise using retractors and Kocher clamps. A 12-mm Hasson trocar is inserted. Pneumoperitoneum is created with a pressure of 12-mm Hg. Two 5-mm trocars are placed on the left in the upper and lower quadrants. An additional port on the right may be added to facilitate dissection. A diagnostic laparoscopy is performed for staging purposes to localize the tumor and inspect the entire abdominal cavity for distant metastases.

The patient's right side is now tilted up and in Trendelenburg position. This way the right colon is exposed. A medial-to-lateral dissection is often easier and strongly recommended. Dissection starts by incising the peritoneum anterior to the right iliac artery and inferior to the terminal ileum to enter both planes of Gerota's fascia and start dissecting them from each other. This guarantees preservation of the mesocolic plane. The incision should be enlarged medially toward the mesenteric root (Fig. 13.1) and lateral toward the cecum (Fig. 13.2). Careful mobilization is now continued cephalad, laterally and medially to separate both planes of Gerota's fascia toward the right transverse colon, the hepatic flexure, and the ascending colon and mobilize the duodenum and the pancreatic head posteriorly (Fig. 13.3). This dissection effectively creates a blind-ending retroperitoneal tunnel below the right mesocolon.

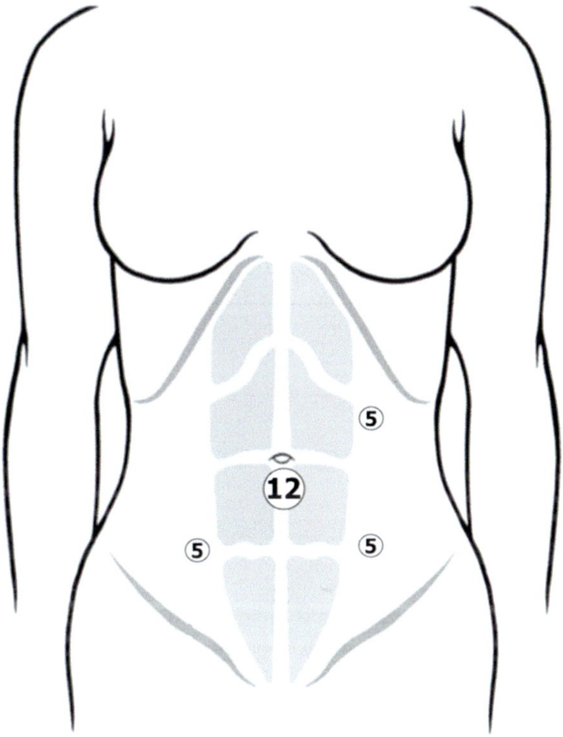

Fig. 13.1 Trocar positions, numbers indicate trocar sizes in mm

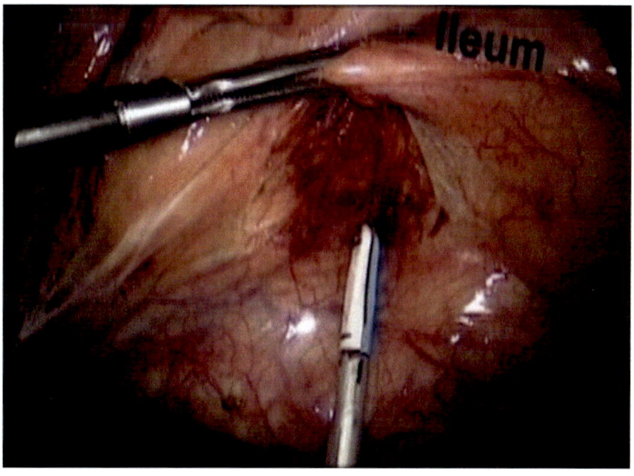

Fig. 13.2 Opening of the peritoneum below the ileocolic vascular bundle

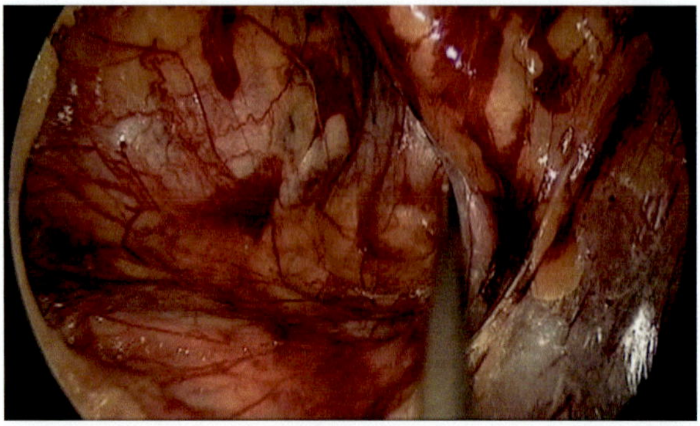

Fig. 13.3 Medial-to-lateral dissection posterior to the right mesocolon and anterior to Gerota's fascia

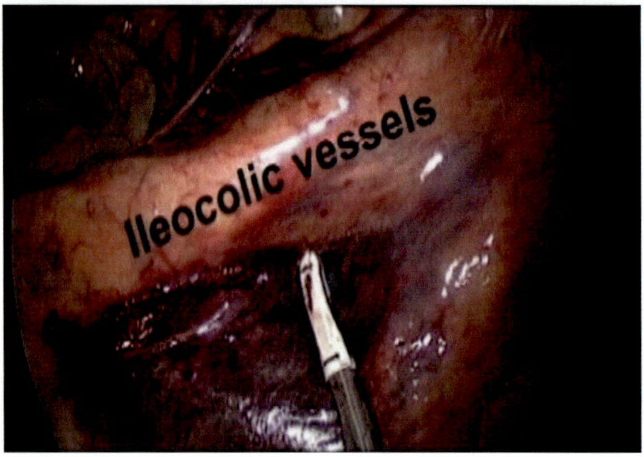

Fig. 13.4 Beginning of medial-to-lateral dissection, with opening of the peritoneum below the ileocolic vascular bundle

Lateral mobilization is now facilitated. This portion of the dissection starts around the cecum and the appendix (Fig. 13.4), and then gradually the lateral suspension of the ascending colon is taken down. Hepatic flexure mobilization is completed by taking down its suspension toward the fatty tissue around the right kidney and the retroperitoneum below the liver. The omentum is gradually taken down until the central transverse colon is reached.

The ileocolic vascular bundle (Fig. 13.5) is exposed by lifting it up laterally close to the cecum. An incision is made medially below it, and a connection is created toward the previously created blind ending located posteriorly. The peritoneum is further incised below the ileocolic vessels toward their origin. The superior mesenteric vein (SMV) is identified and dissected for further central lymph node harvest (Fig. 13.6). The origin of the ileocolic vessels is identified, skeletonized, and divided with the laparoscopic energy device, a laparoscopic stapler or clips. The dissection continues cephalad along the SMV. In a minority of cases, a true right colic artery (Fig. 13.7), originating from the superior mesenteric artery (SMA), is identified and similarly divided. Further central dissection will lead toward the gastrocolic trunk

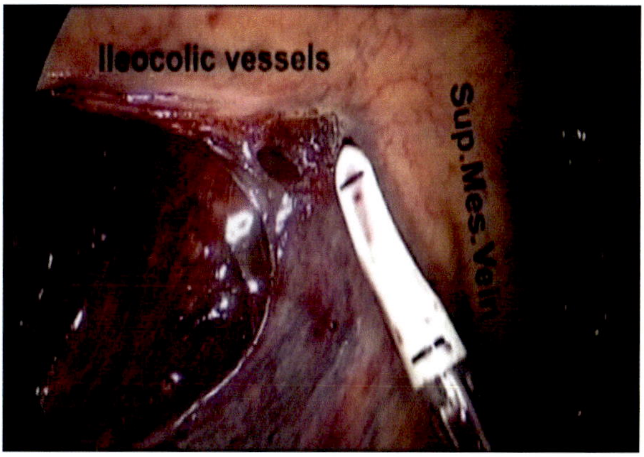

Fig. 13.5 Medial-to-lateral dissection, approaching the superior mesenteric vein

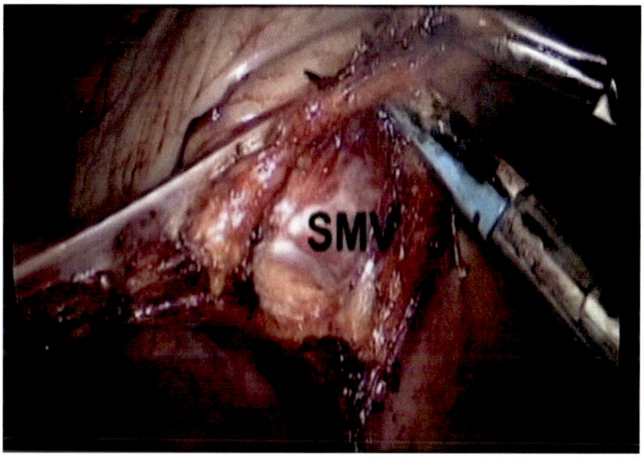

Fig. 13.6 Identification and dissection of superior mesenteric vein

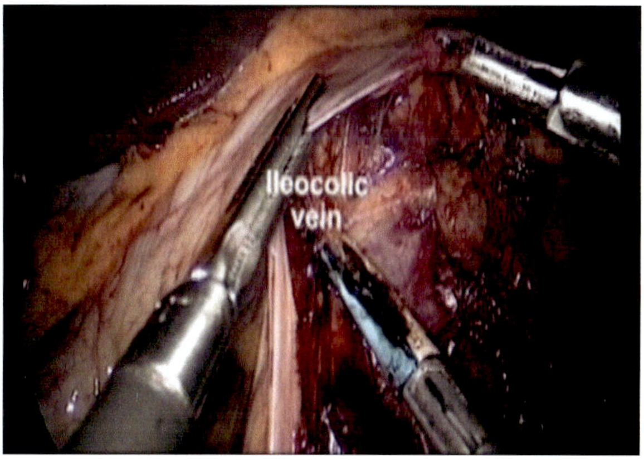

Fig. 13.7 Identification and dissection of superior mesenteric vein

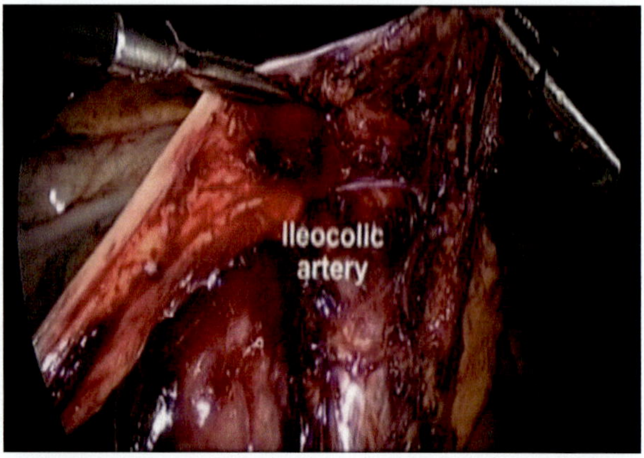

Fig. 13.8 Identification and dissection of ileocolic artery

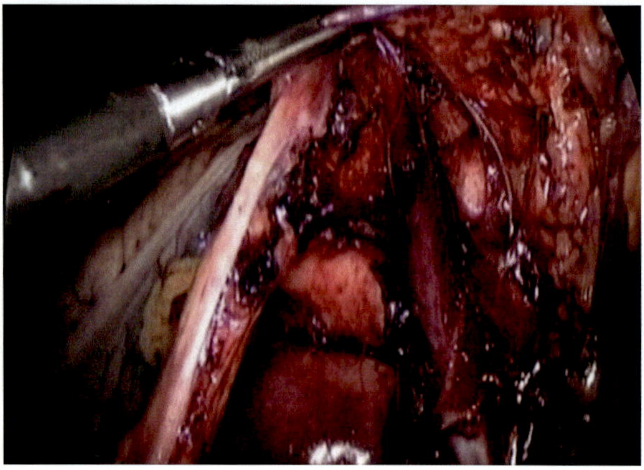

Fig. 13.9 Identification and dissection gastrocolic trunk of Henle

of Henle (Fig. 13.8) where anatomic variations are frequent. In most cases, the right colic vein, superior right colic vein, and right gastroepiploic vein form this trunk, but they may also have separate origins from the SMV. The trunk or the individual veins are sealed and transected centrally. Next, the middle colic vein and artery (Fig. 13.9) are identified. The SMA normally runs posteriorly toward the anatomical left side of the SMV in this region. Central dissection continues along the middle colic vein and artery toward the right branches of both vessels (Fig. 13.10). They are also sealed and transected centrally. The transverse mesocolon may be further transected distally to facilitate mobilization if needed. At this point the central dissection is complete (Fig. 13.11). The bowel is grasped close to the cecum using a laparoscopic bowel grasper. The right ureter stays behind the anterior peritoneal envelope which is never injured or dissected and may be visualized in skinny patients easily.

In laparoscopic right colectomy with extracorporeal anastomosis (ECA), the camera trocar is removed, and a periumbilical incision is made around the left side of the umbilicus to create a mini-laparotomy. A 4- or 5-cm incision is typically adequate. A wound protector is placed, and the mobilized right colon is

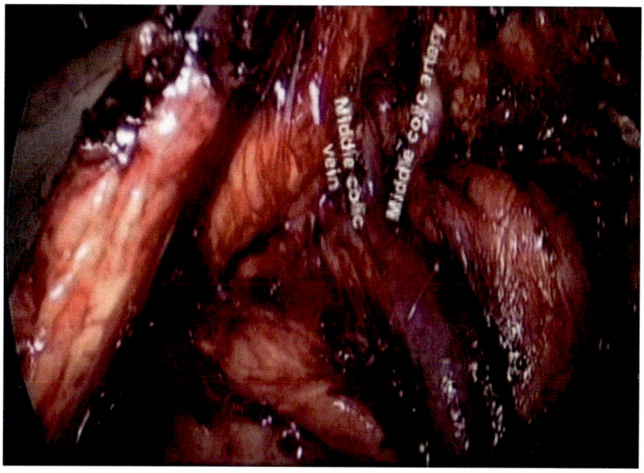

Fig. 13.10 Middle colic trunk

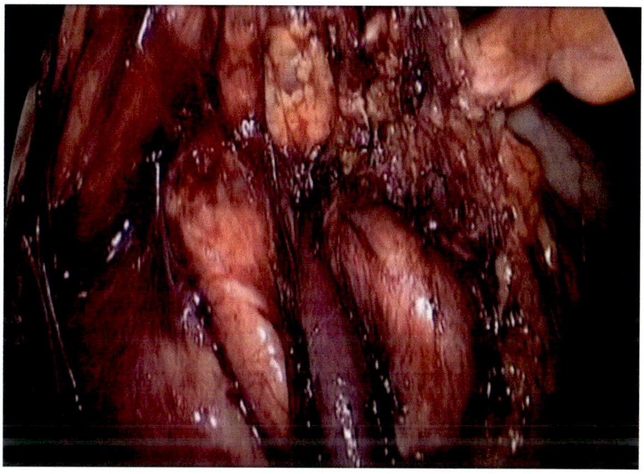

Fig. 13.11 Completion of central vascular dissection. (**a**) Middle colic vein. (**b**) Middle colic artery. (**c**) Pancreas

exteriorized. Alternative extraction sites would be the right lower abdominal trocar site (transverse incision) or a Pfannenstiel incision which may bear a lower risk of hernias, but both alternatives would demand a more comprehensive mobilization of the transverse colon for optimal reach to create a tension-free anastomosis.

Alternatively, laparoscopic right colectomy can be combined with intracorporeal anastomosis (ICA), which facilitates specimen extraction through a Pfannenstiel incision, since extensive mobilization of the transverse colon and terminal ileum is not needed. For detailed techniques of ECA and ICA during laparoscopic and robotic right colectomy, please refer to the chapters on options for ileocolonic reconstruction (Chap. 14) and robotic right-sided colon resection (Chap. 15), respectively.

The position of the tumor is verified by careful palpation. Mesenteric transection is completed toward the ileum and transverse colon at the sites of planned transection. The bowel is divided using a linear stapler. Photo documentation of the specimen may be performed with a ruler next to it. The central transection areas of the major vessels may be marked using sutures of different colors based on institutional availability. The ileocolic anastomosis is performed with proper orientation of the ileum and colon. The oncologic principles of conventional surgery do not change as the omentum is taken off the right transverse colon in cancers proximally to the hepatic flexure and taken along en bloc with the specimen in tumors of the hepatic flexure and right transverse colon.

Operative Technique: Comparison with Lateral-to-Medial Approach

The technique of creating a retroperitoneal tunnel in the medial-to-lateral approach offers several advantages such as a minimized risk of injury to the retroperitoneal envelope which covers the right ureter and the gonadal vessels. Furthermore, the named arteries are clearly visible posteriorly at their origins, and they may be ligated early, proximally, and safely to minimize the risk of bleeding and keeping the small intestine out of the operative field; an early proximal ligation of the mesenteric vessels (observation of no-touch isolation technique) is achieved. By leaving the lateral attachments of the colon intact until the mesenteric division has been carried out, important natural anatomic countertraction is applied to the bowel as the mesentery and bowel are mobilized. Colectomy is facilitated by leaving the lateral attachments intact, and the described anatomic landmarks are highlighted clearly. Only minimal manipulation of the tumor-bearing colon is needed, as most of the colon mobilization and dissection of the mesentery are accomplished before the cecum and ascending colon are freed from their lateral attachments (no-touch isolation technique).

In a lateral-to-medial approach, the tumor-bearing colon is mobilized first. The lateral dissection is started by elevating the colon on its vascular pedicle, and then both planes of Gerota's fascia must be entered laterally and dissected apart from each other. The mesenteric and vascular division is the same as in a medial-to-lateral approach with respect to the principles of CME. The vessels are ligated intra- or extracorporeally in a second step; however, it must be ensured that the superior mesenteric vessels and the origins of the mesenteric vessels are clearly identified and divided at their origins. An assistant has to pull on the tumor-bearing bowel to create traction and countertraction for central exposure of the mesentery and avoid the risk of tearing the colon and mesentery. It is important to note that the mobilized colon and small bowel become more difficult to manage laparoscopic surgery relative to open surgery.

Pitfalls and Troubleshooting

For carcinomas of the hepatic flexure and right transverse colon, an extended right hemicolectomy is indicated. The omentum is not dissected off the colon, but the dissection is continued along the lower edge of the duodenum toward the right aspect of the greater curvature of the stomach. The gastrocolic ligament is transected at the left transverse colon. The middle colic vein and artery are dissected and transected centrally at the level of the SMV and SMA to assure a complete lymphovascular resection. The right branches of the middle colic vessels are also divided. In patients where a tension-free anastomosis may be challenging, such as those who are obese, splenic flexure mobilization in combination with further takedown of the omentum may be beneficial as well as a total laparoscopic approach with intraabdominal bowel transection and creation of an intracorporeal ileocolonic anastomosis (ICA) to avoid tension from an extracorporeal approach (ECA).

In obese patients, the landmarks of dissection are more difficult to find, especially the SMV. In such cases, a laparoscopic lateral-to-medial approach may provide improved exposure. In particularly challenging cases, the laparoscopic colon mobilization may be followed by central mesocolic and lymph node dissection in an open technique through a relatively short midline incision.

If the tumor has not been tattooed and cannot be identified at exploration, intraoperative colonoscopy may be necessary. CO_2 insufflation should be used to minimize dilatation of the colon that will hinder further laparoscopic dissection. If the tumor cannot be localized laparoscopically or endoscopically, conversion to laparotomy and careful palpation of the colon may be necessary. As pointed out previously, a conversion to a hand-assisted approach can facilitate medial-to-lateral mobilization, especially in reoperative and obese cases.

The most frequently described intraoperative complication is bleeding. In order to avoid any vascular injury which may be hazardous especially with SMV, SMA, and middle colic vessels, a very slow and meticulous dissection technique is imperative. The laparoscopic energy devices and instruments used for dissection should be carefully observed to avoid contact with vessels. Especially in obese patients, the visualization may be difficult, and the threshold for conversion should be kept very low. As explained above, in a medial-to-lateral approach, the risk of injury to adjacent organs is low: duodenal adhesions by small ligaments toward the posterior mesocolon should be taken down cautiously. The same applies to adhesions between the pancreatic head and the mesocolon. In cases of previous pancreatitis with firm adhesions, conversion is recommended. The ureter normally stays safely below the surface of the retroperitoneal envelope; whenever possible it should be visualized.

If against expectations from preoperative staging by CT scans a T4 tumor is found at exploration, conversion to open approach for planned en bloc resection is recommended.

There are no data of the learning curve in oncologic laparoscopic right hemicolectomy. However, when possible, the technique of CME should be mastered first in the context of open surgery to better understand variations in the relevant anatomy Also, the laparoscopic expertise required to perform these cases should be advanced, and it may be helpful to practice the procedure first in benign cases, especially adenomas. The retroperitoneal tunnel approach has advantages also when applied in Crohn's disease and may be practiced in such cases first to gain confidence and become familiar with the technique.

Outcomes

Numerous retrospective studies have shown that a laparoscopic oncologic approach for right colon cancer has results comparable to that of open procedures [28] (Table 13.1). The laparoscopic approach to right hemicolectomy, specifically, has

Table 13.1 Studies comparing results of laparoscopic oncologic right hemicolectomy

Author	Year	Country	Study	Patients	Surgery	Lymph nodes harvested	R0 resection	Locoregional recurrences	Systemic recurrence	OS	DFS	DSS
Ozben [28]	2019	Turkey	Retrospective	37 robotic CME	Right colectomy	40 (22–65)	100%	□	□	□	□	□
Siani [29]	2017	Italy	Retrospective	600 lap CME	Right colectomy	27 ± 3	94.5%	6.8%	22.7%	87% (5 years)	78.3% (5 years)	79.5% (5 years)
Wu [30]	2017	China	Retrospective	31 hand-assist CME	Right colectomy	34 (18–91)	□	□	□	□	□	□
Wang [31]	2017	China	Retrospective	172 lap CME	Right colectomy	23.3 ± 9.2		□	□	69.1% (3 years)	81.7% (3 years)	□
Huang [32]	2015	China	Retrospective	53 lap CME 49 open CME	Right colectomy	14 ± 6/13 ± 5 $p = 0.313$	□	0 (2 years)	0 (2 years)	□	□	□
Bae [33]	2014	Korea	Retrospective	128 lap CME 137 open CME	Right colectomy	27 (8–62)/28 (8–79) $p = 337$	□	1.5%/3.6% No difference	6.2%/8.7% No difference	77.8%/90.3% $p = 0.028$ (5 years)	71.8%/83.3% $p = 0.578$ (5 years)	□
Kang [34]	2014	Korea	Retrospective	128 lap CME	Right colectomy	28 (3–88)	□	0	5.4%	□	□	□
Adamina [35]	2012	United States	Retrospective	52 lap CME	Right colectomy	22 (18–29)	100%	0	7.6%	38 (23–54) months	37 (22–46) months	□

Refs. [29–35]

been shown equivalent to the open approach with regard to key oncologic outcome measures. These include the ability to obtain R0 resection with negative resection margins, disease-free and overall survival, lymph node harvest, and incidence of local and systemic recurrence. With experience, some would argue the laparoscopic view provides an advantage over open resection regarding lymph node harvest. With the magnified view provided by the laparoscopic camera, surgical planes can be visualized and dissected with more accuracy and less trauma to surrounding structures.

Conclusions

Laparoscopic right hemicolectomy for malignant disease is a procedure with standardized setup, equipment, and surgical steps leading to short- and long-term results equivalent to open surgery. The principles of high vascular ligation and preservation of the mesocolic planes need to be respected. A low threshold for conversion in challenging cases will keep complication rates low.

References

1. Lacy AM, García-Valdecasas JC, Delgado S, Castells A, Taurá P, Piqué JM, et al. Laparoscopy-assisted colectomy versus open colectomy for treatment of non-metastatic colon cancer: a randomised trial. Lancet. 2002;359(9325):2224–9.
2. McCombie AM, Frizelle F, Bagshaw PF, Frampton CM, Hewett PJ, McMurrick PJ, et al. The ALCCaS trial: a randomized controlled trial comparing quality of life following laparoscopic versus open colectomy for colon cancer. Dis Colon Rectum. 2018;61(10):1156–62.
3. Schlinkert RT. Laparoscopic-assisted right hemicolectomy. Dis Colon Rectum. 1991 Nov;34(11):1030–1.
4. Jacobs M, Verdeja JC, Goldstein HS. Minimally invasive colon resection (laparoscopic colectomy). Surg Laparosc Endosc. 1991;1(3):144–50.
5. Chung CC, Ng DCK, Tsang WWC, Tang WL, Yau KKK, Cheung HYS, et al. Hand-assisted laparoscopic versus open right colectomy: a randomized controlled trial. Ann Surg. 2007;246(5):728–33.
6. Liang JT, Lai HS, Lee PH. Laparoscopic medial-to-lateral approach for the curative resection of right-sided colon cancer. Ann Surg Oncol. 2007;14(6):1878–9.
7. Rotholtz NA, Bun ME, Tessio M, Lencinas SM, Laporte M, Aued ML, et al. Laparoscopic colectomy: medial versus lateral approach. Surg Laparosc Endosc. 2009;19(1):43–7.
8. Remzi FH, Kirat HT, Kaouk JH, Geisler DP. Single-port laparoscopy in colorectal surgery. Color Dis. 2008;10(8):823–6.
9. Maggiori L, Tuech JJ, Cotte E, Lelong B, Denost Q, Karoui M, et al. Single-incision laparoscopy versus multiport laparoscopy for colonic surgery: a multicenter, double-blinded, randomized controlled trial. Ann Surg. 2018;268(5):740–6.
10. Park JS, Choi GS, Park SY, Kim HJ, Ryuk JP. Randomized clinical trial of robot-assisted versus standard laparoscopic right colectomy. Br J Surg. 2012;99(9):1219–26.
11. Akram WM, Al-Natour RH, Albright J, Wu J, Ferraro J, Shanker B-A, et al. A propensity score-matched comparison of intracorporeal and extracorporeal techniques for robotic-assisted right colectomy in an enhanced recovery pathway. The American Journal of Surgery 2018. 2018 Dec;216(6):1095–100.

12. Vogel JD, Eskicioglu C, Weiser MR, Feingold DL, Steele SR. The American society of colon and rectal surgeons clinical practice guidelines for the treatment of colon cancer. Dis Colon Rectum. 2017;60(10):999–1017.
13. COST. A comparison of laparoscopically assisted and open colectomy for colon cancer. N Engl J Med. 2004;350(20):2050–9.
14. Fleshman J, Sargent DJ, Green E, Anvari M, Stryker SJ, Beart RW, et al. Laparoscopic colectomy for cancer is not inferior to open surgery based on 5-year data from the COST Study Group trial. Ann Surg. 2007;246(4):655–62.
15. Green BL, Marshall HC, Collinson F, Quirke P, Guillou P, Jayne DG, et al. Long-term follow-up of the Medical Research Council CLASICC trial of conventional versus laparoscopically assisted resection in colorectal cancer. Br J Surg. 2013;100(1):75–82.
16. Kuhry E, Schwenk WF, Gaupset R, Romild U, Bonjer HJ. Long-term results of laparoscopic colorectal cancer resection. Cochrane Database Syst Rev. 2008;(2):CD003432.
17. Asano H, Kojima K, Ogino N, Fukano H, Ohara Y, Shinozuka N. Postoperative recurrence and risk factors of colorectal cancer perforation. Int J Color Dis. 2017;32(3):419–24.
18. Paquette IM, Varma M, Ternent C, Melton-Meaux G, Rafferty JF, Feingold D, et al. The American Society of Colon and Rectal Surgeons' clinical practice guideline for the evaluation and management of constipation. Dis Colon Rectum. 2016;59(6):479–92.
19. Hohenberger W, Weber K, Matzel K, Papadopoulos T, Merkel S. Standardized surgery for colonic cancer: complete mesocolic excision and central ligation – technical notes and outcome. Color Dis. 2009;11(4):354–64.
20. Kim NK, Kim YW, Han YD, Cho MS, Hur H, Min BS, et al. Complete mesocolic excision and central vascular ligation for colon cancer: principle, anatomy, surgical technique, and outcomes. Surg Oncol. 2016;25(3):252–62.
21. Chang GJ, Rodriguez-Bigas MA, Skibber JM, Moyer VA. Lymph node evaluation and survival after curative resection of colon cancer: systematic review. J Natl Cancer Inst. 2007;99(6):433–41.
22. Wang G, Zhou J, Sheng W, Dong M. Hand-assisted laparoscopic surgery versus laparoscopic right colectomy: a meta-analysis. World J Surg Oncol. 2017;15(1):215.
23. NCCN. NCCN Guidelines Version 3.2018. Colon cancer. Retrieved 1 Oct 2018. From https://www.nccn.org/professionals/physician_gls/pdf/colon.pdf.
24. Offermans T, Vogelaar FJ, Aquarius M, Janssen-Heijnen MLG, Simons PCG. Preoperative segmental localization of colorectal carcinoma: CT colonography vs. optical colonoscopy. Eur J Surg Oncol. 2017;43(11):2105–11.
25. Klinger AL, Green H, Monlezun DJ, Beck D, Kann B, Vargas HD. The role of bowel preparation in colorectal surgery. Ann Surg. 2019 Apr;269(4):671–7.
26. Kiran RP, Murray ACA, Chiuzan C, Estrada D, Forde K. Combined preoperative mechanical bowel preparation with oral antibiotics significantly reduces surgical site infection, anastomotic leak, and ileus after colorectal surgery. Ann Surg. 2015;262(3):416–23.
27. Koller SE, Bauer KW, Egleston BL, Smith R, Philp MM, Ross HM, et al. Comparative effectiveness and risks of bowel preparation before elective colorectal surgery. Ann Surg. 2018;267(4):734–42.
28. Ozben V, Aytac E, Atasoy D, Erenler Bayraktar I, Bayraktar O, Sapci I, et al. Totally robotic complete mesocolic excision for right-sided colon cancer. J Robot Surg. 2019 Feb;13(1):107–14.
29. Siani LM, Lucchi A, Berti P, Garulli G. Laparoscopic complete mesocolic excision with central vascular ligation in 600 right total mesocolectomies: Safety, prognostic factors and oncologic outcome. Am J Surg. 2017;214(2):222–7.
30. Wu QB, Deng XB, Yang XY, Chen BC, He WB, Hu T, et al. Hand-assisted laparoscopic right hemicolectomy with complete mesocolic excision and central vascular ligation: a novel technique for right colon cancer. Surg Endosc Other Interv Tech. 2017;31(8):3383–90.
31. Wang Y, Zhang C, Zhang D, Fu Z, Sun Y. Clinical outcome of laparoscopic complete mesocolic excision in the treatment of right colon cancer. World J Surg Oncol. 2017;15(1):1–6.

32. Huang JL, Wei HB, Fang J, Zheng ZH, Chen TF, Wei B, et al. Comparison of laparoscopic versus open complete mesocolic excision for right colon cancer. Int J Surg. 2015;23:12–7.
33. Bae SU, Saklani AP, Lim DR, Kim DW, Hur H, Min BS, et al. Laparoscopic-assisted versus open complete mesocolic excision and central vascular ligation for right-sided colon cancer. Ann Surg Oncol. 2014;21(7):2288–94.
34. Kang J, Kim IK, Kang SI, Sohn SK, Lee KY. Laparoscopic right hemicolectomy with complete mesocolic excision. Surg Endosc Other Interv Tech. 2014;28(9):2747–51.
35. Adamina M, Manwaring ML, Park K-J, Delaney CP. Laparoscopic complete mesocolic excision for right colon cancer. Surg Endosc. 2012;26(10):2976–80.

Laparoscopic Right Colectomy: Options for Ileocolonic Reconstruction

14

Giovanni Dapri and Marco Montorsi

Introduction and Rationale

The advent of minimally invasive surgery (MIS) has prompted surgeons to develop new techniques and strategies to perform the same surgical steps as in open surgery. During laparoscopic right colectomy, ileocolonic anastomosis has traditionally been performed outside the abdomen through the extraction incision created after completing ileocolonic mobilization and mesenteric transection [1]. The extraction sites most commonly utilized are periumbilical and upper midline incisions which allow the specimen to be extracted with the least amount of transverse colon mobilization and tension on the ileal mesentery and middle colic vessels. Due to their location, these incisions are associated with increased incisional pain relative to lower abdominal incisions, as well as substantial wound complications (infection, hematoma) and a significant incidence of incisional hernias of up to 13% [2, 3].

Over time and with more experience with MIS, surgeons began to perform bowel transection and anastomosis creation intracorporeally. Since the adoption of the endoscopic linear stapler, the ileocolonic anastomosis was created by firing of linear stapler and closing the enterotomy by another firing of the stapler or by intracorporeal suturing. With continued improvement in the surgeon's skills, advances of the technology, and the adoption of robotic surgery, intracorporeal anastomoses have become enabled, and techniques have become standardized [4–6]

G. Dapri (✉)
Saint-Pierre University Hospital, European School of Laparoscopic Surgery, Department of Gastrointestinal Surgery, Brussels, Belgium
e-mail: giovanni@dapri.net

M. Montorsi
Humanitas University, Humanitas Research Hospital, Rozzano, Italy

P. Sylla et al. (eds.), *The SAGES Manual of Colorectal Surgery*,
https://doi.org/10.1007/978-3-030-24812-3_14

Indications and Contraindications

There are few contraindications to laparoscopic right colectomy other than patient-related factors such as inability to tolerate pneumoperitoneum or general anesthesia. During minimally invasive right colectomy, both intracorporeal anastomoses (ICA) and extracorporeal anastomoses (ECA) can be safely performed [2, 3, 7–9]. The main technical differences between intracorporeal and extracorporeal anastomoses include but are not limited to (1) the ability to visualize the mesentery completely to ensure no twisting during anastomotic construction, (2) the ability to create the smallest possible extraction incision and to select an extraction incision in the lower abdomen or off-midline since there is no tension on the ileal or transverse colon mesentery during extraction, (3) improved cosmesis and reduced postoperative pain, and (4) reduced incisional hernia formation, particularly when using a Pfannenstiel incision as the extraction site. Furthermore, in obese patients, the benefits of MIS are further amplified when using intracorporeal anastomotic techniques and further reduce the risk of postoperative wound complications including surgical site infection (SSI), hematoma, and incisional hernia.

For surgeons using robot-assisted MIS, advantages provided by the robotic platform include the availability of a robotic stapler which facilitates insertion and positioning of the stapler, more precise visualization provided by 3D optics, and the enhanced suturing ability provided by the articulating robotic instruments. Ultimately, the choice between intra- or extracorporeal anastomosis during minimally invasive right colectomy is dependent on the surgeon's training, skills, preference, patient-related factors, and costs, taking into account the fact that handsewn anastomosis reduces the cost related to the use of multiple stapler loads.

Principles and Quality Benchmarks

Ileocolonic anastomoses follow the same principles whether performed during right colectomy for benign or malignant indications. For more details on specific laparoscopic techniques during right colectomy, please refer to the chapters on laparoscopic right colectomy for benign (Chap. 2) and malignant (Chap. 13) disease.

Extracorporeal anastomoses are most commonly constructed following the similar methods achieved during open surgery. Most ECA are performed using an antiperistaltic configuration, most commonly referred as side-to-side functional anastomosis. It is critical that enough length of the transverse colon and terminal ileum have been mobilized prior to exteriorization in order to minimize tension on the bowel and its mesentery which can result in tearing or ischemia. In addition, one must ensure that there is no twisting of the mesentery before and during exteriorizing the bowel. The standard strategy is to follow the root of the transected mesentery and mesocolon back to the duodenum and visualize the mesentery lying flat, without twisting. This can be challenging laparoscopically or when performed through a small extraction incision, especially in obese patients.

Extracorporeal anastomoses are created slightly differently as they require the use of a different stapler load/size and possibly the need for suturing the enterotomy close. With stapled antiperistaltic ICA, both ileum and transverse colon are incised at the apex of the antimesenteric side in order to insert the stapler. This is either done by excising the antimesenteric portion of the staple line or opening the bowel 1–2 cm proximal to the staple line. After firing the stapler, the enterocolotomy is closed either by utilizing another firing of stapler or by suturing. There are many options for suturing the enterocolotomy: single vs. double layer, absorbable vs. non-absorbable sutures, and running vs. interrupted suturing. With regard to ensuring that there is no twisting of the mesentery before construction of the ileocolonic anastomosis, it is much easier to visualize the mesentery fully and continuously to ensure that there is no twisting. ICA requires the least amount of transverse colon mobilization and eliminates any potential of tension or ischemia on the middle colic vessels during extraction and anastomotic creation.

Preoperative Planning

During the preoperative work-up of patients with right colon pathology, a fundamental requirement is a complete colonoscopy with confirmation of the location of the tumor. When the tumor is not within the cecum, it is commonly tattooed to allow for visualization at the time of MIS. It is important to clarify with the endoscopist if the tattoo is at the site of the neoplasia, distal, proximal, or both distal and proximal to the lesion, in order to precisely map the tumor's location and plan the extent of the resection. This is particularly important when creating an ICA as there will not be the ability to palpate the bowel until after extraction. When right colectomy is being performed for malignancy, staging CT scans of the chest, abdomen, and pelvis are completed in order to rule out metastatic disease and invasion into adjacent organs that may require en bloc oncologic resection. Patients are prepared for surgery using enhanced recovery protocols including full mechanical bowel preparation, oral antibiotics, cleansing of the skin, and oral carbohydrate loading, among other strategies [10]. The use of mechanical bowel preparation for right colectomy has not been shown to reduce major postoperative complications [11]. That being said, the prepped bowel may be easier to handle utilizing minimally invasive techniques with less risk of spillage during creation of the anastomosis, especially when ICA is performed. For more details on enhanced recovery programs, please refer to Chap. 7 on debunking enhanced recovery protocols in colorectal surgery.

Operative Techniques

Positioning

Laparoscopic right colectomy can be performed using one of two configurations with respect to patient and surgical team positioning on and around the operative room table, respectively. Patients are most commonly placed supine with the surgical team located on the patient's left side, where the surgeon stands in the middle, the scrub nurse to the surgeon's left, and the camera assistant to the surgeon's right (Position A) (Fig. 14.1). Another option is the use of the so-called French positioning, where the patient is placed in supine position with split legs, or alternatively, if a split-leg table is not available, the patient can be placed in low lithotomy position. With this setup, the surgeon stands in between the patient's legs, the camera assistant to the surgeon's right, and the scrub nurse to the right of the camera assistant (Position B) (Fig. 14.2). Typically, the patient will be placed in the slight Trendelenburg position and tilted right-side up for the majority of the operation.

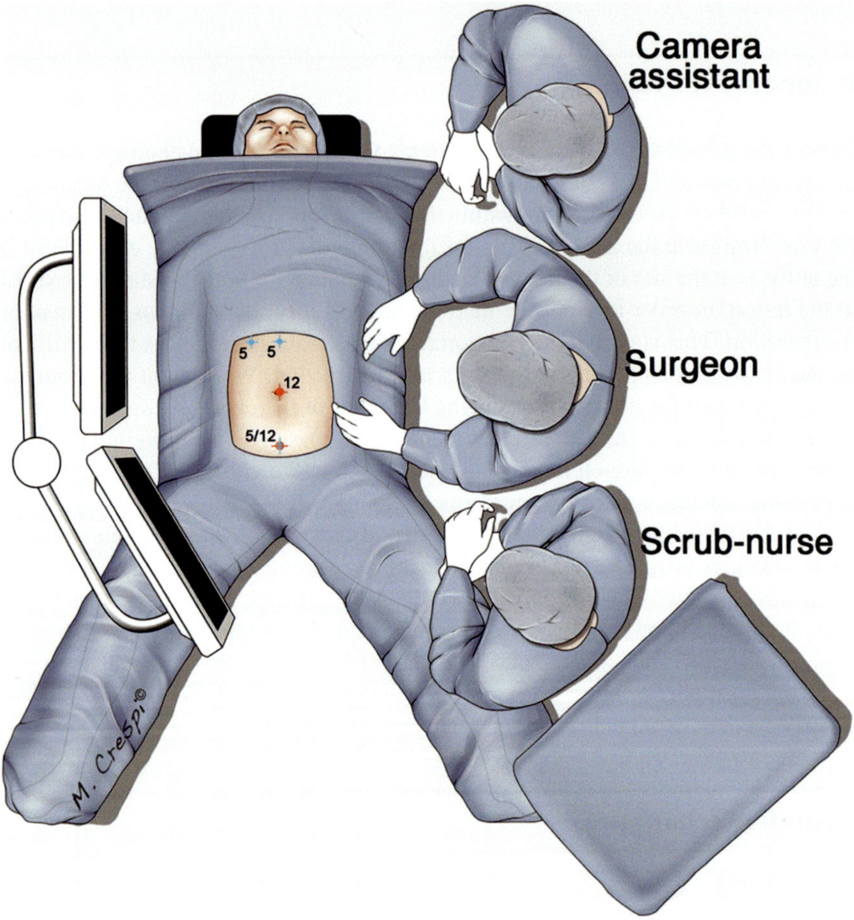

Fig. 14.1 Position A. Trocars positioning with the surgical team on the patient's left. (Copyright © Giovanni Dapri. Illustration by M. Crespi)

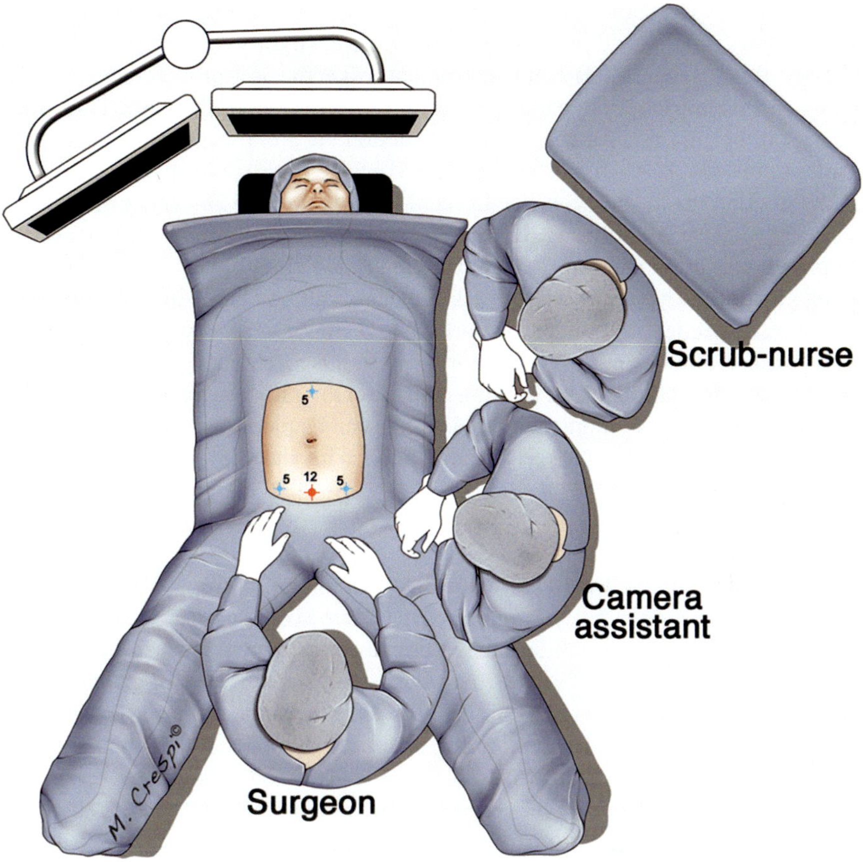

Fig. 14.2 Position B. Trocars positioning with the surgical team between the patient's legs. (Copyright © Giovanni Dapri. Illustration by M. Crespi)

Trocars Placement

There are several options for trocar positioning for laparoscopic right hemicolectomy with planned ECA or ICA. Over time, the surgeon will eventually identify their preferred configuration and alternatives when required based on body habitus, adhesions from prior surgery, and need for additional assist trocars. Most surgeons will place their 12 mm stapler port where they plan to extract the specimen, so that there are fewer incisions at risk for subsequent hernia formation. It is important to mark potential extraction sites at the start of the procedure as after insufflation; the abdominal wall will become distorted.

Position A (Fig. 14.1)

With the patient supine, a 5/12 mm trocar is placed just at the umbilicus for the 5/10 mm scope or endoscopic linear stapler. This trocar site can later be enlarged for specimen extraction via the umbilical incision when ECA is performed. A 5/12 mm trocar is placed in the suprapubic region, slightly to the left of the midline for the surgeon's left-hand instruments like the grasping forceps, or the scope or the endoscopic linear stapler if introduced through this port. This latter trocar will be enlarged for specimen's extraction via a Pfannenstiel incision after completion of ICA. A 5 mm trocar is placed in the epigastrium, slightly to the left of the midline for the surgeon's right-hand instrument, like an energy device and the needle holder for suturing. If needed for added retraction, a 5 mm trocar can be placed along the right mid-clavicular line in the right upper quadrant for the assist grasping forceps. Additional assist trocars can be placed in any number of locations as needed. This is particularly useful in obese patients and in patients with extensive adhesions. When suturing is found to be challenging due to the suboptimal port placement, an existing assist port is firstly recommended. If this is still suboptimal, one or more additional trocars can be placed, so that the surgeon's right and left hands are properly triangulated with the camera targeted on the relevant anatomy.

Position B (Fig. 14.2)
With the patient supine with split-leg or in low lithotomy position, a 12 mm trocar is placed in the suprapubic location for the 10 mm scope and for the endoscopic linear stapler. This trocar will be enlarged for specimen removal via a Pfannenstiel incision, after completion of intracorporeal anastomosis. A 5 mm trocar is placed on the left mid-clavicular line in the left iliac fossa for the surgeon's right-hand instruments like the needle holder for suturing or for the introduction of 5 mm scope at the time of endoscopic stapling. A 5 mm trocar is placed on the right mid-clavicular line in the right iliac fossa for the surgeon's left-hand instruments, like the grasping forceps. If needed for retraction, a 5 mm trocar is placed in the epigastrium, slightly to the left of the midline for the assist grasping forceps.

Options for Ileocolonic Reconstruction

When an ECA is performed, the specimen is extracted through the enlarged trocar site (e.g., 12 mm umbilical trocar). Both the ileum and trasnverse colon are transected extracorporeally using a standard linear stapler, and the specimen is handed off the field. The anastomosis is then created.

When an ICA is performed, following vascular dissection and mobilization of the ileum, right and transverse colon, the distal ileum and the proximal transverse colon are transected intracorporeally using an endoscopic linear stapler. The specimen is then placed above the liver or in the low pelvis and the ICA is created. The specimen will be later extracted through the incision of the surgeon's choice.

Techniques of Intracorporeal and Extracorporeal Ileocolonic Anastomoses

Side-to-Side Stapled Anastomosis

The ileal loop is placed alongside the transverse colon ensuring no twisting of the mesentery. The limbs can be aligned in an isoperistaltic or antiperistaltic configuration, depending on the natural way the bowel lays and surgeon's preference.

In the isoperistaltic anastomotic configuration, an enterotomy is created along the antimesenteric aspect of the ileum 1–2 cm proximal to the stapled end using monopolar cautery or any energy device. The transverse colon is opened as well along its antimesenteric aspect, keeping a 5–8 cm distance from its stapled end (Fig. 14.3). Each arm of a standard or endoscopic linear stapler (with a 45 mm or 60 mm load of the appropriate staple height) is inserted in each limb, and the stapler is closed and fired (Fig. 14.4). The staple line can be visualized through the enterotomy and checked for hemostasis. The enterocolotomy can then be closed by another firing of the stapler or by suturing. With the stapled closure, care must be taken not to narrow the anastomosis or staple across the mesentery to the anastomosis. Authors' preference for sutured closure of the enterocolotomy is a single layer anastomosis by two converging running sutures, using absorbable material (e.g., polydioxanone/PDS 2/0), started at both corners of the anastomosis (Fig. 14.5). There are several options for suture closure of the enterocolotomy based on the surgeon's preference.

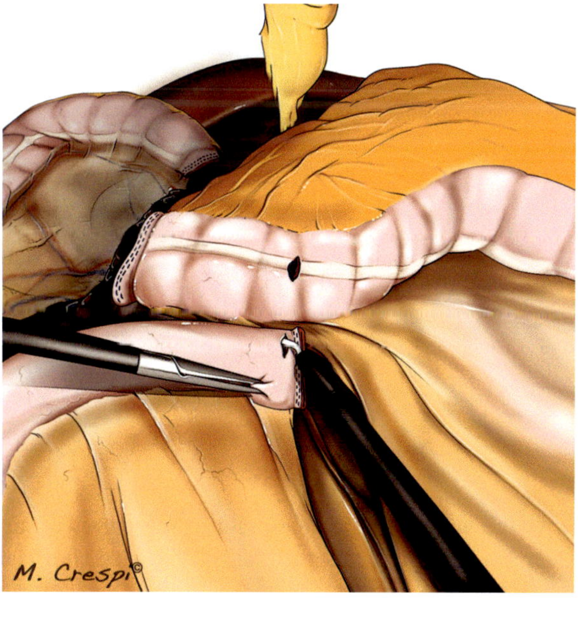

Fig. 14.3 Side-to-side stapled isoperistaltic anastomosis: opening of the viscera. (Copyright © Giovanni Dapri. Illustration by M. Crespi)

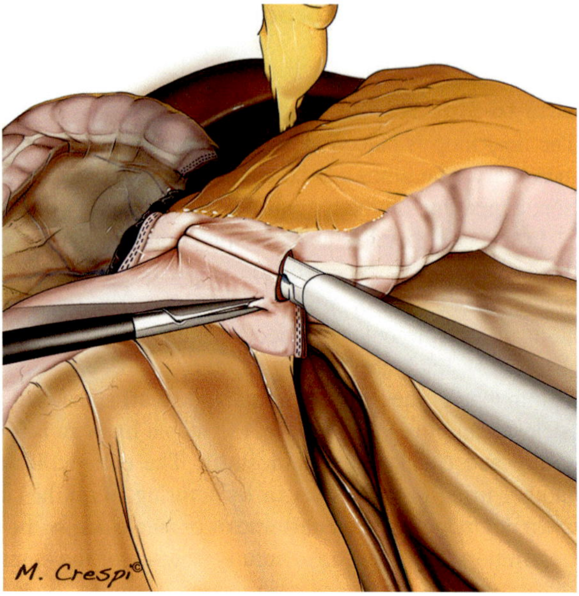

Fig. 14.4 Side-to-side stapled isoperistaltic anastomosis: insertion of the linear stapler. (Copyright © Giovanni Dapri. Illustration by M. Crespi)

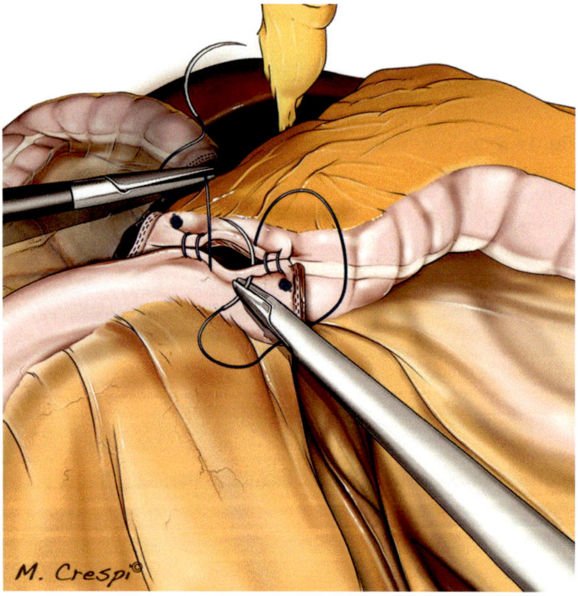

Fig. 14.5 Side-to-side stapled isoperistaltic anastomosis: closure of the enterocolotomy by two running sutures. (Copyright © Giovanni Dapri. Illustration by M. Crespi)

In the antiperistaltic anastomotic configuration, an enterocolotomy is created along the ileum 1–2 cm proximal to its stapled end. The transverse colon is opened close to its stapled end as well (Fig. 14.6). Each arm of a standard or endoscopic linear stapler is inserted in each limb, and the stapler is closed and fired (Fig. 14.7). The enterocolotomy is then closed using two converging running sutures of

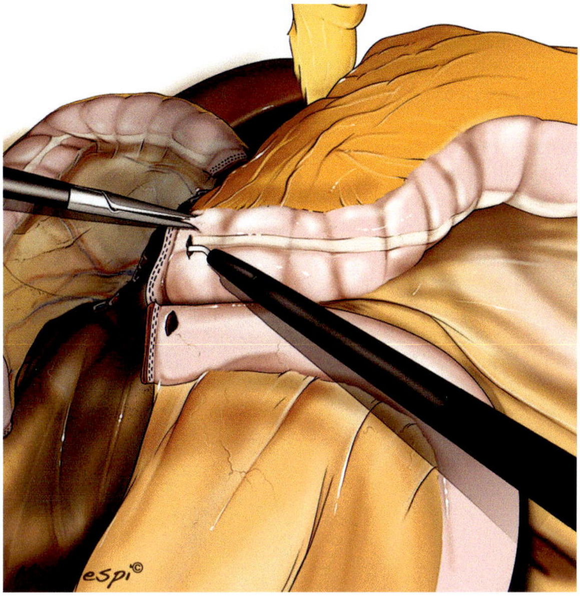

Fig. 14.6 Side-to-side stapled antiperistaltic anastomosis: opening of the bowel. (Copyright © Giovanni Dapri. Illustration by M. Crespi)

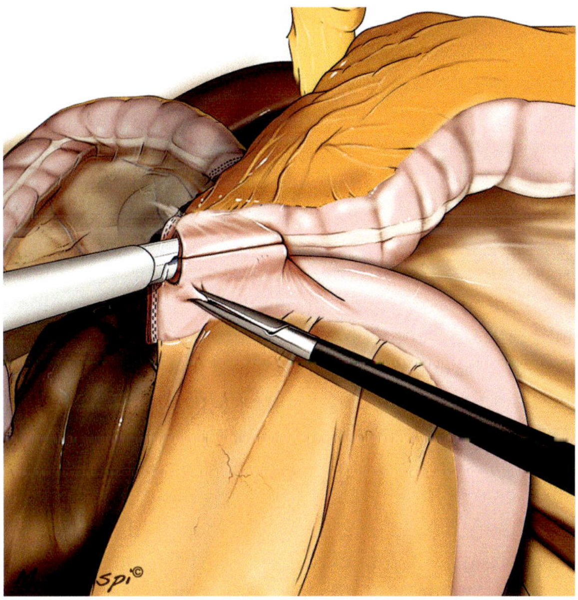

Fig. 14.7 Side-to-side stapled antiperistaltic anastomosis: insertion of the linear stapler. (Copyright © Giovanni Dapri. Illustration by M. Crespi)

absorbable material (e.g., PDS 2/0), started at both corners (Fig. 14.8) or using the other options described above.

An alternative technique during right colectomy with ECA consists in exteriorizing the specimen en bloc with the distal ileum and proximal transverse colon

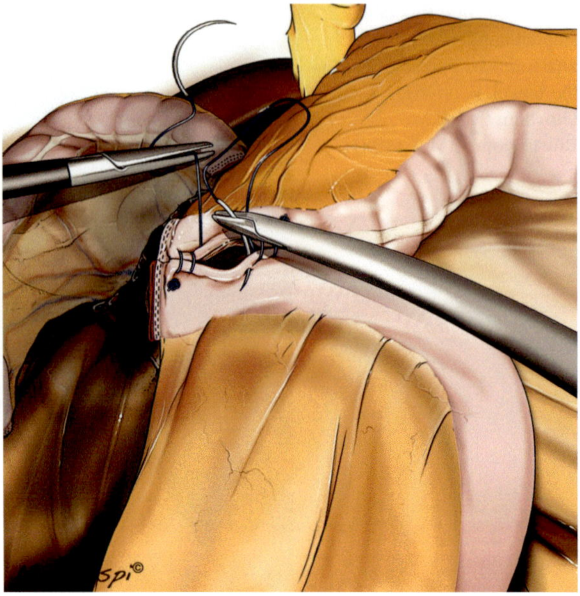

Fig. 14.8 Side-to-side stapled antiperistaltic anastomosis: closure of the enterocolotomy with running sutures. (Copyright © Giovanni Dapri. Illustration by M. Crespi)

without transecting the bowel first. Upon exteriorization, rather than transecting the bowel, the enterotomy and colotomy are made with insertion of the linear stapler and creation of the anastomosis. The enterocolotomy is transected along with the attached ileum and transverse colon using a second load of linear stapler. This approach only requires a total of two stapler loads rather than three to four loads, when the bowel is transected prior to creation of the anastomosis.

Side-to-Side Handsewn Anastomosis

The ileal loop is placed alongside the transverse colon, in either an isoperistaltic or antiperistaltic configuration. A continuous running suture is placed aligning the ileum to the colon using absorbable material (e.g., PDS 2/0) (Fig. 14.9). After completing this first running suture (typically ~5 cm in length), which constitutes the posterior anastomotic layer, a second running suture for the anterior layer is started at the planned apex of the anastomosis. After taking the first bite with the suture, a transverse colotomy and ileal enterotomy are created using monopolar cautery or any energy device (Fig. 14.10). The second running suture is used to construct the anterior layer of the anastomosis. At the opposite corner of the anastomosis, the posterior running suture is continued onto the anterior layer for a few bites in order to oversew the corner of the anastomosis (Fig. 14.11). The two running sutures are then tied together.

Side-to-End Stapled Anastomosis

For this type of anastomosis, the bowel is aligned in an isoperistaltic configuration with the terminal ileum oriented at 90 degrees relative to the transverse colon. The

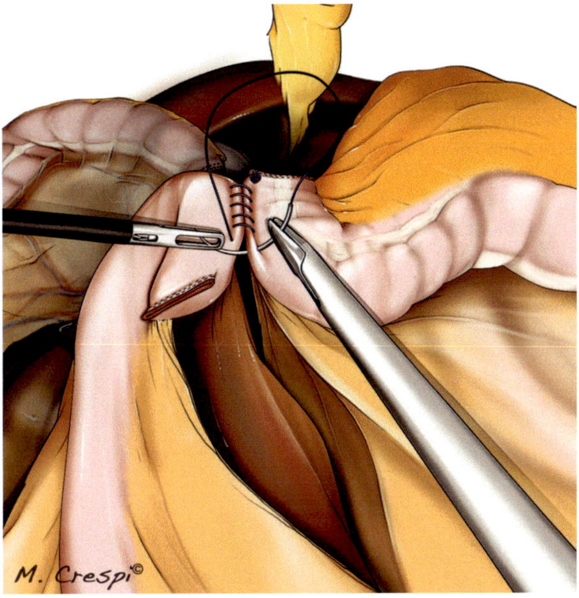

Fig. 14.9 Side-to-side handsewn anastomosis: posterior anastomotic layer completed with the first running suture. (Copyright © Giovanni Dapri. Illustration by M. Crespi)

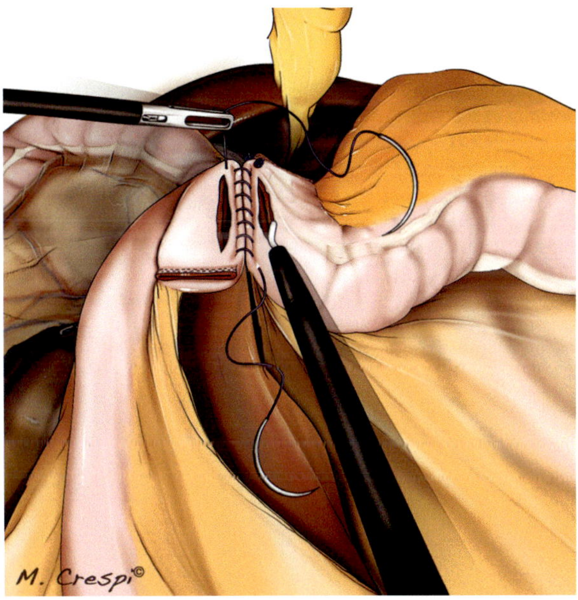

Fig. 14.10 Side-to-side handsewn anastomosis: creation of the enterotomy and colotomy after having started the second running suture for the anterior anastomotic layer. (Copyright © Giovanni Dapri. Illustration by M. Crespi)

ileal loop is placed with its lateral (antimesenteric) side against the stapled end of the transverse colon. The ileum is opened by making an enterotomy close to its stapled end. The transverse colon is also opened close to its stapled end (Fig. 14.12). A standard or endoscopic linear stapler is inserted in each limb and fired (Fig. 14.13). The enterocolotomy is closed by any method previously described (Fig. 14.14).

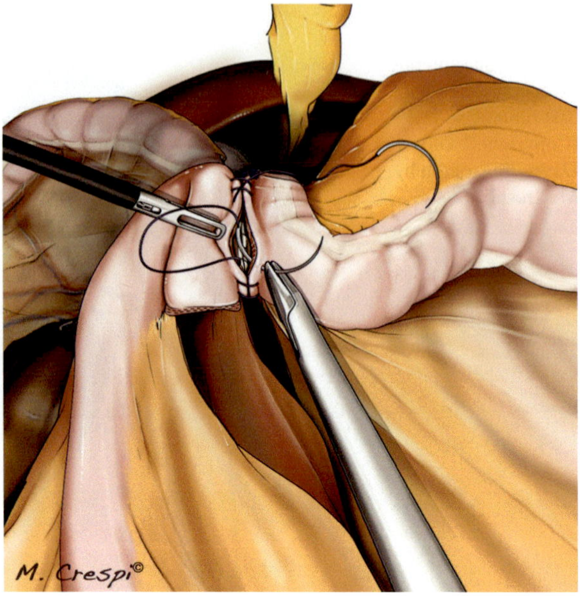

Fig. 14.11 Side-to-side handsewn anastomosis: transition of the posterior running suture to anteriorly, for a few bites, to oversew the corner of the anastomosis. (Copyright © Giovanni Dapri. Illustration by M. Crespi)

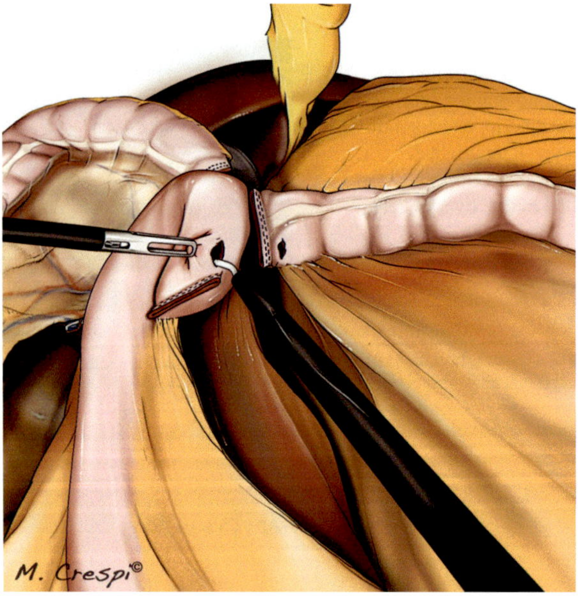

Fig. 14.12 Side-to-end stapled anastomosis: opening of the viscera. (Copyright © Giovanni Dapri. Illustration by M. Crespi)

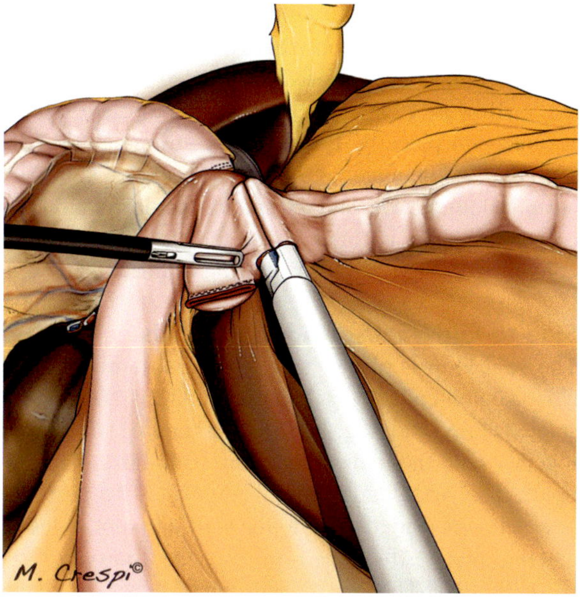

Fig. 14.13 Side-to-end stapled anastomosis: insertion of the linear stapler. (Copyright © Giovanni Dapri. Illustration by M. Crespi)

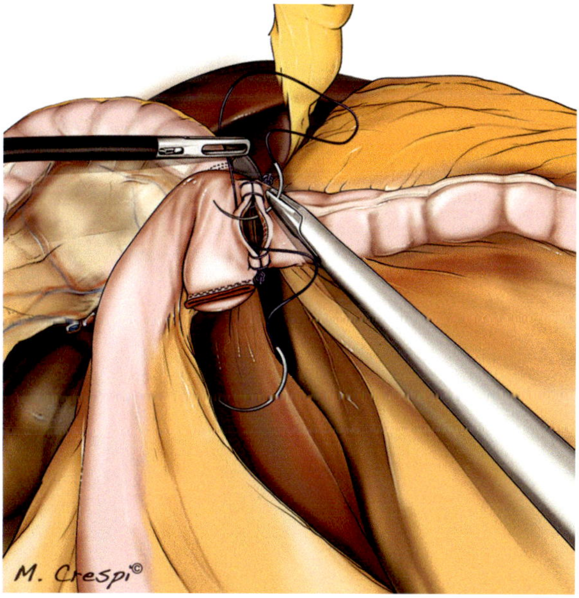

Fig. 14.14 Side-to-end stapled anastomosis: closure of the enterocolotomy by two running sutures. (Copyright © Giovanni Dapri. Illustration by M. Crespi)

An alternative ECA with side-to-end stapled anastomosis, which is popular among few surgeons, consists in the use of a circular stapler to complete a side-to-end ileocolonic anastomosis. The stapled end of the terminal ileum is transected and the anvil of an EEA stapler (of the appropriate size) is inserted in the lumen and secured into place by tying a purse-string suture. A colotomy is made along the transverse colon either at the stapled end or just proximal to it. The EEA stapler is advanced retrograde, and the spike is deployed along the antimesenteric side of the colon. The spike is connected to the anvil and the stapler is closed and fired. The colotomy is transected using a firing of linear stapler.

Side-to-End Handsewn Anastomosis

The ileal loop is placed with its lateral (antimesenteric) side against the stapled closed colon end. A first running suture is started on the ileum, 5–8 cm from its stapled closed end (Fig. 14.15). This running suture is performed bringing the ileum together with the transverse colon, from far to near, toward the stapled end of the ileum. This first running suture constitutes the posterior anastomotic layer. Then, a new suture is started close to the starting point of the posterior layer, to initiate the anterior layer. After the first bite, the transverse colon and ileum are incised (Figs. 14.16). The rest of the anastomosis is created as described previously (Fig. 14.17).

End-to-Side Handsewn Anastomosis

This type of anastomosis replaces the anatomic ileocecal junction and is constructed in an isoperistaltic configuration. The ileal loop is placed with its stapled

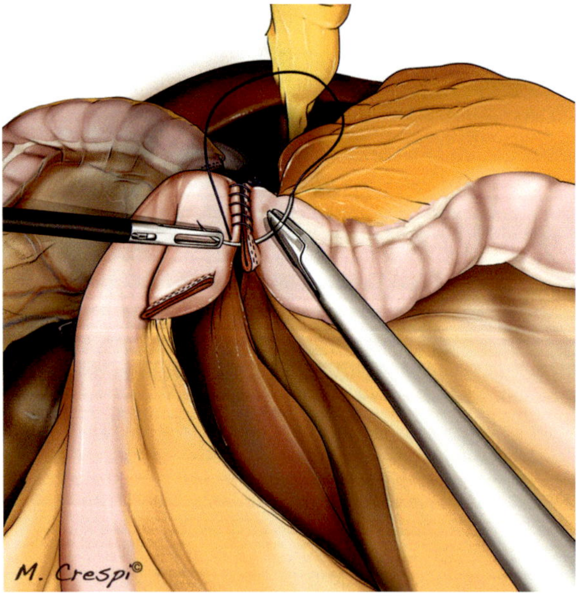

Fig. 14.15 Side-to-end handsewn anastomosis: posterior anastomotic layer completed with the first running suture. (Copyright © Giovanni Dapri. Illustration by M. Crespi)

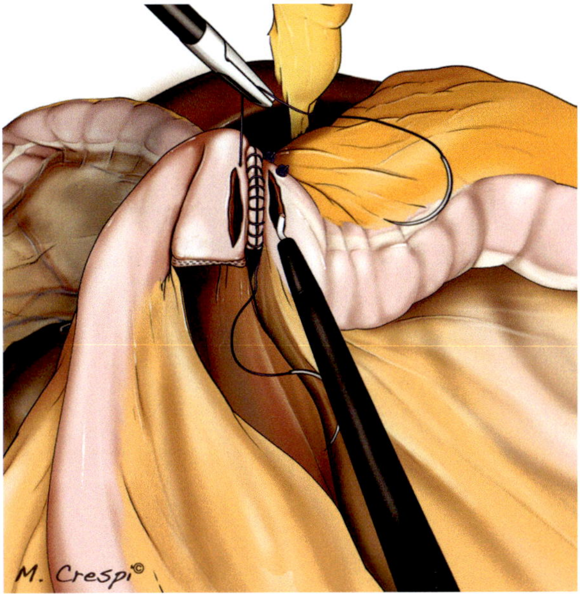

Fig. 14.16 Side-to-end handsewn anastomosis: opening of both transverse colon and ileum, after having started the first bite of the second running suture for the anterior layer. (Copyright © Giovanni Dapri. Illustration by M. Crespi)

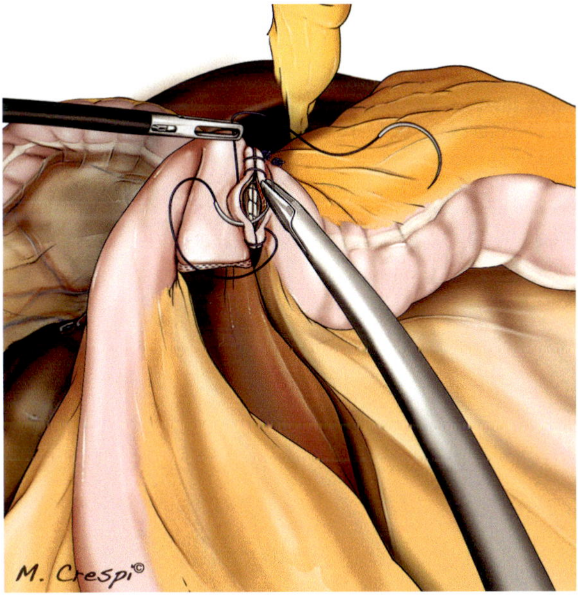

Fig. 14.17 Side-to-end handsewn anastomosis: transition of the posterior running suture to anteriorly, for a few bites, to oversew the corner of the anastomosis. (Copyright © Giovanni Dapri. Illustration by M. Crespi)

closed end against the lateral side of the transverse colon. A continuous running suture is placed aligning the ileum to the colon, using absorbable material (e.g., PDS 2/0) (Fig. 14.18). The rest of the anastomosis is created as described previously (Figs. 14.19 and 14.20).

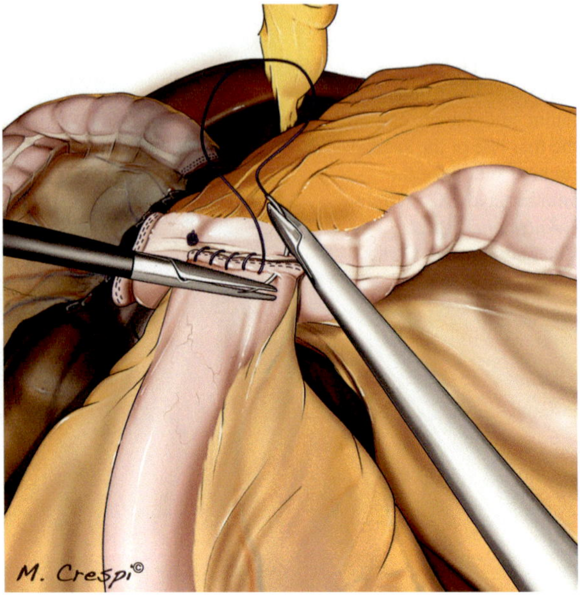

Fig. 14.18 End-to-side handsewn anastomosis: posterior anastomotic layer completed with the first running suture. (Copyright © Giovanni Dapri. Illustration by M. Crespi)

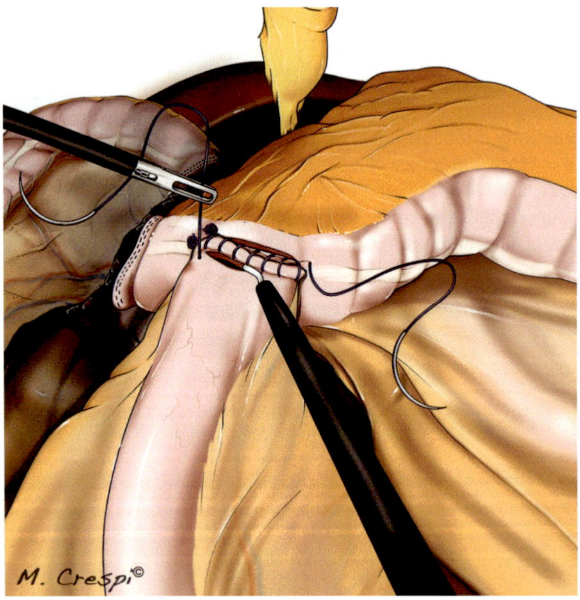

Fig. 14.19 End-to-side handsewn anastomosis: opening of both transverse colon and ileum, after having started the first bite of the second running suture for the anterior layer. (Copyright © Giovanni Dapri. Illustration by M. Crespi)

End-to-End Handsewn Anastomosis

This type of isoperistaltic anastomosis is useful in cases of intestinal obstruction and consequent small bowel dilatation when the ileal diameter is of similar size to the colon. The two linear staple lines, on the ileal end and on the transverse colon end, are placed in front of each other. A posterior running suture is performed from

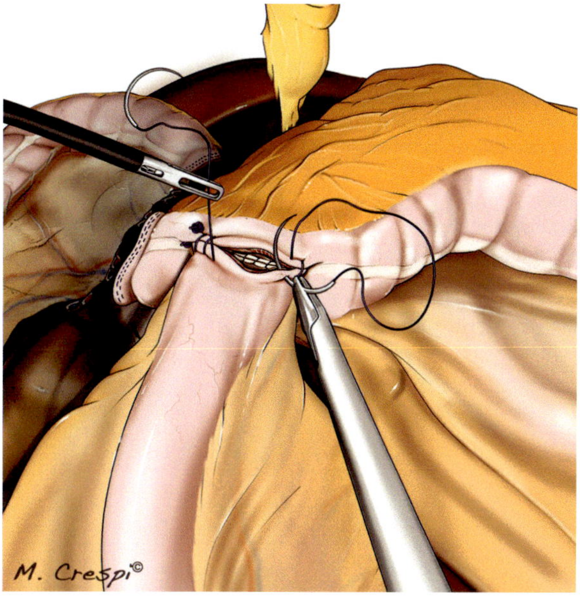

Fig. 14.20 End-to-side handsewn anastomosis: transition of the posterior running suture to anteriorly, for a few bites, to oversew the corner of the anastomosis. (Copyright © Giovanni Dapri. Illustration by M. Crespi)

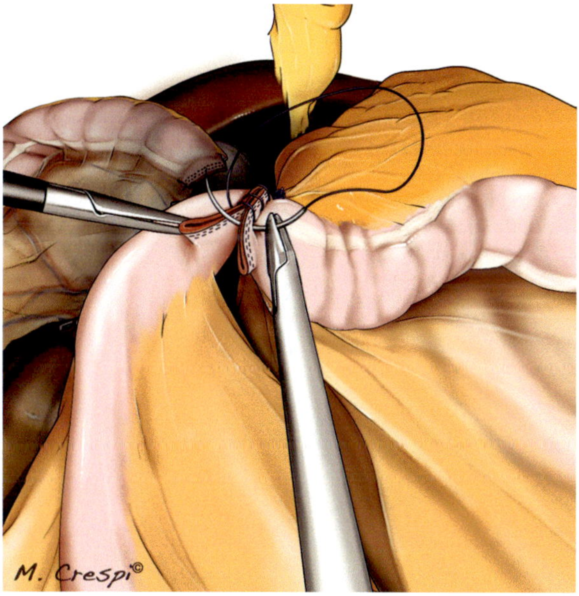

Fig. 14.21 End-to-end handsewn anastomosis: posterior anastomotic layer completed with the first running suture. (Copyright © Giovanni Dapri. Illustration by M. Crespi)

one corner of each limb to the opposite corners (Fig. 14.21). Then, a new running suture (anterior layer) is initiated at one end of the anastomotic apex. After taking the first bite, the colon and ileum can either be opened along the staple line (Fig. 14.22). The anterior layer of the anastomosis is completed as described previously (Fig. 14.23).

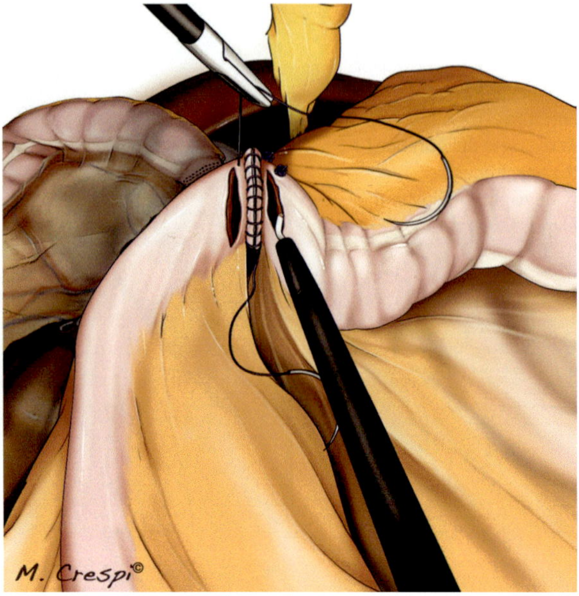

Fig. 14.22 End-to-end handsewn anastomosis: opening of both transverse colon and ileum, after having started the first bite of the second running suture for the anterior layer. (Copyright © Giovanni Dapri. Illustration by M. Crespi)

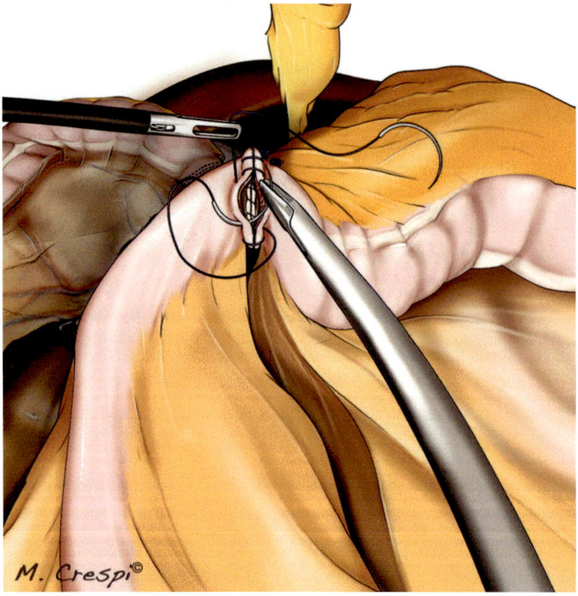

Fig. 14.23 End-to-end handsewn anastomosis: transition of the posterior running suture to anteriorly, for a few bites, to oversew the corner of the anastomosis. (Copyright © Giovanni Dapri. Illustration by M. Crespi)

Pitfalls and Troubleshooting

Twisting of the Anastomosis

With ICA, the choice of anastomotic configuration can be decided upon by observing the natural positioning of the viscera after their transection. Additionally, by being able to fully visualize the abdominal cavity, bowel, and mesentery, twisting and tension are avoided. When an ECA is being constructed, care must be taken during extraction and after bowel transection to avoid twisting. It can often be difficult to visualize the mesentery through the extraction incision. If there is any doubt about twisting prior to performing the anastomosis, the recommendation is to view the mesentery. This can be done while keeping the bowel limbs extracorporeally and placing the camera in one of the lateral ports to visualize the bowel and mesentery.

Operative Time

Although ICA can initially take longer to perform, as the surgeon gains experience, the time needed to create it can eventually equal that of ECA. In addition, there are several facts that will help reduce operative time during ICA: (1) There is less need for full transverse colon and ileal mobilization with ICA as the bowel does not need to be pulled up through the abdominal wall for extraction. This is particularly helpful in obese patients or in patients with prior surgeries where adhesions are a rate-limiting step. (2) Place all sutures required for anastomosis creation/enterocolotomy closure within the abdomen after specimen's transection to minimize the need to keep placing and removing sutures. (3) Stapled closure of the common channel will avoid the need for any suturing. (4) Using clips and barbed sutures or creating a loop at the end of the suture avoids the need to tie knots.

Spillage

During ECA creation, a wound protector is commonly placed prior to specimen's extraction. A sterile field can be created around the bowel prior to making an enterotomy/colotomy. With enough length of bowel mobilized and extracted extracorporeally, non-crushing bowel clamps can be placed on both bowel limbs to prevent enteric flow during enterotomy creation or enterotomy closure. During ICA, there is minimal leakage of intestinal contents because of the pressure generated by the pneumoperitoneum. As discussed earlier, the use of a mechanical bowel preparation can also reduce the possibility of spillage during anastomotic creation. During intracorporeal stapled anastomosis, one must be prepared to handle the contaminated stapler after completion of the stapled anastomosis. A gauze can be inserted into the abdomen (before stapling) and used to cover the stapler upon removal through the trocar. In this way, the fecal contamination of the trocar can be avoided or at least minimized.

Alignment/Ergonomics

Often times after bowel division and aligning the bowel in preparation for ICA, the surgeon realizes that the trocar position is not optimized for ICA. This can either be secondary to suboptimal position of the camera or suboptimal trocar positioning. There are several maneuvers that can help in this scenario:

1. Place a stay suture on the far side of the planned anastomosis, and have the assistant hold it upward toward the abdominal wall, or use a suture passer through the abdominal wall to retract it. This allows for improved traction on the bowel which remains in stable and optimized position for the surgeon. In addition, by pulling up on the bowel in this manner, there is less risk of fecal spillage after enterotomy or during the anastomosis.
2. Although many surgeons prefer to staple through the suprapubic port site as this is the incision that will be upsized for specimen extraction, sometimes it can be challenging to get a good angle to staple the anastomosis from this location. In these cases, stapling from an alternative port (e.g., umbilical port) is recommended.
3. When the ports are found to be too challenging for safe anastomotic creation, the placement of even one additional 5 mm port can solve the problem.
4. If the bowel continues to lay in a position that makes it challenging to safely create an ICA, additional mobilization of the transverse colon and root of ileal mesentery can be done to gain mobility and to optimize positioning.
5. Lastly, when all of the above maneuvers fail, one can always perform an ECA.

Outcomes

Five recent systematic reviews and meta-analyses have compared outcomes of laparoscopic right hemicolectomy performed with extracorporeal versus intracorporeal anastomosis [3, 7–9, 12] (Tables 14.1). None of the meta-analyses demonstrated statistically significant differences in operative time, and only one describes a lower mortality rate [12]. Cirocchi and colleagues [12] reported also less blood loss during ICA, while van Oostendorp and colleagues [3] and Ricci and colleagues [7] demonstrated a reduced short-term morbidity after ICA, including significant reduction in wound infection rates. Wu and colleagues [8], Feroci and colleagues [9], and Cirocchi and colleagues [12] showed a shorter time to first defecation. Ricci and associates [7], Wu and associates [8], and Feroci and associates [9] showed reduced time to first oral intake. The use of analgesics was evaluated by Feroci and coauthors [9] and Cirocchi and coauthors [12], and the ICA was associated to a decreased use. The length of hospital stay was significantly shorter with ICA [3, 7–9]. Cosmetic outcomes were evaluated by Wu and associates [8] and Cirocchi and associates [12], with superior results after ICA. Most notable, ICA was also associated with significantly lower rate of incisional hernia [7] with overall rates 2.3% vs. 13.7% following ICA vs. ECA across 14 matched studies.

Table 14.1 Overview of results from meta-analyses comparing laparoscopic right hemicolectomy performed with intracorporeal versus extracorporeal anastomosis

Study	*N* ICA	*N* ECA	Results
Ricci et al. [7]	864	853	ICA associated with lower: Overall complication rate (27.6% vs 38.4%, $P = 0.01$). Time to first oral intake (WMD −1; 95% CI = −1.59 to −0.41). Length of stay (WMD −1.13; 95% CI = −1.90 to −0.35). Wound infection (4.9% vs 8.9%, $P = 0.03$). Incisional hernia (2.3% vs 13.7%, $P = 0.02$). No differences in anastomotic leak (3.4% vs 4.6%, $P = 0.12$), OR time, blood loss, conversion, reoperation, mortality, analgesia required
Wu et al. [8]	994	963	ICA associated with lower: Length of stay (WMD −1.03, 95% CI −1.57 to −0.48). Time to first bowel movement (WMD −0.65, 95% CI −0.97 to −0.32). Time to liquid diet (WMD −0.87, 95% CI −1.41 to −0.33). No significant differences in intraoperative (OR = 0.75, 95% CI 0.21–2.74) and postoperative complications (OR = 0.74, 95% CI 0.49–1.12), mortality (RR = 0.59, 95% CI 0.19–1.86), and anastomotic leak (OR = 0.77, 95% CI 0.45–1.31)
Van Oostendorp et al. [3]	763	729	ICA associated with lower: Short-term morbidity (OR 0.68, 95% CI 0.49–0.93). Length of stay (WMD −0.77, 95% CI −1.46 to −0.07). Surgical site infection (OR 0.56, 95% CI 0.35–0.88). No significant difference in mortality (OR 0.36, 95% CI 0.09–1.46), anastomotic leak (OR 0.77, 95% CI 0.39–1.49), ileus (OR 0.94, 95% CI 0.57–1.57).
Cirocchi et al. [12]	945 total		ICA associated with lower: Mortality rate (0.34% vs 1.32%, OR 0.52; 95% CI 0.09–3.10), though not statistically significant. No significant difference in anastomotic leak (1.13% vs 1.84%, OR 0.90, 95% CI 0.24–3.10) and intraoperative complications (OR 0.54; 95% CI 0.09–3.24). A meta-analysis of postoperative morbidity was not possible because the data reported in the included studies were too heterogenous
Feroci et al. [9]	202	223	ICA associated with significantly decreased: Time to first flatus (OR = -0.48, 95% CI −0.78 to −0.18). Time to solid diet (OR = -1.00, 95% CI −1.33 to −0.67). Use of analgesics (OR = -1.00, 95% CI −1.34 to −0.66). Length of stay (OR = −0.93, 95% CI −1.79 to −0.07). No significant difference in intraoperative complications (OR 0.84; 95% CI −0.14–5.20), mortality (OR 0.75; 95% CI 0.10–5.93), nonsurgical site complications (OR = 0.79, 95% CI 0.20–3.13), surgical site complications (OR = 0.44, 95% CI 0.14–1.39)

ICA intracorporeal anastomosis, *ECA* extracorporeal anastomosis, *WMD* weighted mean difference, *CI* confidence interval, *OR* odds ratio

Conclusions

The choice of the anastomotic technique during laparoscopic right colectomy depends on the surgeon's preference, as well as patient's anatomy and intraoperative findings. While the literature does not suggest any major differences in outcomes related to these various anastomotic techniques, many suggest decreased wound-related morbidity, better cosmesis, decreased postoperative pain, and incisional hernia rate with ICA.

References

1. Jacobs M, Verdeja JC, Goldstein HS. Minimally invasive colon resection (laparoscopic colectomy). Surg Laparosc Endosc. 1991;1(3):144–50.
2. Stein SA, Bergamaschi R. Extracorporeal versus intracorporeal anastomosis. Tech Coloproctol. 2013;17(Suppl 1):S35–9.
3. van Oostendorp S, Elfrink A, Borstlap W, Schoonmade L, Sietses C, Meijerink J, et al. Intracorporeal versus extracorporeal anastomosis in right hemicolectomy: a systematic review and meta-analysis. Surg Endosc. 2017;31(1):64–77.
4. Lipski D, Dapri G, Himpens J. Completely staple-free hand-sewn laparoscopic anastomosis in colorectal surgery. J Laparoendosc Adv Surg Tech A. 2008;18(2):282–5.
5. Dapri G, Carandina S, Mathonet P, Himpens J, Cadière GB. Suprapubic single-incision laparoscopic right hemicolectomy with intracorporeal anastomosis. Surg Innov. 2013;20:484–92.
6. D'Annibale A, Pernazza G, Morpurgo E, Monsellato I, Pende V, Lucandri G, et al. Robotic right colon resection: evaluation of first 50 consecutive cases for malignant disease. Ann Surg Oncol. 2010;17(11):2856–62.
7. Ricci C, Casadei R, Alagna V, Zani E, Taffurelli G, Pacilio CA, et al. A critical and comprehensive systematic review and meta-analysis of studies comparing intracorporeal and extracorporeal anastomosis in laparoscopic right hemicolectomy. Langenbeck's Arch Surg. 2017;402(3):417–27.
8. Wu Q, Jin C, Hu T, Wei M, Wang Z. Intracorporeal versus extracorporeal anastomosis in laparoscopic right colectomy: a systematic review and meta-analysis. J Laparoendosc Adv Surg Tech A. 2017;27(4):348–57.
9. Feroci F, Lenzi E, Garzi A, Vannucchi A, Cantafio S, Scatizzi M. Intracorporeal versus extracorporeal anastomosis after laparoscopic right hemicolectomy for cancer: a systematic review and meta-analysis. Int J Color Dis. 2013;28(9):1177–86.
10. Tiefenthal M, Asklid D, Hjern F, Matthiessen P, Gustafsson UO. Laparoscopic and open right-sided colonic resection in daily routine practice. A prospective multicentre study within an Enhanced Recovery After Surgery (ERAS) protocol. Color Dis. 2016;18(2):187–94.
11. Moghadamyeghaneh Z, Hanna MH, Carmichael JC, Mills SD, Pigazzi A, Nguyen NT, et al. Nationwide analysis of outcomes of bowel preparation in colon surgery. J Am Coll Surg. 2015;220(5):912–20.
12. Cirocchi R, Trastulli S, Farinella E, Guarino S, Desiderio J, Boselli C, et al. Intracorporeal versus extracorporeal anastomosis during laparoscopic right hemicolectomy – systematic review and meta-analysis. Surg Oncol. 2013;22(1):1–13.

Robotic Right-Sided Colon Resection: Unique Considerations and Optimal Setup

15

Konstantin Umanskiy

Introduction and Rationale

Laparoscopic right colectomy is a commonly performed procedure. While some general surgeons steadfastly reject minimally invasive approach to right colectomy, most general and colorectal surgeons are quite comfortable performing laparoscopic (hand-assist or pure) right hemicolectomy. Below are a few reasons to consider the robotic approach:

1. Gaining experience with robotic colon surgery. Right colectomy is often referred to as a "gateway procedure" because it allows the surgeons who are learning minimally invasive surgery to begin with procedures that are considered "less challenging" [1]. Once surgeons ascend the learning curve, they may expand their clinical portfolio to other, more complex procedures such as left colectomy, low anterior resection, and abdominoperineal resection.
2. Complete mesocolic excision (CME). There is a growing body of literature suggesting that extensive excision of mesocolon at the time of right colectomy, similar to total mesorectal excision of the rectum, can improve lymph node yield and lead to improved oncologic outcomes [2–4]. The CME involves central vascular ligation with complete exposure and lymphadenectomy along the superior mesenteric vessels. This increases the technical demand of minimally invasive surgery in right colon cancer and adds the potential of worsened vascular complications compared to standard right hemicolectomy. Even in the hands of experienced laparoscopists, mastering laparoscopic CME technique has proven to be quite challenging. Robotic surgery may potentially overcome the limitations of straight laparoscopic instruments in CME given its technical features

K. Umanskiy (✉)
University of Chicago, Department of Surgery, Chicago, IL, USA
e-mail: kumanskiy@surgery.bsd.uchicago.edu

P. Sylla et al. (eds.), *The SAGES Manual of Colorectal Surgery*,
https://doi.org/10.1007/978-3-030-24812-3_15

such as instrument stability, enhanced dexterity of wristed instruments, and improved 3D visualization.
3. Intracorporeal anastomosis (ICA) is a compelling reason to adopt the robotic technique for right colectomy [5]. With its advantages of wristed instruments and easier intracorporeal suturing, intracorporeal robotic anastomosis may become easier to perform and may gain popularity. With adoption of ICA, surgeons are able to move the specimen extraction site away from periumbilical midline region and toward the pubis using a small muscle-splitting Pfannenstiel incision. This likely contributes to decreased pain, lower rates of wound complications, and incisional hernia that have been reported in some comparative studies of laparoscopic right colectomy performed with intracorporeal vs. extracorporeal anastomosis [6, 7].
4. With popularization of da Vinci Xi® (Intuitive Surgical, Sunnyvale, CA, USA) surgical robot, which is capable of rotating its base, single docking total abdominal colectomy is now feasible [8]. Learning the technical steps of right colectomy could enable surgeons to seamlessly incorporate right colectomy into total abdominal colectomy or other multiquadrant procedures [9].

Indications and Contraindications

Any patient who is a candidate for minimally invasive procedure could be considered for robotic colectomy. Morbid obesity, a relative contraindication to laparoscopic approach, could be one of the reasons to consider robotic approach instead of conventional laparoscopy. During conventional laparoscopy in morbidly obese individuals, the thick abdominal wall may cause significant torqueing of the instruments, reduce precision and accuracy of movements, and lead to instrument malfunction or even breakage. Robotic platform is uniquely suited to overcome these disadvantages and reduce physical and psychological strain on the surgeon [10]. The remote center on the ports reduces trocar site torque and instrument strain. The robotic approach also allows smooth, controlled movements with variable degree of scaling and built-in tremor reduction. Furthermore, construction of robotic intracorporeal anastomosis could eliminate the need for additional dissection to exteriorize the bowel for anastomosis. This, thereby, would reduce unnecessary traction on the tissue and minimize the length of the incision. Absolute contraindications to robotic surgery are similar to those of laparoscopy and include surgical scenarios resulting hemodynamic compromise and inability to tolerate pneumoperitoneum. Relative contraindications to robotic right colectomy include intestinal obstruction, significant intra-abdominal adhesions, large lesions, or fistulizing lesions.

Principles and Quality Benchmarks

Most of the principles of the robotic right colectomy for benign and malignant disease are based on the well-established laparoscopic approach [11] and are described in detail in chapters on laparoscopic right colectomy for benign (Chap. 2) and malignant

(Chap. 13) indications in this textbook. There is a consensus in the literature that the medial to lateral approach is the preferred approach during laparoscopic and robotic surgery. Robotic right colectomy is compared to the laparoscopic approach based on quality metrics such as operative time, rate of conversion to open surgery, blood loss, procedural complications, early and long-term morbidity rates, incidence of incisional hernia, and short and long-term oncologic outcomes (R0 resection, lymph node yield, local and distant recurrence rates, and long-term survival).

Preoperative Planning, Patient Workup, and Optimization

Specific preoperative planning for robotic right colectomy should include detailed review of computer tomographic (CT) imaging, particularly the relationship of the tumor to surrounding structures such as the liver, gallbladder, duodenum, right kidney/ureter, and adrenal gland. Preoperative planning should also consider points for potential transection of the colon and ileum as well as planning for the extraction site and type of anastomosis (intracorporeal vs. extracorporeal) to be performed. If the tumor is not visible on imaging and has not been tattooed at the time of initial colonoscopy, a preoperative colonoscopy should be performed to identify and mark the lesion. Alternatively, intraoperative colonoscopy could be performed prior to commencing the procedure, but even with the CO_2 insufflation, the colon and small bowel can become distended, obscuring the operative field.

Operative Setup

The patient is placed in a supine or lithotomy position. The patient is secured to the operating table with the help of a Pink Pad® (Xodus Medical, New Kensington, PA, USA) or similar anti-sliding device, with both arms tucked at bedside. The patient is placed in slight Trendelenburg position, and tilted right side is up. Upon initial exploration of the abdomen, unless the da Vinci Xi® system (Intuitive Surgical, Sunnyvale, CA, USA) is used in combination with the OR table equipped with an integrated table motion functionality, the small bowel is retracted to the left upper quadrant laparoscopically prior to docking the robot. Table motion functionality allows changes in OR table position with the robot being fully docked. The robotic arms will automatically adjust their position as table position changes [12]. If a da Vinci Si® or X® system (Intuitive Surgical, Sunnyvale, CA, USA) is used or if the integrated table motion is not available with Xi robot, there can be no changes in table position or the robot's position without first undocking the robotic arms.

General Considerations for Port Placement and Docking

In the early stages of adoption of the robotic approach for right colectomy, surgeons may consider replicating the steps of laparoscopic procedure using similar port configuration and steps of the procedure. This allows the surgeon to begin the procedure laparoscopically, dock the robot, but have the option of converting back to laparoscopy at any time during the case. Familiar port placement may reduce surgeon's anxiety, decrease operative time and make adoption of robotic technology easier. As the surgeon's proficiency increases, ports can be placed to accommodate a potential extraction site, optimize intracorporeal anastomosis, and cluster near the pubic region where it is more cosmetically favorable [13]. Because of the mechanical differences between da Vinci Si, da Vinci X, and da Vinci Xi robots, port placement varies. There are no strict rules for robotic port placement, and many surgeons arrive to their own preferred configuration. When considering port placement, one must ensure an optimal camera view, trocar spacing to minimize external collisions, and adequate reach of the operating instruments to the targeted field.

da Vinci Si® and X® Setup (Intuitive Surgical, Sunnyvale, CA, USA)

The da Vinci Si and newer X models use the similar general mechanical architecture; however, the da Vinci X features upgraded arms and instruments of the Xi model.

After pneumoperitoneum is established, a 12 mm camera port is placed either supraumbilically or 2–3 cm to the left of the midline to decrease the incidence of incisional hernias related to the a midline location [14]. The larger (stapler) port could be placed at the proposed extraction site. Location and position of the hepatic flexure should be noted. Ports placed too far laterally on the left side may not have sufficient reach and excursion for dissection and retraction of colon at hepatic flexure. While some surgeons use robotic camera from the beginning of the case, others find da Vinci Si camera to be too cumbersome and heavy to be used as a laparoscope. The da Vinci X camera, on the other hand, is 8 mm in diameter and significantly smaller and lighter than Si's, making it easier to be used as a laparoscope. The da Vinci X camera can be inserted into any of the robotic cannulas and connected to any of the robotic arms.

Instrument cannulas are placed under direct laparoscopic or robotic camera vision. These additional ports should be triangulated in relation to the target anatomy with instrument ports approximately 10–20 cm from the target anatomy (Figs. 15.1 and 15.2). Five mm assistant ports (non-robotic instrument cannulas) should be placed as needed. Most surgeons who use the Si system for right colectomies dock the robot over the right side (over right shoulder). General principles of docking are the same between Si and X machines. When docking the patient's cart, the distance of the robot from the OR table is determined by the camera arm's "sweet spot." The camera port, target anatomy, and patient cart should be in a straight line to maximize range of motion of the robotic arms, though side docking is also a widely used option.

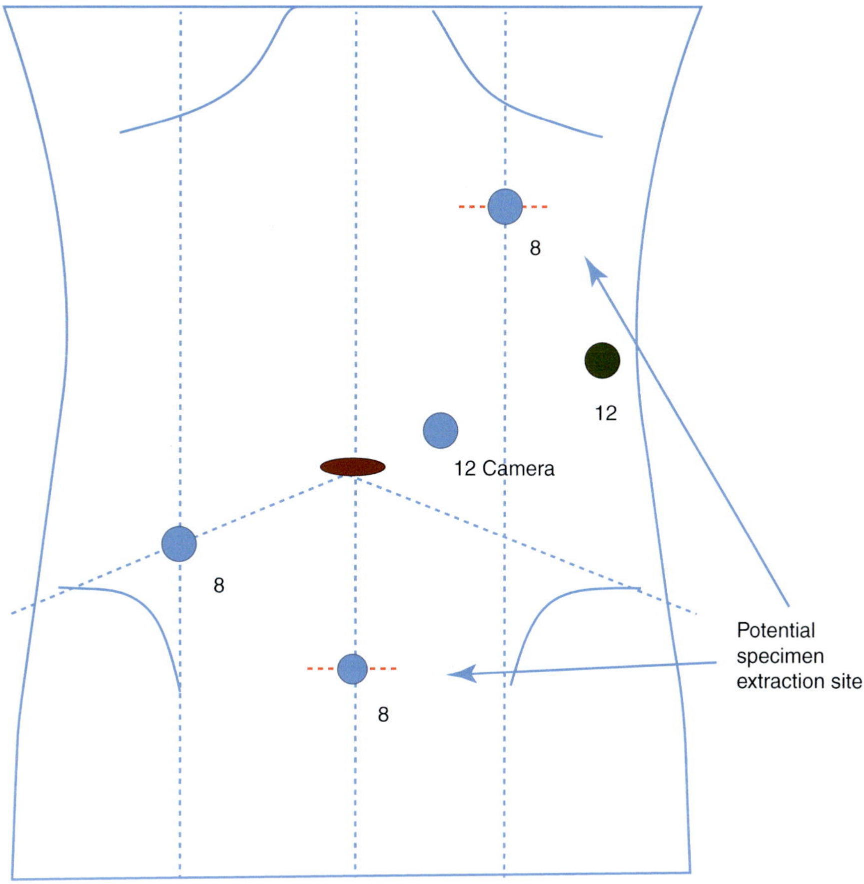

Fig. 15.1 Port placement for da Vinci Si® or da Vinci X® (Intuitive Surgical, Sunnyvale, CA, USA) right colectomy

da Vinci Xi® Setup (Intuitive Surgical, Sunnyvale, CA, USA)

The da Vinci Xi has sleeker arms with an extra joint for movement, which allows for closer arm positioning without concern for external collisions. The Xi instruments are longer than Si, and the camera is the same as the one used for da Vinci X (8 mm). Port placement for robotic right colectomy with the Xi system is in a diagonal line from a point to the left of the costal margin cephalad to the suprapubic region caudally (Fig. 15.3). Alternatively Xi ports can be clustered within the suprapubic region to improve cosmetic outcomes (Fig. 15.4). Most surgeons dock the Xi robot directly over the right side of the operating table.

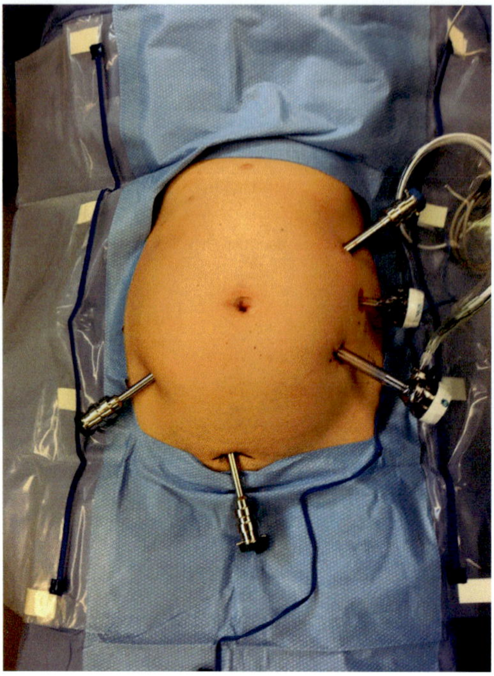

Fig. 15.2 Operative photograph demonstrating port placement for da Vinci Si® or da Vinci X® (Intuitive Surgical, Sunnyvale, CA, USA) right colectomy. (Photo courtesy of Dr. Craig Johnson, Tulsa, Oklahoma)

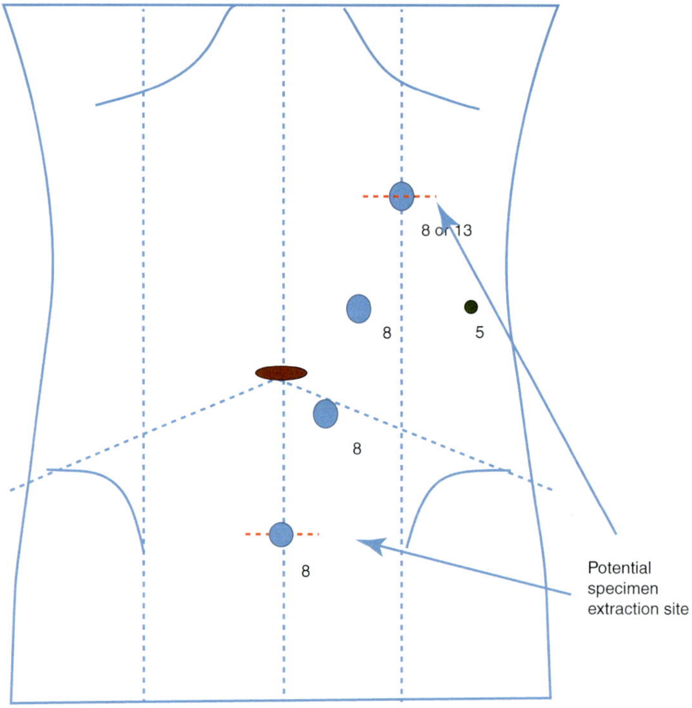

Fig. 15.3 Port placement for da Vinci Xi® (Intuitive Surgical, Sunnyvale, CA, USA) right colectomy

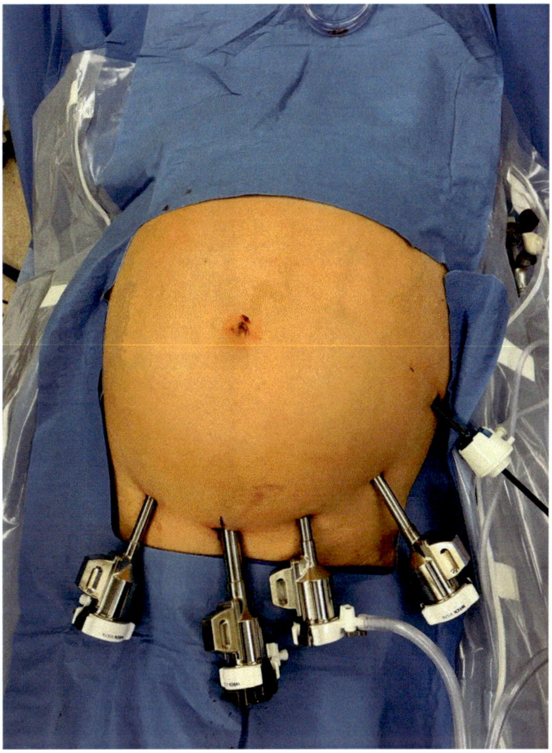

Fig. 15.4 Alternative port placement for da Vinci Xi® (Intuitive Surgical, Sunnyvale, CA, USA) robotic right colectomy. (Courtesy of Dr. Craig Johnson, Tulsa, Oklahoma)

Operative Technique: Surgical Steps

The abdomen is inspected laparoscopically to determine the feasibility of minimally invasive resection and to identify the extent of disease. The patient is placed in slight Trendelenburg position with the right side tilted up. This allows for the small bowel to be displaced to the left upper quadrant, exposing the cecum, terminal ileum, and right colon mesentery. The omentum is retracted over the liver. We prefer to use a robotic hook cautery on the left robotic arm, while other surgeons prefer to use robotic shears and a bipolar fenestrated grasper on the right robotic arm. Other surgeons will use either two instruments for the left hand or two for the right hand and swap them as needed. For example, two left-hand instruments could be a tip up/stapler and a fenestrated bipolar and one right-hand scissors/vessel sealer/needle driver. Depending on the surgeon's comfort, training, and experience, an additional robotic port can be used for the swappable instrument. We typically proceed with a medial to lateral approach. If medial to lateral approach is not feasible because of anatomic variant or inability to expose the ileocolic pedicle, a lateral to medial approach can be used.

The cecum is grasped and retracted laterally, caudally, and anteriorly exposing the ileocolic pedicle. In most individuals, the second portion of duodenum can be visualized through a thin layer of parietal peritoneum. In the setting of visceral obesity, however, these anatomic landmarks may be more difficult to identify

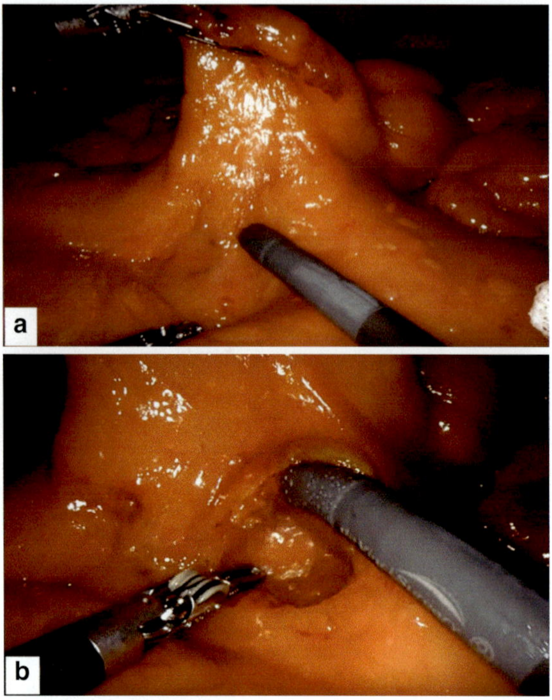

Fig. 15.5 (**a**, **b**) The ileocolic pedicle is retracted and placed under tension (**a**). The plane between the right colon mesentery and the retroperitoneum is dissected bluntly, and the second portion of the duodenum is identified (**b**). (Courtesy of Daniel Popowich, MD)

(Fig. 15.5a). The peritoneum inferior and posterior to the ileocecal pedicle is opened sharply, and blunt dissection is carried out along the retroperitoneal plane (Fig. 15.5b). Next, the ileocolic pedicle is controlled. The ileocolic artery is carefully dissected close to its origin (Fig. 15.6a). While visualizing the duodenum, the artery is ligated and divided using a suitable device (Fig. 15.6b). Available methods include vascular endostapling, clips, bipolar energy, or suture ligation with the robotic system. The robotic technique has been successfully applied to complete mesocolic excision (CME) for right-sided colon cancers. In this approach, the ileocolic vessels are dissected and ligated near their origin. Dissection continues cephalad along the ventral aspect of the superior mesenteric vein (SMV). While following embryological planes between the mesocolon and retroperitoneal structures, mesenteric dissection is extended up to the root of the right colic vessels and middle colic vessels. Depending on the location of the mass, one or both of the above vessels are divided at their origin. After transection of the terminal ileum, the remainder of the operation proceeds in the conventional fashion with mobilization of the colon from the gastrocolic ligament and from its lateral attachments.

The table is tilted to reverse Trendelenburg position to mobilize the hepatic flexure, although this is not mandatory, and often single docking is usually suitable. The omentum and transverse colon are retracted caudally thereby exposing the hepatocolic ligament. For this step, unless da Vinci Xi with table motion is used, the instruments may need to be removed and the robotic arms temporarily undocked from the ports before changing the OR table position. The transverse colon is retracted caudally and the hepatocolic ligament is divided with energy device to control the

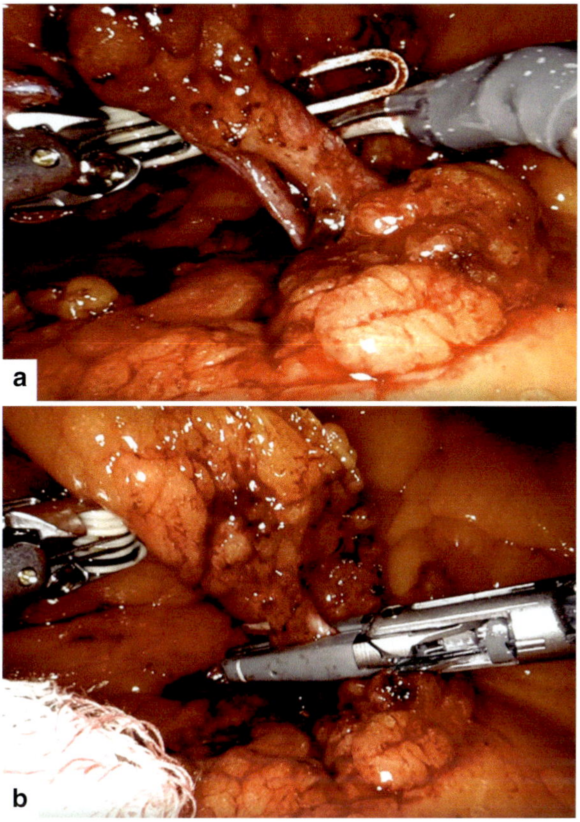

Fig. 15.6 (**a**, **b**) The ileocolic artery and vein are dissected (**a**). The ileocolic artery is divided using the robotic vessel sealer (**b**). (Courtesy of Daniel Popowich, MD)

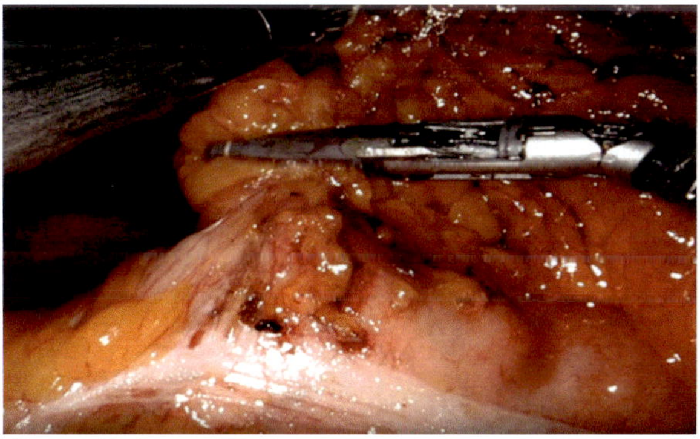

Fig. 15.7 Division of the hepatocolic ligament. The mentum is dissected off the proximal transverse colon. (Courtesy of Daniel Popowich, MD)

blood vessels within the ligament (Fig. 15.7). The dissection is continued toward the hepatic flexure, and the final attachments of the colon to the retroperitoneum are divided. The first and second portions of the duodenum should be visualized and protected. If necessary, the gastrocolic ligament is divided to achieve additional mobilization of transverse colon.

Depending on the surgeon's skill and complexity of the procedure, the terminal ileum and its mesentery and transverse colon with its mesocolon are divided with

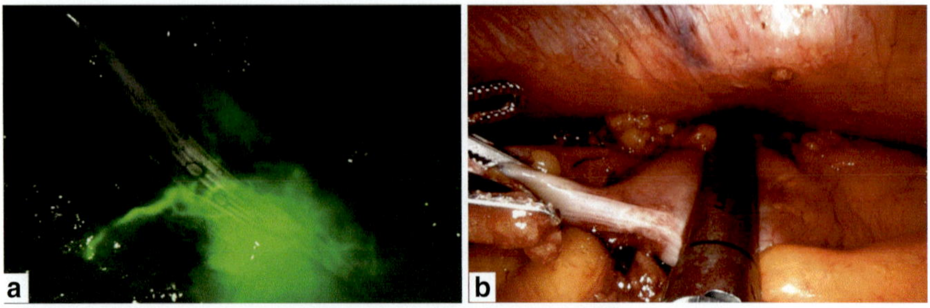

Fig. 15.8 (**a**, **b**) Following complete mesocolic excision, bowel perfusion is assessed using ICG perfusion and FireFly fluorescence imaging (**a**). After confirming the level of vascular demarcation, the proximal colon is divided with the robotic stapler (**b**). (Courtesy of Daniel Popowich, MD)

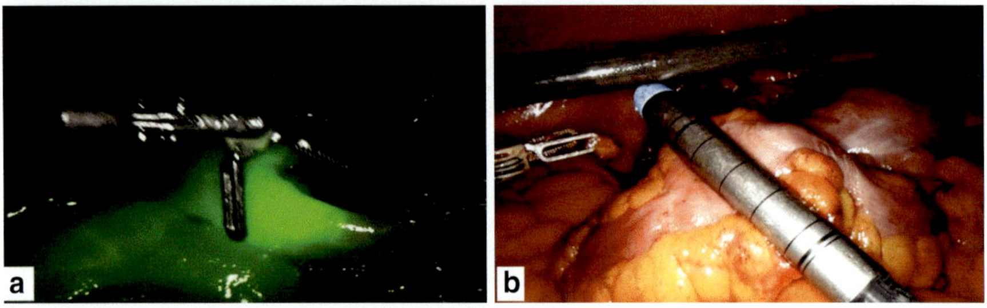

Fig. 15.9 (**a**, **b**) Following mobilization of the terminal ileum mesentery, ICG perfusion confirms the level of vascular demarcation along the small bowel (**a**) which is divided with the robotic stapler at that level (**b**). (Courtesy of Daniel Popowich, MD)

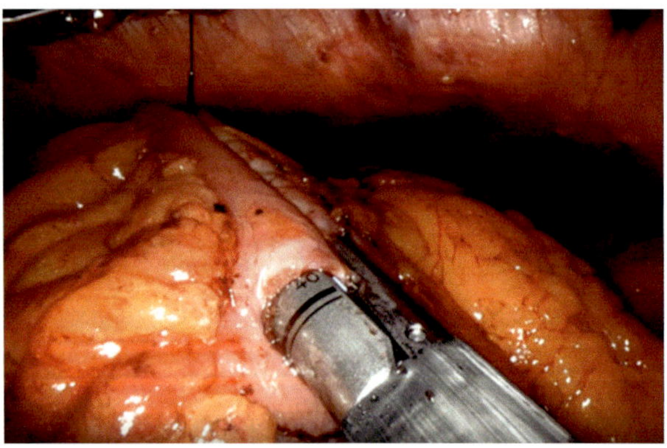

Fig. 15.10 An enterotomy is made along the terminal ileum and the transverse colon, and the robotic stapler is inserted to complete stapled side-side isoperistaltic anastomosis. (Courtesy of Daniel Popowich, MD)

the robotic bipolar energy device and/or stapler (Figs. 15.8a, b and 15.9a, b). An intracorporeal anastomosis can be constructed robotically with removal of the specimen through either a Pfannenstiel incision or by extending left upper quadrant 12 mm stapler trocar (Figs. 15.10 and 15.11). For more details on how to perform laparoscopic intracorporeal anastomosis, please refer to Chap. 14 on option for ileocolonic reconstruction.

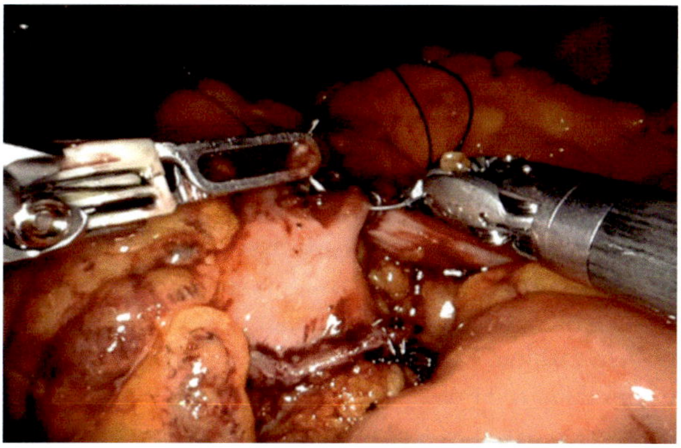

Fig. 15.11 The common enterotomy is closed using intracorporeal robotic suturing to complete the ileocolonic anastomosis. (Courtesy of Daniel Popowich, MD)

Alternatively, the remainder of the operation can be performed via an open approach. After the robot is undocked, the incision for a camera port is extended superiorly to create a small midline mini-laparotomy. The mobilized right colon is then exteriorized through this incision and resected. A standard extracorporeal side-to-side ileocolic anastomosis is created.

Pitfalls and Troubleshooting

1. Incorrect port placement. This could result in external collisions, limited reach, or instrument excursion. An attempt at repositioning the arms or adjusting the Flex joints on Xi should be made. If the setup remains suboptimal, the surgeon should consider placing another robotic cannula in a more favorable location on the abdomen.
2. Motion scaling. Most da Vinci machines have their default scaling set to "fine." For right colectomy, fine scaling may result in excessive need for clutching; therefore, we prefer to use "normal" scaling.

Common Errors and Intraoperative Difficulties (Anatomic Landmarks)

1. Failure to identify the correct plane during medial to lateral dissection. Initial incision posterior to ileocolic pedicle does not always lead to a correct bloodless retroperitoneal plane. If the plane of dissection appears bloody, it is recommended to enter the plane in a different location distal or proximal along the ileocolic pedicle.
2. Division of the ileocolic artery using energy device without clear identification of the duodenum. In the event of bleeding from the ileocolic artery following division, attempt at controlling the artery could result in injury to the duodenum.
3. Failure to fully mobilize terminal ileal attachments could result in limited mobility of the transected terminal ileum and tension on the anastomosis.
4. Excessive traction on the transverse colon during exteriorization of the specimen could result in avulsion of middle colic vein at its confluence with the SMV.

Management of Intraoperative Complications: Tips and Tricks, Salvage, and When to Convert

1. Rapid control of intraoperative hemorrhage is one of the essential skills in robotic surgery. Unless a major vascular injury has occurred, an attempt at robotic control of hemorrhage should be made. It is imperative to communicate with the OR team and especially bedside assistant in a calm and clear fashion. An assistant can operate the suction, apply pressure on a vessel, and introduce a mini-laparotomy pad. A bipolar energy device should be used in controlled and precise fashion since careless bites can result in injury to nearby organs, such as duodenum, or worsen the hemorrhage. Suture ligature, ties, clips, or stapler can be considered as alternatives. Most importantly, the surgeon must exercise judgment and consider converting to laparoscopy, hand-assist laparoscopy, or open approach if several attempts at control of the hemorrhage have been made without success. It is ill-advised to struggle robotically to control intraoperative hemorrhage, especially in the early phases of learning of robotic technique.
2. Organ injury may occur during dissection in the vicinity of the duodenum, liver, and gallbladder. Injury to the right ureter and gonadal vessels is rare during right colectomy. If the correct retroperitoneal plane is developed during medial to lateral dissection, identification of right ureter and gonadal vessels is not required. However, if the psoas muscle is exposed, the plane of dissection is likely too posterior. In this circumstance right ureter needs to be positively identified to assure that it has not been lifted with ascending mesocolon. If injury to the organ is identified, a skilled colleague should be asked to assist with repair. The repair should be carried out robotically only if the surgeon is absolutely confident in their skill to complete the task. An example of repair suitable for robotic approach is a small defect in the second portion of the duodenum that can be repaired with suture closure.
3. If the decision to convert has been made, it does not necessarily mean that a surgeon should convert right away. For example, in the cases of severe terminal ileal of Crohn's disease where dense phlegmon is deemed not amenable to robotic mobilization, the surgeon may still consider taking down hepatic flexure and mobilize ascending colon robotically. This way the incision may be created in the lower midline or in the right lower quadrant to specifically address terminal ileal disease and eliminate the need for cephalad extension of the incision. For more details, refer to the chapter on advanced laparoscopic right colectomy techniques in Crohn's disease and preoperative ileocolonic resection.

Outcomes

The comparison of outcomes between laparoscopy and robotic right colectomy is summarized in Table 15.1. In a recent meta-analysis by Solaini and colleagues [15], operative time was found to be significantly longer for robotic colectomy procedures in the pooled analysis (standard mean difference (SMD) – 0.99; 95% CI – 1.4

Table 15.1 Comparison of outcomes between laparoscopic and robotic right colectomy

First author	Study type	Study period	Study design	Number of patients LRC/RRC	Operative time (min) LRC/RRC	Complication rate (%) LRC/RRC	Total hospital cost ($) LRC/RRC
Casillas [18]	Single center	2005–2012	Prospective	110/52	79/143	35/17 ($p = 0.03$)	Not reported
Trastulli [5]	Multicenter	2005–2014	Retrospective	40/102	208/287	20/22.5	Not reported
Davis [17]	Multicenter	2009–2011	Retrospective	207/207	179/247	LRC = RRC	16,396/18,515
Dolejs [19]	Multicenter	2012–2014	Retrospective	6521/259	133/173	22/ 22	Not reported
Lujan [6]	Single center	2009–2015	Retrospective	185/89	Not reported	25.8/32.6	Not reported
de'Angelis [20]	Single center	2012–2015	Retrospective	50/30	204/200	0/1	Not reported

LRC laparoscopic right colectomy, *RRC* robotic right colectomy to −0.6, $p < 0.001$), while the rate of conversion was less in the robotic group (RR 1.7; 95% CI 1.1–2.6, $p = 0.02$). There was a trend toward higher lymph node yield during robotic right colectomy than for laparoscopic right colectomy (23.4 versus 24.3), $p = 0.057$. Postoperative complications, morbidity, and mortality were similar between the two procedures. Return of bowel function, as determined by passage of flatus, was earlier in robotic group (SMD 0.85 days; 95% CI 0.16–1.54, $p = 0.016$). The incidence of other complications such as anastomotic leak, postoperative hemorrhage, ileus, wound infection, abdominal abscess, and incisional hernia was similar between the groups.

Robotic colectomy is considered feasible and safe in regard to oncologic outcomes. Spinoglio and colleagues [3] reported results of their study of 100 consecutive patients who underwent robotic CME. With a median follow-up period of 48.5 months (range, 24–114 months), the survival rates were 94.5% for disease-specific (DSS), 91.4% for disease-free survival (DFS), and 90.3% for overall survival. The DSS rates were 100% for stage 1 cancer, 97.1% for stage 2 cancer, and 89.3% for stage 3 cancer. The disease-free survival rates were 100% for stage 1 cancer, 94.3% for stage 2 cancer, and 78.2% for stage 3 cancer. The overall survival rates were 95% for stage I, 91.7% for stage II, and 86.3% for stage III cancer. The anastomotic leak rate was 1%.

The cost of robotic surgery for right colectomy remains higher than laparoscopy [16, 17]. The pooled mean surgery-related costs was higher in the robotic group ($5953; 95% CI 2223–9684) than in the laparoscopic one ($3930; 95% CI 1733–6127; $p = 0.051$) [15].

Conclusions

Robotic right colectomy is considered to be feasible and safe procedure with postoperative morbidity and mortality rates similar to the laparoscopic approach, among surgeons who have overcome their learning curve. Specific surgical complications such as anastomotic leak, postoperative hemorrhage, postoperative ileus, wound infections, and abdominal abscess are similar between the two procedures.

References

1. deSouza AL, Prasad LM, Ricci J, Park JJ, Marecik SJ, Zimmern A, et al. A comparison of open and robotic total mesorectal excision for rectal adenocarcinoma. Dis Colon Rectum. 2011;54(3):275–82.
2. Ozben V, Baca B, Atasoy D, Bayraktar O, Aghayeva A, Cengiz TB, et al. Robotic complete mesocolic excision for right-sided colon cancer. Surg Endosc. 2016;30(10):4624–5.
3. Spinoglio G, Marano A, Bianchi PP, Priora F, Lenti LM, Ravazzoni F, et al. Robotic right colectomy with modified complete mesocolic excision: long-term oncologic outcomes. Ann Surg Oncol. 2016;23(Suppl 5):684–91.
4. Spinoglio G, Bianchi PP, Marano A, Priora F, Lenti LM, Ravazzoni F, et al. Robotic versus laparoscopic right colectomy with complete mesocolic excision for the treatment of colon

cancer: perioperative outcomes and 5-year survival in a consecutive series of 202 patients. Ann Surg Oncol. 2018 Nov;25(12):3580–6.
5. Trastulli S, Coratti A, Guarino S, Piagnerelli R, Annecchiarico M, Coratti F, et al. Robotic right colectomy with intracorporeal anastomosis compared with laparoscopic right colectomy with extracorporeal and intracorporeal anastomosis: a retrospective multicentre study. Surg Endosc. 2015;29(6):1512–21.
6. Lujan HJ, Plasencia G, Rivera BX, Molano A, Fagenson A, Jane LA, et al. Advantages of robotic right colectomy with intracorporeal anastomosis. Surg Laparosc Endosc Percutan Tech. 2018;28(1):36–41.
7. Harr JN, Juo YY, Luka S, Agarwal S, Brody F, Obias V. Incisional and port-site hernias following robotic colorectal surgery. Surg Endosc. 2016;30(8):3505–10.
8. Jimenez-Rodriguez RM, Quezada-Diaz F, Tchack M, Pappou E, Wei IH, Smith JJ, et al. Use of the Xi robotic platform for total abdominal colectomy: a step forward in minimally invasive colorectal surgery. Surg Endosc. 2019;33(3):966–71.
9. Protyniak B, Jorden J, Farmer R. Multiquadrant robotic colorectal surgery: the da Vinci Xi vs Si comparison. J Robot Surg. 2018;12(1):67–74.
10. Harr JN, Luka S, Kankaria A, Juo YY, Agarwal S, Obias V. Robotic-assisted colorectal surgery in obese patients: a case-matched series. Surg Endosc. 2017;31(7):2813–9.
11. Formisano G, Misitano P, Giuliani G, Calamati G, Salvischiani L, Bianchi PP. Laparoscopic versus robotic right colectomy: technique and outcomes. Updat Surg. 2016;68(1):63–9.
12. Morelli L, Palmeri M, Guadagni S, Di Franco G, Moglia A, Ferrari V, et al. Use of a new integrated table motion for the da Vinci Xi in colorectal surgery. Int J Color Dis. 2016;31(9):1671–3.
13. Lee HJ, Choi GS, Park JS, Park SY, Kim HJ, Woo IT, et al. A novel robotic right colectomy for colon cancer via the suprapubic approach using the da Vinci Xi system: initial clinical experience. Ann Surg Treat Res. 2018;94(2):83–7.
14. Samia H, Lawrence J, Nobel T, Stein S, Champagne BJ, Delaney CP. Extraction site location and incisional hernias after laparoscopic colorectal surgery: should we be avoiding the midline? Am J Surg. 2013;205(3):264–7; discussion 8
15. Solaini L, Bazzocchi F, Cavaliere D, Avanzolini A, Cucchetti A, Ercolani G. Robotic versus laparoscopic right colectomy: an updated systematic review and meta-analysis. Surg Endosc. 2018;32(3):1104–10.
16. Park JS, Choi GS, Park SY, Kim HJ, Ryuk JP. Randomized clinical trial of robot-assisted versus standard laparoscopic right colectomy. Br J Surg. 2012;99(9):1219–26.
17. Davis BR, Yoo AC, Moore M, Gunnarsson C. Robotic-assisted versus laparoscopic colectomy: cost and clinical outcomes. JSLS. 2014;18(2):211–24.
18. Casillas MA Jr, Leichtle SW, Wahl WL, Lampman RM, Welch KB, Wellock T, et al. Improved perioperative and short-term outcomes of robotic versus conventional laparoscopic colorectal operations. Am J Surg. 2014;208(1):33–40.
19. Dolejs SC, Waters JA, Ceppa EP, Zarzaur BL. Laparoscopic versus robotic colectomy: a national surgical quality improvement project analysis. Surg Endosc. 2017;31(6):2387–96.
20. de'Angelis N, Lizzi V, Azoulay D, Brunetti F. Robotic versus laparoscopic right colectomy for colon cancer: analysis of the initial simultaneous learning curve of a surgical fellow. J Laparoendosc Adv Surg Tech A. 2016;26(11):882–92.

Advanced Laparoscopic Right Colectomy Techniques for Crohn's and Reoperative Surgery

16

Alexander John Greenstein and Barry Salky

Introduction and Rationale

Crohn's disease (CD) surgery, both primary and revisional, may present unique challenges for the surgeon. Because there is currently no cure for CD, recurrent disease after prior resection is relatively common. The risk of endoscopic and surgical recurrence increases with time. Documented recurrence rates are 20–25% at 5 years and approximately 50% at 10 years [1]. Not all of these patients will require surgery, but as recurrence tends to mimic the original presentation, many of these patients will require repeat resections over their lifetime. This is one of the main reasons a minimally invasive approach is particularly advantageous in this population, as it may lessen the incidence of abdominal wall hernia. Another relevant advantage of a laparoscopic approach is the reduction in abdominal adhesions following resection which potentially could make subsequent surgery less demanding. Multiple articles have documented decreased adhesions and decreased adhesive obstructions following laparoscopic surgery [2, 3].

Although simple fibrostenotic CD is typically easy to manage laparoscopically, the surgical complexity of resections increases dramatically in the setting of severe inflammatory and fistulizing disease. While similar difficulties may be encountered during surgery for cancer and/or diverticulitis, these complicating factors are more commonly encountered in CD, particularly in right sided disease. Surgeons should be prepared to encounter these findings and plan their surgical approach accordingly. There is evidence from several large retrospective series that complex CD can

A. J. Greenstein (✉)
Mount Sinai Hospital, Department of Surgery and Health Policy, New York, NY, USA
e-mail: alexander.greenstein@mountsinai.org

B. Salky
Mount Sinai Hospital, Department of Surgery, New York, NY, USA

P. Sylla et al. (eds.), *The SAGES Manual of Colorectal Surgery*,
https://doi.org/10.1007/978-3-030-24812-3_16

be approached safely and effectively laparoscopically, with reduced hospital stay and comparable or fewer complications including decreased adhesions and decreased adhesive obstructions relative to open surgery [4–7]. We will discuss these various scenarios in detail below. All surgeons taking care of these patients should be familiar with advanced laparoscopic techniques, especially for those with recurrent disease.

Indications and Contraindications

Indications for laparoscopic revisional surgery for CD are the same as for primary CD and including medically refractory fibrostenotic, fistulizing disease, and recurrent inflammatory disease with abscess or phlegmon. Absolute contraindications to a laparoscopic approach include hemodynamic instability or other medical conditions precluding tolerance of pneumoperitoneum and intestinal perforation with diffuse intraabdominal spillage. Relative contraindications include intestinal obstruction with massive abdominal distention and severely decreased working space and/or friability of the bowel wall. If it is safe to defer surgery, a period of nasogastric tube decompression, bowel rest, and parenteral nutrition is highly recommended in order to facilitate a laparoscopic approach in these patients.

Reoperation in the setting of multiple prior abdominal surgeries, while feasible, requires a change in strategy with respect to establishing safe intraabdominal access, planned steps of the procedure, and manipulating the bowel. Achieving adequate exposure and evaluating the bowel proximal and distal to the pathology can be challenging in the setting of dense adhesions. Careful review of preoperative imaging is critical in order to determine the best intraoperative strategy. High BMI in the setting of reoperative or Crohn's surgery is not a contraindication to laparoscopy, and we would consider it to actually create an even stronger indication for surgery as these patients stand to benefit even more from a minimally invasive approach.

Principles and Quality Benchmarks

The primary guiding principle for all surgery in CD is bowel conservation. This is especially the case in patients with multifocal disease and those who require recurrent resections. Although the goal of the resection is to remove the diseased segment, resection to microscopically negative margins has not been shown to decrease the rate or time to recurrence or increase quality of life. Strictureplasty should be considered when appropriate, especially in multifocal disease, i.e., multiple narrow segments over a long span of bowel. Avoidance of intestinal leak is also critical to reduce bowel loss. As fistulizing disease is common in CD, it is important to spare the normal bowel attached to the diseased bowel whenever possible. In general, almost all internal connections can be divided laparoscopically using endoscopic linear staplers. This will decrease the extent of bowel that is resected and decrease the size of the extraction incision as well. During reoperative ileocolic resection, identification of the duodenum and ureter and meticulous lysis of adhesions are paramount.

Preoperative Planning, Patient Work-Up, and Optimization

As bowel conservation is key to the success of resection for primary or recurrent CD, the preoperative work-up is critical in determining the planned surgical procedure. A thorough review of prior operative reports will provide details regarding the extent and location of all prior resections and/or strictureplasties, length of small bowel removed and of small bowel remaining, as well as type of anastomosis previously created. Recent CT and MR enterography (CTE/MRE) can be very helpful to define the anatomy of the diseased segments as well as "occult" areas that may not be clinically significant or visualized on endoscopy may dramatically affect the operative plan. We have found it very useful to review these with experienced radiologists preoperatively. We also highly recommend a preoperative colonoscopy on all patients. Ileosigmoid fistulas are common, and it is helpful to evaluate the sigmoid mucosa prior to dividing the fistula. While CD typically affects the ileum, it is possible to have sigmoid disease concurrently which would make a double resection mandatory.

For patients in whom fecal diversion is anticipated, preoperative marking of stoma sites by an enterostomal therapist is critical for improved function and quality of life. If an enterostomal nurse is not available, it is critical that the patient is marked in the office or even in the preoperative area the day of surgery. We recommend that the patient be examined while sitting up, standing, and lying down in order to identify a location away from creases, scars, and belt line and ensure that it is in an area that the patient is able to see (i.e., not below a large pannus). We recommend marking patients preoperatively even if a stoma is not definitively planned for as operative conditions may determine the need for one and marking the patient on the operating room table will lead to unsatisfactory results. A thorough discussion between the physician and the patients/family and GI doctor is also helpful in managing short- and long-term expectations regarding disease control and potential need for reoperation.

Physiological optimization is required in all elective patients with CD. Nutrition and anemia should be corrected as much as the clinical condition will allow. There is some debate about the impact of new biologics and anti-tumor necrosis factor (TNF) medications on postoperative infectious complications and on the safest time interval between the last dose and surgery. While some studies have shown that preoperative use of infliximab does not increase postoperative complication rates, others have suggested worse outcomes with newer biologic agents such as vedolizumab especially when used within 3 months of surgery [8–12].

In general, if possible, most of these medications should be stopped at least 2 weeks prior to surgery. Unfortunately it may not be possible to wean these patients completely from their immunosuppression as their disease may worsen and their clinical condition may deteriorate prior to surgery. In our own experience, with the exception of steroids, recent use of biologics has not been found to increase postoperative morbidity.

Operative Setup

In general, if an ileosigmoid fistula is not present and a left colectomy, sigmoid, or rectosigmoid resection is not required, the patient is placed supine, with arms tucked at the sides. It is key to protect against all potential nerve injury sites, including the brachial plexus. A urinary drainage catheter is always placed, as is an orogastric tube. Preoperative antibiotic dosing is performed within 1 hour of the incision. All patients have sequential compression devices (SCDs) on and functioning during the operation, and many surgeons prefer to give the first perioperative dose of subcutaneous heparin at this time. For right-sided disease, the surgeon and assistant stand on the patient's left, and the OR nurse and video monitor are on the patient's right. If an ileosigmoid fistula is present or a left colectomy and sigmoid/anterior resection is required, the patient is placed in low lithotomy position utilizing stirrups with the thighs flexed in such a manner as to not impede the abdominal instruments and allow access to the anus for potential endoscopic evaluation and stapler placement. As the patient is frequently placed in steep, head down position, some type of fixation to the OR table is highly recommended (belts, pink pad, bean bag, tape).

There are multiple laparoscopic energy devices available, and each one of them is adequate for dissection and vessel division. Mechanical hemostatic devices are available as well. Each surgeon tends to have their preferred device for vessel sealing, and we have found no difference in outcome with any of them. It is important to be familiar with whichever device is being used, especially regarding troubleshooting. None of these devices are infallible during dissection or mesenteric division especially with thick, friable Crohn's mesentery.

Operative Technique: Surgical Steps Including Pitfalls and Troubleshooting

Abdominal Entry and Trocar Placement

Safe intraabdominal access is essential to decreasing complications at the earliest phase of the operation. There are multiple methods to gain access to the abdomen in previously operated patients, none of which have shown superiority with respect to avoiding injury. Whichever method is used, we would not place the first trocar through a previous scar as the chance of bowel adhesions under a scar is high. We prefer an open (Hasson) approach or use of an optical viewing trocar at Palmer's point in the left upper quadrant. Following entry, the abdominal wall under the original trocar is visualized to ensure a through and through bowel injury has not occurred. On occasion, several entry sites will be attempted in order to gain safe

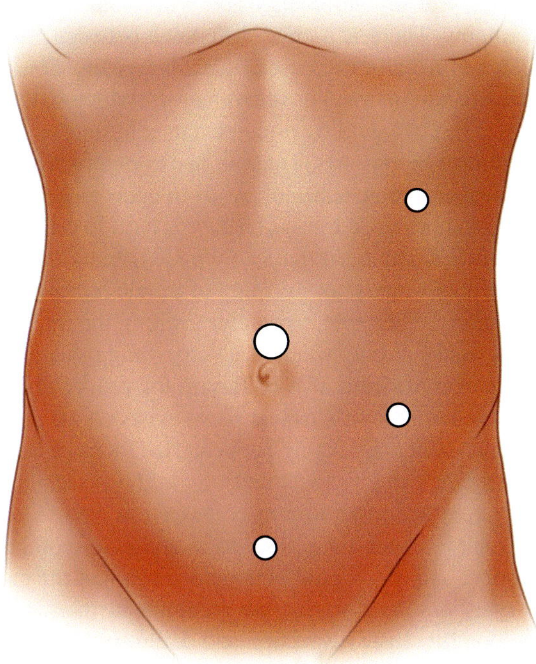

Fig. 16.1 Laparoscopic port setup: three 5 mm ports and a 12 mm port

access. In general, we like to approach the pathology further away. Whenever possible, 5 mm trocars should be preferentially used, with a 12 mm trocar reserved for the use of an endoscopic stapler and preferably placed in planned extraction sites. Additional 5 mm trocars should be added as necessary in order to optimize visualization and exposure. Please see Fig. 16.1 for typical port placement. We prefer the use of a 5 mm camera as this allows the camera to be placed in different trocar locations during adhesiolysis and disease mobilization.

Adhesiolysis and Intestinal Dissection

The extent and density of adhesions can vary significantly from case to case. It is for this reason that we believe that diagnostic laparoscopy should be performed in every patient before committing to an open operation. In some cases, minimal adhesions are found, and laparoscopic reoperative resection will be as straightforward as primary resection. In Crohn's patients, it is thought that this may be due to their chronic immunosuppression. More typically, however, extensive laparoscopically lysis of adhesions and bowel mobilization will be needed to expose anatomic landmarks and the pathology. Even if the case is ultimately converted to open due to inability to fully expose the pathology, the size of the extraction may be reduced by having mobilized the bowel proximal and distal to the pathology laparoscopically. Surgeons should be familiar with multiple techniques for safe adhesiolysis.

In general, sharp "cold" dissection with endoshears is safer than using monopolar cautery or bipolar energy and will avoid inadvertent burn injury and delayed enterotomy. There is a clear difference between "filmy" adhesions (nonvascular), which can usually be teased apart and easily transected, and "dense" adhesions which are vascularized or inflammatory, which will not separate without sharp dissection. The two guiding principles in adhesiolysis are preventing bowel injury and maintaining hemostasis. Traction and counter-traction principles are just as important in laparoscopic adhesiolysis as in open surgery. However, the amount of counter-traction provided by an assistant is hard to estimate and control. Serosal tearing to bowel wall can occur passively by assistant traction on the bowel against a point of fixation. Overzealous grasping of friable bowel can result in partial- or full-thickness tearing. Therefore, we prefer limiting the traction applied by the assistant and use the assistant only when necessary during this phase of the operation. The other important consideration is to stay in the proper dissection plane. When dissecting off the abdominal wall, a clear plane exists on the parietal peritoneum. It tends to be avascular. When dissecting between two loops of bowel or two loops of mesentery, it is important to go slowly and stay in the avascular plane. If bleeding occurs, it is most likely due to an improper dissection plan. After extensive adhesiolysis, it is important to check for serosal tears and enterotomies prior to moving on with the resection, and this should be repeated again at the end of the procedure. If there is any question about injury, we recommend marking the area with a suture or an endoloop for closer inspection and definitive suture repair later during the case.

Complex Crohn's Disease Resection

As with any other complex surgery, mastery of the anatomy and careful dissection techniques are required to identify anatomic landmarks during complex or reoperative right colectomy such as the right ureter, kidney, and duodenum. Laparoscopic reoperative surgery for CD follows the same steps as for primary resection. Differences include identification of the prior anastomosis and its mesentery and careful mobilization of the anastomosis from surrounding structures, which is usually complicated by fibrosis, acute or chronic inflammation, and/or fistulas. Once mobilized fully, the planned resection of the anastomosis and adjacent diseased bowel and construction of a new ileocolonic anastomosis is performed. As most patients have had the retroperitoneum exposed previously, repeat dissection and identification of landmarks is often more challenging, especially in the setting of scarring, fibrosis, abscesses, phlegmons, and fistulas. Rather than dissecting the mesentery using a medial to lateral approach during reoperative right colectomy, a lateral to medial approach may facilitate ureteral identification and avoid inadvertent injury. This is particularly useful in CD where the mesentery can be very thickened and friable and not suitable to be taken safely via a minimally invasive approach with an energy device.

Additionally, in reoperative Crohn's disease with prior resection, the mesentery to the diseased bowel may not be readily identifiable until after full mobilization of the diseased segment and therefore best to be divided after lateral to medial mobilization.

Crohn's Abscess, Phlegmon, and Mass

Intraperitoneal, pelvic, or retroperitoneal abscess formation remains a serious complication of Crohn's fistulizing disease. Assuming that the collection is greater than 5 cm and there is a safe window on imaging, preoperative drainage under radiological control is standard of care. If percutaneous drainage is not possible, preoperative or simultaneous surgical aspiration may be necessary. Eventually, the diseased segment and source of the abscess requires resection.

After successful drainage of intraabdominal or retroperitoneal abscess and return to optimal health, resection of the associated segment of bowel may be attempted laparoscopically. We recommend waiting approximately 3 months to allow for the inflammatory changes to resolve and the patient to be medically and nutritionally optimized. Conversion, or hand-assisted laparoscopy with a smaller incision may be necessary in the most difficult cases, but we typically begin with a pure laparoscopic approach even in the setting of a large phlegmon. The prevailing goal in these cases is to mobilize the phlegmonous mass in order to exteriorize it through as small an incision as possible (midline or off-midline). We generally approach this using a lateral to medial approach given the thickened mesentery that tends to accompany a Crohn's mass and the difficulty manipulating it.

Often the hepatic flexure, even if previously mobilized, is not diseased and is an optimal place to begin a lateral to medial dissection. After mobilizing the hepatic flexure, we continue the lateral to medial dissection down toward the ileocolic angle. Unfortunately, the area with greatest inflammation often tends to be adjacent to the confluence of the ureter and iliac vessels. Appropriate use of blunt dissection is paramount to a successful mobilization of the disease and avoidance of collateral damage. Our instrument of choice is the suction-irrigating device (which allows for simultaneous clearance of blood or purulence) or laparoscopic peanut which can serve as a replacement for open finger fracture dissection. A bipolar or ultrasonic device should be available to lyse scar tissue when determined safe. Eventually, the scar will need to be penetrated leaving the mesentery of the ileocolic region, and the mass can be mobilized medially. If one enters a retroperitoneal plane, one must be careful to remain superficial and anterior to the ureter. Ureteral catheters with and without the use of lighted devices or indocyanine green (ICG) can be used at the surgeon's discretion for ureteral identification.

Crohn's Fistula

Ileosigmoid and ileorectal fistulae are relatively common in patients with fistulizing disease. One large case series estimated the prevalence of internal fistulizing disease at 6% for all CD patients and, of those, 19% possessed fistulas from the ileum to the sigmoid colon [13]. In these fistulae, the inflamed terminal ileum most commonly adheres to the medial aspect of the sigmoid colon, which is usually otherwise healthy, but on occasion there is disease of both the terminal ileum and sigmoid colon. Because of this, dealing with the sigmoid side of the fistula can involve either simple division across the fistulous tract with resection of only the diseased ileocolic segment or en bloc resection. While simple ileosigmoid fistulae can often be approached laparoscopically, fistulae low in the sigmoid colon or more distal in the region of the rectouterine or rectovesical pouch may require a hand-assisted or open approach.

In the event of a simple ileosigmoid fistula, after mobilization of the right colon and sigmoid, it should be possible to lift the Crohn's mass and sigmoid anteriorly and superiorly in order to identify the tract from the ileum to the sigmoid. After it has been dissected out and thinned out as much as possible, it should be possible to laparoscopically place an endoscopic linear stapler loaded with a 60-mm-long purple, green, or black load through an appropriately sized port and staple across the fibrous tract (Figs. 16.2a, b1, c1 and 16.3a–c). The sigmoid will fall gently aside leaving the right colon and ileum which can then be resected and anastomosed. Complex ileosigmoid fistulae which require double resection (Fig. 16.2a, b2, c2) may be able to be performed by a pure laparoscopic approach, but often their complexity may require conversion. Again, we recommend trying to mobilize as much as possible laparoscopically or try hand-assisted techniques prior to converting as this can reduce the size of the incision and still greatly benefit the patient.

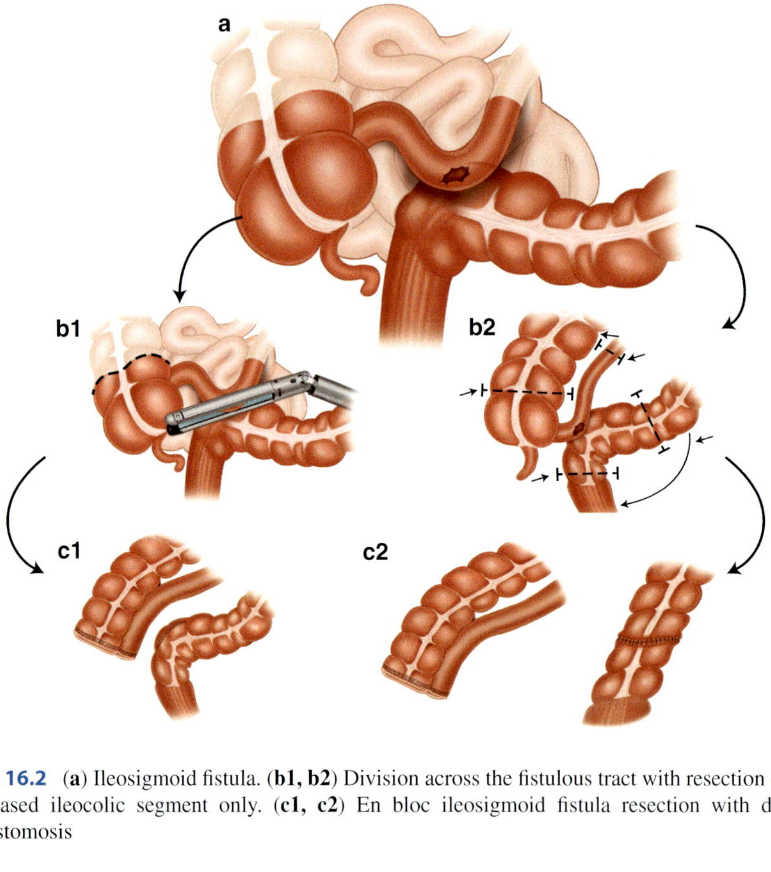

Fig. 16.2 (**a**) Ileosigmoid fistula. (**b1, b2**) Division across the fistulous tract with resection of the diseased ileocolic segment only. (**c1, c2**) En bloc ileosigmoid fistula resection with double anastomosis

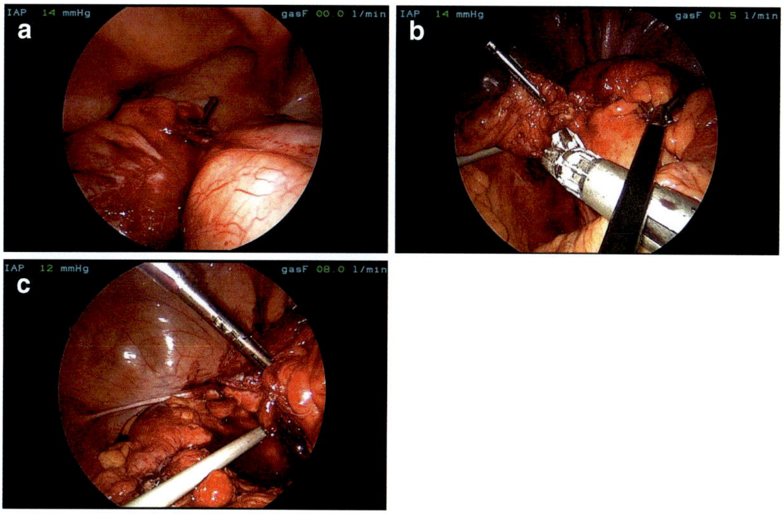

Fig. 16.3 (**a**–**c**) Crohn's ileosigmoid fistula. The endoscopic stapler is used to transect across the fistula with ileocolic resection and preservation of the sigmoid

Difficult Crohn's Mesentery

As discussed previously, the friable and thickened Crohn's mesentery presents a unique challenge, as often the standard energy devices are not adequate to seal the vessels. For this reason, we recommend mobilizing the diseased bowel first to lift the mesentery off the retroperitoneum prior to mesenteric division. Once the diseased bowel is mobilized, a decision is made whether to transect the mesentery intracorporeally or extracorporeally. If the mesentery appears thin and pliable and amenable to division with an energy device, laparoscopic transection can be attempted. Additionally, the mesentery further away from the bowel wall may be thinner and more amenable to standard division with an energy device. In these situations, a high ligation and mesenteric division similar to that for oncologic resections is recommended. There are many devices well equipped to deal with intracorporeal mesenteric division. These include ultrasonic, bipolar, mechanical (staplers and clips), and monopolar electric devices. All can be utilized to divide the mesentery and control bleeding. When these fail, the surgeon needs to be ready with a backup plan which may include laparoscopic suturing or temporary pressure control and conversion to open.

If the mesentery appears to be very bulky and is deemed to be at risk for bleeding after transection with a bipolar device, then it may be safer to perform mesenteric division in an extracorporeal fashion. By mobilizing the diseased and adjacent normal bowel, at least the extraction incision will be smaller than if approached open to start. When in doubt, and if there are questions about vascular control, performing this portion of the procedure in an open fashion is safer. When ready to extract and divide mesentery, we make a periumbilical incision, place a wound protector, and exteriorize the diseased bowel. Occasionally, the Crohn's mass is too large to fit through the small extraction site, so the skin incision may need to be enlarged. It is critical that one maintains control of the proximal portion of the mesenteric vessels during exteriorizing the bowel and mesenteric transection in order to reduce arterial bleeding and/or hematoma formation. After exteriorization, one can place a soft bowel clamp toward the root of the mesentery and use the bipolar device on the more distal portion of the vessel. Even with this technique, it is not uncommon to require multiple 2-0 Vicryl sutures in a figure-of-eight fashion or horizontal mattress fashion in order to control bleeding vessels after attempted control with an energy device or even clamp and tie technique. With the specimen already exteriorized, resection and anastomosis will follow mesenteric transection through this incision.

Ileocolonic Reconstruction

After the mesentery has been divided intracorporeally, one can then decide whether to make an intracorporeal or extracorporeal anastomosis. In addition to the patient's pathology, the surgeon's comfort and proficiency plays a role in this decision, and we will outline both approaches in the next two sections. The benefits of an intracorporeal anastomosis include but are not limited to the need for more limited mobilization of the bowel as it does not need to be exteriorized until after division. Ability to place the extraction site at any location, preferably Pfannenstiel or off midline/planned stoma site, as this is associated with decreased pain and decreased subsequent hernia formation.

Intracorporeal Anastomosis

Our preferred intracorporeal ileocolic anastomotic technique is as follows [14]. Once the mesentery and specimen have been divided, the two ends of the bowel are aligned in an isoperistaltic fashion (antiperistaltic is another option), after the mesentery is visualized at its base. This is an important maneuver to ensure there is no twisting of the anastomosis. If this step is followed, it is impossible to twist the anastomosis. Stay sutures are often placed to help align the bowel and to help with manipulation during stapler placement. Once the intestine is aligned, an enterotomy is made in both the proximal and distal bowel. We prefer to do this with cutting current electrocautery, but ultrasonic devices can be used. If the intestine is dilated from obstruction, a laparoscopic "bulldog" clamp can be placed on the proximal side at least 10 cm up from the planned anastomosis to prevent spillage. Often, however, the pressure of the pneumoperitoneum is enough to prevent enteric spillage. Once the enterotomies are made, an endoscopic linear stapler is placed into each limb of the intestine and fired to create the side-to-side anastomosis. A 60 mm load is preferred but a 45 mm is acceptable. We prefer a purple load, but vascular or thicker loads may be required based on the condition of the bowel and surgeon preference (Fig. 16.4). At this point, the inside staple line is checked for bleeding. Any bleeding must be controlled now before the common enterotomy is closed. We

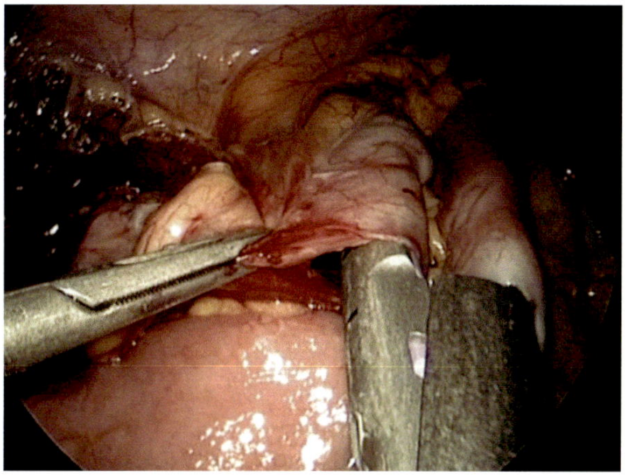

Fig. 16.4 Intracorporeal anastomosis: stapling and creating of a common channel

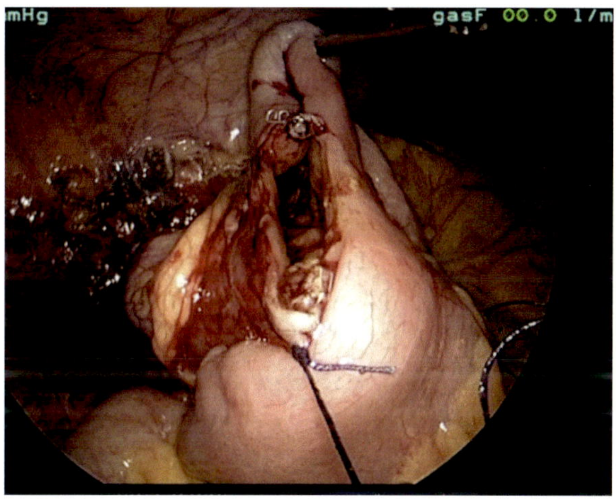

Fig. 16.5 Intracorporeal anastomosis: suturing close the common enterotomy

prefer bipolar energy to control bleeding points on the metal staple line, but this can also be controlled by monopolar cautery, clips or suture ligation.

The options for enterotomy closure are largely dictated by surgeon preference. We prefer a 2-layer closure with an inner absorbable and outer permanent suture. In our experience, this is preferably with 2-0 Vicryl for the inner layer and 3-0 Prolene for the seromuscular outer layer. The use of a single-layer closure, of barbed sutures, and of stapled closure has all been validated. When starting the first/inner layer, we recommend that the surgeon sew away from oneself laparoscopically and toward oneself in open procedures (Fig. 16.5). The reason for this is that it allows the surgeon to place the sutures at right angles to the bowel easier than if sewing toward oneself. This also ensures that the innermost portion of the common channel is completely closed. This can often become difficult to see if sewing toward oneself on the inner layer as that area will have less exposure as the suture progresses closer to the near corner. As suturing can be perceived as a difficult task, the common channel can be stapled closed using an endoscopic stapler. However, if a stapler is used to close the enterotomy, extreme care must be taken to not include the mesentery or to narrow the anastomosis.

Extracorporeal Anastomosis

In order to minimize anastomotic leaks, our preferred approach when performing an extracorporeal anastomosis is to "oversew" the anastomotic staple lines. After the specimen has been resected, the end of the ileum is aligned with the proximal colon in an antiperistaltic side-to-side fashion. We first lay down a posterior continuous 3-0 silk back row on the taenia of the colon and adjacent to the mesentery of the small bowel (Fig. 16.6a). Enterotomies are then made by

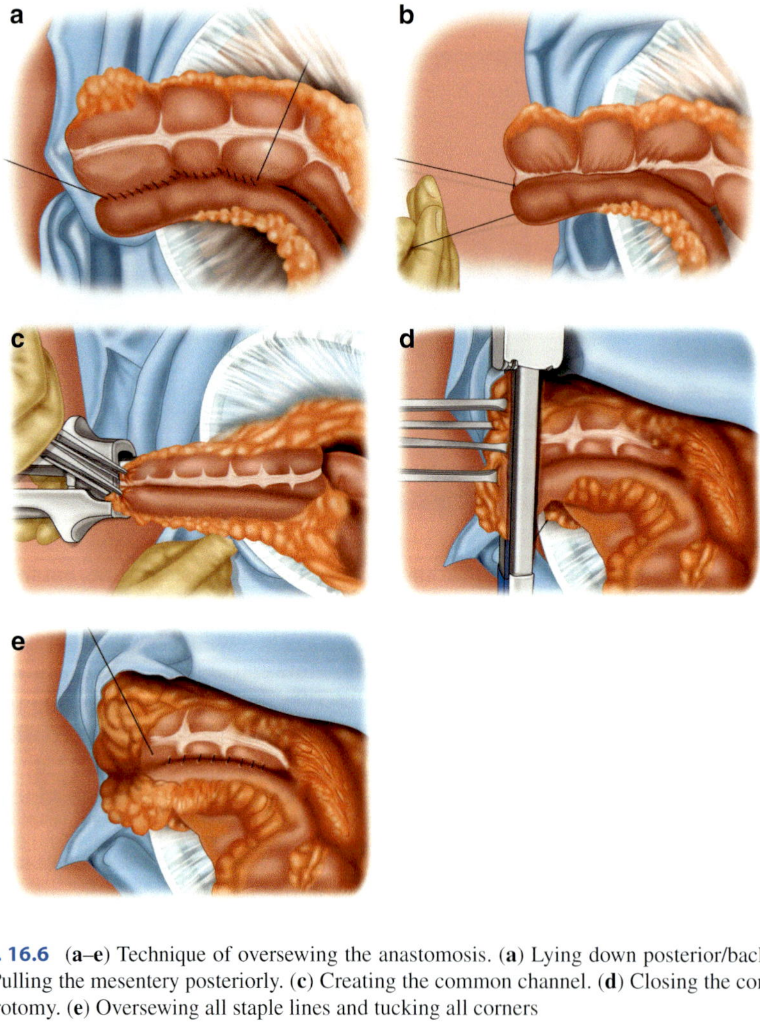

Figs. 16.6 (**a**–**e**) Technique of oversewing the anastomosis. (**a**) Lying down posterior/back row. (**b**) Pulling the mesentery posteriorly. (**c**) Creating the common channel. (**d**) Closing the common enterotomy. (**e**) Oversewing all staple lines and tucking all corners

excising the anti-mesenteric corners of the staple lines on the bowel. The row of silk sutures is then pulled posteriorly so as to remove the mesentery away from the staple line (Fig. 16.6b), and a linear stapler (typically 80 mm) is placed to create the common channel (Fig. 16.6c). A second linear stapler load is used to close the enterotomy (Fig. 16.6d), and then all staple lines are oversewn and covered with running 3-0 silk suture (Fig. 16.6e). For more details and alternative techniques, please refer to Chap. 14 on options for ileocolonic reconstruction.

Pitfalls and Troubleshooting

Entry

Avoid previous scars. Use either optical trocars or open Hasson techniques depending on expertise of the surgeon. After subsequent trocar placement, always look back at the original trocar and the abdominal wall to make sure a through and through or occult injury has not occurred. In the unoperated abdomen, a Veress needle has also been shown to be a safe entry as well.

Adhesiolysis

Use sharp dissection whenever possible. Beware of the "aggressive" assistant. Traction injuries from graspers are common in laparoscopic surgery. If there is troublesome bleeding during adhesiolysis, it is likely that the wrong surgical plane has been entered. Stop the dissection and correct the plane of dissection. After adhesiolysis, always go back and visualize the areas lysed to be sure a bowel injury has not occurred. If there is any suspicion of injury, repair is indicated. If there is any question, exteriorization of the segment is advised.

Duodenum and Right Ureter

It is critical that these two structures be clearly identified during mobilization of the right colon. The best plane for proximal transverse colon mobilization is right on the duodenum, and we advise that a sweeping-blunt technique be used when possible with minimal energy use. Any injury or potential injury to either of these structures must be immediately addressed.

Thickened Mesentery

This has been discussed in detail above. Bleeding can be profuse from inflamed mesentery; therefore, suturing skills should be obtained before tackling difficult mesenteric dissection via minimally invasive techniques. Consider higher ligation as in cancer cases as the mesentery tends to be thinner in this area compared to immediately adjacent to the bowel wall. Laparoscopic or open figure of 8 or horizontal mattress sutures placed while the mesentery is compressed and controlled can get the patient and surgeon out of a difficult situation. Mechanical staplers do not work well on the thickened mesentery, and in general, they should be avoided unless the jaws will close easily around the vessels.

Anastomotic Problems

Keeping the anastomotic leak rate low is important. In order to avoid twisting the anastomosis, the base of the mesentery must be identified and the edge of the mesentery traced up to the cut end of the bowel. At the completion of the anastomosis, it should look correctly oriented. If there is any doubt as to that, we strongly recommend that the anastomosis be redone.

Postoperative Issues

In general, the patients look well, and they are ambulating the first evening or certainly the next day. The WBC can be elevated, but it is highly unusual for that to last more than a day or two. There are some studies that suggest following CRP is a more predictive value in assessing for postoperative complications such as anastomotic leak. It is not uncommon to have a low-grade temperature for a day or two, but not more than that. While a little nausea is common, vomiting is not. The abdomen can, of course, be a little tender for the first day or two, but usually not more than that. If the patient does not adhere to these clinical parameters, it is likely that there is something wrong. We have a very low threshold to take the patient back to the OR for a diagnostic laparoscopy to make sure that the anastomosis is intact. An early CT of the abdomen in our experience almost never tells the real picture of what is happening in the abdomen. Additionally, if there is high clinical concern over the patient's status, there are very few findings on CT that absolve the concern and prevent return to the OR. When returning to the OR, we prefer a laparoscopic approach to asses for anastomotic leak or occult bowel injury or bleeding as most can be dealt with in this manner. It is a mistake to wait until the patient is overtly ill before returning them to the OR.

Ileostomy and Conversion

Temporary ileostomies are occasionally needed. Decisions for end or loop stoma creation should be definitively made preop based on the patient's overall condition. This is often based on patient-related factors such as nutritional status, lab values and immunosuppressive medications, and recent weight loss. Occasionally the decision to create a stoma is made based on intraoperative conditions such as finding an abscess, dilated/thickened proximal bowel, residual diseased bowel, and/or the need for double resections. Marking the patient preoperatively is mandatory to avoid the issue of improper stoma creation if the decision is made based on unplanned operative findings. We believe that the anastomosis should be perfect in appearance, or it should be revised. We do not divert to compensate for a suboptimal anastomosis.

The threshold to conversion to open or hand-assist will vary based on the surgeon's experience and expertise with advanced skills. We strongly believe in preemptive conversion rather than reactive conversion, especially in cases where there is failure to progress due to difficulties identifying the correct anatomical planes of key landmarks. Prompt conversion will avoid injury and reduce intraabdominal spillage with associated septic complications.

Outcomes

Increasingly, laparoscopic resection has been used to treat patients with Crohn's disease and for those requiring reoperative surgery, and this has been validated by several articles that depict good results. Prospective randomized, retrospective, database studies and meta-analyses have all shown short- and long-term benefits of laparoscopic surgery in comparison with open surgery. Short-term benefits include reduced morbidity, expedited recovery, and lower cost, while significant long-term benefits include fewer small bowel obstructions and incisional hernias [6, 15–21]. CD recurrence rates, not surprisingly, are unchanged by laparoscopic surgery. They are essentially equivalent to that of open surgery and remain high [22, 23]. Please see Table 16.1 for a listing of some of these studies.

Clearly, laparoscopic resections are possible, even likely, in Crohn's and reoperative surgery given a certain level of expertise. Considering the incidence of recurrent disease and surgery in these patients, an initial laparoscopic approach is indicated [24]. There are also several studies that have been published which analyze laparoscopic surgery for recurrent Crohn's versus primary Crohn's disease. They essentially demonstrate that laparoscopic surgery can be performed safely on recurrent patients with minimal difference in postoperative complications in comparison with primary Crohn's patients [25–28].

With regard to "oversewing" the anastomosis, a retrospective comparative study at our institution has revealed that the use of this technique for our Crohn's patients led to a significant reduction in major anastomotic complications – a compilation of anastomotic leak, intraabdominal abscess, small bowel obstruction, and anastomotic bleed [29]. Even in the setting of acute abscess or phlegmon, if a carefully constructed anastomosis is created, it is not necessary to create an end ileostomy or diverting loop ileostomy for these cases. There are currently many retrospective papers debating the relative merits of different configurations of ileocolic anastomoses – end-to-end, side-to-side – as well as different types of handsewn anastomoses [30]. A full discussion of this is beyond the scope of this chapter, but there are no good randomized prospective trials indicating advantage of any one technique [31]. We recommend that the individual surgeon perform the anastomosis that they are most comfortable with.

As for intracorporeal anastomosis, several papers and meta analyses have been published so far stressing the feasibility and safety in colorectal surgery. The use of intracorporeal anastomosis should lead to the reduction of incision length, allow for off-midline or Pfannenstiel incisions to decrease postoperative pain, lower incisional hernia rate, and eliminate the need for bowel exteriorization for anastomosis, which could be particularly difficult in the presence of thick and short mesentery and involve the risk of bowel torsion [32–34]. There is a decreased wound infection risk with intracorporeal anastomosis as well, primarily because there is minimal contamination at the extraction site. All specimens are removed in a bag or with wound protection, and typically through a Pfannenstiel incision. Our data have shown a statistically significant decrease in narcotic use as well [14]. Other studies

Table 16.1 Lap vs open ICR for Crohn's disease

Author	Year	*N* (%Lap)	Term	Type	Short-term results	Long-term results
Milsom [20]	2001	60 (52% lap)	Short	Prospective randomized	Lap with significant decrease in minor complications and significantly better lung function	N/A
Maartense [19]	2006	60 (505 lap)	Short	Prospective randomized	Lap with significant decrease in complications (10% vs 33%), LOS (−2 days), and costs	N/A
Lee [6]	2011	1917 (34% lap)	Short	Database (NSQIP)	Lap with significant decrease in major (0.629) and minor complications (0.576), significant decrease in LOS (−1.08 days)	N/A
Aytac [21]	2012	52 (50% lap)	Short	Case-matched retrospective	No statistical difference in overall morbidity and reoperation rate. Lap with significant decrease LOS	N/A
Young-Fadok [16]	2001	66 (50% lap)	Short	Case-matched retrospective	Lap with significant decrease in LOS (−3 days) and costs ($3373)	N/A
Bergamaschi [18]	2003	92 (42% lap)	Short and long	Retrospective	Lap with significant decrease in LOS (−5.6 days) but longer OR time (80 min)	No significant difference in 5-year recurrence (approx 28%)
Lowney [23]	2005	113 (56% lap)	Long	Retrospective	N/A	No significant difference in 5-year recurrence
Heimann [24]	2017	750 (33% lap)	Long	Retrospective	N/A	Hernia rate higher for open (10.8%) than lap (8.4%) but not significantly different
Patel [17]	2013	2519 (N/A)	Short and long	Meta-analysis	Lap with significant decrease in complications (0.71)	No significant difference recurrence. Hernia rate significantly lower for lap(RR =0.24)

LOS length of hospital stay, *RR* relative risk

Table 16.2 Intracorporeal versus extracorporeal results for ileocolic resection

Author	Year	*N* (%IC)	Term	Type	Patient characteristics	Short-term results	Long-term results
Grams [14]	2009	105 (51%)	Short	Retrospective	Crohn's patients	ICA with significantly less narcotic usage, LOS, morbidity	N/A
Vignali [39]	2017	128 (50%)	Short and long	Case matched retrospective	Obese patients with colorectal disease	ICA with significantly earlier bowel function	ICA with significantly less (8% vs 25%) incisional hernia at 2 years
Martinek [38]	2018	453(51%)	Short	Propensity score matched cohort.	Crohn's and obese colon cancer	ICA with significantly lower SSI rates and less morbidity (5.1% vs 12.8%)	N/A
Milone [37]	2014	512 (56%)	Short	Propensity score matched case-control study	Colon cancer	ICA with significantly lower minor complication rate 0.63)	N/A
Cirocchi [35]	2012	945 (N/A)	Short	Meta-analysis	All	No significant difference in leak rate and morbidity	N/A

ICA intracorporeal anastomosis, *ECA* extracorporeal anastomosis, *SSI* surgical site infection, *LOS* length of hospital stay

that have looked at right colonic intracorporeal anastomosis for various indications with no adverse effect on complications, anastomotic leak, or reoperation rates and particularly good results appear to be present for intracorporeal anastomosis in the setting of obesity [14, 35–39]. See Table 16.2.

Conclusion

Primary and reoperative surgery in Crohn's disease is common. The preoperative evaluation is important so as to have an exact diagnosis of the type and extent of the disease including mapping of fistulas and abscesses. Even if the patient has had multiple, previous open surgeries, an attempt at laparoscopy is worthwhile for the patient and will reduce both short- and long-term outcomes. While intracorporeal anastomosis has several advantages, the technical demand and additional time it takes to complete laparoscopically has lead thus far to limited widespread usage among surgeons. For some surgeons, the robotic platform may make the creation of an intracorporeal anastomosis easier and is described in other chapters. If an extracorporeal anastomosis is to be performed, oversewing the anastomosis can reduce anastomotic complications and can be considered.

References

1. Frolkis AD, Dykeman J, Negron ME, Debruyn J, Jette N, Fiest KM, et al. Risk of surgery for inflammatory bowel diseases has decreased over time: a systematic review and meta-analysis of population-based studies. Gastroenterology. 2013;145(5):996–1006.
2. Burns EM, Currie A, Bottle A, Aylin P, Darzi A, Faiz O. Minimal-access colorectal surgery is associated with fewer adhesion-related admissions than open surgery. Br J Surg. 2013;100(1):152–9.
3. Hull TL, Joyce MR, Geisler DP, Coffey JC. Adhesions after laparoscopic and open ileal pouch-anal anastomosis surgery for ulcerative colitis. Br J Surg. 2012;99(2):270–5.
4. Chand M, Siddiqui MR, Gupta A, Rasheed S, Tekkis P, Parvaiz A, et al. Systematic review of emergent laparoscopic colorectal surgery for benign and malignant disease. World J Gastroenterol. 2014;20(45):16956–63.
5. Holder-Murray J, Marsicovetere P, Holubar SD. Minimally invasive surgery for inflammatory bowel disease. Inflamm Bowel Dis. 2015;21(6):1443–58.
6. Lee Y, Fleming FJ, Deeb AP, Gunzler D, Messing S, Monson JR. A laparoscopic approach reduces short-term complications and length of stay following ileocolic resection in Crohn's disease: an analysis of outcomes from the NSQIP database. Color Dis. 2012;14(5):572–7.
7. Pini-Prato A, Faticato MG, Barabino A, Arrigo S, Gandullia P, Mazzola C, et al. Minimally invasive surgery for paediatric inflammatory bowel disease: personal experience and literature review. World J Gastroenterol. 2015;21(40):11312–20.
8. Colombel JF, Loftus EV Jr, Tremaine WJ, Pemberton JH, Wolff BG, Young-Fadok T, et al. Early postoperative complications are not increased in patients with Crohn's disease treated perioperatively with infliximab or immunosuppressive therapy. Am J Gastroenterol. 2004;99(5):878–83.
9. Subramanian V, Pollok RC, Kang JY, Kumar D. Systematic review of postoperative complications in patients with inflammatory bowel disease treated with immunomodulators. Br J Surg. 2006;93(7):793–9.
10. Marchal L, D'Haens G, Van Assche G, Vermeire S, Noman M, Ferrante M, et al. The risk of post-operative complications associated with infliximab therapy for Crohn's disease: a controlled cohort study. Aliment Pharmacol Ther. 2004;19(7):749–54.
11. Nasir BS, Dozois EJ, Cima RR, Pemberton JH, Wolff BG, Sandborn WJ, et al. Perioperative anti-tumor necrosis factor therapy does not increase the rate of early postoperative complications in Crohn's disease. J Gastrointest Surg. 2010;14(12):1859–65; discussion 65–6.
12. Lightner AL, McKenna NP, Tse CS, Raffals LE, Loftus EV Jr, Mathis KL. Postoperative outcomes in vedolizumab-treated Crohn's disease patients undergoing major abdominal operations. Aliment Pharmacol Ther. 2018;47(5):573–80.
13. Levy C, Tremaine WJ. Management of internal fistulas in Crohn's disease. Inflamm Bowel Dis. 2002;8(2):106–11.
14. Grams J, Tong W, Greenstein AJ, Salky B. Comparison of intracorporeal versus extracorporeal anastomosis in laparoscopic-assisted hemicolectomy. Surg Endosc. 2010;24(8):1886–91.
15. Tan JJ, Tjandra JJ. Laparoscopic surgery for Crohn's disease: a meta-analysis. Dis Colon Rectum. 2007;50(5):576–85.
16. Young-Fadok TM, HallLong K, McConnell EJ, Gomez Rey G, Cabanela RL. Advantages of laparoscopic resection for ileocolic Crohn's disease. Improved outcomes and reduced costs. Surg Endosc. 2001;15(5):450–4.

17. Patel SV, Patel SV, Ramagopalan SV, Ott MC. Laparoscopic surgery for Crohn's disease: a meta-analysis of perioperative complications and long term outcomes compared with open surgery. BMC Surg. 2013;13:14.
18. Bergamaschi R, Pessaux P, Arnaud JP. Comparison of conventional and laparoscopic ileocolic resection for Crohn's disease. Dis Colon Rectum. 2003;46(8):1129–33.
19. Maartense S, Dunker MS, Slors JF, Cuesta MA, Pierik EG, Gouma DJ, et al. Laparoscopic-assisted versus open ileocolic resection for Crohn's disease: a randomized trial. Ann Surg. 2006;243(2):143–9; discussion 50–3.
20. Milsom JW, Hammerhofer KA, Bohm B, Marcello P, Elson P, Fazio VW. Prospective, randomized trial comparing laparoscopic vs. conventional surgery for refractory ileocolic Crohn's disease. Dis Colon Rectum. 2001;44(1):1–8; discussion -9.
21. Aytac E, Stocchi L, Remzi FH, Kiran RP. Is laparoscopic surgery for recurrent Crohn's disease beneficial in patients with previous primary resection through midline laparotomy? A case-matched study. Surg Endosc. 2012;26(12):3552–6.
22. Malireddy K, Larson DW, Sandborn WJ, Loftus EV, Faubion WA, Pardi DS, et al. Recurrence and impact of postoperative prophylaxis in laparoscopically treated primary ileocolic Crohn's disease. Arch Surg. 2010;145(1):42–7.
23. Lowney JK, Dietz DW, Birnbaum EH, Kodner IJ, Mutch MG, Fleshman JW. Is there any difference in recurrence rates in laparoscopic ileocolic resection for Crohn's disease compared with conventional surgery? A long-term, follow-up study. Dis Colon Rectum. 2006;49(1):58–63.
24. Heimann TM, Swaminathan S, Greenstein AJ, Greenstein AJ, Khaitov S, Steinhagen RM, et al. Can laparoscopic surgery prevent incisional hernia in patients with Crohn's disease: a comparison study of 750 patients undergoing open and laparoscopic bowel resection. Surg Endosc. 2017;31(12):5201–8.
25. Hasegawa H, Watanabe M, Nishibori H, Okabayashi K, Hibi T, Kitajima M. Laparoscopic surgery for recurrent Crohn's disease. Br J Surg. 2003;90(8):970–3.
26. Chaudhary B, Glancy D, Dixon AR. Laparoscopic surgery for recurrent ileocolic Crohn's disease is as safe and effective as primary resection. Color Dis. 2011;13(12):1413–6.
27. Pinto RA, Shawki S, Narita K, Weiss EG, Wexner SD. Laparoscopy for recurrent Crohn's disease: how do the results compare with the results for primary Crohn's disease? Color Dis. 2011;13(3):302–7.
28. Tavernier M, Lebreton G, Alves A. Laparoscopic surgery for complex Crohn's disease. J Visc Surg. 2013;150(6):389–93.
29. Widmar M, Cummings DR, Steinhagen E, Samson A, Barth AR, Greenstein AJ, et al. Oversewing staple lines to prevent anastomotic complications in primary ileocolic resections for Crohn's disease. J Gastrointest Surg. 2015;19(5):911–6.
30. Kono T, Fichera A, Maeda K, Sakai Y, Ohge H, Krane M, et al. Kono-S anastomosis for surgical prophylaxis of anastomotic recurrence in Crohn's disease: an international multicenter study. J Gastrointest Surg. 2016;20(4):783–90.
31. European Society of Coloproctology Collaborating G. The impact of stapling technique and surgeon specialism on anastomotic failure after right-sided colorectal resection: an international multicentre, prospective audit. Color Dis. 2018;20(11):1028–40.
32. Scatizzi M, Kroning KC, Borrelli A, Andan G, Lenzi E, Feroci F. Extracorporeal versus intracorporeal anastomosis after laparoscopic right colectomy for cancer: a case-control study. World J Surg. 2010;34(12):2902–8.
33. Magistro C, Lernia SD, Ferrari G, Zullino A, Mazzola M, De Martini P, et al. Totally laparoscopic versus laparoscopic-assisted right colectomy for colon cancer: is there any advantage in short-term outcomes? A prospective comparative assessment in our center. Surg Endosc. 2013;27(7):2613–8.
34. Lee KH, Ho J, Akmal Y, Nelson R, Pigazzi A. Short- and long-term outcomes of intracorporeal versus extracorporeal ileocolic anastomosis in laparoscopic right hemicolectomy for colon cancer. Surg Endosc. 2013;27(6):1986–90.

35. Cirocchi R, Trastulli S, Farinella E, Guarino S, Desiderio J, Boselli C, et al. Intracorporeal versus extracorporeal anastomosis during laparoscopic right hemicolectomy - systematic review and meta-analysis. Surg Oncol. 2013;22(1):1–13.
36. Milone M, Angelini P, Berardi G, Burati M, Corcione F, Delrio P, et al. Intracorporeal versus extracorporeal anastomosis after laparoscopic left colectomy for splenic flexure cancer: results from a multi-institutional audit on 181 consecutive patients. Surg Endosc. 2018;32(8):3467–73.
37. Milone M, Elmore U, Di Salvo E, Delrio P, Bucci L, Ferulano GP, et al. Intracorporeal versus extracorporeal anastomosis. Results from a multicentre comparative study on 512 right-sided colorectal cancers. Surg Endosc. 2015;29(8):2314–20.
38. Martinek L, You K, Giuratrabocchetta S, Gachabayov M, Lee K, Bergamaschi R. Does laparoscopic intracorporeal ileocolic anastomosis decreases surgical site infection rate? A propensity score-matched cohort study. Int J Color Dis. 2018;33(3):291–8.
39. Vignali A, Elmore U, Lemma M, Guarnieri G, Radaelli G, Rosati R. Intracorporeal versus extracorporeal anastomoses following laparoscopic right colectomy in obese patients: a case-matched study. Dig Surg. 2018;35(3):236–42.

Part IV

Left-Sided Resections

Laparoscopic Left and Sigmoid Colectomy for Malignant Disease

17

Melissa I. Chang and Evangelos Messaris

Introduction and Rationale

Colon and rectal cancer represents the third most common cancer in men and the second in women worldwide. Furthermore, it is the fourth leading cause of cancer death in the world [1]. The incidence of colorectal cancer varies by geographic region with Europe having the highest incidence followed by North America, Australia, Latin America, and Africa. In addition, there is an increasing incidence of colon cancer in patients younger than 50 years old [2]. The majority of colon cancers are located in the left side of the colon [1]. The mainstay treatment for non-metastatic colon cancer is surgical resection. The surgical approach to a left or sigmoid resection has evolved over time from the traditional open approach to hand-assisted laparoscopy, multi-port laparoscopy, single-port laparoscopy, and more recently robotic surgery.

With the publication of the COST trial in 2004 [3, 4], laparoscopic surgery for colon resection has been applied to the treatment of colon cancer. This study demonstrated the short-term benefits of laparoscopy including faster return of bowel function, shorter hospital length of stay, and less narcotic use. Importantly, the 3-year oncologic results between the laparoscopic and open groups were equivalent. These findings have been confirmed by two additional international, multicenter, prospective randomized trials: the UK CLASICC trial published in 2007 and 2013 [5, 6] and the European COLOR trial published in 2009 [7].

M. I. Chang (✉)
Saint Joseph Mercy Hospital Ann Arbor, Department of Surgery, Ypsilanti, MI, USA
e-mail: melissa_chang@ihacares.com

E. Messaris
Beth Israel Deaconess Medical Center, Department of Surgery, Harvard University Medical School, Boston, MA, USA

P. Sylla et al. (eds.), *The SAGES Manual of Colorectal Surgery*,
https://doi.org/10.1007/978-3-030-24812-3_17

Indications and Contraindications

All patients with colon cancer should be considered candidates for a laparoscopic approach. Locally advanced tumors can be a relative contraindication for laparoscopic resection. Cases with T4a tumors (tumor growing into the surface of the visceral peritoneum) can be approached laparoscopically with caution and if R0 resection can be achieved. Extreme caution should be used for T4b lesions, where the tumor has grown into or has attached to other organs or structures. For cases requiring multi-visceral resections, laparoscopy is not supported [8].

Other relative contraindications for the laparoscopic approach are many prior abdominal surgeries, extreme morbid obesity precluding tolerance of pneumoperitoneum, and severe obstructive lung disease. The surgeon's experience is a key factor in determining whether each case can be completed laparoscopically or an early conversion to the open approach can be the most beneficial for the patient.

Principles and Quality Benchmarks

The National Comprehensive Cancer Network provides the recommended principles of surgical resection for colon cancer [9]. These principles can be used in any surgical approach: open, laparoscopic, or robotic. These principles include obtaining:

1. Adequate proximal and distal margin (5 cm).
2. Adequate lymphadenectomy (≥12 lymph nodes). High ligation of the feeding vessels is the preferred method of lymph node dissection. The lymph nodes at the origin of the feeding vessel should be marked to be identified on pathologic examination. The concept of high versus low ligation of the primary feeding pedicle has been controversial in the literature; however, the goal remains to clear all regional lymph nodes to obtain the minimum lymph nodes necessary for adequate pathologic evaluation.
3. Clinically positive lymph nodes outside the field of resection should be removed. Positive lymph nodes left behind are considered an R2 resection. The concept of a total mesorectal excision (TME) in certain cases also applies to the resection of colon and its mesentery along the fascial planes or the complete mesocolic excision (CME). Although CME has been associated with higher postoperative complication rates, it has shown to increase lymph node harvest with longer vascular ligation, increased resection of extranodal tumor deposits, and increased upstaging, resulting in improved locoregional control and survival in certain cases. Its use remains controversial.
4. On an individualized basis, young patients (<50 years) or patients that are suspected to have Lynch syndrome need to be considered for more extensive resections.
5. The laparoscopic approach should be cautiously used in locally advanced cancers (T4) or cases that present with contained perforation or obstruction.

Preoperative Planning, Patient Workup, and Optimization

The first step in the management of a patient with a left-sided colonic mass is to establish tissue diagnosis of the malignancy. Colonoscopy should be complete with confirmed evaluation of the ileocecal valve. Furthermore, it is paramount to use any localizing technique for any unresected or incompletely resected lesions or suspicious lesions that were resected. Placement of an endoscopic clip or endoscopic tattooing proximal and distal to the tumor in three separate areas around the circumference of the colon wall will facilitate subsequent intraoperative localization of the tumor. Accurate tumor localization preoperatively is imperative for a successful resection as manual palpation is not possible in laparoscopy or in cases where the tumor has been completely removed endoscopically.

After the diagnosis of left-sided colon cancer has been established, the patient will undergo clinical staging. A carcinoembryonic antigen (CEA) blood level and a computed tomography of the chest, abdomen, and pelvis with intravenous and oral contrast will be needed to rule out distant metastatic disease. Positive emission tomography is not recommended as a first-line imaging study.

Preoperative Optimization

Preoperative optimization of patients with colon cancer is known to improve surgical outcomes and consequently oncologic outcomes. Patient optimization should be focused in five modifiable factors: functional status, nutrition, anemia, tobacco use, and glycemic control. There are programs that can improve with exercise the patient's functional status and decrease the hospital and rehabilitation length of stay [10]. Prehabilitation before elective surgery is to be considered for patients undergoing elective colorectal surgery with multiple comorbidities or significant deconditioning. Several screening tools can be used for nutritional assessment [11]. Malnourished patients will have to improve their sarcopenia in order to be able to undergo surgery without severe postoperative complications [12]. Anemia has been associated with poor postoperative outcomes. Iron supplementation is the preferred treatment, but sometimes it requires a long period of time to restore the hemoglobin levels, and that is time that cancer patients do not have. In cases of severe anemia, preoperative transfusions of packed red blood cells may be required, although low perioperative anemia has not been associated with worse long-term oncologic outcomes in patients with colon cancer [13]. Tobacco use has been associated with poor outcomes after any abdominal operation. Any patient that is scheduled for an elective colectomy for colon cancer should be enrolled in a smoking cessation program [14]. Poor glycemic control is associated with higher wound complications and infectious complications after surgery. Euglycemia in the perioperative period is important to avoid such infectious complications [15].

Mechanical bowel preparation has been a controversial issue over the past decade, but most of the studies on left-sided resections have concluded that mechanical and antibiotic bowel preparation is associated with a lower surgical site infection rate and in some studies with a lower anastomotic leak rate. All left-sided resections should undergo combined bowel preparation with mechanical cleansing and oral antibiotics [16].

Accelerated Recovery Pathway

The American Society for Colon and Rectal Surgery (ASCRS) Clinical Practice Guidelines Committee [17] and members of the Society of American Gastrointestinal and Endoscopic Surgeons (SAGES) Surgical Multimodal Accelerated Recovery Trajectory Enhanced Recovery Task Force and Guidelines Committee have joined together to produce guidelines, written and approved by both the ASCRS and SAGES [18]. The combined ASCRS/SAGES panel worked together to develop the statements in the following guidelines for the care of patients undergoing colon and rectal resections in order to have an accelerated recovery. Appropriate preoperative counseling should include discussion of milestones and discharge criteria, ileostomy education and marking, and counseling on dehydration avoidance. Just before surgery a clear-liquid diet may be continued up to 2 hours before surgery, and carbohydrate loading should be encouraged in nondiabetic patients.

Mechanical bowel preparation plus oral antibiotic bowel preparation before colorectal surgery is the preferred preparation and is associated with reduced complication rates. Furthermore, for distal rectosigmoid lesions, the addition of two fleet enemas may optimize cleansing. Optimizing bowel preparation is critical should intraoperative localization be required through endoscopic evaluation.

During the operation, a bundle of measures should be in place to reduce surgical site infections. A multimodal, opioid-sparing, pain management plan should be used and implemented before the induction of anesthesia, and antiemetic prophylaxis should be guided by preoperative screening for risk factors for postoperative nausea and vomiting. Preemptive, multimodal antiemetic prophylaxis should be used in all at-risk patients. Maintenance infusion of crystalloids should be tailored to avoid excess fluid administration and volume overload. Balanced chloride-restricted crystalloid solutions should be used as maintenance infusion in patients undergoing colorectal surgery, and in specific high-risk patients with significant intravascular losses, the use of goal-directed fluid therapy is recommended. The routine use of intra-abdominal drains and nasogastric tubes for colorectal surgery should be avoided, and early and progressive patient mobilization is associated with shorter length of stay. Intravenous fluids should be discontinued in the early postoperative period after recovery room discharge, and patients should be offered a regular diet immediately after elective colorectal surgery. Urinary catheters should be removed within 24 hours of elective colonic or upper rectal resection when not involving a colovesical fistula. Please refer to Chapters 7 and 8 on bowel preparation in colorectal surgery and enhanced recovery protocols in colorectal surgery for additional details.

Operative Technique: Surgical Steps

Before induction of anesthesia, the patient receives 5000 units of unfractionated heparin subcutaneously. In addition, the patient has at least knee-length compression stockings and sequential compression device prophylaxis. The patient is positioned and secured in the lithotomy position with both arms tucked and padded to avoid any neurovascular injury during operative positioning. An overview of the involved anatomy is provided in Fig. 17.1. Concerning port placement, they should be based on surgeon approach and preference. An example of port placement is provided in Fig. 17.2. As this is a multi-quadrant procedure, placement of the camera port is most optimal at the apex of pneumoperitoneum, which is typically in the midline either just above or below the umbilicus. Placement of the 12 mm port that can be used for the laparoscopic stapler can be either in the right lower quadrant or the suprapubic area.

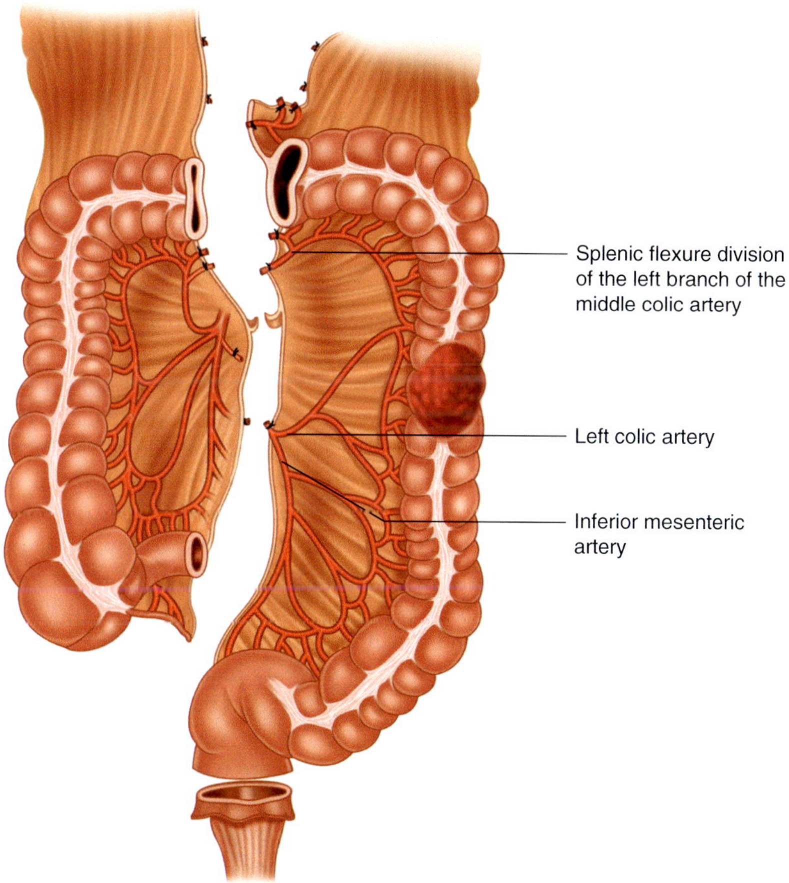

Fig. 17.1 Left colectomy anatomy

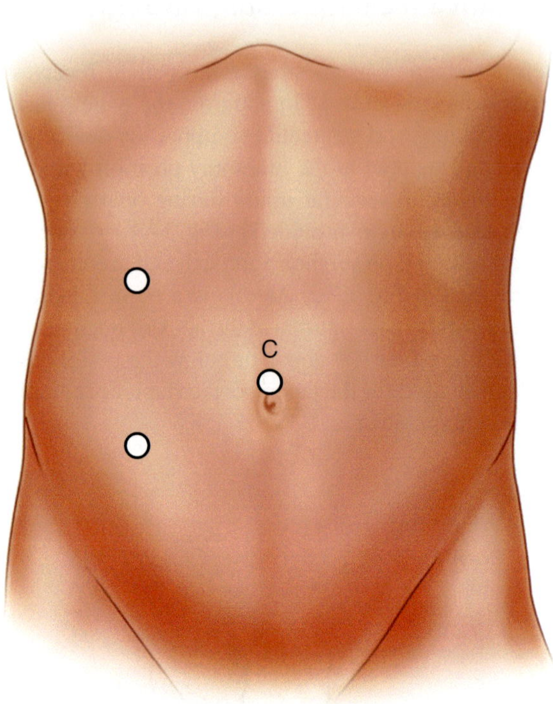

Fig. 17.2 Laparoscopic left colectomy ports

The first step after establishing pneumoperitoneum and port placement is to explore the abdomen to rule out any metastatic disease and identify the lesion in the colon. The patient is positioned in steep Trendelenburg with right tilt so that the left side is up, and the small bowel is swept to the right to expose the left colon mesocolon. The superior rectal artery is then identified at the level of the sacral promontory. This is facilitated by retracting and tenting the superior rectal artery to the anterior abdominal wall to trace to its origin and opening the peritoneum from below the sacral promontory to the inferior mesenteric artery (IMA) origin on the aorta. The retroperitoneum is swept posteriorly until the left ureter is identified and protected as shown in Fig. 17.3. The IMA is isolated and ligated (can use clips, energy device, stapler, and vessel loop) as shown in Fig. 17.4. The inferior mesenteric vein (IMV) is then identified by separating the mesentery from the retroperitoneum to the inferior border of the pancreas. The IMV is then isolated and ligated (can use clips, energy device, stapler, and vessel loop) as shown in Fig. 17.5. The sigmoid colon and descending colon are retracted medially to free all the lateral attachments along the white line of Toldt, and the omentum is reflected cephalad to the transverse colon to expose the transverse colon and splenic flexure. In order to mobilize the splenic flexure, the superficial peritoneal plane between the omentum and transverse colon is opened toward the midline to enter the lesser sac, and the splenic flexure is then retracted medially and caudally to divide the peritoneal attachments to the inferior border of the pancreas. The

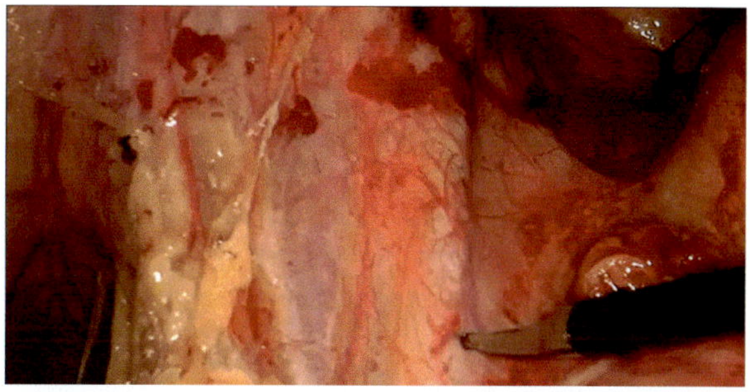

Fig. 17.3 Identifying the left ureter

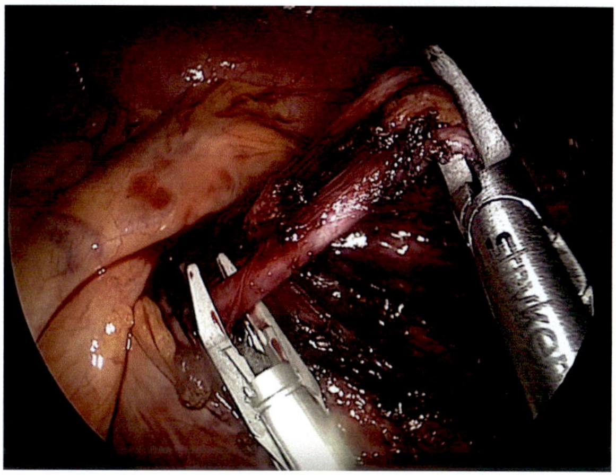

Fig. 17.4 High ligation of the inferior mesenteric artery

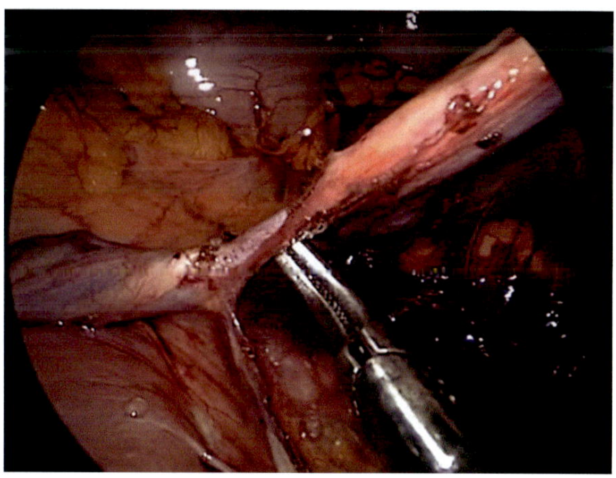

Fig. 17.5 High ligation of the inferior mesenteric vein

splenocolic ligament is divided. By detaching the mesocolon off the kidney at Gerota's fascia, the last attachments of the colon can be taken down sharply to achieve complete mobilization of the splenic flexure.

The identification of the proximal and distal points of transection can be performed with the assistance of indocyanine green enhanced fluorescence as shown in

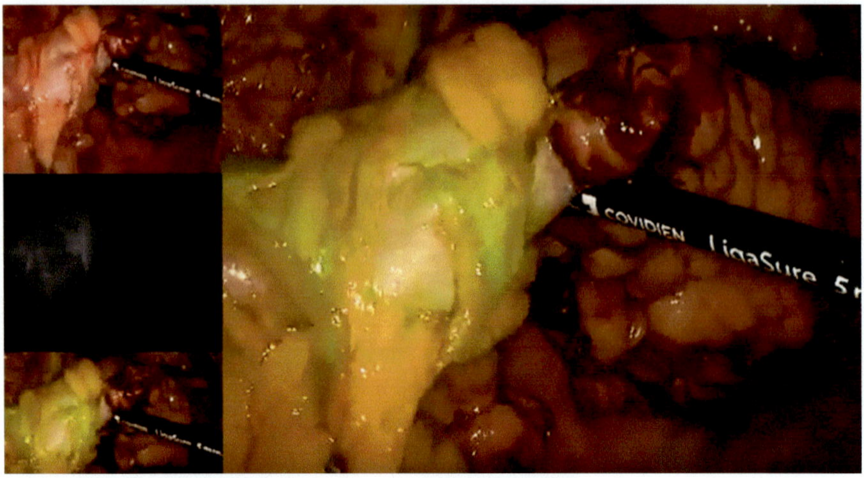

Fig. 17.6 Perfusion assessment

Fig. 17.6. An intracorporeal transection of the rectosigmoid junction is performed with the laparoscopic stapler at the confluence of the taenia coli. The specimen can be extracted through an extended off midline lower-quadrant trocar site (such as the 12 mm trocar site) or a suprapubic (Pfannenstiel) incision, a technique that is associated with a lower hernia rate.

The descending colon can be transected at least 5 cm proximal to the tumor, and the anvil of a circular stapler can then be secured in the colon with a purse-string suture. The perineal operator then inserts the circular stapler transanally and deploys the pin through the midportion of the staple line of the rectal stump to complete an end-to-end colorectal anastomosis. An alternative approach would be to perform a side-to-end colorectal anastomosis by placing the anvil through the anti-mesocolic border of the descending colon. In either case, the anastomotic rings are checked for intactness and sent to pathology as additional proximal and distal margin. An air leak test of the anastomosis is performed with endoscopic assessment under laparoscopic visualization. Before closing, reassess if any unexpected findings during the surgery would warrant an unplanned diverting ostomy or placement of a drain. Several randomized trials and a meta-analysis suggest that routine use of drains for left colectomy is not recommended [19].

Pitfalls, Troubleshooting, and Special Considerations

Difficulty Identifying the Ureter

The left ureter should be clearly identified and safely dissected free of the left colon mesentery prior to the division or the IMA or the IMV. A ureteral stent may be inserted at the discretion of the surgeon. To help facilitate identification, these maneuvers may be taken in a step-wise fashion: access the retroperitoneum at the level of the superior rectal artery at the sacral promontory, identify the IMV, and open the medial aspect of the peritoneum to develop a plane in the retroperitoneum. Dissection can proceed caudally until the sacral promontory to identify the ureter. As an alternative to locate the ureter, mobilize the colon in a lateral to medial fashion to completely expose it, utilize a hand port, or convert to open to directly palpate for the ureter.

Difficulty with Reach

Resection of a proximal left colon lesion (splenic flexure, proximal descending) may require division of both branches of the middle colic artery to allow the proximal transverse colon to reach the rectal stump for anastomosis. The division of the left colic artery, marginal, and the middle colic vessels can lead to poor perfusion of the remaining transverse colon and can lead either to evident intraoperative colonic ischemia or to an under-perfused colorectal anastomosis with associated complications such as anastomotic leak, stricture, and segmental narrowing of the transverse colon. In cases where the transverse colon does not have adequate blood supply or cannot reach the rectum, if maintenance of the right colon is preferred, a retroileal right colon to rectum anastomosis may be performed versus an extended right colectomy with an ileosigmoid or ileorectal anastomosis.

Locally Advanced Tumors

As mentioned earlier in this chapter, T4a tumors can be approached laparoscopically with caution and can be completely removed. When there is clear invasion of an adjacent organ by a T4b tumor, conversion to an open approach is recommended [8]. En bloc resection of the colon and involved organ should be performed with the goal of achieving R0 resection.

When to Consider Conversion

The surgeon should consider conversion to a different approach if there is failure to progress over a significant period of time. Furthermore, excessive bleeding, unexpected organ injury, significant amount of adhesions, and difficulty in obtaining a high ligation of the vessels should prompt the surgeon to consider changing the surgical approach either to open or to another laparoscopic technique that can assist with solving the occurring problem. Strategies that can enhance the surgeon's ability to deal with intraoperative difficulties or complications would include the placement of additional ports or hand assistance. If these strategies fail, the case should be converted to open surgery.

Table 17.1 Prospective, randomized controlled trials comparing laparoscopic versus open surgery for colorectal cancer

Trial (year)	*N* (lap:open)	Postoperative complications (%)	30-day mortality	5-year DFS (%); *p*-value	5-year OS (%); *p*-value
COST (2004, 2007)	435:437	19:19%	<1:1%	69.2:68.4% ($p = 0.94$)	76.4:74.6% ($p = 0.93$)
CLASICC (2007, 2013)	526:268	33:32%	4:5%	77.0;89.5% ($p = 0.589$)	82.7:78.3 ($p = 0.78$)
COLOR (2009)	627:621	21:20%	1:2%	74.2:76.2 ($p = 0.19$)[a]	81.8:84.2 ($p = 0.21$)[a]
Australasian (2012)	290:297	NA	NA	72.7:71.2% ($p = 0.70$)	77.7:76.0% ($p = 0.64$)
JCOG0404 (2017)	529:528	10:13%	0:<1%	79.3:79.7%	91.8:90.4%

DFS disease-free survival, *OS* overall survival, *NA* not available
[a]3-year period vs. 5 year

Outcomes

Laparoscopic colectomy for colon cancer has been found to have short-term benefits relative to open surgery and to be as safe and efficacious as open surgery. The COST trial published in 2004 was the initial large multicenter study group with almost 900 patients randomized to either open or laparoscopic approaches, with no differences found in overall survival or disease-free survival [3, 4]. This was followed by the UK CLASICC trial in 2005 and the European COLOR trial in 2009 which echoed similar findings [5–7]. More recently, the Australian Laparoscopic Colon Cancer Study trial conducted across Australia and New Zealand in 2012 and the Japanese JCOG0404 trials have continued to demonstrate and uphold the short-term benefits for the laparoscopic approach without differences in long-term overall survival, disease-free survival, and recurrence rates [20, 21]. The results of these five trials are summarized in Table 17.1.

While participants in the COST trial were required to have performed at least 20 laparoscopically assisted colectomies with a conversion rate of less than 21%, other publications have suggested that the learning curve in laparoscopic colorectal surgery ranges from 20 to 70 cases [22–28]. In Tekkis and colleagues, the learning curve for laparoscopic left colectomy, based on operative time, conversion to open, postoperative complications, and readmission rates, was calculated as 62 cases [28]. While laparoscopic left colectomy continues to be a technically challenging procedure, studies have shown that operative autonomy can be mastered in a structured training protocol in a specialized surgical fellowship [29, 30].

Conclusions

While laparoscopic approach for left-sided and sigmoid colon cancers can achieve similar oncologic outcomes in the setting of faster return of bowel function and shorter length of hospital stay, performing a complete oncologic resection, including a proximal and distal margin of >5 cm and an adequate lymphadenectomy of >12 regional lymph nodes, is paramount in patient outcome. Special attention and consideration should be taken based on patient and tumor characteristics to determine if the patient is a candidate for a laparoscopic approach.

References

1. Arnold M, Sierra MS, Laversanne M, Soerjomataram I, Jemal A, Bray F. Global patterns and trends in colorectal cancer incidence and mortality. Gut. 2017;66(4):683–91.
2. Bailey CE, Hu CY, You YN, Bednarski BK, Rodriguez-Bigas MA, Skibber JM, et al. Increasing disparities in the age-related incidences of colon and rectal cancers in the United States, 1975-2010. JAMA Surg. 2015;150(1):17–22.
3. Clinical Outcomes of Surgical Therapy Study Group, Nelson H, Sargent DJ, Wieand HS, Fleshman J, Anvari M, et al. A comparison of laparoscopically assisted and open colectomy for colon cancer. N Engl J Med. 2004;350(20):2050–9.
4. Fleshman J, Sargent DJ, Green E, Anvari M, Stryker SJ, Beart RW Jr, et al. Laparoscopic colectomy for cancer is not inferior to open surgery based on 5-year data from the COST Study Group trial. Ann Surg. 2007;246(4):655–62.
5. Jayne DG, Guillou PJ, Thorpe H, Quirke P, Copeland J, Smith AM, et al. Randomized trial of laparoscopic-assisted resection of colorectal carcinoma: 3-year results of the UK MRC CLASICC Trial Group. J Clin Oncol. 2007;25(21):3061–8.
6. Green BL, Marshall HC, Collinson F, Quirke P, Guillou P, Jayne DG, et al. Long-term follow-up of the Medical Research Council CLASICC trial of conventional versus laparoscopically assisted resection in colorectal cancer. Br J Surg. 2013;100(1):75–82.
7. Colon Cancer Laparoscopic or Open Resection Study Group, Buunen M, Veldkamp R, Hop WC, Kuhry E, Jeekel J, et al. Survival after laparoscopic surgery versus open surgery for colon cancer: long-term outcome of a randomised clinical trial. Lancet Oncol. 2009;10(1):44–52.
8. Klaver CEL, Kappen TM, Borstlap WAA, Bemelman WA, Tanis PJ. Laparoscopic surgery for T4 colon cancer: a systematic review and meta-analysis. Surg Endosc. 2017;31(12):4902–12.
9. https://www.nccn.org/professionals/physician_gls/default.aspx.
10. Lee CHA, Kong JC, Ismail H, Riedel B, Heriot A. Systematic review and meta-analysis of objective assessment of physical fitness in patients undergoing colorectal cancer surgery. Dis Colon Rectum. 2018;61(3):400–9.
11. Hennessey DB, Burke JP, Ni-Dhonochu T, Shields C, Winter DC, Mealy K. Preoperative hypoalbuminemia is an independent risk factor for the development of surgical site infection following gastrointestinal surgery: a multi-institutional study. Ann Surg. 2010;252:325–9.
12. Marimuthu K, Varadhan KK, Ljungqvist O, Lobo DN. A meta-analysis of the effect of combinations of immune modulating nutrients on outcome in patients undergoing major open gastrointestinal surgery. Ann Surg. 2012;255:1060–8.
13. Wilson MJ, van Haaren M, Harlaar JJ, Park HC, Bonjer HJ, Jeekel J, et al. Long-term prognostic value of preoperative anemia in patients with colorectal cancer: a systematic review and meta-analysis. Surg Oncol. 2017;26(1):96–104.
14. Sørensen LT. Wound healing and infection in surgery: the pathophysiological impact of smoking, smoking cessation, and nicotine replacement therapy: a systematic review. Ann Surg. 2012;255(6):1069–79.
15. Tanner J, Padley W, Assadian O, Leaper D, Kiernan M, Edmiston C. Do surgical care bundles reduce the risk of surgical site infections in patients undergoing colorectal surgery? A systematic review and cohort meta-analysis of 8,515 patients. Surgery. 2015;158(1):66–77.
16. Scarborough JE, Mantyh CR, Sun Z, Migaly J. Combined mechanical and oral antibiotic bowel preparation reduces incisional surgical site infection and anastomotic leak rates after elective colorectal resection: an analysis of colectomy-targeted ACS NSQIP. Ann Surg. 2015;262(2):331–7.

17. Carmichael JC, Keller DS, Baldini G, Bordeianou L, Weiss E, Lee L, et al. Clinical practice guidelines for enhanced recovery after colon and rectal surgery from the American Society of Colon and Rectal Surgeons and Society of American Gastrointestinal and Endoscopic Surgeons. Dis Colon Rectum. 2017;60:761–84.
18. McClane J, Feldman LS, Steele SR. Clinical practice guidelines for enhanced recovery after colon and rectal surgery from the American Society of Colon and Rectal Surgeons and Society of American Gastrointestinal and Endoscopic Surgeons. Dis Colon Rectum. 2017;60(8):761–84.
19. Zhang HY, Zhao CL, Xie J, Ye YW, Sun JF, Ding ZH, et al. To drain or not to drain in colorectal anastomosis: a meta-analysis. Int J Colorectal Dis. 2016;31(5):951–60.
20. Bagshaw PF, Allardyce RA, Frampton CM, Frizelle FA, Hewett PJ, McMurrick PJ, et al. Long-term outcomes of the australasian randomized clinical trial comparing laparoscopic and conventional open surgical treatments for colon cancer: the Australasian Laparoscopic Colon Cancer Study trial. Ann Surg. 2012;256(6):915–9.
21. Kitano S, Inomata M, Mizusawa J, Katayama H, Watanabe M, Yamamoto S, et al. Survival outcomes following laparoscopic versus open D3 dissection for stage II or III colon cancer (JCOG0404): a phase 3, randomised controlled trial. Lancet Gastroenterol Hepatol. 2017;2(4):261–8.
22. Senagore AJ, Ma L, Mackeigan JM. What is the learning curve for laparoscopic colectomy? Am Surg. 1995;61:681–5.
23. Simons AJ, Anthone GJ, Ortega AE, Franklin M, Fleshman J, Gesi WP, et al. Laparoscopic-assisted colectomy learning curve. Dis Colon Rectum. 1995;38:600–3.
24. Wishner JD, Baker JW Jr, Hoffman GC, Hubbard GWII, Gould RJ, Wohlgemuth SD, et al. Laparoscopic-assisted colectomy. The learning curve. Surg Endosc. 1995;9:1179–83.
25. Agachan F, Joo JS, Sher M, Weiss EG, Nogueras JJ, Wexner SD. Laparoscopic colorectal surgery. Do we get faster? Surg Endosc. 1997;11:331–5.
26. Schlachta CM, Mamazza J, Seshadri PA, Cadeddu M, Gregoire R, Poulin EC. Defining a learning curve for laparoscopic colorectal resections. Dis Colon Rectum. 2001;44:217–22.
27. Dincler S, Koller MT, Steurer J, Bachmann LM, Christen D, Buchmann P. Multidimensional analysis of learning curves in laparoscopic sigmoid resection: eight-year results. Dis Colon Rectum. 2003;46:1371–9.
28. Tekkis PP, Senagore AJ, Delaney CP, Fazio VW. Evaluation of the learning curve in laparoscopic colorectal surgery: comparison of right-sided and left-sided resections. Ann Surg. 2005;242:83–91.
29. Li JC, Hon SS, Ng SS, Lee JF, Yiu RY, Leung KL. The learning curve for laparoscopic colectomy: experience of a surgical fellow in an university colorectal unit. Surg Endosc. 2009;23:1603–8.
30. Waters JA, Chihara R, Moreno J, Robb BW, Wiebke EA, George VV. Laparoscopic colectomy: does the learning curve extend beyond colorectal surgery fellowship? JSLS. 2010;14(3):325–31.

Laparoscopic Left and Sigmoid Colectomy: Options for Colonic and Colorectal Reconstruction

18

Matthew G. Mutch

Introduction and Rationale

This chapter will focus on the construction of colorectal anastomosis after laparoscopic resection of the left and sigmoid colon or low anterior resection. Therefore, anastomoses of the colon to anywhere on the rectum ranging from the upper rectum to the level of the pelvic floor will be covered. Indications and contraindications for performing an anastomosis, types of anastomoses, options for exteriorization of the colon, anastomotic assessment, and recognizing and managing intraoperative anastomotic complications will be discussed. Surgical technique and judgment are paramount for a successful anastomosis as this is one of the most important aspects of the entire operation. The primary goals for restoring intestinal continuity are to maintain the patient's quality of life and avoid the associated complications of an anastomosis such as leak, bleeding, and stricturing.

Indications and Contraindications

An anastomosis can be performed after any left-sided resection provided that the sphincter complex remains intact. The decision to perform an anastomosis in a given patient involves several factors that are related to the specific circumstances of the operation. There are no absolute contraindications to performing an anastomosis, but there are several relative contraindications. Reasons to avoid restoring intestinal continuity during an elective colon resection include patient preference, preoperative history of fecal incontinence, hemodynamic instability during the

M. G. Mutch (✉)
Washington University School of Medicine, Department of Surgery, Section of Colon and Rectal Surgery, St. Louis, MO, USA
e-mail: mutchm@wustl.edu

P. Sylla et al. (eds.), *The SAGES Manual of Colorectal Surgery*,
https://doi.org/10.1007/978-3-030-24812-3_18

surgery, poor tissue quality, or risk factors for anastomotic leak that make not performing anastomosis a prudent decision. These concepts highlight the importance of surgeon decision-making during each individual operation. The utilization of a diverting stoma is also an issue that impacts a surgeon's decision to perform an anastomosis, and this possibility should be discussed with the patient preoperatively.

Principles and Quality Benchmarks

The general principles of a healthy anastomosis are (1) ensuring adequate blood supply, (2) utilization of healthy bowel, (3) adequate mobilization to avoid tension on the anastomosis, and (4) assessment of the mechanical integrity of the anastomosis. An anastomosis can be created with handsewn, stapled, or compression techniques. Techniques for creating an anastomosis have evolved significantly since the advent of stapling devices. Staplers have increased the surgeon's ability to preserve the sphincter and avoid a permanent colostomy. This chapter will only cover stapled anastomoses, but many of the types of anastomotic constructions are applicable to handsewn anastomosis. Compression anastomoses will not be covered because these techniques are not widely used.

Anastomotic leak is one of the most devastating complications for patients undergoing restorative procedures. The causes of anastomotic leaks are multifactorial, and identification of clear and consistent risk factors has been difficult. Unquestionably, however, surgeon decision-making and technique are paramount to a successful reconstruction. General factors related to the risk of an anastomotic leak include those associated with the patient, disease process, surgeon, and location of the anastomosis. A surgeon's ability to predict an anastomotic leak is limited. Several authors have attempted to develop predictive models for anastomotic leak using such variables as comorbidities, operative events, and operative complexity with marginal success [1]. Specific risk factors for anastomotic leak will be discussed below.

Preoperative Planning, Patient Work-Up, and Optimization

The majority of preoperative planning is centered on the disease process and the extent of resection required to appropriately manage the patient. This is the time to discuss the risks associated with the anastomosis and to understand the patient's bowel function, continence, overall functional status, and their associated comorbidities. It is also prudent to discuss the various situations in which a temporary diverting ileostomy or colostomy may be required. If there is a reasonable likelihood that the patient will leave the operating room with a stoma, it is imperative to have the patient see an enterostomal therapist for education and marking prior to the day of surgery.

Operative Setup

Once the colon has been mobilized, the decision for resection, extraction, and anastomosis must be made. The choices for resection include intracorporeal division of the colon and rectum with endoscopic staplers, intracorporeal division of the rectum with exteriorization, and open division of the proximal colon or exteriorization of the colon with extracorporeal division of both ends of the bowel. The approach is really a matter of surgeon preference as long as the principles of the resection can be maintained. Intracorporeal division of the bowel allows for the smallest extraction site and allows for the extraction site to be off the midline, whereas extracorporeal division typically requires the extraction site to be in the midline, suprapubic position so that the rectum may be divided in an open fashion.

Laparoscopic division of the rectum can be challenging because of the depth of the pelvic, port placement, and limitations of the endoscopic staplers. Ideally, the rectum is divided at a right angle with a single firing of the stapler, but that is not always possible. It is recommended to use an articulating endoscopic stapler, and the length of stapler is predicated on the size of the pelvis. Given the relative thickness of the rectum, a thicker load stapler may be preferred. Dividing the rectum below the peritoneal reflection becomes much more difficult because of the challenge to get the stapler across it at a right angle. As a result, multiple firing may be required. Some surgeons may use a shorter stapler and utilize two staple firings to divide the rectum. It is important to keep in mind that the risk of anastomotic leak increases when three or more staple firings are needed to divide the rectum [2]. A suprapubic port may be a good alternative to allow for stapling the rectum in an anterior to posterior fashion at the pelvic floor. Alternatively, a suprapubic midline or Pfannenstiel incision can be utilized to divide the rectum with an open stapler. In either case, the associated mesorectum is divided at a right angle to the rectum with the energy source of choice.

The colon can be extracted and exteriorized via an upper or lower midline incision, Pfannenstiel incision, or a left lower quadrant muscle-splitting incision. The use of an upper midline and left lower quadrant incision requires the incision to be closed and the anastomosis to be performed laparoscopically. With a lower midline or Pfannenstiel incision, the anastomosis can be carried out either laparoscopically or open under direct visualization. Once the incision is made, a wound protector should be used as there are clear data supporting a decreased incidence of wound infections and to protect the wound from tumor implantation for cancer cases [3]. Wound protectors can be capped or twisted and clamped in order to reestablish pneumoperitoneum.

Whether the colon and its mesentery are divided intracorporeally or extracorporeally, the proximal colon must be assessed for adequate perfusion. This can be accomplished in several ways such as flashing the marginal artery, observing bright red blood from the cut edge of the colon, or utilization of indocyanine green fluorescence imaging. The technique used for the anastomosis will dictate how the colon is divided and prepared.

Operative Technique: Surgical Steps

End to End Anastomosis

An end to end anastomosis is the most common type of anastomosis between the colon and rectum. This typically is described as a double-stapled technique as the rectum is divided with a linear stapler and the end to end anastomosis is created across this staple line using a circular stapler. To prepare the proximal colon, a purse string is placed to secure the stapling anvil. A purse string can be placed with either a disposable device, a reusable device using a 2-0 monofilament suture on a Keith needle, or as a handsewn purse string. The key concept is to ensure the edges of the colotomy are everted and that the purse string is complete and secure. For a hand-sewn purse string, a running Connell stitch is best to ensure these principles are met (Fig. 18.1a, b). It allows for full-thickness bites circumferentially around the lumen of the proximal colon. When using a disposable device, be aware that the staples securing the purse string only grab the serosa with or without the underlying muscularis, so it is very important to ensure the mucosal edges are everted to adequately secure the entire bowel edge around the post of the anvil when cinching the purse string down. It is up to the surgeon to "clean" tissue from the colon at the level of the anvil. The goal of this would be to minimize fat within the staple line, to identify diverticula that could be caught in the circular staple line, and to ensure a complete purse string. If a diverticulum is identified that may fall within the staple line, it is drawn up into the anvil with a stitch. A full-thickness stitch is placed just proximal to the diverticulum, and the suture is then tied around the post of the anvil. This maneuver allows the diverticula to be drawn up and out of the staple line. This is important as these colonic diverticula are false diverticula, so they only contain mucosa and serosa. After the anvil has been securely placed, the anastomosis can be performed.

It is at the surgeon's discretion whether to perform the anastomosis under pneumoperitoneum or open via the laparotomy incision. For the laparoscopic approach, the proximal colon and anvil are returned to the peritoneal cavity, and the fascia is definitively closed. Alternatively, with an extraction site in the suprapubic position, the creation of the anastomosis can be performed under direct visualization. The advantage of this open approach is the ease of management of any difficulties or complications associated with the anastomosis – these will be discussed in the Pitfalls and Troubleshooting section.

With either approach, the end to end anastomosis (EEA) stapling cartridge is passed transanally to the top of the rectal stump. The flat end of the stapler should be advanced so that the top of the rectal stump is splayed out flat across the device (Fig. 18.2a). This is to ensure that there are no rectal folds or redundant mucosa incorporated into the staple line. Once it is flush at the top of the rectal stump, the spike of the stapler should be deployed (Fig. 18.2b). The spike can pass through the rectal wall either just posterior or anterior to the staple line or even directly through the staple line. With the spike fully deployed, the anvil should be joined with the spike after confirming the proximal colon is properly oriented and not twisted. The anvil is then cinched down under direct visualization to ensure there is no extra tissue

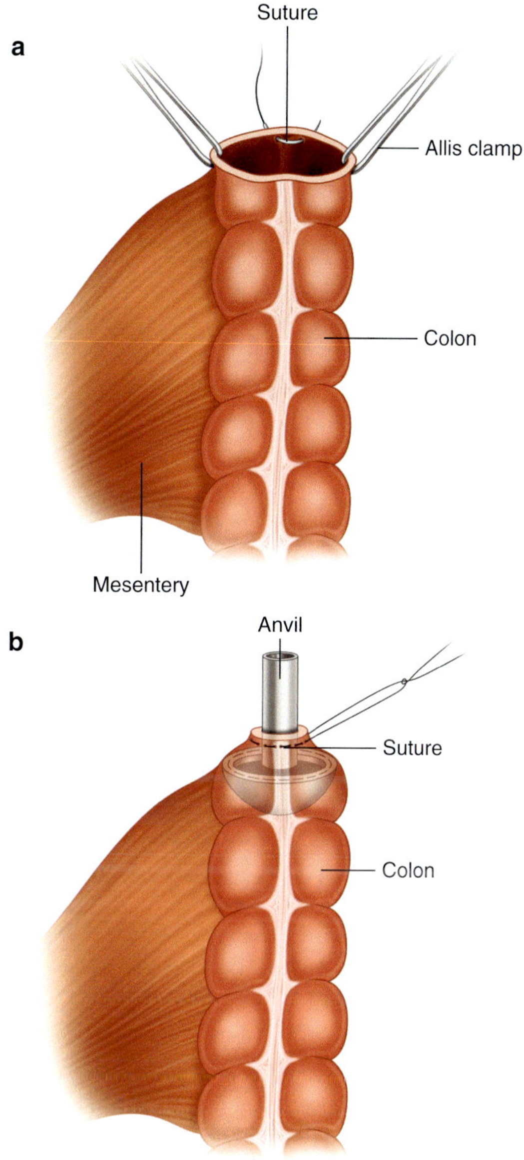

Fig. 18.1 (**a**) Placement of a handsewn purse string in the colostomy. (**b**) Cinching down of the purse string with the stapling anvil in place

(e.g., vagina, bladder) incorporated into the staple line and make sure the proximal purse string remains intact (Fig. 18.2c). Once the stapler is fired and extracted, the anastomotic doughnuts should be inspected for completeness. A complete doughnut is intact circumferentially and includes all layers of the bowel wall – mucosa, muscularis, and serosa. The final step in creating a secure anastomosis involves assessing that the anastomosis is airtight and intact, which will be discussed below.

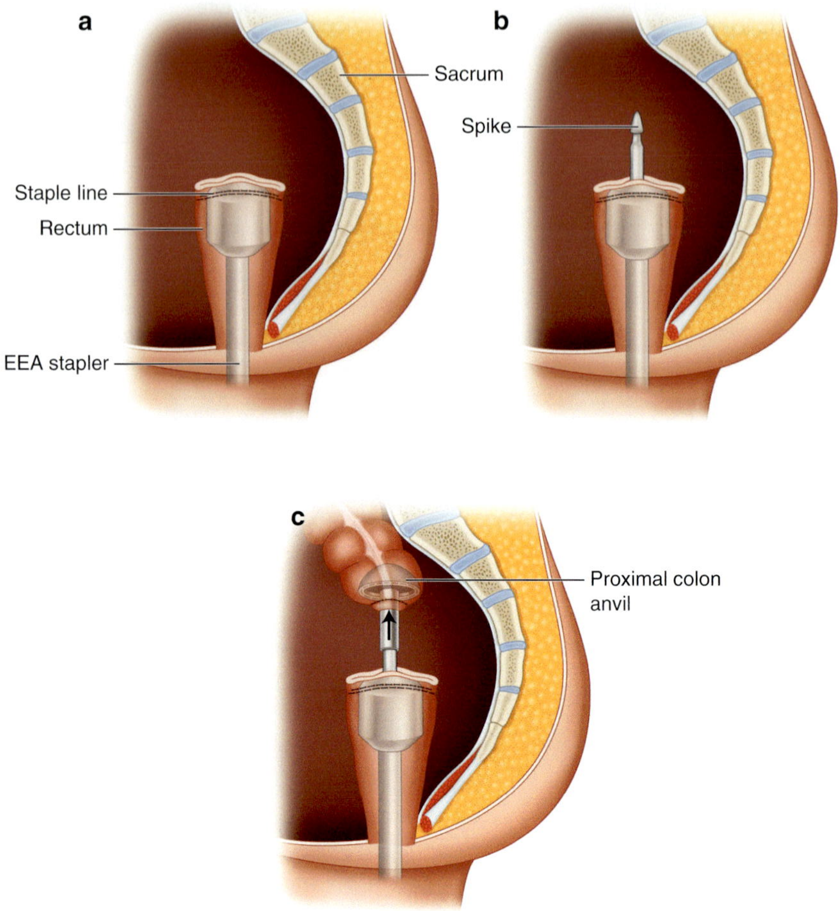

Fig. 18.2 (**a**) Sagittal view of the pelvis and rectum. EEA stapler passed to the top of the rectal stump. (**b**) EEA stapler with the spike deployed. (**c**) The anvil is attached to the EEA staple cartridge

End to Side Anastomosis

An end to side anastomosis is variation of an end to end that does not require the placement of a purse string. It can be used for any level of rectal anastomosis. For this technique, the colon is divided sharply, and the colotomy is opened. The anvil is passed into the lumen via the end colotomy (Fig. 18.3a). The spike is then brought out through the antimesenteric wall roughly 3–4 cm proximal to the colotomy and secured in position with a clamp (Fig. 18.3b). The colotomy is then re-approximated with Allis clamps and closed with a firing of linear stapler (Fig. 18.3c). It is critical to ensure that the anvil is brought out through the colonic

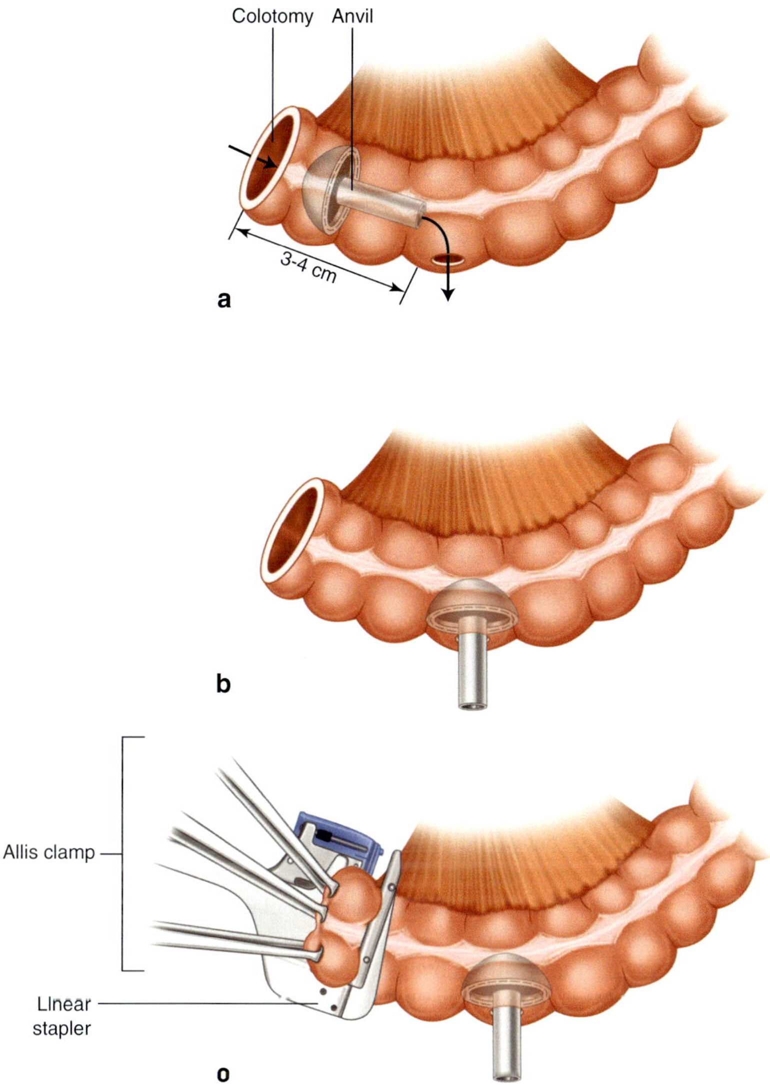

Fig. 18.3 (**a**) The stapling anvil is passed through the open colotomy at the end of the colon. (**b**) The anvil is brought out the antimesenteric border of the colon 3–4 cm proximal to the end colostomy. (**c**) The end colotomy is closed by approximating it with Allis clamps and stapling with a linear stapler

wall proximal enough to ensure that the linear staple line is not incorporated into the circular staple line and that there is enough tissue (>2 cm) between the circular and linear staples lines to maintain perfusion to this bridge of tissue. Once the placement of the anvil is complete, the anastomosis is created using the same technique as described above.

Colonic J Pouch

Proctectomy with reconstruction has a very profound impact on a patient's bowel function. Therefore, surgeons have developed several reservoir or neorectum procedures for anastomosis within 5 cm of the anal verge. Utilization of a reservoir above 5 cm often results in increased difficulties with evacuation. Options for reconstruction after proctectomy include a straight colorectal anastomosis (described under end to end anastomosis), colonic J pouch, transverse coloplasty, and the Baker anastomosis (described under end to side anastomosis). Functionally, the colonic J pouch has better immediate outcome, but after 2 years all of the types of reconstruction have similar functional outcomes [4]. Using a reservoir for an anastomosis above 5 cm may result in difficulties with evacuation. Anastomosis at the pelvic floor will require division of the inferior mesenteric artery at its origin, division of the inferior mesenteric vein at the inferior boarder of the pancreas, and complete mobilization of the splenic flexure to ensure adequate length for the proximal colon to reach the pelvic floor. For the best functional outcomes, it is recommended that soft, pliable descending colon be used for the anastomosis. Utilization of stiff, thickened sigmoid colon will result in decreased compliance of the neorectum and may increase the chances of developing low anterior resection syndrome.

A colonic J pouch is constructed to be 5 cm in length. A larger reservoir is associated with evacuation difficulties. The colon is divided with a linear stapler, and staple line may be oversewn to prevent a leak at the tip of the J. A colotomy is made on the antimesenteric border 5 cm proximal to the transecting staple line (Fig. 18.4a). One fork of the stapler is passed up the proximal limb, and the other fork is passed up the distal limb. The stapler is then reassembled, and the bowel wall is rotated so that the stapler will fire down the antimesenteric boarder of the colon (Fig. 18.4b). It is important to ensure that all epiploic appendages are excluded from the staple line. Once the stapler is removed, a handsewn purse string in a Connell fashion is placed at the colotomy. The EEA stapling anvil is placed into the colotomy, and purse string is cinched down (Fig. 18.4c). The anastomosis is then created by passing the stapling device transanally and deploying the spike through the rectal stump. The anvil is then connected to the stapling cartridge ensuring proper orientation of the left colon. As the stapler is cinched down, the anterior tissues (prostate and bladder in a male and the vagina in a female) must be elevated and confirmed to be free of the EEA staple line before firing. Given the complexity of J pouch and the low anastomosis, most surgeons would recommend proximal diversion.

Transverse Coloplasty

A transverse coloplasty is an acceptable alternative to a colonic J pouch when the pouch will not fit into the pelvis. Reasons that a J pouch will not fit into the pelvis include a bulky mesentery and or a narrow pelvis. Construction of the coloplasty begins with sharp division of the proximal colon, placement of a purse string, and

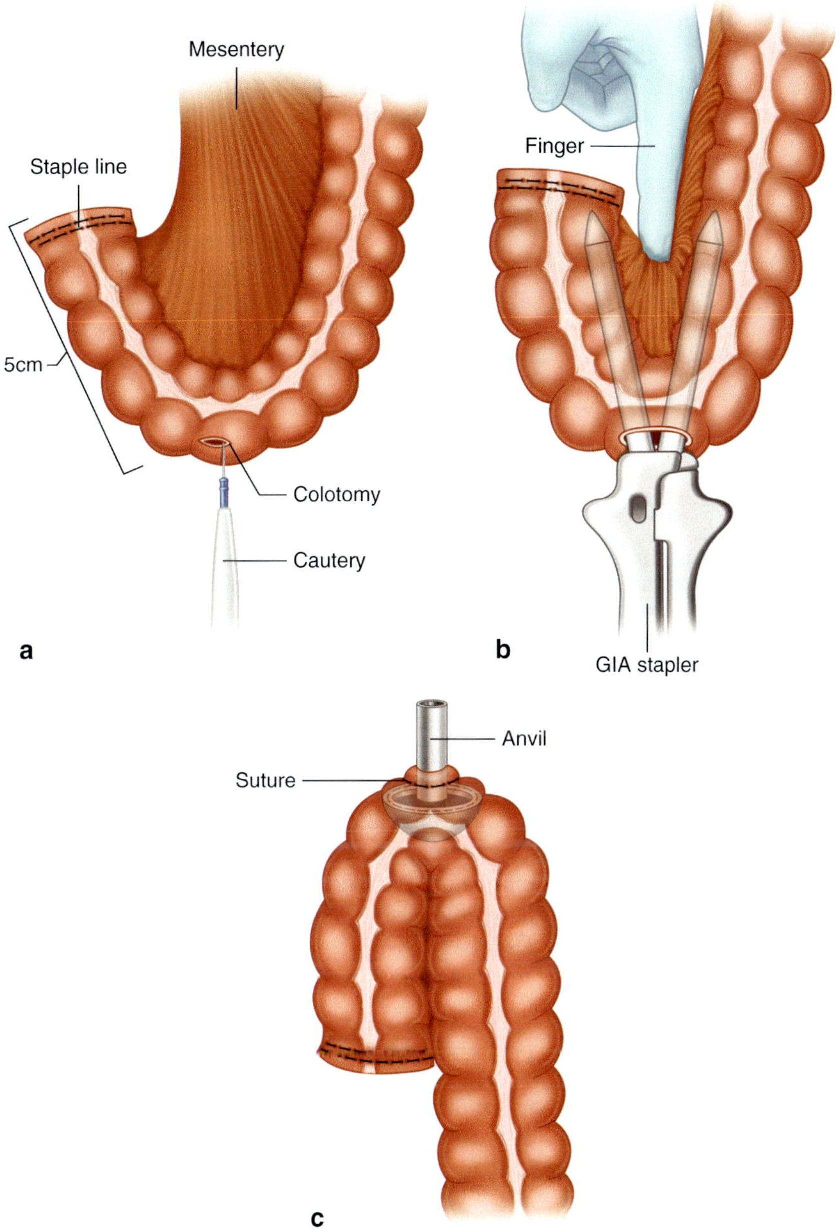

Fig. 18.4 (**a**) Creation of colonic j pouch. A 5 cm limb is measured, and a colotomy is made at the apex of the pouch on the antimesenteric border. (**b**) A GIA stapler is used to create the pouch. The finger is used to get the mesentery out of the staple line so the staple line is antimesenteric to antimesenteric. (**c**) A purse string is placed using a handsewn technique

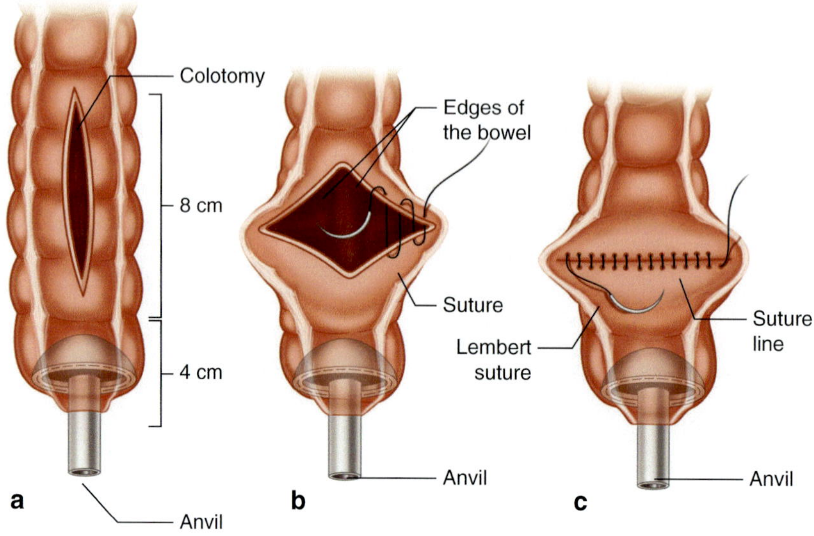

Fig. 18.5 (**a**) The anvil is in place in the distal colotomy and secured with a handsewn purse string. The measurement for the placement and extent of the colotomy are shown. (**b**) The colotomy is open with electrocautery. The first layer is closed in a transverse fashion with a running suture. (**c**) The colotomy closure is reinforced with a second layer of Lembert sutures

securing of an EEA stapling anvil. On the antimesenteric border of the colon and 4 cm proximal to the anvil, an 8 cm colotomy is created and extended proximally (Fig. 18.5a) The longitudinal colotomy is then closed in a transverse direction in a handsewn fashion (Fig. 18.5b). A 3-0 monofilament suture is for the first layer. Beginning at one of the corners, a running Connell stitch is used to close the colotomy, and the second layer of imbricating Lembert stitches are placed to reinforce the suture line (Fig. 18.5c). With the coloplasty completed, an end to end anastomosis is completed as previously described.

Baker's Anastomosis

This is the same anastomosis as that described in the end to side technique. When constructed as an anastomosis at 5 cm or less from the anal verge, functional outcome falls in between that for a colonic J pouch and a transverse coloplasty.

Anastomotic Assessment

Once the anastomosis is created, it must be appropriately assessed to ensure that it is intact. Proper assessment has three components: (1) inspection of the anastomotic doughnuts, (2) air leak testing, and (3) direct intraluminal visualization of the anastomosis. The proximal and distal anastomotic doughnuts should be intact circumferentially with all three layers of the bowel. The management of incomplete doughnuts is addressed below. Inspection of the anastomosis itself can occur with either rigid proctoscopy or flexible endoscopy. With either technique, the pelvis is filled with normal saline, and the bowel is manually occluded proximal to the anastomosis. The endoscope is then introduced transanally into the rectum, air is insufflated to distend the anastomosis, and the pelvis is examined for the presences of air bubbles. The management of an anastomosis that is leaking air bubbles is described below. During or after the air leak test, the endoscope is used to directly evaluate the anastomosis. The anastomosis is examined for completeness, bleeding, and perfusion. For more details on techniques to assess the integrity and perfusion of left-sided anastomoses, please refer to Chap. 29 on minimizing colorectal anastomotic leaks.

Pitfalls and Troubleshooting

Unable to Pass Stapler to the Top of the Rectal Stump

The longer the rectal stump, the more difficult it can be to get the EEA stapler to navigate past all of the rectal folds and get the stapler head flush against the transverse staple line. Adhesions or scarring of rectum may make it difficult in which case further mobilization of the rectum will be beneficial. This may require mobilization below the peritoneal reflection. The upper rectal folds or a narrowed upper rectum may also prevent passage of the stapler. The use of EEA sizers may help flatten out the folds or dilate a narrowed rectum because of their oval shape, and this will help to facilitate the passage of the flat or square face of the stapler head. If this is unsuccessful, then the rectum needs to be divided again at the level to where the stapler can easily be passed.

Rectal Stump Blowout

A disruption of the transverse staple line on the rectum can be one of the most frustrating situations because it often happens at the end of a long case. Poor tissue quality, thickened rectum, and traumatic rupture from passing the stapler are all causes of the rectal staple line falling apart. If this occurs in the upper rectum, it is easily rectified by dividing the rectum a few centimeters below the previous staple line. If this is due to a thicken rectum, it may be helpful to use a longer staple height when stapling across the rectum or dividing the rectum a level where it is the softest. When the disruption of the staple line occurs in the rectum below the peritoneal reflection, salvaging the rectum becomes much more complicated. The first step is to mobilize the rectum to the pelvic floor circumferentially. This will maximize the chances that another stapler can be fired across the rectum. If you are unable to re-staple the rectum laparoscopically, conversion with a suprapubic incision is warranted. This will allow the rectal stump to be grasped with clamps and re-stapled with an open linear stapler. If it is not possible to staple across the rectal stump, there are two remaining options. The first option is a handsewn purse string on the rectal stump. All of the staples must first be removed. The purse string can be placed intraabdominally from an open or laparoscopic approach. With the use of a 2-0 monofilament suture, a purse string is sewn in a full-thickness Connell fashion. This can be particularly challenging because of limitations of the laparoscopic instrumentation, and because visualization from an open approach is poor at best. A second option is to place the purse string transanally. With the patient in the lithotomy position, the legs are frog-legged in the stirrups to expose the anus. The anus in then everted with Lone Star retractor. An operating anoscopy is passed into the anal canal, and the purse string is then placed in the same fashion as above. In either the transabdominal or transanal technique, the stapler is inserted into the rectum, and the spike is deployed before the purse string is cinched down. The purse string is then tied around the spike of the stapler, ensuring that the rectal wall is securely and circumferentially drawn into the stapler. The ultimate fallback for when the rectal stump cannot be salvaged is a mucosectomy with a handsewn coloanal anastomosis. This will work for all the described types of reconstruction. Once again, the patient is placed in high lithotomy position to expose the anal canal. The anal canal is everted with a Lone Star retractor. If the top of rectal stump is visible and easily accessed, the staple line is excised, and the anastomosis is created. Otherwise, a mucosal incision is made circumferentially 1–2 cm above the dentate line. The submucosal plane is developed and dissected in a cephalad fashion, and eventually the dissection becomes full thickness resecting the rest of the rectal stump. The idea is to preserve as much of the internal sphincter as possible. With the dissection completed, the first sutures are placed in the rectum at the 12, 3, 6, and 9 o'clock positions. The sutures are placed from inside the lumen to the outside, and the needles are left on the suture. Next the proximal colon is grasped transanally and delivered into the anal canal. The sutures are then sutured to the proximal colon in an outside to inside fashion, so the knots for each suture are inside the lumen. Each quadrant is then completed with full-thickness, interrupted sutures.

Positive Air Leak Test of the Anastomosis

The assessment of the anastomosis entails inspection of the anastomotic doughnuts and air leak testing of the anastomosis as described above. As a result, there are four different scenarios that can arise (Fig. 18.6): (1) complete doughnuts with an airtight anastomosis, (2) complete doughnuts with air leaking from the anastomosis, (3) incomplete doughnuts with an airtight anastomosis, and (4) incomplete doughnuts with air leaking from the anastomosis. Each component of the scenarios impacts the management of the anastomosis. The ideal is intact doughnuts with an airtight anastomosis. However, if the doughnuts are incomplete or there is an air leak at the anastomosis, this will require further management. The presence of complete doughnuts with an air leaking from the anastomosis is managed based on the

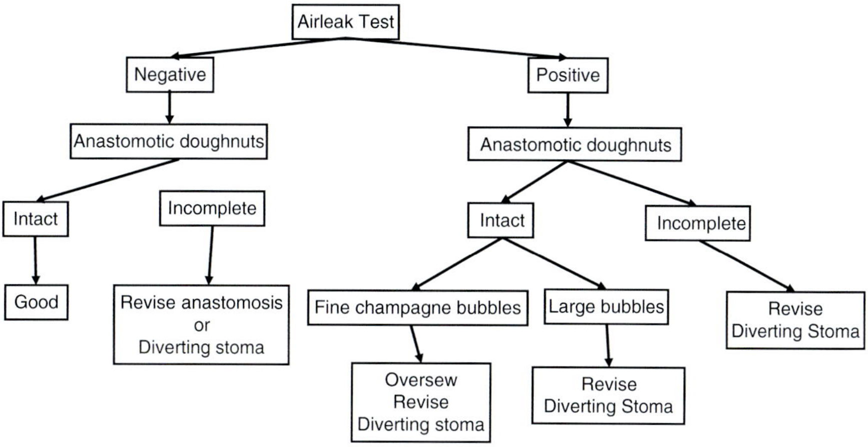

Fig. 18.6 Algorithm for managing a positive air leak test

size of the air bubbles leaking and the source can be clearly visualized. Small "champagne" bubbles for the anterior half of the anastomosis that can be visualized can be managed by placing Lembert stitches across the anastomosis. The placement of multiple stitches along the anastomosis is recommended as a single suture is not adequate. If the small "champagne"-type bubbles cannot be seen, consider proximal diversion or revision of the anastomosis by taking it down and recreating it. If the bubbles are large with an obvious defect in the staple line, this needs to be managed with revision of the anastomosis. However, if the anastomosis is low and can be accessed transanally, the anastomosis can be repaired transanally with proximal diversion. When the doughnuts are incomplete with an airtight anastomosis, this anastomosis should be protected with proximal diversion, or it should be revised because it cannot be guaranteed that the anastomosis is full thickness. For an anastomosis with incomplete doughnuts and leaking air, it should be taken down and re-created as proximal diversion alone is unlikely to be sufficient. For more details on techniques to manage intraoperative air leak and other anastomotic complications, please refer to Chap. 30 on how to salvage the failed anastomosis.

Staple Line Bleeding

With routine use of endoscopic assessment of the anastomosis, it is easy to identify and manage bleeding from the anastomosis. It is important to use CO_2 insufflation so the colon and rectum do not remain distended. If a site of bleeding is identified, it can be managed with endoscopic clips or injection with epinephrine or coagulated. Caution with epinephrine is needed as to not over-inject, causing issues with local perfusion and with caution with electrocoagulation as not to cause extensive thermal injury to the anastomotic tissue. If transanal or endoscopic attempts at controlling the bleeding fails, direct suture ligation of anastomotic bleeding can be achieved using a transanal endoscopic platform (TEM/TAMIS), assuming the anastomosis can be reached.

Inadequate Reach of the Colonic Conduit

Ensuring the proximal colon has adequate reach for a well-perfused and tension-free anastomosis is critical to ensure proper healing. The first steps to provide adequate length for the colon to reach the top of the rectal stump include high ligation of the inferior mesenteric artery at its origin, ligation of the inferior mesenteric vein adjacent to the ligament of Treitz near the inferior border of the pancreas, and full mobilization of the splenic flexure with division of the attachment to the inferior border of the pancreas to the midline. If there is still inadequate length to reach the rectal stump, then additional maneuvers will be required, which will be presented in a step-wise progression. First, complete mobilization of the transverse colon from the omentum and the attachments within the lesser sac especially the stomach. This mobilization should extend to the hepatic flexure. Second, the colon may be brought down the right side of the abdomen and passed through a window on the small bowel side of the ileocolic pedicle. This is an avascular window, and by bringing the colon through this window, it is the shortest path and prevents the colon from coursing over the terminal ileum (Fig. 18.7). Third, the middle colic vessels can be ligated in a sequential fashion. If the colon maintains perfusion from one of the remaining branches of the middle colic vessels, bringing the colon down the right side as described above is often adequate to reach into the pelvis. Finally, if perfusion to the distal colon or there is still not enough length, then resection of the distal portion of the colon to a point where the prefusion to the remaining colon is depend upon the ileocolic pedicle will be needed. To get adequate length, complete mobilization of the right colon and the proximal colon can be brought into the pelvic either via the window in the ileal mesentery described above or with the use of Deloyer's technique. The Deloyer's technique involves complete mobilization of the right colon and its mesentery off the retroperitoneum. The proximal colon is then rotated counterclockwise 180, so the colon is brought down the patient's right side, and the cecum ends up in the right upper quadrant (Fig. 18.8a, b).

Outcomes

Anastomotic Leak

An anastomotic leak is one of the most dreaded complications associated with colorectal resections. Its occurrence has significant impact on the patient's recovery, bowel function, cancer-related outcomes, and may ultimately result in a permanent stoma. These are multifactorial events, and the literature is full of reports detailing potential risk factors. The literature has several limitations that impact our ability to accurately identify true and consistent risk factors such as

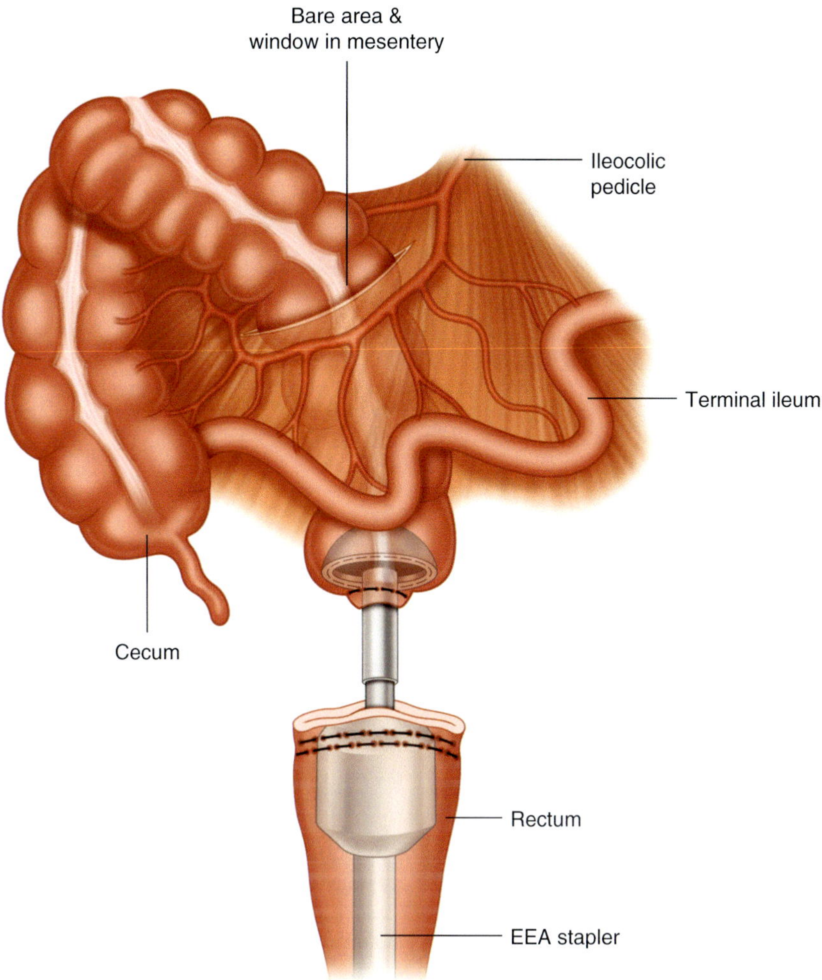

Fig. 18.7 When there is difficulty getting the proximal colon to reach easily into the pelvis, the colon can be brought down the right side and passed through a window on the ileal side of the ileocolic pedicle

retrospective study designs, relatively low incidence of anastomotic leaks, varying definitions of a leak, and selection bias based on inability to account for surgeon decision of when not to create an anastomosis. Having said all of that, there are a handful of factors that have consistently been shown to impact the rate of anastomotic leak (Box 18.1). The site of the anastomosis does have an impact. Any anastomosis of the colon to the rectum has a higher rate of leak when compared to ileocolic anastomosis and small bowel anastomosis [5]. Additionally, the level of the anastomosis from the anal verge has an impact as anastomoses <5 cm from the anal verge have a six times greater risk of an anastomotic leak than anastomoses

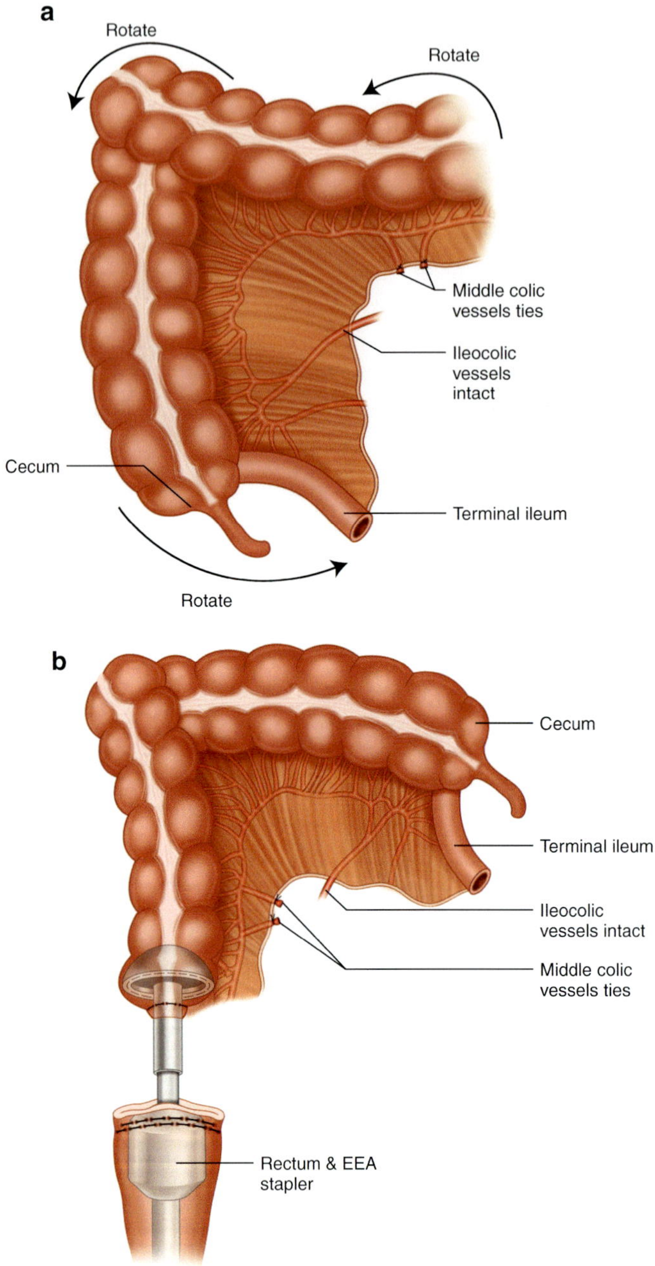

Fig. 18.8 (**a**, **b**) The Deloyer's technique. (**a**) The right colon and transverse colon are in situ with the middle colic vessels have been ligated. The arrows demonstrate that the end of the colon and cecum are rotated counterclockwise 180. (**b**) The right colon and transverse colon are completely mobilized and rotated counterclockwise 180. This results in placing the cecum in the RUQ and the end of the colon in the pelvis

Box 18.1 Risk Factors for an Anastomotic Leak

Site of anastomosis:
- Colorectal > ileorectal > ileocolic > small bowel
- Height of colorectal anastomosis:
  - <5 cm from anal verge
  - Male gender
  - BMI >30
- Complexity of procedure:
  - Combined procedures
  - Excessive operative time
  - Excessive blood loss
  - Intraoperative adverse event
- Malnutrition
- Smoking
- Crohn's disease
- Failure to perform an air leak test

above that level [6]. The complexity of the patient and operative procedure influences the risk of an anastomotic leak. For example, prolonged operative times of >200 minutes, combined procedures, and need for blood transfusions have been shown to be associated with an increased risk of leak by factors of 3.4, 3.7, and 3.1 times, respectively [7]. Specific patient-related factors that have been found to increase the risk of anastomotic leak include male gender, a body mass index (BMI) >30 who are having an anastomosis below the peritoneal reflection, steroid use, and smoking [8, 9]. Based on the German Rectal Cancer Trial that compared preoperative vs postoperative radiation therapy, there was no difference in the rate of anastomotic leak between the two groups [10]. After the introduction of early recovery after surgery protocols, there has been a flurry of articles examining the association between NSAID usage and anastomotic leaks [11–14]. There does appear to be some associated increased risk, but these studies have been retrospective. As a result, they lack detailed information such as accurate usage from a timing and dosage perspective, and there are many confounding factors in the study populations such as comorbidities, steroid use, and emergent and elective surgery. Thus, it is difficult to draw firm conclusions, so routine usage in ERAS protocols remains common practice. Finally, one of the most effective preventative measures for anastomotic leak is the use of preoperative bowel preparation with a mechanical component and oral antibiotics. Using colon and rectal surgery-specific NSQIP (National Surgical Quality Improvement Program) data, Scarborough and colleagues demonstrated a significantly lower rate of leak with a mechanical and oral antibiotic prep (2.8%) compared to mechanical prep only (4.2%), oral antibiotics only (5.5%), and no prep (5.7%) ($p = 0.001$) [15]. Therefore, it is recommended that all patients undergoing elective colon and rectal surgery receive a mechanical and oral antibiotic preparation.

Anastomotic Assessment

Anastomotic assessment at the time of surgery is critical for a successful anastomosis. There are two components to the assessment. Air leak testing assesses that the staple line is airtight, and direct visualization provides the ability to confirm an intact staple line, gross perfusion to both ends of the bowel, and to manage bleeding from the staple line. The benefit of routine anastomotic testing is a decrease in the chances that the anastomosis leaks. The state of Washington through their Surgical Care and Outcomes Assessment Program demonstrated a 75% reduction in the anastomotic leak rate for hospitals that performed routine testing (defined as >90% of cases) compared to hospitals that did not routinely test their anastomosis [OR 0.23 (95% CI 0.05–0.99] [16]. Management of specific anastomotic complications is discussed above. The assessment can be performed with either flexible endoscopy or rigid proctoscopy, and some will advocate instilling the rectum with betadine versus air. It is also essential to clearly document your findings in the operative note.

Bowel Function for Reconstruction After Low Anterior Resection

Bowel function changes significantly for patients after proctectomy. Low anterior resection syndrome (LARS) occurs in 25–80% of patients and is characterized by stool frequency, urgency, clustering, and/or emptying problems. In order to improve bowel function after proctectomy for anastomosis within 5 cm of the anal verge, surgeons have utilized all of the reconstruction techniques described above. In 2007, Fazio and colleagues published the first results from a prospective randomized trial comparing colonic J pouch, transverse coloplasty, and straight coloanal anastomosis [4]. They reported that the colonic J pouch had significant improvement in number of bowel movements, fragmentation, and incontinence, but there was no difference between coloplasty and straight anastomosis. However, after 2 years there was no difference in quality of life score between all three groups. In a more recent multicenter prospective randomized trial comparing end to side, colon J pouch, and straight anastomosis, it demonstrated no difference in composite evacuation and incontinence scores at any time point [17]. The composite evacuation score included data on the use of medications, difficulty emptying, need for digitation to empty, feeling of incomplete evacuation, need for straining, and time required to evacuate. Putting these studies together, the determination for the type of reconstruction after proctectomy remains up to surgeon preference. There does appear to be some early benefit for the use of a colonic J pouch, but any difference is lost after 2 years. Therefore, patients with concern for difficulty managing their bowels, fecal incontinence, or an anastomosis below 5 cm may be best served by a colonic J pouch.

Temporary Fecal Diversion

Utilization of fecal diversion for high-risk anastomoses is beneficial in reducing the incidence of leak and managing the leak when it occurs. There are several multicenter, prospective randomized trials demonstrating a decreased leak rate after low anterior resection for rectal cancer. In 2007, a trial from Sweden reported a reduced leak rate with either a diverting ileostomy of colostomy of 10.3% or 28% without diversion ($p < 0.001$) for anastomosis below 5 cm [18]. These findings have been confirmed by more recent study by Mrak and colleagues [19]. They demonstrated improved leak rate for those patient with diverting stomas [5.8% compared to 16.3% ($p = 0.04$)]. Both studies also demonstrated a decreased rate of urgent reoperation when a leak does occur, thus suggesting greater ease of managing a leak.

Diversion with either a loop ileostomy vs loop colostomy is acceptable. Each type of stoma has positives and negatives. Loop ileostomies are easy to manage and easy to reverse but have a higher rates of dehydration and pouching difficulties [20]. In contrast, loop colostomies have a higher rate of prolapse, herniation, and morbidity after closure. It remains surgeon preference for utilizing a diverting ileostomy versus colostomy. For more details on optimizing stoma function and quality of life, please refer to Chap. 36 on best practices in planned and unplanned stoma creation.

Conclusion

Anastomotic creation after left-sided colon or rectal resection is technically demanding and its critical aspect of a successful operation. The principles of a healthy anastomosis include utilization of healthy bowel, adequate perfusion to the bowel, adequate mobilization of the colon to ensure no tension, and assessment of the anastomosis. The type of reconstruction for the anastomosis is up to surgeon discretion as there appears to be little benefit of one type of reconstruction over another. Surgeons should be familiar with potential risk factors associated with leaks and capable of identifying and managing intraoperative anastomotic complications as their decision-making at the time of the operation is critical for a successful outcome.

References

1. Rojas-Machado SA, Romero-Simó M, Arroyo A, Rojas-Machado A, López J, Calpena R. Prediction of anastomotic leak in colorectal cancer surgery based on a new prognostic index PROCOLE (prognostic colorectal leakage) developed from the meta-analysis of observational studies of risk factors. Int J Color Dis. 2016;31(2):197–210.
2. Jim JH, Kim HY, Lee IK, Oh ST, Kim JG, Lee YS. Intra-operative double-stapled colorectal or coloanal anastomosis complications of laparoscopic low anterior resection for rectal cancer: double-stapled anastomotic complication could result in persistent anastomotic leakage. Surg Endosc. 2015;(11):3117–24.
3. Cheng KP, Roslani AC, Sehha N, Kueh JH, Law CW, Chong HY, et al. ALEXIS O-Ring wound retractor vs conventional wound protection for the prevention of surgical site infections in colorectal resections(1). Color Dis. 2012;14(6):e346–51.
4. Fazio VW, Zutshi M, Remzi FH, Parc Y, Ruppert R, Fürst A, et al. A randomized multicenter trial to compare long-term functional outcome, quality of life, and complications of surgical procedures for low rectal cancers. Ann Surg. 2007;246(3):481–8.

5. Telem DA, Chin EH, Nguyen SQ, Divino CM. Risk factors for anastomotic leak following colorectal surgery: a case-control study. Arch Surg. 2010;145(4):371–6.
6. Lipska MA, Bissett IP, Parry BR, Merrie AE. Anastomotic leakage after lower gastrointestinal anastomosis: men are at a higher risk. ANZ J Surg. 2006;76(7):579–85.
7. Buchs NC, Gervaz P, Secic M, Bucher P, Mugnier-Konrad B, Morel P. Incidence, consequences, and risk factors for anastomotic dehiscence after colorectal surgery: a prospective monocentric study. Int J Color Dis. 2008;23(3):265–70.
8. Gendall KA, Raniga S, Kennedy R, Frizelle FA. The impact of obesity on outcome after major colorectal surgery. Dis Colon Rectum. 2007;50(12):2223–37.
9. Midura EF, Hanseman D, Davis BR, Atkinson SJ, Abbott DE, Shah SA, et al. Risk factors and consequences of anastomotic leak after colectomy: a national analysis. Dis Colon Rectum. 2015;58(3):333–8.
10. Sauer R, Becker H, Hohenberger W, Rödel C, Wittekind C, Fietkau R, et al. Preoperative versus postoperative chemoradiotherapy for rectal cancer. N Engl J Med. 2004;351(17):1731–40.
11. Hakkarainen TW, Steele SR, Bastaworous A, Dellinger EP, Farrokhi E, Farjah F, et al. Nonsteroidal anti-inflammatory drugs and the risk for anastomotic failure: a report from Washington State's Surgical Care and Outcomes Assessment Program (SCOAP). JAMA Surg. 2015;150(3):223–8.
12. Saleh F, Jackson TD, Ambrosini L, Gnanasegaram JJ, Kwong J, Quereshy F, et al. Perioperative nonselective non-steroidal anti-inflammatory drugs are not associated with anastomotic leakage after colorectal surgery. J Gastrointest Surg. 2014;18(8):1398–404.
13. Kotagal M, Hakkarainen TW, Simianu VV, Beck SJ, Alfonso-Cristancho R, Flum DR. Ketorolac use and postoperative complications in gastrointestinal surgery. Ann Surg. 2016;263(1):71–5.
14. Bakker N, Deelder JD, Richir MC, Cakir H, Doodeman HJ, Schreurs WH, et al. Risk of anastomotic leakage with nonsteroidal anti-inflammatory drugs within an enhanced recovery program. J Gastrointest Surg. 2016;20(4):776–82.
15. Scarborough JE, Mantyh CR, Sun Z, Migaly J. Combined mechanical and oral antibiotic bowel preparation reduces incisional surgical site infection and anastomotic leak rates after elective colorectal resection: an analysis of colectomy-targeted ACS NSQIP. Ann Surg. 2015;262(2):331–7.
16. Kwon S, Morris A, Billingham R, Frankhouse J, Horvath K, Johnson M, et al. Routine leak testing in colorectal surgery in the Surgical Care and Outcomes Assessment Program. Arch Surg. 2012;147(4):345–51.
17. Marti WR, Curti G, Wehrli H, Grieder F, Graf M, Gloor B, et al. Clinical outcome after rectal replacement with side-to-end, Colon-J-Pouch, or straight colorectal anastomosis following total mesorectal excision: a Swiss prospective, randomized, multicenter trial (SAKK 40/04). Ann Surg. 2019;269(5):827–35.
18. Matthiessen P, Hallböök O, Rutegård J, Simert G, Sjödahl R. Defunctioning stoma reduces symptomatic anastomotic leakage after low anterior resection of the rectum for cancer: a randomized multicenter trial. Ann Surg. 2007;246(2):207–14.
19. Mrak K, Uranitsch S, Pedross F, Heuberger A, Klingler A, Jagoditsch M, et al. Diverting ileostomy versus no diversion after low anterior resection for rectal cancer: a prospective, randomized, multicenter trial. Surgery. 2016;159(4):1129–39.
20. Rondelli F, Reboldi P, Rulli A, Barberini F, Guerrisi A, Izzo L, et al. Loop ileostomy versus loop colostomy for fecal diversion after colorectal or coloanal anastomosis: a meta-analysis. Int J Color Dis. 2009;24(5):479–88.

Robotic Left-Sided Colon Resections: Unique Considerations and Optimal Setup

19

Mark Karam Soliman and Ovunc Bardakcioglu

Introduction and Rationale

It is widely accepted that compared with open operations, minimally invasive abdominal surgery is superior in nearly every aspect: reduced pain, faster return of bowel function, reduced length of hospital stay, lower overall cost of care, improved cosmesis, lower hernia rates, and quicker return to work [1]. This holds true for most laparoscopic operations and is therefore the reason that the laparoscopy has become the gold standard for a large part of elective and emergent operations. The same clinical benefits are seen in patients undergoing minimally invasive colorectal operations but with the added benefit of equivalent oncologic benefits and a trend towards improved cancer-related survival in at least one randomized controlled trial (RCT) comparing open and laparoscopic resection for colon cancer [2]. However, despite the known benefits and widespread availability of laparoscopy [3], adoption has remained relatively low, with rates of laparoscopic colectomy reaching 55.4% based on the most recent data from the National Inpatient Sample database [4, 5]. The adoption is low even considering an increase in worldwide prevalance of left-sided colonic pathology [6]. Slow adoption can be partly explained by the complexity of colorectal operations, which require control and ligation of one or more major vascular pedicles, mastery of the relevant anatomical landmarks, careful dissection and manipulation of tumor specimens, and familiarity with all the steps required to construct an adequate anastomosis.

M. K. Soliman (✉)
Colon and Rectal Clinic of Florida, University of Florida, Orlando, FL, USA

Colorectal Surgery, AdventHealth Central Florida, Orlando, FL, USA
e-mail: mark.soliman@crcorlando.com

O. Bardakcioglu
Division of Colorectal Surgery, Department of Surgery, University of Nevada at Las Vegas School of Medicine, Las Vegas, NV, USA
e-mail: ovunc.bardakcioglu@unlv.edu

P. Sylla et al. (eds.), *The SAGES Manual of Colorectal Surgery*,
https://doi.org/10.1007/978-3-030-24812-3_19

Continued advances in minimally invasive technologies have led to the development of robotic platforms in the hope that the ergonomic benefits of a robotic platform, combined with wristed instruments and 3D visualization, would help mitigate some the technical challenges of laparoscopy, thereby increasing adoption of minimally invasive surgery (MIS) while reducing conversion rates. This rise in pathology has likewise encouraged surgeons to incorporate instruments and technology to bridge the gaps that laparoscopic surgery was unable to fill.

This chapter will describe various techniques and strategies for robotic left-sided colonic resections, with emphasis on best practices based on tumor location and tumor pathology.

Indications and Contradictions

There are no absolute contraindications to a robotic approach for left-sided colorectal resection. In fact, in recent years, absolute contraindications to minimally invasive approaches in "high-risk" patients have been challenged, such as prior abdominal surgery and obesity [7]. Authors now advocate for the use of minimally invasive surgery when possible, even in "high-risk" patients based on the benefits derived from reduced physiologic stress and postoperative morbidity. Similarly, robotic colorectal operations may also be offered to all patients undergoing left-sided colon resections. Relative contraindications to robotic surgery include the following:

- Hemodynamic instability
- Inability to tolerate insufflations: e.g., due to cardiopulmonary disease
- Inability to access the abdominal cavity safely: e.g., intense adhesive burden from previous surgery, intraperitoneal mesh placement
- Inability to adequately insufflate: e.g., abdominoplasty, bowel obstruction causing over distension of bowel
- Tumor-related issues: e.g., size of tumor larger than incision required for laparotomy, local extension into adjacent structures that would require a multidisciplinary approach where other surgical teams are not proficient in reconstructive procedures using a minimally invasive approach

Principles and Quality Benchmarks

The critical steps to be completed during minimally invasive resection of malignant and benign left-sided pathology are outlined below.

Malignant Diseases

1. Dissection along embryologic planes of the parietal and visceral peritoneal layer to the root of the mesentery and avoiding retroperitoneal structures and the left ureter (complete mesocolic excision)

2. Identification and dissection of the inferior mesenteric artery (IMA) with selective ligation of the IMA at its origin or just distal to the junction of the left colic artery resulting in adequate lymph node yield for malignant diseases (minimum of 12 lymph nodes)
3. Adequate proximal and distal tumoral margins of healthy, non-affected colon of 5–10 cm
4. Adequate colonic mobilization with technical ability for complete splenic flexure mobilization and high ligation of the inferior mesenteric vein (IMV) if necessary for a tension-free anastomosis

Benign Diseases

1. Definition of the appropriate extent of the resection as defined by the nature of the disease: for example, for a resection in diverticulitis cases, it is necessary to precisely identify and divide the colon at the rectosigmoid junction (coalescence of the teniae) to avoid retaining distal sigmoid colon with an increased risk of recurrent diverticulitis.
2. Proximal division of the colon where the bowel is healthy.
3. Definition of an appropriate degree of devascularization: Unless there is strong confirmation about the benign nature of the disease, the same oncological vascular dissection should be performed as for known malignant disease; if the disease is confirmed to benign, a less aggressive and blood supply-sparing dissection may be sufficient as the lymph node harvest is not of relevance.

Preoperative Planning, Patient Workup, and Optimization

Patients with left-sided pathologies are – like for any major surgical intervention – evaluated for relevant comorbidities and optimized accordingly. Special attention is paid to obese patients, where a thorough pulmonary evaluation is needed to rule out underlying diseases such as chronic obstructive pulmonary disease which can be associated with difficulties with ventilation during prolonged periods in Trendelenburg position.

Computer tomography of the chest, abdomen, and pelvis is obtained for tumor staging. It further provides important strategic information about pathology itself as well as about the configuration of the colon, its redundancy, and the level of the splenic flexure.

Preoperative complete colonoscopy or alternative colon evaluation is necessary to exclude secondary pathology and possible for tattooing if the tumor location is not otherwise reliably defined.

Individual hospital and institutional specific enhanced recovery protocols determine further preoperative optimization. These frequently include prehabilitation, nutritional supplements, patient education, and bowel preparation with oral antibiotics.

Operative Setup

Patient Positioning

The patient is placed in the modified lithotomy position with both arms tucked in neutral position along the torso. The legs are placed in stirrups such that they can be moved from a 0-degree angle at the hip level to an elevated position when access to the anus is needed.

To minimize sliding when the patient is placed in steep Trendelenburg position, an anti-sliding pad should be used. Alternatively, a beanbag with respective external stabilizers may be helpful. Shoulder brackets should be used with caution to avoid damage to the brachial plexus. The patient is further secured to the table by means of safety straps across the upper chest. Testing the various positions before prepping the patient may be helpful to identify instabilities.

Room Setup

It is important to optimize the limited space and arrange the various items in the room, such as operating table, towers, robot, accessory equipment, room lights, anesthesia equipment, sterile trays, colonoscopy cart, etc. The arrangement needs coordination in such a fashion that adequate space is available to access the robotic arms and execute an unrestricted and sterile exchange of instruments once the patient is prepped and draped.

The assistant surgeon will be on the right side of the patient and can help with instrument changes, retraction, suctioning, and irrigation as needed. The scrub tech is also on the right side next to the assistant surgeon.

Operative Technique

Trocar Placement

Planning the trocar outline should take into consideration the extent of the planned colon dissection, the midpoint between the most proximal and the most distal point, the optimal site for an accessory port as well as the specimen extraction site. Trocar sites should be marked onto the patient's skin using a sterile pen after draping. Abdominal access, CO_2 insufflation and initial camera insertion are completed in the usual fashion using safe practice guidelines.

Si® Robot (Intuitive Surgical, Sunnyvale, CA, USA)

When using the Si system, the ports should be placed along a curve and be approximately 20 cm away from the target and 10 cm apart in order to avoid clashing of the robotic arms. The ports/arms are labeled C for the camera and 1, 2, and 3 for trocars going right to the left. The specimen extraction and anvil insertion site may be planned at one of the existing ports or as a separate small Pfannenstiel incision in the suprapubic region.

A typical trocar setup for a robotic low anterior resection (LAR) is illustrated in Fig. 19.1a. The camera is placed through a periumbilical 12 mm laparoscopic trocar. A 12 mm robotic trocar (arm 1) is placed in the right lower quadrant making sure not to injure the inferior epigastric vessels. A more medial position facilitates access to the deep pelvis, whereas a more lateral position is appropriate if the extent of the dissection ends at the pelvic inlet. One 8 mm robotic trocar (arm 2) is placed in the left upper quadrant on the midclavicular line between ribs and the iliac crest, and another 8 mm trocar (arm 3) is placed in the left lower quadrant (position 3A). For splenic flexure mobilization, a right upper quadrant 8 mm trocar may temporarily be used for arm 3 (position 3B). An accessory 5 mm port is placed in the right upper quadrant to be used by the bedside assistant.

Figure 19.1b shows a modification of the trocar outline when the entire left side (left and sigmoid colon) is the target of the operation.

Xi® Robot (Intuitive Surgical, Sunnyvale, CA, USA)

For the Xi system, the ports have a different layout and should be placed on a straight line from left upper to right lower quadrant. The slope of the line may be steeper if the splenic flexure needs to be taken down and flatter if that step is not anticipated. The space between arms should be an equal distance of 6–8 cm. In contrast to the previous setting, the ports/arms in the Xi are labeled as 1–4 from left

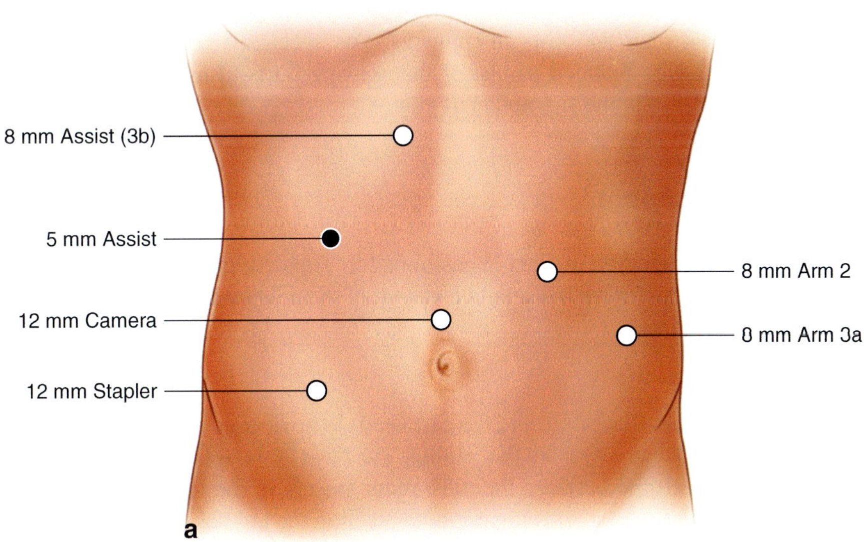

Fig. 19.1 (**a**) Robotic sigmoid Si port placement for anticipated splenic flexure takedown. (**b**) Robotic left/sigmoid colectomy, da Vinci Xi® (Intuitive Surgical, Sunnyvale, CA, USA) port placement

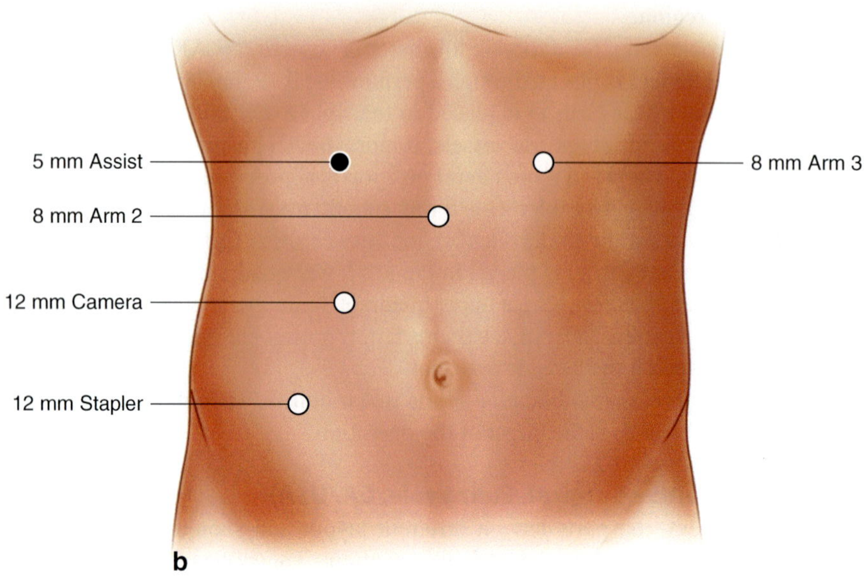

Fig. 19.1 (continued)

to right (Fig. 19.2). The standard robotic port including the one for the camera is 8 mm; stapler insertion requires a 12 mm port (typically arm 4) with an 8 mm reducer when used for the other instruments. The specimen extraction and anvil insertion site may be planned as one of the existing ports or as a separate small Pfannenstiel incision in the suprapubic region.

Docking of the Robot

After trocar placement, the patient is positioned in Trendelenburg and with the left side up just enough to move the small bowel out of the pelvis and expose the root of the left colon mesentery.

Si Robot

The Si robot has less flexibility, and the cart needs to be docked in an oblique angle (approximately 30 degrees) from the left hip. The base of the robotic cart is aligned parallel to a virtual line between the most outer trocars in the left flank and right lower quadrant (Fig. 19.1a). It is important to position the left leg in the stirrup such that it will not interfere with the robotic arm movements after the patient is positioned in Trendelenburg position and tilted to the right. The Si system will allow reasonable access to two quadrants involved in the operation. If the ports are configured for a lower pelvic operation, access to the pelvis and a portion of the left

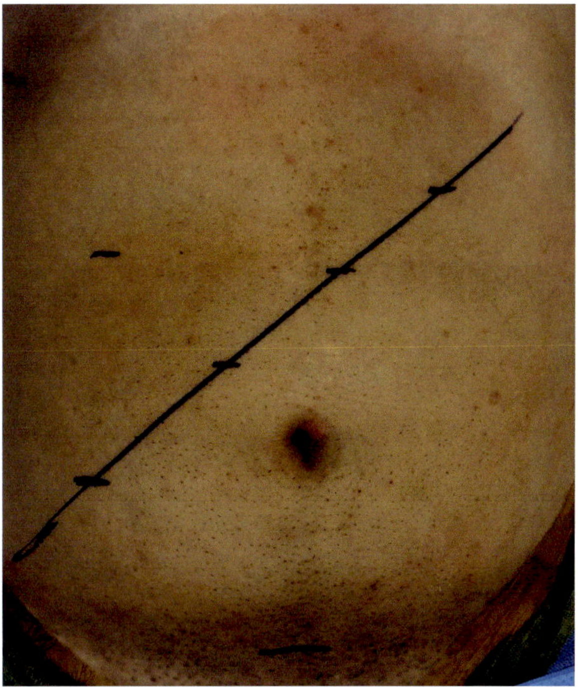

Fig. 19.2 Optimal trocar outline for left colectomy using the da Vinci Xi® system (Intuitive Surgical, Sunnyvale, CA, USA) (Courtesy of Andreas Kaiser, MD)

hemi-abdomen will be possible without repositioning. If the splenic flexure needs to be mobilized, three options exist: [1] arm 3a is undocked and rotated into the 3b position (Fig. 19.1a), [2] the robotic cart may need to be redocked over the left shoulder, or [3] the splenic flexure is mobilized laparoscopically. Once the Si robot has been docked, it needs to be manually targeted to the area of interest.

Xi Robot

As the Xi robot has a central boom that allows for 360 degrees rotation, it can be docked from any direction, typically though from the left. First, the boom is centered and then docked to the camera port (arm 3) only. The camera is inserted and pointed at the surgical target. The boom and the other arms are automatically optimized using the integrated targeting function. The other arms are docked and adequately spaced.

Instrument Insertion

Instruments should be carefully inserted, best under visual control or by testing the direction first by means of a nontraumatic laparoscopic peanut. With either system, the right hand typically controls an energy device (monopolar scissors, hook, or bipolar vessel sealer) through the right lower quadrant port. The left hand directs two retracting instruments (fenestrated bipolar forceps, Cadiere forceps or tip up, fenestrated graspers). These instruments are frequently adjusted utilizing the foot switch to allow for optimal traction and countertraction. Much of the exposure is achievable without the assistant surgeon and is considered one of the major benefits of robotic compared to laparoscopic approaches.

CME Dissection of the Colon Mesentery and Isolation of the Mesenteric Root

When the goal is to perform an oncological resection, the procedure follows the same steps as described for the laparoscopic approach. Please refer to Chap. 11 on Principles of Complete Mesocolic Excision (CME) for Colon Cancer.

Depending on the location of the pathology and whether left colectomy is performed for benign or malignant indications, different levels of vascular dissection are needed. The dissection usually commences with retracting the rectosigmoid colon upwards to tent up the inferior mesenteric artery (IMA) pedicle towards the anterior abdominal wall (Fig. 19.3). The two robotic arms from the left side and a laparoscopic grasper through the assistant trocar can be utilized to achieve optimal tension on the peritoneum. This will allow CO_2 dissection to better identify the dissection planes defined by embryological anatomy. Wide scoring of the peritoneum overlying the base of the left colon mesentery starts at the peritoneal groove on the right side of the lateral mesorectum and continues towards the inferior border of the inferior mesentery artery (Fig. 19.4). Subsequent adjustment of the robotic arms with lifting the rectosigmoid colon and by passive upwards retraction with the instrument shafts from beneath the colon wall will expose the areolar tissue between the sigmoid colon mesentery and all retroperitoneal structures. This dissection continues from medial to lateral until the IMA and inferior mesenteric vein (IMV) are completely mobilized, the left ureter is identified close to the mesenteric root, the hypogastric nerves identified and preserved, and the lateral peritoneal reflection is

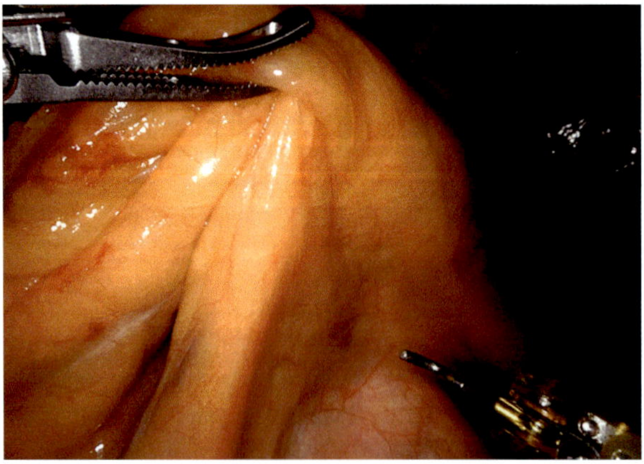

Fig. 19.3 Rectosigmoid junction being tented anteriorly exposing the IMA pedicle

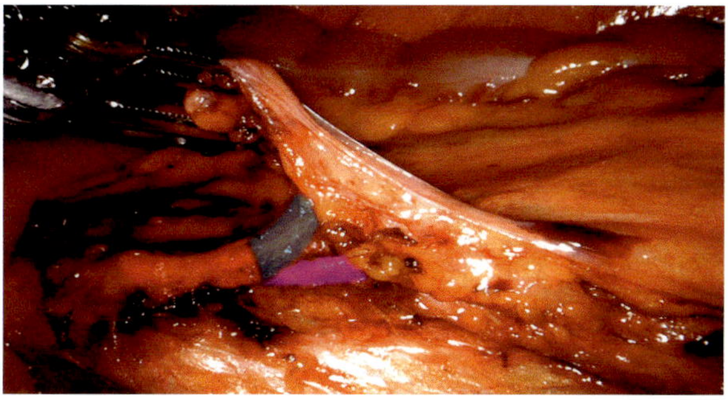

Fig. 19.4 Red masking indicates IMA takeoff from aorta. Blue masking indicates left colic artery. Purple masking indicates superior hemorrhoidal artery. Note the close proximity of the bifurcation relative to the root of the IMA

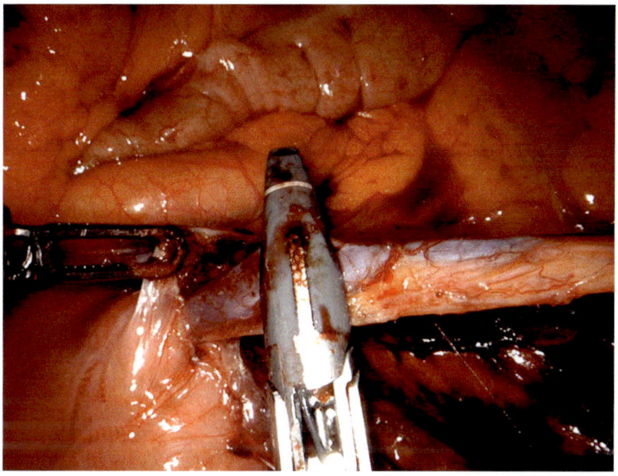

Fig. 19.5 View of the IMV prior to its division. Note that division is at the inferior border of the pancreas and the fourth portion of the duodenum

reached. The dissection is performed along the embryological planes of the visceral and parietal peritoneum to yield an intact mesocolon (complete mesocolic excision).

At this point, the decision has to be made whether the IMV will be ligated next to the artery or higher near the duodenum (see Fig. 19.5, which demonstrates high ligation of the IMV). This step is most commonly used during low anterior resection (LAR) and will be described in detail in Chap. 24 on Robotic Low Anterior Resection. The entire pedicle is encircled, and high ligation of the IMA and IMV is performed with the robotic vessel sealer or stapler after being individually dissected and skeletonized. Alternatively, the left colic artery can be preserved and ligation of the superior rectal artery only performed just distal to its runoff.

With few exceptions, it is recommended to follow the natural planes regardless of the indication for left colectomy. The ability to consistently and intentionally dissect, isolate, and divide the IMA, left colic artery, and superior rectal artery is invaluable and mandatory for malignant disease. Even for confirmed benign disease, dissection along these planes is often easier and less bloody than dissecting through the mesentery. In addition, a high ligation increases colon mobility which is needed for lower anastomoses.

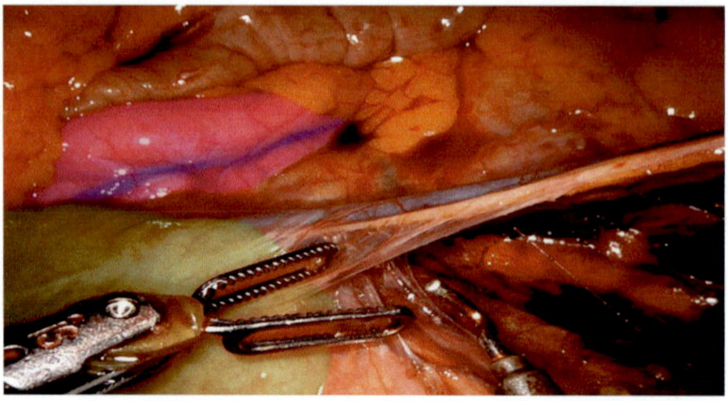

Fig. 19.6 Magenta masking indicates the pancreatic body with the splenic vein at its inferior border. Green masking indicates the duodenal-jejunal junction with IMV diving deep to it. Note the close proximity of the transverse colon to the body of the pancreas

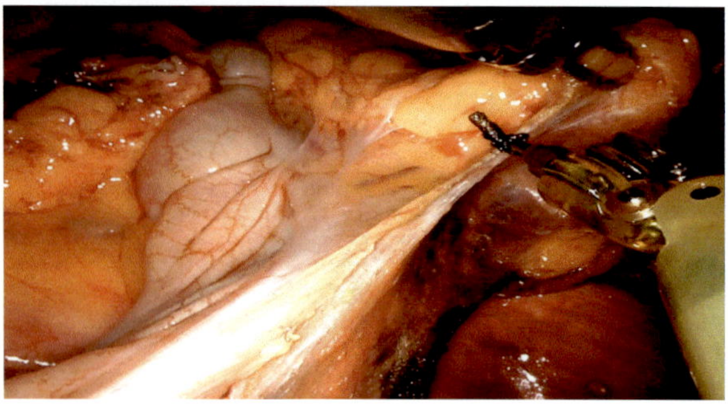

Fig. 19.7 Omentocolic attachments being divided during the final steps of splenic flexure mobilization

A non-anatomic "wedge resection" along the bowel wall may on occasion be preferable in proven benign disease with severely altered anatomy (Crohn's colitis, severe diverticulitis) and is technically facilitated using vessel sealing devices. For more details and techniques, please refer to Chap. 5 on Laparoscopic Left Colon Resection for Complex Inflammatory Bowel Disease.

The dissection continues with a medial to lateral mobilization of the descending colon mesentery off Gerota's fascia. If the splenic flexure is mobilized for a tension-free anastomosis, the inferior border of the distal pancreas should be recognized to maintain the dissection plane anteriorly (Fig. 19.6). The sigmoid and descending colon is now retracted medially to divide a thin remaining layer of peritoneum along the line of Toldt. This dissection is continuous from lateral to medial for the splenocolic ligament. Alternatively, the lesser sac is entered from medially, and the omentum and splenocolic ligament are divided starting from the distal transverse colon (Fig. 19.7). Upon complete mobilization of the descending colon and the splenic flexure, the peritoneum lateral to the rectosigmoid junction is scored, and a window is created using blunt dissection along the posterior wall of the colon. This allows transection of the rectosigmoid colon with a robotic stapler through the right lower quadrant port. The remaining mesentery is divided to the planned proximal transection. Bowel perfusion can be assessed with indocyanine green injection and the fluorescence imaging mode of the robotic camera. For additional details on perfusion assessment for left-sided anastomoses, refer to Chap. 29 on Minimizing Colorectal Anastomotic Leaks.

Extracorporeal Anastomosis

Multiple extraction sites can be selected for extracorporeal anastomosis and mostly used are a Pfannenstiel or a lower midline incision. A small wound protector is inserted prior to specimen exteriorization to help reduce the risk of wound infection. The anvil of the EEA stapler is placed into the descending colon and secured with a purse string suture. An end-to-end or end-to-side anastomosis to the rectum is then created with the EEA stapler.

Intracorporeal Anastomosis

The robotic approach simplifies intracorporeal anastomosis (ICA), which has the benefits of moving the specimen extraction sites off the midline to decrease the risk of incisional hernia. The most commonly used extraction site is an extension of the right lower quadrant stapler port. A small wound protector is placed after enlarging the 12 mm trocar site, and the anvil of the EEA stapler is placed intra-abdominally.

For a side-to-end anastomosis, an enterotomy is created on the specimen side, i.e., just distal to the planned level of transection on the proximal colon. The anvil can be manipulated spike-first through the anterior wall of the descending colon. The spike is pushed laterally through the proximal bowel wall after incising the wall over the tip of the anvil. The anvil spike should be located approximately 5 cm above the planned transection site on the proximal colon. The initial enterotomy is closed with a running suture to avoid spillage of content from the specimen. The colon is transected with the robotic stapler just proximal to this closure.

Alternatively, a true end-to-end anastomosis can be created as well. The bowel is transected with the stapler first, the proximal staple line is excised, and a purse string suture is placed. The anvil (secured with a string) is inserted backwards with the tip aiming distally, and the purse string is tied.

Pitfalls, Intraoperative Difficulties, and Complications

Instrument Collisions

Instrument collisions are frequently related to suboptimal trocar placement too close to each other in relation to the target. The idea of laparoscopic triangulation should always be the underlying principle for trocar placement. It is always recommended that the surgeon walks from the console to the bedside to inspect and analyze the reason for the collisions. If the adjustment of the robotic arms and elbow joints do not improve the instrument movement, the surgeon should not hesitate to consider repositioning the trocars.

Inadequate Colon Length and Morbid Obesity

Morbid obesity and inadequate colon length can go hand in hand due to thickened and foreshortened mesentery. The short and fatty mesentery makes it significantly difficult to safely identify, isolate, and divide the inferior mesenteric artery/vein, left colic vessels, and superior rectal artery. In addition, small bowel loops tend to slide back into the surgical field and cannot be kept out of the pelvis and away from the mesenteric root for adequate visualization of the inferior mesenteric pedicle. Furthermore, the steep Trendelenburg position might not be tolerated from the anesthesia perspective when the massive weight pushes onto the diaphragm. At the same time, benefits of a minimal invasive approach are more pronounced in the morbidly obese specifically as it relates to the abdominal wall and wound complications.

Achieving additional colon length can be achieved using multiple strategies. High ligation of the IMA close to the junction to the aorta will help relieve tension on the descending colon after the descending colon mesentery is mobilized from the retroperitoneum and Gerota's fascia. The next step consists in ligation of the IMV close to the duodenum, followed by medial to lateral splenic flexure mobilization over the inferior border of the pancreas. Care must be taken to avoid avulsion and interruption of the marginal artery along the entire colon. If there is still inadequate length, the omentum is taken off the transverse colon; the middle colic vessels may have to be sacrificed unless the plan of an anastomosis is abandoned. In any such challenging case, it is helpful to check the perfusion of the colon with the integrated fluorescence imaging technology using intravenous injection of indocyanine green.

These are difficult situations that require experience and sound clinical judgment as it relates to the implications of further vascular division, including that of the middle colic vessels. Rather than blindly continue, this may be a moment to reconsider the goals and progress of the surgery and evaluate whether conversion to laparoscopy or an open approach would be justified.

Bleeding

Bleeding is often related to non-anatomical tissue and mesenteric dissection. Precise dissection is easier to perform due to the three instrument traction, countertraction, and dissection. Clear identification and circumferential dissection of all major vessels is paramount before attempted division. If bleeding is encountered at the mesenteric root, a third arm is helpful to immediately occlude proximally, while the other instruments can help suction and identify the exact source. Repeat attempt at controlling the proximal vessel can be attempted, but early conversion and laparotomy is sometimes mandatory before massive blood loss ensues. Surgeons and operating room teams should be prepared and trained for emergent robotic undocking for vascular injuries.

Anastomotic Leak

Intraoperative anastomotic leaks are almost always due to technical difficulties and complications. Even though genuine failure of the EEA stapler can occur, more often leaks are due to technical issues. Proximal colon anvil placement could be impaired from a loose proximal purse string suture, incorporation of a diverticulum, or uneven bowel wall thickness from the suture placement. It is important to recognize a suboptimal purse string suture and redo it, or alternatively place the anvil through the antimesenteric wall of the colon and perform a side-to-end anastomosis (Baker type).

Distally, the passage of the EEA stapler through the rectum can cause unrecognized serosal or even full-thickness injuries of the rectal wall often seen anteriorly. It is advised not to force the stapler through the rectum but rather perform a limited rectal mobilization, specifically posteriorly. Posterior rectal mobilization straightens out the rectum and allows the stapler to advance more easily.

An alternative is to place the spike through the anterior rectum distal and away from the blind staple line for an end-to-side stapled anastomosis (reversed Baker Type).

If the anastomosis is found to be suboptimal or faulty, as evidenced by either a positive air leak test, incomplete anastomotic doughnut, or endoscopic inspection, the options are (1) to reinforce the anastomosis (with/without diversion), (2) to redo the entire anastomosis, or (3) to abandon the anastomosis and convert to a Hartmann's procedure.

Outcomes

Several studies have been published examining the outcomes for robotic versus laparoscopic versus open colectomy in patients undergoing resection for both malignant and benign disease [8–10]. In general, robotic and laparoscopic surgery take longer than open operations, but they are both associated with improved short-term outcomes, shorter length of stay, fewer 30-day complications, and equivalent long-term oncologic results. In a comprehensive meta-analysis analyzing 40 peer-reviewed studies with varying study designs, Sheng and colleagues [9] compared robotic surgery to laparoscopic surgery in oncologic resections. They noted that blood loss, complication rate, mortality rate, bleeding rate, and ileus rate were all lowest in the robotic group. The authors also demonstrated that wound infection rate for laparoscopic resections was lowest, but this was statistically similar to the robotic group. Notably, both minimally invasive approaches were superior to the open approach with regard to reducing wound infections.

Table 19.1 Comparative studies of robotic vs. laparoscopic left-sided colorectal resections

Benefits	Robotic (references)	Laparoscopic (references)	No difference (references)
Decreased conversion to open	13, 18, 20		
Shorter length of stay	18, 19, 24		20, 23
Increased lymph node harvest	16		
Improved rectal cancer TME quality	15, 16, 20		
Decreased pain	14		23
Faster return of GI function	17		23
Reduced hernia rates	15		
Shorter operative time		19, 21, 22, 24	20

Table created with the positive benefits in the left-handed column with supporting articles referenced using their respective approach

Fewer conversions to open surgery are also a clear benefit of left-sided robotic colonic resections [10]. Robotic colorectal surgery has been associated with a nearly 50% reduction in open conversion when compared to equivalent laparoscopic operations (15.1 vs. 7.6%, $p < 0.001$) [11]. These lower conversions translate into improved clinical outcomes such as decreased length of stay, fewer 30-day complications, and a reduction in overall cost of care [11]. Alva and colleagues has performed an exhaustive review of the currently published data regarding clinical outcomes in laparoscopic versus robotic colorectal surgical cases and is summarized in Table 19.1 [12].

Conclusions

A robotic approach to a sigmoid and left colectomy has several technical advantages compared to a laparoscopic approach. The addition of a third surgeon-controlled instrument arm allows optimal traction and countertraction. In combination with improved stable and 3D visualization and wristed instruments, consistent dissection along embryologic and anatomic planes and precise visualization, mapping, and dissection of the left-sided mesenteric vessels allow consistent oncologic resections for malignant disease. Intracorporeal anastomosis is facilitated allowing off midline extraction of the specimen with decreased incisional hernia rates.

References

1. Lacy AM, García-Valdecasas JC, Delgado S, Castells A, Taurá P, Piqué JM, et al. Laparoscopy-assisted colectomy versus open colectomy for treatment of non-metastatic colon cancer: a randomised trial. Lancet. 2002;359(9325):2224–9.
2. Lacy AM, Delgado S, Castells A, Prins HA, Arroyo V, Ibarzabal A, et al. The long-term results of a randomized clinical trial of laparoscopy-assisted versus open surgery for Colon cancer. Ann Surg. 2008;248(1):1–7.

3. Blackmore AE, Ching MT, Tang CL. Evolution of laparoscopy in colorectal surgery: an evidence-based review. World J Gastroenterol. 2014;20(17):4926–33.
4. Abu Gazala M, Wexner S. Adoption rates for laparoscopy in colorectal surgery: why are they lagging behind? Ann Laparosc Endosc Surg. 2018. http://ales.amegroups.com/article/view/4625/5418.
5. Yeo HL, Isaacs AJ, Abelson JS, Milsom JW, Sedrakyan A. Comparison of open, laparoscopic, and robotic colectomies using a large National Database: outcomes and trends related to surgery center volume. Dis Colon Rectum. 2016;59:535–42.
6. Bharucha A, Parthasarathy G, Ditah I, Fletcher J, Ewelukwa O, Pendlimari R, et al. Temporal trends in the incidence and natural history of diverticulitis: a population-based study. Am J Gastroenterol. 2015;110(11):1589–96.
7. Marks J, Kawun U, Hamdan W, Marks G. Redefining contraindications to laparoscopic colorectal resection for high-risk patients. Surg Endosc. 2008;22(8):1899–904.
8. Ragupathi M, Ramos-Valadez DI, Patel CB, Haas EM. Robotic-assisted laparoscopic surgery for recurrent diverticulitis: experience in consecutive cases and a review of the literature. Surg Endosc. 2011;25(1):199–206.
9. Sheng S, Zhao T, Wang X. Comparison of robot-assisted surgery, laparoscopic-assisted surgery, and open surgery for the treatment of colorectal cancer: a network meta-analysis. Medicine (Baltimore). 2018;97(34):e11817.
10. Bhama AR, Obias V, Welch KB, Vandewarker JF, Cleary RK. A comparison of laparoscopic and robotic colorectal surgery outcomes using the American College of Surgeons—National Surgical Improvement Program (ACS-NSQIP) database. Surg Endosc. 2016;30:1576–84.
11. Cleary RK, Mullard AJ, Ferraro J, Regenbogen SE. The cost of conversion in robotic and laparoscopic colorectal surgery. Surg Endosc. 2018;32(3):1515–24.
12. Alva S. Laparoscopic vs robotic surgery in colorectal cases. World J Laparosc Surg. 2018;11(1):43–7.

Key Steps During Hartmann's Procedures to Facilitate Minimally Invasive Hartmann's Reversal

20

Alan E. Harzman and Syed Husain

Introduction and Rationale

Hartmann's creation (colectomy with closed rectosigmoid stump and end colostomy) is a commonly performed surgical procedure in emergency colorectal surgical practice. The most common indication for this procedure is perforation or obstruction of the distal colon or rectum, typically secondary to diverticulitis or a neoplastic process. Other indications include uncontrolled inflammatory bowel disease involving the rectum and anal canal or dehiscence of a previously performed colorectal anastomosis. Irrespective of the underlying etiology, the overwhelming majority of Hartmann's procedures are usually performed in an urgent or semi-urgent setting. Given the emergent nature of these operations, surgeons are typically focused on addressing the acute situation at hand, and measures to facilitate Hartmann's closure are often ignored.

Hartmann's closure has been historically associated with a high complication rate attributable to the technical complexity of this operation [1]. For this reason, many patients with Hartmann's pouches are never offered a reversal [2]. While there is a plethora of evidence indicating that a laparoscopic approach ameliorates

The authors would like thank the members of the SAGES Colorectal Surgery Masters Program Collaboration Facebook Group for their recommendations regarding this chapter.

A. E. Harzman (✉) · S. Husain
The Ohio State University, Department of Surgery, Columbus, OH, USA

Ohio State University Wexner Medical Center, Division of Colon and Rectal Surgery, Columbus, OH, USA
e-mail: Alan.Harzman@osumc.edu; Syed.Husain@osumc.edu

P. Sylla et al. (eds.), *The SAGES Manual of Colorectal Surgery*,
https://doi.org/10.1007/978-3-030-24812-3_20

many complications associated with Hartmann's closure [3, 4], there has been underutilization of this technique, and the adoption of minimally invasive techniques for Hartmann's closure has lagged behind that observed for other colorectal procedures [5].

In this chapter, we discuss the measures that can be undertaken at the time of Hartmann's creation to potentially rectify common difficulties experienced during closure. We believe that adaption of these techniques can lead to improved stoma reversal rates and facilitate utilization of laparoscopic technique for Hartmann's reversal.

Indications and Contraindications

There are no absolute contraindications to the operative maneuvers discussed below. Hemodynamic instability can be considered a relative contraindication as most of these measures can lead to prolongation of operative time. Operating surgeons should use their judgment to determine the appropriateness of the measures in an unstable patient where an expeditious laparotomy may prove more beneficial than maneuvers to facilitate a future operation. Given that many patients will never have the colostomy closed, it is also unwise to focus strictly on facilitating colostomy closure. The ideal is creating a good colostomy that the patient could keep forever while setting up for a future closure if possible.

Principles and Quality Benchmarks

Timing of Hartmann's Reversal

The need to resist patient's demands for an expeditious stoma reversal cannot be overstated. Stoma reversal is almost never an urgent operation, and it is important to permit a sufficient interval between the index operation and stoma reversal to allow time for the thick vascularized adhesive bands to evolve into avascular, filmy adhesions. We recommend an interval of at least 6 months between Hartmann's creation and reversal, both to minimize trouble with adhesions at the second operation and to allow the patient to return to an otherwise normal physiologic state.

Impact of Laparoscopic Hartmann's Procedure

In the authors' opinion, the most important maneuver to minimize complications and ensure successful Hartmann's reversal is to perform Hartmann's operation laparoscopically. Laparoscopy has been proven to be associated with less adhesion formation than an open approach in a variety of surgical settings [6]. With the emergence of literature favoring "straight" laparoscopy, hand-assisted laparoscopic colectomy has been largely supplanted by straight laparoscopy. Despite its shortcomings hand assistance may be particularly useful during emergency Hartmann's creation for acute, complicated diverticulitis, where presence of inflammation and abscess formation may preclude successful completion of the case using a straight laparoscopic technique. This is particularly true when most of the case can be accomplished laparoscopically, but one portion of the case, such as dissection of a phlegmon tightly adherent to the left pelvic side wall or retroperitoneum or takedown of a colovesical fistula, can be performed more safely and expeditiously using direct hand palpation, dissection, and retraction. When needed, conversion from laparoscopic to hand assist or to open should be done prior to creating a significant injury or greatly prolonging operative time.

In cases where a laparoscopic approach is abandoned due to hemodynamic instability or colonic dilation precluding safe visualization of operative field, use of an adhesion barrier should be considered. While adhesion barriers have never been tested in this particular clinical setting, there is plenty of evidence that they result in significant reduction in adhesions in a variety of surgical settings comparable to Hartmann's [7, 8] creation. Another step that can minimize adhesions is the restoration of peritoneal lining by careful peritoneal approximation during midline incision closure. Finally, placing omentum under the midline laparotomy incision can minimize adhesions between the anterior abdominal wall and underlying small bowel loops which can present a challenge during Hartmann's closure.

Operative Technique: Surgical Steps

The following are techniques to aid later laparoscopic stoma closure, broken down by the steps of the original Hartmann's operation.

- Opening
  - Perform a laparoscopic Hartmann's procedure when possible.
- Resection
  - Proximal extent: Resect only what is required, and do not mobilize the splenic flexure unless absolutely required to form the colostomy. This will allow it to be newly mobilized at the stoma closure and maximum length obtained.
  - Distal extent: For inflammatory disease such as diverticulitis, dividing just distal to the inflammation leaves sigmoid colon and therefore decreases the chance that the rectosigmoid will retract into the pelvis. However, the remaining sigmoid will then need to be resected at the time of stoma closure. Therefore, the authors would divide at the rectosigmoid junction (where the tinea splay out) at the first operation. Do not, though, divide lower than that unless absolutely necessary. Certainly do not divide at or distal to the anterior peritoneal reflection if the goal is to close the stoma later. Doing so makes the rectal stump exceptionally difficult to identify and dissect from the vagina and bladder.
  - Do not divide the IMA or the superior hemorrhoidal vessels, and do not violate the mesorectal plane. Save the holy plane to use to find the rectum later.

  - Avoid topical procoagulants as a means of hemostasis, especially on the rectal stump staple line. These can cause a great deal of inflammation and scarring.
- Stoma creation
  - As above, avoid mobilizing the splenic flexure unless required to create a good stoma.
  - Remember that for many patients the stoma will be permanent.
  - Making a large trephine in the fascia may increase the risk of parastomal hernia. However, it may also allow the patient to regain bowel function more quickly than a tight stoma. A large parastomal hernia can make stoma closure difficult, although a small hernia can make it easier to dissect the stoma from the abdominal wall.
  - Wrap an adhesion barrier around the stoma before closing when feasible.
  - For more details regarding optimizing stoma formation, please refer to Chap. 36 on best practices in planned and unplanned stoma creation.
- Dealing with the rectal stump and pelvis
  - Place dyed, nonabsorbable sutures on the staple line on the rectal stump. These can be placed through the corners of the staple line or through the peritoneum immediately adjacent to them (Fig. 20.1a, b).
  - Some surgeons use those sutures to tack the rectal stump to the anterior abdominal wall. The authors prefer to tack them to the peritoneum along the sacral promontory, medial to the ureters. This does not require a particularly long stump and does not create any space that could create an internal hernia.
  - Cut the sutures 3–5 cm long to make them easier to find at the time of stoma closure.
- Closing
  - Thoroughly explore and irrigate the abdomen.

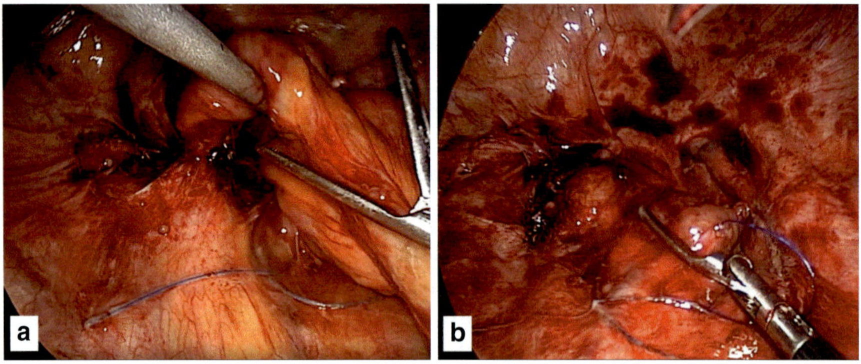

Fig. 20.1 (**a**, **b**) Intraoperative identification of the suture marking the rectal stump during laparoscopic Hartmann's reversal. (**a**) The suture can be identified, but the rectal stump is tightly adherent to a loop of small bowel that is partially covering it. (**b**) Following dissection of the small bowel loop, the rectal stump is exposed. (Both: Courtesy of Dan Popowich, MD)

- Leave a drain in the pelvis to prevent accumulation of contaminated fluid and subsequent abscess formation in the pelvis.
- Bring the omentum down to underlie the incision. If possible, place the tip in the pelvis to prevent the small bowel from adhering to the pelvis or rectal stump.
- If the operation is done open, use an adhesion barrier under the midline wound and in the pelvis.
- Close the peritoneum as part of the fascial closure. The goal of this is to minimize the raw surface area for abdominal wall adhesions to form.
- Leave the skin open to lower the rate of wound infection and therefore the rate of hernia formation and/or dehiscence.

• Postoperative course
  - Ensure that the patient has fully recovered from the first operation. This includes returning to work and all normal activities.
  - Wait at least 6 months before attempting stoma reversal. Stoma reversal may be possible at 3 months, but adhesions will continue to transition from inflammatory to flimsy between 3 and 6 months. A failed attempt at stoma closure will make any further attempt exponentially harder, so it is better to wait the full 6 months.
  - Some patients are told after Hartmann's procedure that their stoma is not reversible. When this is true, it is imperative to clearly dictate the reasons and explain them to the patient. It is incumbent on the surgeon closing a stoma created by someone else to understand what was done at the first operation and to know which if any of the above maneuvers were performed.

Pitfalls and Troubleshooting

It is imperative to discuss the reasons why even experienced laparoscopic surgeons often opt to perform Hartmann's reversal using an open technique. The technical challenges deterring laparoscopic Hartmann's closure or prompting conversion to open technique include the following issues discussed below.

Adhesions

Since many Hartmann's operations are performed to treat distal colonic or rectal perforations, these procedures are often complicated by significant peritoneal contamination leading to peritonitis and abscess formation which in turn result in significant adhesion formation (Fig. 20.2). The fear of hostile adhesions often represents the major deterrent to laparoscopic closure of a colostomy. Thus it is imperative to suction out any residual blood, purulence or fecal material from the peritoneal cavity at time of Hartmann's creation. Furthermore, copious peritoneal irrigation with warm saline should be undertaken to decrease the burden of peritoneal contamination.

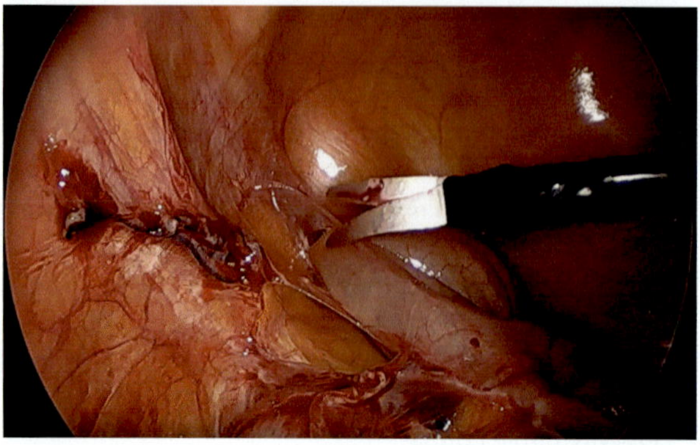

Fig. 20.2 Adhesions of small bowel loops to Hartmann's pouch require careful lysis of adhesions. Identification of the rectal stump is facilitated by visualization of the marking suture that was placed at the original operation. (Courtesy of Dan Popowich, MD)

Presence of a Large Ventral Wall Hernia

Given the contaminated nature of these cases, many Hartmann's creations are associated with incisional complications ultimately leading to incisional hernias [9]. A large ventral or parastomal hernia can present a daunting task especially if laparoscopic reversal is planned. Utilization of a laparoscopic approach at the time of initial stoma creation obviates the need for a large abdominal incision. Whether this reduction in incision length translates into a lower incidence of incisional hernia remains a topic of debate. It is quite plausible, however, that the incisional hernias occurring at a laparoscopic extraction site are much smaller and easier to manage than those occurring after a generous midline laparotomy. In addition, the skin of the midline wound should be left open at the time of Hartmann's operation if there is significant contamination. Wound infection, even those that can be managed by "popping out a few staples," can lead to incisional hernia formation. Certainly efforts to avoid wound dehiscence and evisceration will also contribute to reduced incisional hernias. Avoiding a large abdominal wall fenestration for stoma exteriorization can also minimize the risk of parastomal hernia. On the other hand, prophylactic mesh placement to avoid parastomal hernia is not indicated unless one is certain that the stoma will not be closed later. For additional details, please refer to Chap. 37 on prophylactic mesh placement during laparoscopic stoma creation.

Difficult Rectal Stump Dissection

Identification and dissection of the rectal stump represents another component of Hartmann's reversal that can prove to be quite challenging. The rectal stump often tends to adhere to the lateral pelvic wall in close proximity to ureters and major pelvic vessels. In other cases, the rectal stump forms dense adhesions to the bladder or female genital organs leading to a quite tedious dissection at time of reversal. Copious pelvic irrigation with removal of purulent/fecal material can minimize these adhesions. Furthermore, interposition of omentum between the rectal stump and pelvic organs can also facilitate rectal stump dissection at time of closure. Finally, it is very important to preserve as much rectum as possible at the time of Hartmann's creation. A long rectal stump lends itself to easy identification at time of reversal. Barring malignant cases where it is important to achieve a distal resection margin, rectal division should be carried out as close to the pathology as possible. Every attempt should be made to avoid violation of mesorectal planes as this can lead to dense posterior adhesions which make identification and dissection of rectal stump very difficult at time of closure.

Rectal Stump Retraction

In addition to forming adhesions to the surrounding structures, the divided rectum often retracts into the pelvic cavity leading to "bunching up" of the rectal stump. A retracted rectal stump frequently folds upon itself creating sharp angles which can be very difficult to negotiate with the rigid EEA stapler. This inability to advance the EEA stapler to the end of the rectal stump can lead to the creation of an inadvertent end-to-side rather than end-to-end colorectal anastomosis. While most of the end-to-side anastomoses have excellent functional results, the rectal blind pouch can sometimes lead to bacterial stasis with its attendant issues. Worse yet, adhesions of the vagina or bladder to the retracted stump can lead to inadvertently incorporating them into the anastomosis. Retraction of the rectal stump into the pelvic cavity can be prevented by leaving a long rectal stump and tacking the stapled end to the anterior abdominal wall or retroperitoneum with the help of an anchoring stitch.

Inability to Accomplish a Tension-Free Anastomosis

Inadequate proximal colonic length often prompts surgeons to convert to an open technique to be able to accomplish tension-free anastomosis. Often, this situation is due to extensive mobilization of left colon and splenic flexure at the index operation. We advocate limiting left colonic mobilization to the bare minimum required for exteriorization of the colonic end for stoma creation. Splenic flexure dissection is typically discouraged unless absolutely necessary for exteriorization.

Outcomes

There are no outcome data for the specific techniques described above. Chapter 21 covers the procedure of minimally invasive Hartmann's reversal, for which there are data that are cited there and in the references below. However, the authors of those studies do not specifically identify what steps they or other surgeons took in the initial operation.

Conclusion

There are multiple strategies during stoma creation that can maximize the possibility of a minimally invasive stoma closure. Most of these are also relevant to open stoma closure as well. However, the surgeon must also remember that many stomas will never be closed, so making stoma closure easier should not come at the cost of a good initial stoma. Nor should it significantly prolong the first operation and delay getting a sick patient out of the operating room safely.

References

1. Roig JV, Cantos M, Balciscueta Z, Uribe N, Espinosa J, Rosello V, et al. Hartmann's operation: how often is it reversed and at what cost? A multicentre study. Color Dis. 2011;13(12):e396–402.
2. Hallam S, Mothe BS, Tirumulaju R. Hartmann's procedure, reversal and rate of stoma-free survival. Ann R Coll Surg Engl. 2018;100(4):301–7.
3. Brathwaite S, Kuhrt M, Yu L, Arnold M, Husain S, Harzman AE. Retrospective evaluation of laparoscopic versus open Hartmann's reversal: a single-institution experience. Surg Laparosc Endosc Percutan Tech. 2015;25(5):e156–8.
4. Arkenbosch J, Miyagaki H, Kumara HM, Yan X, Cekic V, Whelan RL. Efficacy of laparoscopic-assisted approach for reversal of Hartmann's procedure: results from the American College of Surgeons National Surgical Quality Improvement Program (ACS-NSQIP) database. Surg Endosc. 2015;29(8):2109–14.
5. Brathwaite S, Latchana N, Esemuede I, Harzman A, Husain S. Risk factors for surgical site infection in open and laparoscopic Hartmann closure: a multivariate analysis. Surg Laparosc Endosc Percutan Tech. 2017;27(1):51–3.
6. Mais V. Peritoneal adhesions after laparoscopic gastrointestinal surgery. World J Gastroenterol. 2014;20(17):4917–25.
7. Kumar S, Wong PF, Leaper DJ. Intra-peritoneal prophylactic agents for preventing adhesions and adhesive intestinal obstruction after non-gynaecological abdominal surgery. Cochrane Database Syst Rev. 2009;1:CD005080.
8. Metwally M, Watson A, Lilford R, Vandekerckhove P. Fluid and pharmacological agents for adhesion prevention after gynaecological surgery. Cochrane Database Syst Rev. 2006;2:CD001298.
9. Timmermans L, Deerenberg EB, Lamme B, Jeekel J, Lange JF. Parastomal hernia is an independent risk factor for incisional hernia in patients with end colostomy. Surgery. 2014;155(1):178–83.

Laparoscopic and Robotic Hartmann's Reversal: Strategies to Avoid Complications

21

David A. Kleiman and Steven A. Lee-Kong

Introduction and Rationale

Approximately 65% of the population over age 65 develop sigmoid diverticulosis [1]. Of those, approximately 20% will develop diverticulitis during their lifetime, requiring some type of medical or surgical intervention [2]. The management of diverticulitis accounts for nearly $2.7 billion in healthcare-related costs within the United States annually and is a common indication for emergency surgery [3].

Current clinical practice guidelines recommend emergent surgery for acute diverticulitis in patients with peritonitis or for those in whom non-operative management of diverticulitis has failed [2]. A Hartmann's procedure, which involves segmental sigmoid colectomy with creation of an end colostomy and a blind-ending distal rectal stump, was initially described for the management of acute malignant large bowel obstructions in 1923 [4]. It has since become the widely accepted standard surgical treatment of sigmoid diverticulitis in the emergent setting, particularly for Hinchey III and IV disease (Fig. 21.1). It remains an attractive option to many surgeons because by not creating a colorectal anastomosis, operative times are shorter, there is usually no need to perform a splenic flexure mobilization, and there is no risk of anastomotic complications (leakage or bleeding). However, the real morbidity of a Hartmann's procedure is often associated with the subsequent reversal operation. Since Hartmann's reversal can require a reoperative laparotomy, there can be significant associated risks, including surgical site infections,

D. A. Kleiman
Division of Colon and Rectal Surgery, Lahey Hospital and Medical Center, Burlington, MA, USA

Tufts University School of Medicine, Boston, MA, USA
e-mail: David.kleiman@lahey.org

S. A. Lee-Kong (✉)
New York Presbyterian Hospital, Columbia University, New York, NY, USA
e-mail: Sal116@cumc.columbia.edu

P. Sylla et al. (eds.), *The SAGES Manual of Colorectal Surgery*,
https://doi.org/10.1007/978-3-030-24812-3_21

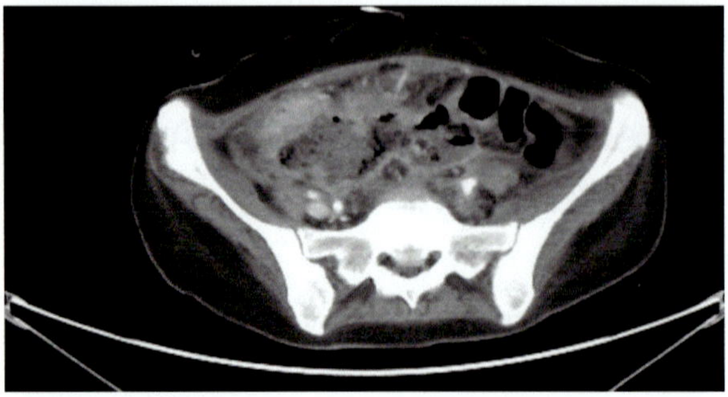

Fig. 21.1 Fecal peritonitis

hernia formation, injury to adjacent organs, anastomotic complications, and risks associated with general anesthesia. In fact, up to 45% of patients who undergo a Hartmann's procedure are never reversed, oftentimes due to fear of these complications or other significant comorbid conditions which can complicate an otherwise elective operation [4, 5].

The morbidity associated with a traditional open Hartmann's reversal has led many surgeons to explore minimally invasive options. However, there are significant inherent challenges to this approach, generally related to the fact that the initial surgery may have been performed via an open approach. These patients may present with significant intra-abdominal contamination, resulting in dense intra-abdominal adhesions. Patients' comorbid conditions may also make a minimally invasive approach challenging. However, in well-selected patients, a minimally invasive approach can be performed safely with low perioperative morbidity and may help increase stoma reversal rates.

In this chapter, we will discuss indications and contraindications of minimally invasive Hartmann's reversal and key aspects of preoperative evaluation and describe general steps of a minimally invasive technique.

Indications and Contraindications

A minimally invasive Hartmann's reversal may be considered in any patient undergoing the procedure. Ideal candidates are those whose initial operation was performed through either a limited laparotomy incision (i.e., a lower midline below the umbilicus) (Fig. 21.2) or a hybrid laparoscopic/open resection (i.e., laparoscopic hand-assisted via Pfannenstiel incision), although any patient considered suitable for laparoscopy may be a candidate [6].

While there are no absolute contraindications to minimally invasive Hartmann's reversal, two factors that are most likely to limit the successful completion of a minimally invasive approach are intra-abdominal adhesions and patient comorbidity. Obesity has been identified as an independent risk factor for complications in patients undergoing Hartmann's reversal [7]. Patients with a BMI ≥ 30 kg/m^2 are at increased risk of morbidity, surgical site infection, and need for diverting ileostomy

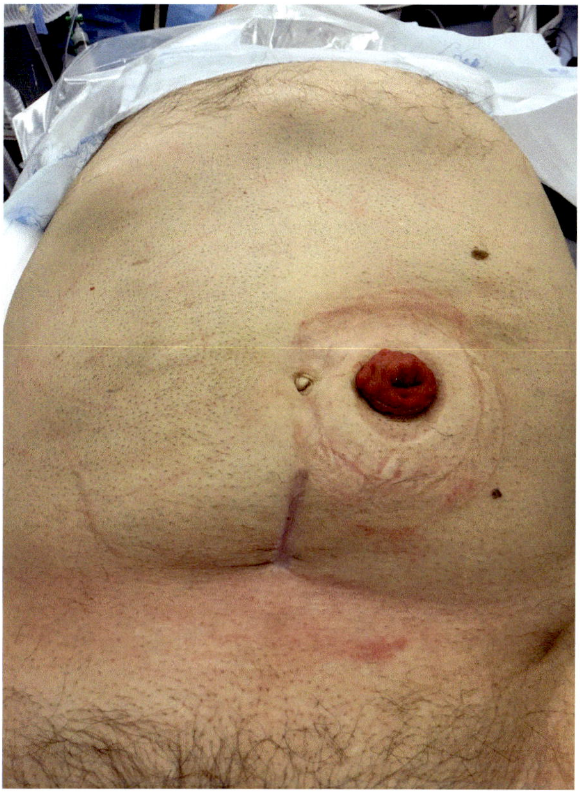

Fig. 21.2 Straightforward abdominal access

creation. While minimally invasive surgery may help ameliorate some of these risks, the technical challenges faced in obese patients can still make minimally invasive Hartmann's reversal difficult. Surgeons often recommend obese patients to lose weight prior to elective surgery. However, many patients find this difficult. Consultation with a dietician, weight loss specialist, or bariatric surgery program should be considered preoperatively.

Patients who suffered medial sigmoid perforations resulting in a large amount of purulent or feculent peritonitis at the index operation are more likely to have extensive lower abdominal or pelvic adhesions, making a minimally invasive approach challenging. Similarly, patients with long midline laparotomy incisions extending well above and below the umbilicus may have limited domain for safe laparoscopic entry into the abdomen (Fig. 21.3). Patients who have had multiple open surgeries in the past may experience difficulties with safe laparoscopic abdominal entry.

Laparoscopic Hartmann's reversal can require extended periods of time in steep Trendelenburg position, particularly if extensive pelvic dissection is required. Patients with significant congestive heart failure, chronic obstructive pulmonary disease, and morbid obesity may not be able to tolerate this positioning, precluding a minimally invasive approach.

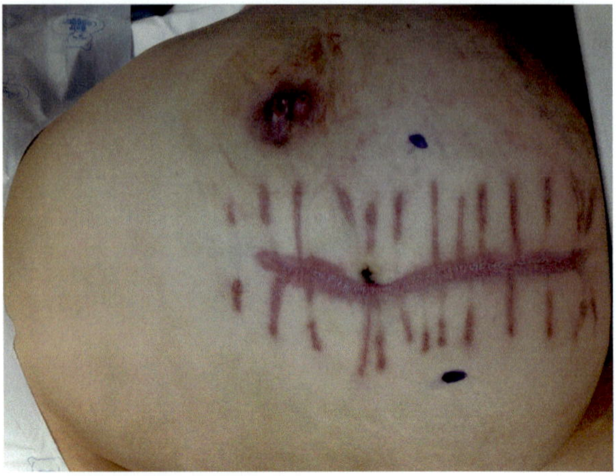

Fig. 21.3 Difficult abdominal access

Principles and Quality Benchmarks

The key steps to a successful minimally invasive Hartmann's reversal include the following:

1. Safe laparoscopic lysis of intra-abdominal adhesions
2. Takedown of the colostomy without injuring the colon
3. Sufficient mobilization of the splenic flexure and descending colon (often needed)
4. Identification, mobilization, and preparation of the rectal stump for creation of the anastomosis
5. Performance of a tension-free colorectal anastomosis.

Preoperative Planning, Patient Workup, and Optimization (Box 21.1)

Most Hartmann's procedures are performed emergently with little or no preoperative planning. In contrast, a Hartmann's reversal is an elective procedure. Careful and thoughtful preoperative assessment and planning is essential. Often, this is an excellent opportunity to complete aspects of the preoperative workup that ideally

Box 21.1 Preoperative Checklist Prior to Hartmann's Reversal

[ ] Review operative report
[ ] Review pathology
[ ] Colonoscopy
[ ] Water-soluble enema of rectal stump
[ ] Physical exam (assess sphincter function)
[ ] Medical/cardiac clearance
[ ] Ureteral stents

would have been performed prior to the original sigmoid colectomy. For example, recent colonoscopy reports should be reviewed. If one was not recently performed, this should be considered. Thorough cardiopulmonary assessments should be performed as part of the preoperative workup.

Review Operative Report

Whenever possible, the original operative report of the Hartmann's procedure should be carefully reviewed. Details such as the degree of abdominal contamination, bleeding, and any pre-existing adhesive disease may predict how hostile the abdomen will be during colostomy closure. It is also important to note where the distal margin of resection is and which, in any, major mesenteric vessels were ligated. Additional information such as whether suture tags were left on the end of rectal stump may also be helpful.

Review Pathology Report

The pathology report from the original surgery should be reviewed to ensure that there was no incidental cancer diagnosis or evidence of inflammatory bowel disease at the original operation.

Colonoscopy (Colon and Rectal Stump)

If the patient has not had a recent colonoscopy, this should be performed prior to Hartmann's closure. This should include evaluation of the remaining colon through the colostomy as well as the rectal stump. If the patient is up to date with colonoscopy (i.e., within the past year), then at a minimum a flexible sigmoidoscopy of the rectal stump should be performed to assess the health of the stump and to ensure that it is not structured or obstructed by inspissated mucus or stool. For patients in whom the indication for Hartmann's procedure was colorectal cancer, endoscopy should be performed to rule out persistent or recurrent cancer in the rectal stump. The length of the rectal stump is important to know prior to attempt at colostomy closure, as a short stump may impart poorer functional outcomes after closure. Distensibility of the rectum, which may be poor due to a fibrosing pelvic process from sepsis, may also portend poorer functional outcomes.

A water-soluble contrast enema of the rectal stump is also helpful to ensure that the staple line at the top of the stump is intact and that there are no sinus tracts to adjacent organs.

Assessment of Sphincter Function

A detailed history can reveal if the patient had any degree of fecal incontinence prior to them developing perforated diverticulitis. A digital rectal exam should be performed to assess the patient's sphincter function prior to Hartmann's reversal. If the patient has poor sphincter function, then he or she should be counseled on the expected functional outcomes of reversal, and the option of keeping a permanent colostomy should be discussed. Anorectal manometry may also be considered, although not necessary, if there are any concerns about sphincter function. Patients with long-standing fecal diversion may have impaired function, and this should be clearly discussed with the patient prior to attempts at reversal.

Cross-Sectional Imaging

Although not essential, review of any available cross-sectional imaging (prior to or after the original sigmoid colectomy) should be performed. This may help define relevant anatomy, as well as identify potential anatomic issues that may arise at the time of colostomy reversal. For example, large uterine fibroids may limit access to the pelvis for rectal dissection and anastomosis. Tracing the course of the ureters may also be possible, allowing for anticipation of potential areas of injury during the surgery. This may also reveal parastomal and/or midline hernias that can be addressed simultaneously with the takedown operation.

Ureteral Stents

Bilateral ureteral stents should be considered to assist with intraoperative identification of the ureters and help ensure that they are protected. Patients with Hinchey III or IV diverticulitis often have dense fibrosis in the lower abdomen and pelvis, making intraoperative identification of the ureters challenging.

Operative Setup

A variety of minimally invasive and hybrid techniques are possible based on equipment availability and surgeon preference. As for all colorectal surgery procedures, straight laparoscopic, single-incision laparoscopic, laparoscopic hand-assisted, and robotic-assisted techniques have all been described. There is no single approach that will work for everyone, so the surgeon should remain adaptable and able to alter the surgical approach based on the intraoperative findings.

Regardless of which minimally invasive technique is chosen, there are a few common themes in preparing for the procedure. The patient should be positioned on the operating table with access to the anus to allow for passage of a transanal stapling device or intraoperative endoscopy. Our preference is supine on a split-leg table, but modified lithotomy position is also acceptable (Figs. 21.4 and 21.5). Both arms should be tucked, if possible, to allow both the surgeon and the first assistant to stand cephalad on either side of the patient facing toward the pelvis. The patient should lie on a nonskid mat (our preference is either a bean bag or foam mat), and a shoulder strap should be utilized to secure the patient to the operating table to prevent sliding with steep positioning.

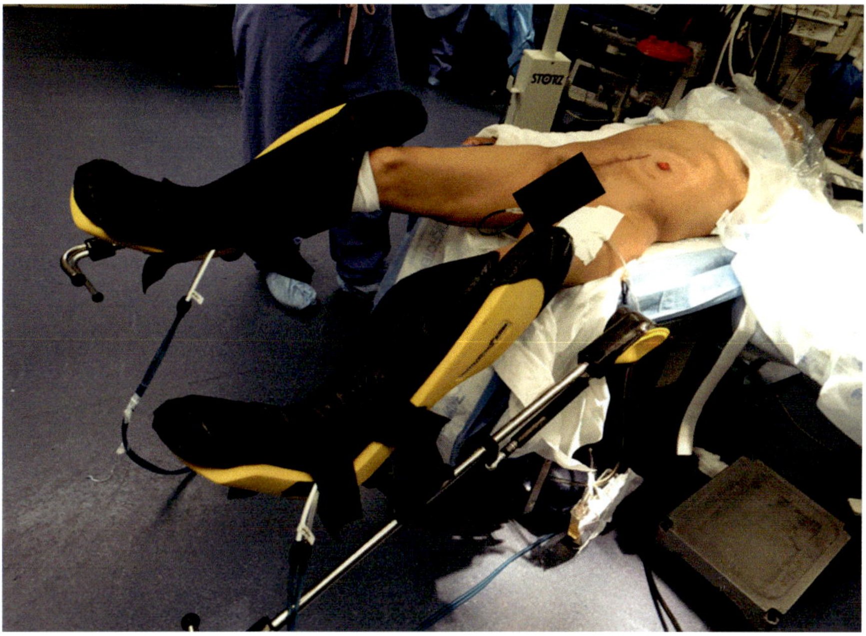

Fig. 21.4 Lithotomy position

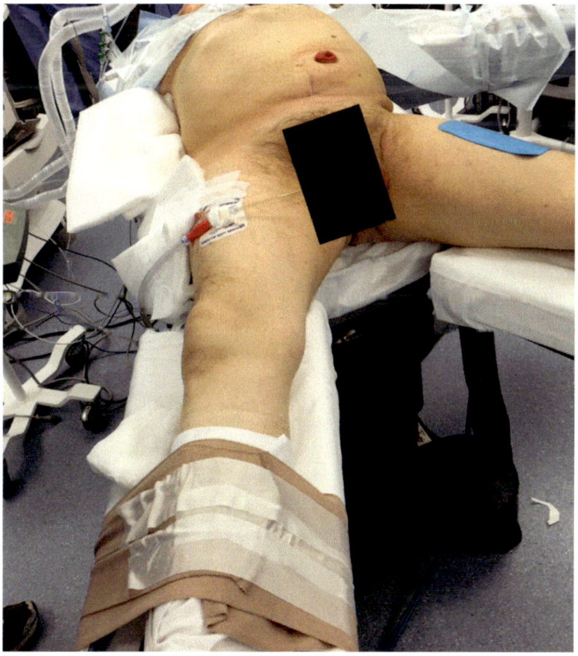

Fig. 21.5 Split-leg position

Robotic-assisted Hartmann's reversal should be reserved for surgeons both trained and comfortable using currently available robotic platforms. The DaVinci Si® or Xi® platforms (Intuitive Surgical, Sunnyvale, CA, USA) are the most widely available. Port placement strategies in general follow conventions unique for each platform. For the DaVinci Si, placing the cannulae in the right abdomen at least 8 cm apart in a "C" configuration is most helpful. One can take down the end colostomy at the beginning of the procedure, or once it is determined intraoperatively, that safe colostomy reversal is possible. For the DaVinci Xi system, the authors find it helpful to place the cannulae in a nearly straight vertical line along the right abdomen. The arm docked closest to the pelvis should be able to accommodate an endoscopic stapler, should division of the rectal stump be necessary. The Xi platform has the added advantage of intraoperative table motion, which can aid in operating in more than one abdominal quadrant comfortably (Fig. 21.6).

For both Si and Xi platforms, intra-abdominal adhesions are typically assessed and managed laparoscopically before the robot is docked. Availability of laparoscopic scissors with monopolar energy is helpful during this portion of the procedure and adds minimal additional cost to the case. Once the robotic trocars are safely inserted, the patient is positioned in steep Trendelenburg position with right side down. The small bowel and omentum are lifted out of the pelvis into the right upper quadrant.

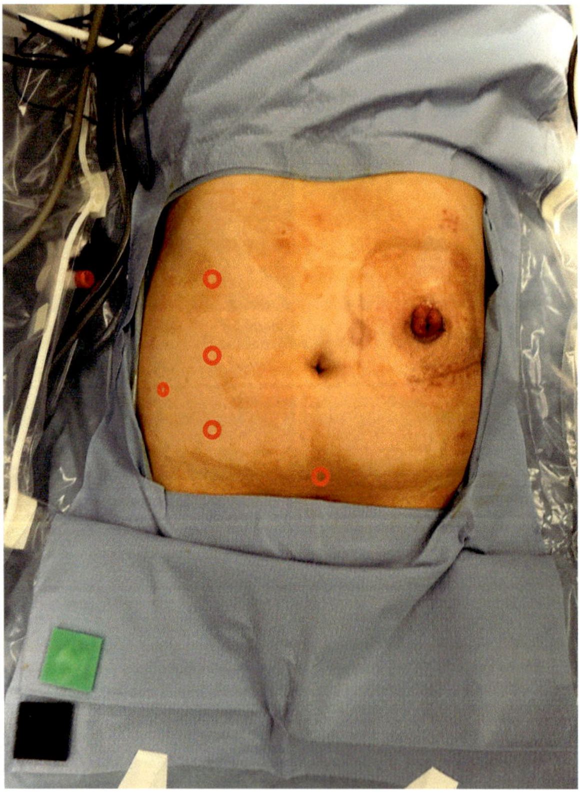

Fig. 21.6 Xi robotic port placement

The authors find it helpful to do this laparoscopically prior to docking the robot. The table is then lowered as low as it can go, and the robot is docked from the patient's left side. If "targeting" is used on the Xi platform to help align the robotic arms, the authors prefer to target the left pelvic inlet, as this typically allows for comfortable reach from the splenic flexure to the pelvis. If the colon proximal to the splenic flexure requires mobilization, the surgeon should be prepared to undock and re-dock as necessary. This can be easily accomplished with the Xi by simply rotating the boom and retargeting. However, with the Si platform, the patient cart may need to be moved to the patient's right side. This can be quite burdensome and is often an indication for conversion to a laparoscopic or open approach. The bedside assistant is positioned on the patient's right side. A sitting stool is provided so that the assistant can comfortably access the ports while staying below the level of the moving robotic arms.

Single-incision laparoscopic surgery (SILS)-assisted Hartmann's reversal can also be considered, if the surgeon is appropriately trained and comfortable. Those who perform SILS procedures often gain abdominal access by first taking down the end colostomy and placing the SILS port at this location. Proponents advocating for this technique report the advantage of avoiding the adhesions often present in the midline from prior laparotomy. The use of an angled or flexible-tip laparoscope can be very helpful to overcome the difficulty encountered with the use of straight laparoscopic instruments and their close proximity. As the vast majority of surgeons do not perform SILS procedures, there are no reliable data examining SILS Hartmann's reversal.

Operative Technique: Surgical Steps

There are many nuances of technique that will vary depending on surgeon preference and the minimally invasive approach that is selected. Here, we will describe the general steps of any minimally invasive Hartmann's resection. These basic steps can be performed using any minimally invasive technique.

The first challenge is to safely gain entry into the peritoneal cavity and establish pneumoperitoneum. This can be quite challenging depending on the degree of intra-abdominal adhesions and is a common reason for early conversion. In general, we allow the patients' previous incision to guide our site of abdominal entry. We try to avoid entering the abdomen directly through a previous incision, as one is likely to encounter dense adhesions immediately underneath. If the patient has a lower midline or Pfannenstiel scar, then a supraumbilical direct cutdown ("Hasson") technique is a good option. If their scar extends above and below the umbilicus, then an off-midline entry site may be better suited. For off-midline entry, our preference is to use a Veress needle in the left upper quadrant at Palmer's point (two fingers below the costal margin at the genu of the rib) (Fig. 21.7). Once pneumoperitoneum has been achieved, a 5 mm laparoscopic camera is advanced through the abdominal wall inside a clear 5 mm trocar so that the surgeon can observe each layer of the abdominal wall as the trocar passes through it until the abdominal cavity is safely entered.

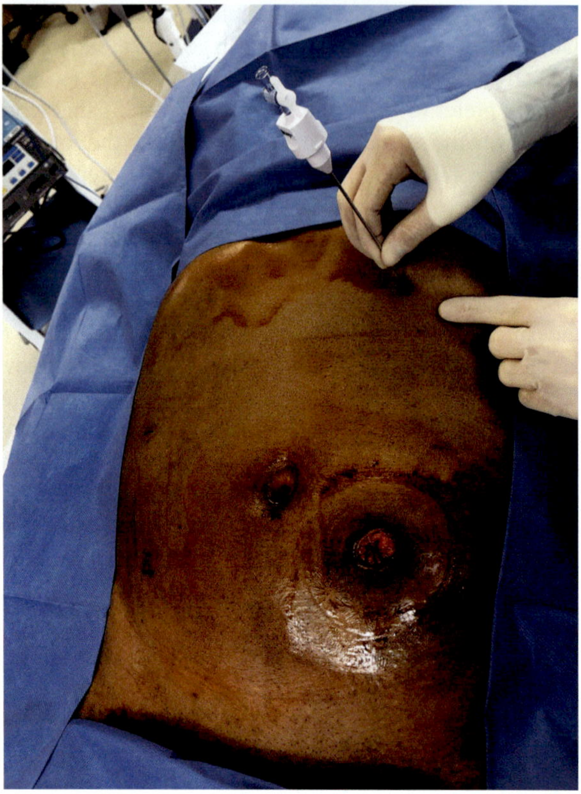

Fig. 21.7 Veress needle entry

Oftentimes, taking down the colostomy with early placement of the anvil into the proximal colon may be the safest and "fastest" approach for entering the abdomen. A balloon trocar or a wound protector with a cap can be subsequently placed. This is an ideal strategy for those who prefer a single-incision laparoscopic approach, whereby the same incision is used for specimen extraction.

Once pneumoperitoneum is established and the first trocar has been placed, we first assess for visceral organ injury due to port placement. Next, a quick survey of the abdominal cavity is performed to assess the burden of the adhesive disease and make a decision as to whether the procedure can safely be performed with minimally invasive techniques. If yes, then additional trocars should be placed.

We then proceed with complete laparoscopic adhesiolysis. This can be quite tedious depending on the density of adhesions. Often patients who have had severe peritonitis from the inciting diverticular process will form difficult to manage adhesive disease. We find that delaying Hartmann's reversal for 3 to 6 months allows for improvement in the adhesive burden and may help facilitate a minimally invasive approach. The surgeon needs to remain patient and flexible and may need to alter their usual trocar placement in order to handle the pattern of adhesions that are encountered. The rectal stump is then mobilized and inspected. Once we confirm that the rectal stump is suitable for creation of a colorectal anastomosis, we then

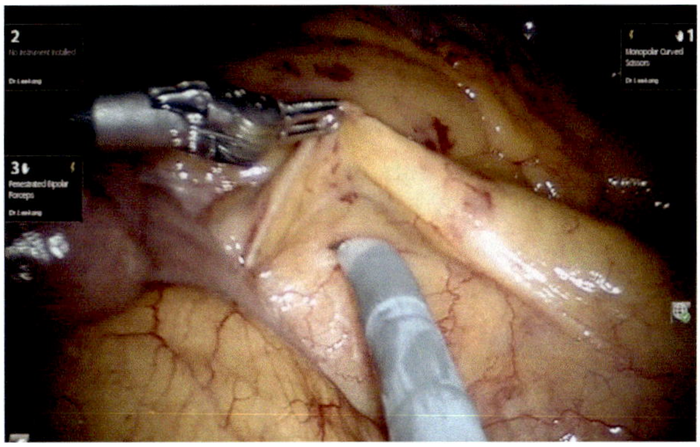

Fig. 21.8 Medial to lateral mobilization of splenic flexure

proceed with taking down the colostomy. Great care is taken not to damage the colon within the abdominal wall so that it can be used for creation of the anastomosis. The mucocutaneous junction will need to be trimmed from the colostomy-bearing segment prior to use in creating the anastomosis. The anvil of an end-to-end circular stapler is then secured in place to the end of the descending colon with a purse-string suture. The colon is then delivered back into the abdomen, and pneumoperitoneum is reestablished. A small wound protector can be placed through the colostomy site and then sealed with a cap or by twisting it in order to reestablish pneumoperitoneum. Alternatively, if a hand-assisted technique is used, the cap of the Gelport device can simply be replaced. The left colon and splenic flexure are then fully mobilized to ensure a tension-free anastomosis. We find that mobilization of the splenic flexure by starting at the inferior mesenteric vein (IMV) is very helpful (Fig. 21.8). Creating a plane between the mesocolon and the retroperitoneum underneath the IMV allows access to a "virginal plane" that has been undisturbed by the previous peritonitis.

A colorectal anastomosis is then performed in the typical fashion. An air leak test can be performed by using a laparoscopic suction irrigator to submerge the anastomosis while occluding the proximal colon with an atraumatic grasper.

Pitfalls and Troubleshooting

The timing of Hartmann's reversal is largely surgeon dependent, with most advocating for a delay of several months from the index operation. This allows for reduction in the postoperative and/or postinfection inflammation seen after emergency surgery. While patients may push for early colostomy reversal for convenience, allowing for some delay may provide for lessening of the degree of adhesions and facilitate the reversal. Reversal is typically delayed by 2–3 months, although this may be delayed by 6 months or more in cases of delayed wound closure, malnutrition, or other long-lasting sequelae of intra-abdominal sepsis.

Adhesions make minimally invasive Hartmann's reversal technically challenging. Access to an experienced assistant can be invaluable during these difficult cases. Having a senior-level trainee or partner available may help reduce frustration and operative time.

Conversion from a minimally invasive to open approach should not be considered failure. The goal of the operation is successful reversal of the colostomy, and the operation should only be considered a failure if the rectal stump cannot be salvaged and reversal is not possible. Oftentimes, this decision to convert to open is made relatively early in the course of the operation. Dense intra-abdominal or pelvic adhesions may preclude adequate visualization. If the surgeon is comfortable with laparoscopic or robotic adhesiolysis, this can be attempted once adequate port placement has been achieved. Hasson entry in the supraumbilical midline or initial colostomy takedown and port placement via this aperture are both reasonable strategies for safe abdominal entry.

Minimally invasive Hartmann's reversal operations can be complicated by nuisance bleeding caused by management of intra-abdominal or pelvic adhesions. The use of a laparoscopic suction irrigator can help evacuate blood, which may obscure your view of the operative field. Alternatively, introduction of a sponge or laparotomy pad into the abdomen can be helpful for the evacuation of blood or clot. This can also be used to clean the laparoscope should the lens become soiled during the operation.

Should splenic flexure mobilization become necessary, a medial to lateral approach can be performed. Incising the peritoneum beneath the IMV and entering the retromesenteric plane at this location may allow for easier flexure takedown. Peritonitis from perforation and prior surgery may make lateral to medial mobilization of the left colon and splenic flexure difficult. Taking advantage of the "virginal" retromesenteric plane may facilitate flexure mobilization and avoid potential injury to the colon conduit.

Even with complete mobilization of the splenic flexure, sufficient reach may not be achieved in all cases. This can happen if a significant portion of the left colon had been resected at the index operation or if the remaining left colon is diseased, ischemic, or otherwise unusable. In such scenarios, the transverse mesocolon may not be long enough to allow a tension-free anastomosis between the distal transverse colon and the rectum. While one option would be to abort the procedure and remature the end colostomy, one can consider mobilization and counterclockwise rotation of the right colon with anastomosis of the right or proximal transverse colon to the rectum (Deloyers procedure). The transverse colon is sacrificed during this procedure to allow for right colon to rectum anastomosis. The blood supply to the right colon must, obviously, be carefully preserved. A variation of this is the Turnbull procedure, in which a window is created in an avascular portion of the terminal ileal mesentery allowing the proximal colon to be passed in a retroileal fashion to the colorectal anastomosis.

Dense pelvic inflammation may hamper attempts at mobilization of the rectal stump. At times, the stump can become completely retroperitonealized, making initial identification difficult. Having an assistant pass an EEA sizer or large bougie transanally may help in identification of the top of the stump and may help define the course of the rectum in the pelvis. Once identified, entering the presacral space, which is seldom violated at the original operation, may allow for easier mobilization of the rectum. This dissection is usually begun at the sacral promontory. Ureteral catheters can be helpful in identification of the ureters at this level. Resection of the fibrotic proximal rectal stump is often required, to allow anastomosis to soft, pliable rectum.

Outcomes

The literature outlining the clinical outcomes of minimally invasive Hartmann's reversal continues to evolve. While the proportion of patients who never undergo colostomy closure remains high, it appears that more reversal surgeries are being performed using minimally invasive techniques.

Several studies have examined outcomes of laparoscopic Hartmann's reversal, which are summarized in Table 21.1. Pei and colleagues examined national trends and outcomes in laparoscopic colostomy reversal using the American College of Surgeons National Surgical Quality Improvement Program (ACS-NSQIP) [9]. By 2014, up to 74% of reversal surgeries were performed laparoscopically, with an annual increase of 2.87% per year during the study period. Laparoscopic reversal was associated with shorter hospital length of stay and lower overall complication rates when compared to open surgery.

Table 21.2 summarizes several studies that compared outcomes of laparoscopic and open Hartmann's reversal. Most studies demonstrated slightly shorter operative times and shorter length of stay in the laparoscopic group compared to open. However, since these studies were not randomized, selection bias likely skewed the laparoscopic group toward less challenging cases.

Arkenbosch and colleagues examined the same database, identifying patients undergoing Hartmann's reversal between 2005 and 2012 [12]. Only 17.6% of patients underwent a laparoscopic procedure. Patients in this group tended to have a lower BMI, shorter operations, and a lower overall morbidity. Rates of

Table 21.1 Outcomes of laparoscopic Hartmann's reversal

Year	Author	Data source	Conversion rate (%)	Major findings in laparoscopic reversal over open reversal
2018	Park [8]	Single institution	49	Lower morbidity, shorter LOS
2018	Pei [9]	ACS-NSQIP	N/A	% of laparoscopic reversal increased over time
2017	Brathwaite [10]	ACS-NSQIP	N/A	Less SSI, shorter LOS
2017	Horesh [11]	Multi-institution	27.2	N/A
2015	Arkenbosch [12]	ACS-NSQIP	N/A	Lower morbidity, shorter LOS
2014	Richards [13]	Multi-institution	64	N/A
2013	Lin [7]	Single institution	47	Lower morbidity

Table 21.2 Comparison of laparoscopic vs. open Hartmann's reversal

Year	Author	Number of patients		Operative time (min)		Length of stay (days)		Complication rate (%)		Surgical site of infection (%)	
		Lap	Open	Lap	Open	Lap	Open	Lap	Open	Lap	Open
2018	Horesh [14]	56	204	NR	NR	10.9	11.8	46	47	36	38
2018	Kwak [6]	17	12	212.5	251.8	11.7	14.8	29.4	41.7	24	17
2015	Arkenbosch [12]	732	3416	187.6	190.4	5	6	18.4	27	14	19
2014	Yang [15]	43	64	276	242	6.7	10.8	19	38	7	5
2013	de'Angelis [16]	28	28	171.1	235.8	6.7	11.2	10.7	27.8	0	33.3

reoperation, incisional and organ space surgical site infection, and sepsis were also lower in the laparoscopic group. A similar study by Brathwaite and colleagues demonstrated identical results [10].

Despite increased experience and comfort with minimally invasive techniques including robotic surgery, conversion rates of Hartmann's reversal remain high, and they have not yet been consistently demonstrated to have decreased over time. It is not yet clear what impact the introduction of robotics will have on conversion rates since very limited data are currently available on this.

Conclusion

Minimally invasive Hartmann's reversal is often a challenging operation, requiring careful patient selection and preoperative planning. Advanced training in minimally invasive colorectal surgery is essential in achieving acceptable outcomes and limiting complications. Rates of conversion to open surgery remain high but should not be interpreted as a failure. Successful completion of minimally invasive surgery is associated with lower postoperative morbidity and shorter length of hospital stay. Surgeons should be comfortable with the various minimally invasive techniques available, applying them as applicable. A significant learning curve for minimally invasive colorectal surgery exists, and this should be kept in mind prior to attempting laparoscopic or robotic Hartmann's reversal surgery.

References

1. Comparato G, Fanigliulo L, Aragona G, Cavestro GM, Cavallaro LG, Leandro G, et al. Quality of life in uncomplicated symptomatic diverticular disease: is it another good reason for treatment? Dig Dis. 2007;25(3):252–9.
2. Feingold D, Steele SR, Lee S, Kaiser A, Boushey R, Buie WD, et al. Practice parameters for the treatment of sigmoid diverticulitis. Dis Colon Rectum. 2014;57(3):284–94.
3. Bailey MB, Davenport DL, Procter L, McKenzie S, Vargas HD. Morbid obesity and diverticulitis: results from the ACS NSQIP dataset. J Am Coll Surg. 2013;217(5):874–80 e1.
4. Steinemann DC, Stierle T, Zerz A, Lamm SH, Limani P, Nocito A. Hartmann's procedure and laparoscopic reversal versus primary anastomosis and ileostomy closure for left colonic perforation. Langenbecks Arch Surg. 2015;400(5):609–16.

5. Royo-Aznar A, Moro-Valdezate D, Martín-Arévalo J, Pla-Martí V, García-Botello S, Espín-Basany E, et al. Reversal of Hartmann's procedure: a single-centre experience of 533 consecutive cases. Colorectal Dis. 2018;20(7):631–8.
6. Kwak HD, Kim J, Kang DW, Baek SJ, Kwak JM, Kim SH. Hartmann's reversal: a comparative study between laparoscopic and open approaches. ANZ J Surg. 2018;88(5):450–4.
7. Lin F, Boutros M, Da Silva GM, Weiss EG, Lu XR, Wexner SD. Hartmann reversal: obesity adversely impacts outcome. Dis Colon Rectum. 2013;56:83–90.
8. Park W, Park WC, Kim KY, Lee SY. Efficacy and safety of laparoscopic Hartmann colostomy reversal. Ann Coloproctol. 2018;34(6):306–11.
9. Pei KY, Davis KA, Zhang Y. Assessing trends in laparoscopic colostomy reversal and evaluating outcomes when compared to open procedures. Surg Endosc. 2018;32:695–701.
10. Brathwaite S, Latchana N, Esemuede I, Harzman A, Husain S. Risk factors for surgical site infection in open and laparoscopic Hartmann closure: a multivariate analysis. Surg Laparosc Percutan Tech. 2017;27(1):51–3.
11. Horesh N, Lessing Y, Rudnicki Y, Kent I, Kammar H, Ben-Yaacov A, et al. Considerations for Hartmann's reversal and Hartmann's reversal outcomes-a multicenter study. Int J Colorectal Dis. 2017;32(11):1577–82.
12. Arkenbosch J, Miyagaki H, Kumara HM, Yan X, Cekic V, Whelan RL. Efficacy of laparoscopic-assisted approach for reversal of Hartmann's procedure: results from the American College of Surgeons National Surgical Quality Improvement Program (ACS-NSQIP) database. Surg Endosc. 2015;29:2109–14.
13. Richards CH, Roxburgh CS, Scottish Surgical Research Group (SSRG). Surgical outcome in patients undergoing reversal of Hartmann's procedures: a multicentre study. Colorectal Dis. 2015;17(3):242–9.
14. Horesh N, Lessing Y, Rudnicki Y, Kent I, Kammar H, Ben-Yaacov A, et al. Comparison between laparoscopic and open Hartmann's reversal: results of a decade-long multicenter retrospective study. Surg Endosc. 2018;32:4780–7.
15. Yang PF, Morgan MJ. Laparoscopic versus open reversal of Hartmann's procedure: a retrospective review. ANZ J Surg. 2014;84:965–9.
16. de'Angelis N, Brunetti F, Memeo R, Batista da Costa J, Schneck AS, Carra MC, et al. Comparison between open and laparoscopic reversal of Hartmann's procedure for diverticulitis. World J Gastrointest Surg. 2013;5(8):245–51.

Principles of Rectal Cancer Management: Preoperative Staging, Neoadjuvant Treatment, Basic Principles of TME, and Adjuvant Treatment

22

Emmanouil Pappou and Martin R. Weiser

Introduction and Rationale

Rectal cancer was considered incurable up until the eighteenth century, when techniques to remove the rectum were developed. With innovations in anesthesia and the advent of aseptic technique, proctectomy became more radical and aggressive. In 1908, William Ernest Miles described his technique of a combined abdominal and perineal resection (APR) with en bloc removal of all associated lymph nodes in upward, lateral, and downward directions (cylindrical concept), introducing the basis for curative rectal cancer surgery. The widespread acceptance of Miles' APR represented an acknowledgment that cancer surgery should be based on anatomical and biological principles. In 1910, the American surgeon Donald Balfour described a technique of anterior resection with construction of a primary end-to-end anastomosis, which didn't gain acceptance, as it was thought that this operation was not radical enough. However, Miles' concept concerning the spread and recurrence of rectal cancer was subsequently proven wrong when Cuthbert Dukes, an English pathologist at St. Mark's Hospital, demonstrated that downward and lateral spread from rectal cancer was overestimated by Miles, as the majority of metastatic lymph nodes were either parallel to or proximal to the level of the primary tumor. This observation initiated the historical shift to sphincter-saving procedures. Claude Dixon, surgical chair at the Mayo Clinic, reported in 1948 a mortality rate of 2.6%

E. Pappou
Department of Surgery, Memorial Sloan Kettering Cancer Center, Cornell University, New York, NY, USA
e-mail: pappoue@mskcc.org

M. R. Weiser (✉)
Department of Surgery, Stuart H.Q. Quan Chair in Colorectal Surgery, Vice Chair for Education and Faculty Development, Memorial Sloan Kettering Cancer Center, Cornell University, New York, NY, USA
e-mail: Weiser1@mskcc.org

P. Sylla et al. (eds.), *The SAGES Manual of Colorectal Surgery*,
https://doi.org/10.1007/978-3-030-24812-3_22

and a 5-year survival of 64% with anterior resection, establishing the technique as an accepted treatment for upper and middle rectal cancers. The understanding in the 1970s that a distal margin of 1–2 cm did not compromise survival or local control initiated the shift from APR to anterior resection even for low-rectal tumors. Circular stapling devices, first conceived in Russia and introduced in the United States by Steichen and Ravitch, revolutionized rectal surgery by facilitating the creation of low colorectal anastomoses in a safe and expeditious manner while reducing the risk of anastomotic leakage. Interest in lateral tumor spread was renewed when Quirke and Dixon found that there was a high predictive value of the involvement of the circumferential resection margin (CRM) for the subsequent development of local recurrence and poor survival. Bill Heald popularized a low anterior resection technique he termed "total mesorectal excision" (TME), which involves en bloc resection of the tumor and mesorectum using sharp dissection under direct vision and along embryologically defined surgical planes, resulting in decreased rates of positive lateral margins and lower rates of local recurrence. This approach became the gold standard in rectal cancer surgery, along with the principle of autonomic nerve preservation (hypogastric nerves, inferior hypogastric plexus, and pelvic splanchnic nerves), which was initiated in Japan by Hojo and Moriya and promoted in the United States by Warren Enker.

Although at present the primary treatment of rectal cancer is centered on surgical resection, chemotherapy and radiation have become increasingly important. The concept of neoadjuvant therapy for rectal cancer was first introduced in the 1920s, when significant tumor response was noted following implantation of radon seeds directly into rectal tumors. As surgery became safer and the limitations of contact radiation (the only radiation treatment modality at that time) became apparent, the use of radiation as a primary treatment declined. After it became apparent that the outcomes of radical surgery were suboptimal, investigators in Europe and the United States explored utilizing neoadjuvant radiotherapy and chemoradiotherapy, and eventually the benefits of administering radiotherapy in the preoperative period in reducing local recurrence rates were demonstrated. Subsequent studies suggested that the oncologic benefits of neoadjuvant radiotherapy and good surgical technique were additive, not compensatory, with regard to pelvic control. Several large trials have since shown the benefit of preoperative radiotherapy combined with chemotherapy, and consensus guidelines since the 1990s have established trimodal therapy – chemotherapy, radiation, and surgery – as the standard of care for locally advanced rectal cancer.

Preoperative Staging

Assessment of the extent of disease at the time of diagnosis is important because clinical stage dictates treatment decisions. The preoperative staging of rectal cancer follows the clinical TNM system, based on the depth of tumor penetration in the rectal wall, presence of involved regional lymph nodes, and presence of distant metastatic disease. However, the preoperative assessment of rectal cancer goes beyond determination of clinical tumor stage; it includes the distance of the tumor from the anal verge, its relationship to the sphincter complex and the levator muscles, the proximity of the tumor to the mesorectal fascia, the involvement of surrounding structures (e.g., prostate, bladder, vagina), and the presence of extramural venous invasion.

A complete history and physical examination are essential components of the initial preoperative evaluation. The physician should inquire about changes in bowel habits, rectal bleeding, control of flatus and stool, obstructive symptoms, recent weight loss or anorexia, and sacral or sciatic pain. A detailed family history should also be taken to rule out the possibility of a hereditary cancer syndrome.

The physical exam should focus on the presence of abdominal masses, inguinal lymphadenopathy, and palpable rectal masses. A careful digital rectal exam should be performed, noting the resting anal tone, anal squeeze, and length of the surgical anal canal. If a mass is encountered, its orientation, quality (hard vs. soft, mobile vs. fixed), and distance both from the anal verge and more importantly from the sphincter complex (anorectal ring) should be noted. A hard mass in the pouch of Douglas felt on digital rectal exam may indicate peritoneal carcinomatosis.

The lumen of the rectum should be examined with either a rigid proctoscope or flexible sigmoidoscopy, although tumor location is most accurately measured by rigid proctoscopy. This allows for accurate assessment of tumor orientation, location in relation to the rectal folds (proximal, middle, and distal Houston's valves), circumferential involvement, proximal and distal extent of the tumor, and whether the tumor is obstructing or near-obstructing. If the diagnosis of invasive cancer has not yet been confirmed, additional biopsies should be taken.

Laboratory studies including complete blood count, coagulation parameters, chemistry panel, and carcinoembryonic antigen (CEA) level are generally obtained prior to start of treatment.

Whenever possible, the patient should have a full colonoscopy because synchronous polyps and synchronous colorectal cancers are present in up to 30% and up to 5.3% of rectal cancer patients, respectively. If a full colonoscopy is not possible at the outset, it can be attempted after tumor downsizing by neoadjuvant therapy. Alternatives include CT colonography (virtual colonoscopy) and intraoperative palpation of the colon. In cases where a complete colonoscopy is not feasible prior to an operation, a short-interval surveillance colonoscopy should be performed 3–6 months after surgery.

Accurate pretreatment locoregional staging is needed to assess the depth of tumor penetration through the rectal wall as well as the presence of suspiciously enlarged regional lymph nodes. The two most commonly utilized imaging modalities for locoregional staging are endorectal ultrasound (ERUS) and magnetic resonance imaging (MRI).

ERUS is used to evaluate the depth of tumor invasion through the rectal wall and to detect any enlarged adjacent mesorectal lymph nodes; it is most useful for staging early-stage, T1–T2 rectal cancers. The main advantages of ERUS are its low cost and ability to distinguish between Tis, T1, and T2 tumors (Fig. 22.1a–d). However, it has a relatively short focal range, is inferior at evaluating the mesorectal fascia, and cannot assess pelvic lymph nodes that are remote from the rectum. It is also limited by operator skill and is associated with a substantial learning curve.

Rectal MRI (specifically high-resolution T2-weighted images including a narrow field of view of the rectum) provides the best assessment of the rectal wall and perirectal fat and is considered the best modality for distinguishing T2–T4 tumors (Fig. 22.2a, b). It provides high tissue resolution and excellent anatomical depiction of the rectum, the mesorectum, the mesorectal fascia, the levator muscles, other pelvic structures adjacent to the tumor, and possible extramural venous invasion. Advanced functional sequences such as diffusion-weighted imaging permit the quantification of tumor biologic processes such as microcirculation, vascular

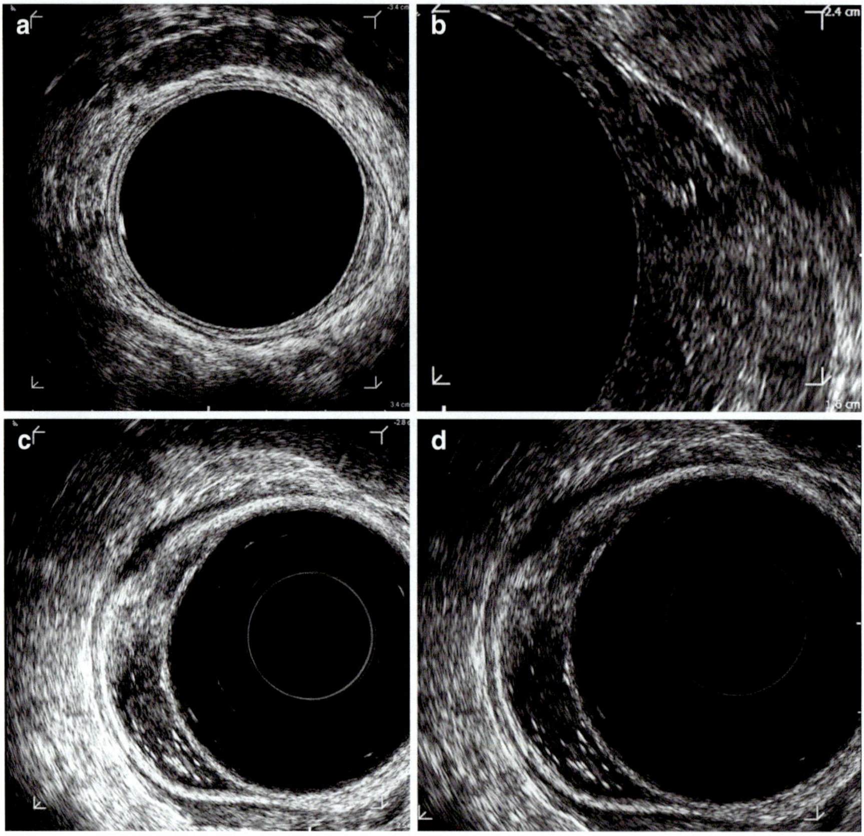

Fig. 22.1 (**a**–**d**) Endorectal ultrasound in rectal cancer staging. The sonographic 5-layer structure of the rectal wall consists of 3 hyperechoic layers (interface between the balloon and mucosa, submucosa, and perirectal fat/serosa) separated by 2 hypoechoic layers (muscularis mucosa and muscularis propria). Lesions are T staged as uT0/uTis when the mass is within the hypoechoic M. mucosa layer, as uT1 when invading the hyperechoic submucosal layer, and as uT2 if they cause a distinct break in the submucosal layer and invade into the hypoechoic muscularis propria layer. (All images used with permission of Springer Nature from Valinluck Lao and Fichera [53].)

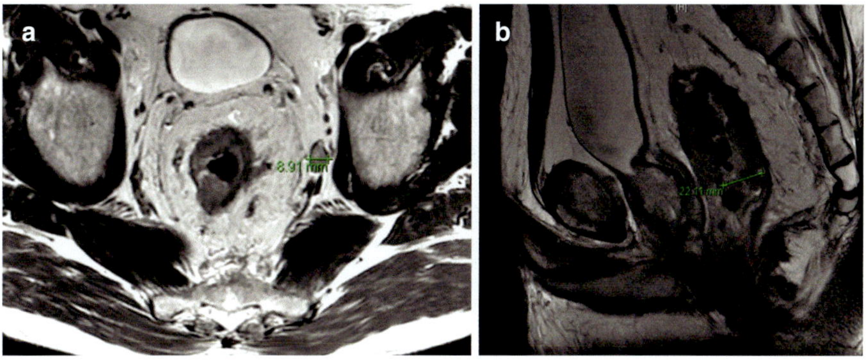

Fig. 22.2 (**a**, **b**) Magnetic resonance imaging in rectal cancer staging. Routine use of rectal MRI in the context of a multidisciplinary assessment of rectal cancer has been used to plan neoadjuvant therapy and surgery and has been shown to reduce the incidence of positive circumferential margins. Axial and sagittal views of a locally advanced rectal cancer are shown, depicting extramural venous invasion and enlarged obturator lymph nodes

permeability, and tissue cellularity and are useful in the assessment of response to neoadjuvant therapy. However, it is often difficult to distinguish the submucosa from the muscularis propria on MRI, and therefore differentiating T1 and T2 tumors can be difficult, and overstaging can occur. Tumor distance from the mesorectal fascia is highly predictive of achieving a negative CRM; it has prognostic implications for local recurrence and patient survival and has become one of the most important parameters in the preoperative evaluation. The excellent accuracy of MRI in delineating the mesorectal fascia – producing results comparable to those of histological analysis – was demonstrated by a large European multicenter trial known as the MERCURY study, in which 349 patients underwent preoperative MRI assessment, followed by TME surgery. MRI was found to be accurate within 0.5 mm, with a specificity of 92%, in predicting a clear CRM [1]. MRI with a rectal cancer protocol has become more widely available and has replaced ERUS as the primary imaging modality used for the locoregional staging of rectal cancer, although ERUS remains useful for staging of early T1–T2 tumors.

The National Accreditation Program for Rectal Cancer (NAPRC) that was developed through a collaboration with the Commission on Cancer (CoC), a quality program of the American College of Surgeons, considers rectal MRI the standard for the pretreatment staging of rectal cancer. ERUS can be used in addition to rectal MRI for small rectal lesions (T1/T2) to improve accuracy of T staging.

A CT scan of the chest, abdomen, and pelvis with oral and intravenous contrast should be obtained to exclude distant metastases, which are present in up to 20% of patients at the time of diagnosis. PET-CT is not routinely used for initial staging.

Indications and Contraindications

One of the difficulties in constructing algorithms and guidelines for treatment of rectal cancer is that treatment decisions must take into account multiple variables,

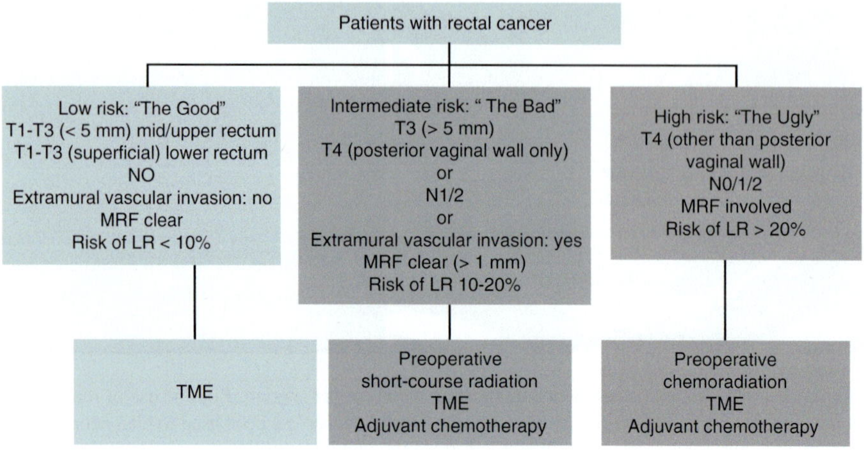

Fig. 22.3 European model of stratification for patients with rectal cancer based on magnetic resonance imaging. Abbreviations: MRF, mesorectal fascia; LR, local recurrence; TME, total mesorectal excision. (Source: Ferrari and Fichera [54]. Published under the terms of the Creative Commons CC License.)

including tumor location, fixation, circumferential involvement of the rectum, the tumor's relation to the pelvic floor muscles, pelvic morphology, clinical stage, presence of symptoms and degree of obstruction, presence and location of metastases, continence status, prior treatments, and patient preferences. It is virtually impossible to create straightforward guidelines that account for all of these factors. At present, the clinician caring for patients with rectal cancer must be able to tailor recommendations for therapy based on the characteristics of the tumor, and the patient, and have a firm grasp of the rationale and the existing data supporting any proposed treatment plan.

In a number of European countries, treatment decisions are based on MRI findings of tumor aggressiveness including the proximity of the primary tumor to the mesorectal fascia, the depth of tumor invasion, the presence of metastatic lymph nodes, and the presence of venous invasion (Fig. 22.3). While this algorithm is intuitive, its utility has not been yet evaluated in prospective trials [2]. A simplified version of the National Comprehensive Cancer Network guidelines for locally advanced rectal cancer is also shown (Fig. 22.4).

Local Excision for Early-Stage Rectal Cancer

Transanal endoscopic surgery for rectal cancer is covered in Chap. 39 in more detail. Historically, local excision was associated with high recurrence rates; however, the advent of accurate preoperative staging, tumor downstaging following neoadjuvant therapy, and the development of new surgical techniques such as transanal endoscopic microsurgery and transanal minimally invasive surgery have resulted in increased interest in local excision. Currently, the National Comprehensive Cancer

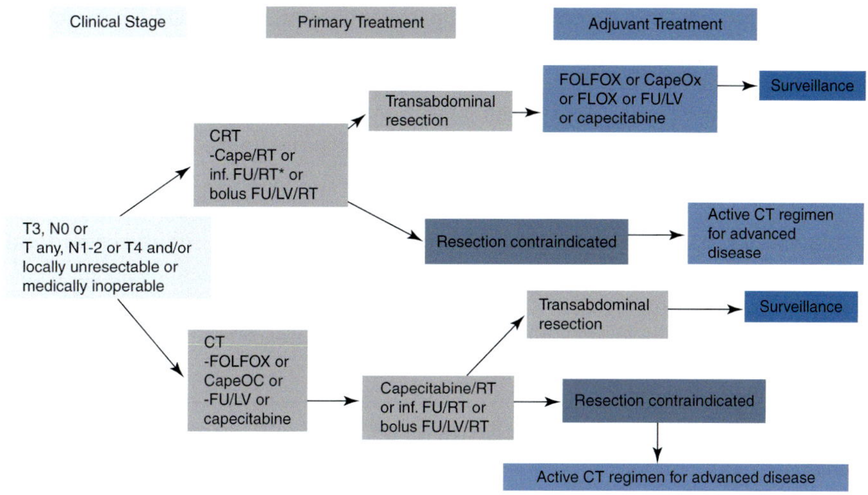

Fig. 22.4 A simplified version of the National Comprehensive Cancer Network algorithm for locally advanced rectal cancer. Abbreviations: CRT, chemoradiation; CT, chemotherapy Cape, capecitabine; RT, radiation therapy; CapeOx, capecitabine plus oxaliplatin; inf., infusional; FLOX, bolus fluorouracil, leucovorin, and oxaliplatin; FOLFOX, infusional fluorouracil, leucovorin, and oxaliplatin; FU, fluorouracil; LV, leucovorin

Network (NCCN) guidelines state that candidates for full-thickness local resection include patients with Tis and T1 tumors up to 3 cm that are well to moderately differentiated, occupy less than one-third of the rectal lumen's circumference, and are located within 8 cm from the anal verge. Any local resection that results in a final margin less than 1 mm or that demonstrates high-risk features for lymph node metastasis, such as lymphovascular invasion, poor differentiation, tumor budding, or penetration of the lower third of the submucosa in the final pathology specimen, should be followed by a formal proctectomy.

Radiotherapy in Combination with Local Excision

Preoperative chemoradiation can be used in combination with local excision for selected patients. A number of retrospective studies have shown good local control rates in patients treated with preoperative chemoradiation in combination with local excision. These studies primarily evaluated patients who were not candidates for radical excision or patients who declined proctectomy. A retrospective study conducted at MD Anderson Cancer Center reported outcomes in patients with T3 rectal cancer treated with preoperative radiation (45–52.5 Gy) and concurrent fluorouracil [3]. Of the 47 treated with local excision, 49% had a pathologic complete response (pCR), and 36% had microscopic residual disease after chemoradiation. The 10-year actuarial risk of local recurrence was 10.6%, in comparison with 7.6% in a cohort of 473 patients treated with TME at the same institution. Similarly, a retrospective study conducted in Korea showed a 5-year rate of local relapse-free survival of 89% in 27 patients with mostly T3 rectal cancer treated with preoperative chemoradiation and local excision [4]. Another retrospective study conducted in the United States reported outcomes in 44 patients with T2–T3 rectal cancer treated with preoperative chemoradiation and full-thickness local excision [5]. Pathologic complete responses were seen in about 43% of patients. The results of all these studies should be interpreted with great caution given their small size and retrospective nature. Careful selection of patients likely contributed to these results, as suggested by the high proportion of patients with pCR. At this point, the combination of preoperative chemoradiation and full-thickness local excision for T1–T3 rectal cancer appears appropriate only for patients who are medically unfit for proctectomy or who refuse radical surgery. Prospective randomized studies are needed to validate the long-term safety of this approach [6].

Principles and Quality Benchmarks of Total Mesorectal Excision

This chapter will focus on the principles of complete TME for mid- or low-rectal tumors. For tumors of the rectosigmoid or upper rectum, the mesorectal excision should be extended to 5 cm distal to the lower edge of the tumor, and the mesorectum should be divided perpendicular to the axis of the rectum (Fig. 22.5). As some of the distal mesorectum is left in the pelvis along with the distal rectal stump, this operation is known as tumor-specific TME (TSME), to distinguish it from the complete TME, and is covered in Chap. 23. Radical proctectomy with complete TME remains the gold standard for locally advanced mid- to low-rectal cancer. Surgical treatment of rectal cancer is aimed at eradicating the primary tumor and its lymphatic drainage by en bloc removal of the rectum and the mesorectum, following well-defined anatomical planes. TME requires sharp dissection under direct vision along the areolar tissue plane situated between the visceral and parietal layers of the endopelvic fascia. A sharp dissection along the mesorectal plane is associated with a higher probability of achieving a negative CRM, lower risk of bleeding from inadvertent tearing of the presacral veins, and reduced risk of injuring the hypogastric and pelvic nerves. The basic principles of TME are as follows:

1. Sharp dissection circumferentially around the mesorectum along an avascular areolar plane between the visceral and parietal layers of the endopelvic fascia.
2. Identification and preservation of the autonomic nerve plexus that controls bladder and sexual function.
3. Prevention of tearing of the mesorectum, especially posteriorly when dividing the rectosacral fascia.
4. Achieving a CRM that is macroscopically clear of tumor. If the tumor extends to the CRM, a more extensive resection is necessary. This would include removal of a portion of the parietal layer of the endopelvic fascia and any additional anatomic structures involved by tumor.

The quality of TME surgery is reflected in the appearance and integrity of the mesorectum in the removed specimen (Fig. 22.6). Quirke and colleagues have described a grading system that classifies rectal cancer specimens according to

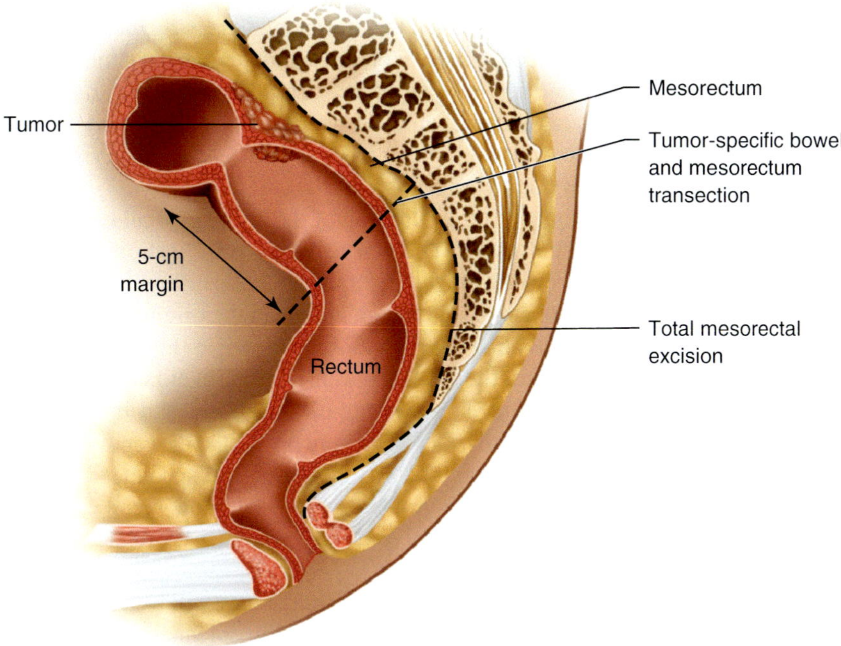

Fig. 22.5 In tumor-specific TME for high rectal cancers, the rectum and mesorectum are divided perpendicularly to the rectal wall 5 cm below the level of the tumor. For mid- and low-rectal tumors, complete TME is performed, removing the entire mesorectum to the level of the levator muscles. (Used with permission of Springer Nature from Hakiman et al. [55].)

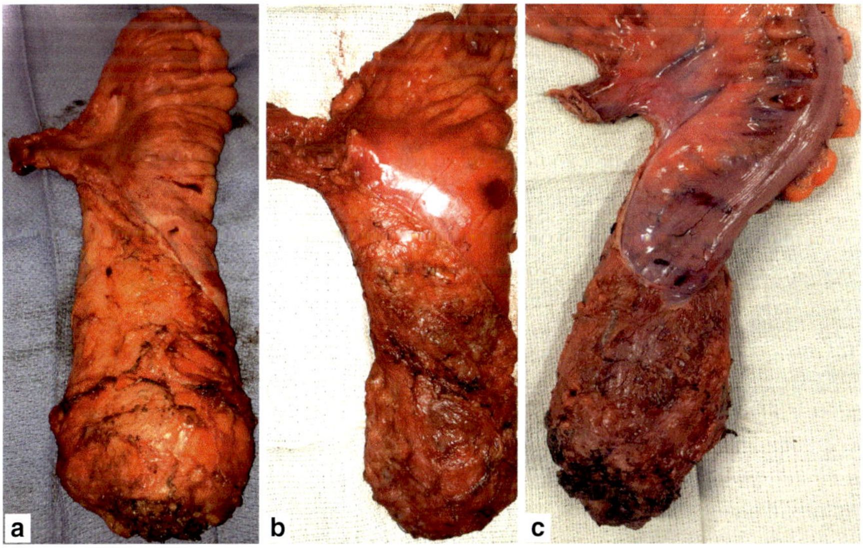

Fig. 22.6 Grading of removed rectal cancer specimens. (**a**) demonstrates the posterior surface of an intact mesorectum consistent with a complete TME grade. (**b**) demonstrates superficial defects in the posterior mesorectum consistent with a near-complete TME grade. (**c**) demonstrates a specimen with incomplete TME grade, with exposed muscularis propria. (All images courtesy of Patricia Sylla, MD.)

whether the surgeon has dissected outside the mesorectal fascia in the correct plane (mesorectal excision plane) or has violated the mesorectum, leaving mesorectal tissue behind the pelvis following either a plane within the mesorectum (intra-mesorectal excision plane) or directly on the muscularis propria (muscularis propria excision plane) [7]. The macroscopic quality of mesorectal excision completeness has been found to be an independent predictor of local recurrence and survival, even in patients with an uninvolved CRM [8].

Adequate lymphadenectomy requires division of the lymphovascular pedicle at the origin of the superior rectal vessels. This can be achieved by ligation of the inferior mesenteric artery distally to the branching of the left colic artery (low ligation), or in cases where clinically suspicious nodes are present at the origin of the inferior mesenteric artery (IMA), by dividing the IMA close to its origin (high ligation). We routinely perform high ligation of the IMA at our institution. In either case, all sigmoidal branches should be included in the surgical specimen, and therefore the colon should ideally be proximally divided at the junction of the descending and the sigmoid colon, incorporating the sigmoid colon in the surgical specimen. As distal tumor extension along the rectal wall is limited for mid- and low-rectal cancers, a distal margin of 1–2 cm of normal rectal wall is considered adequate for most tumors.

Patients with low-rectal cancer <5 cm from anal verge may still be treated with a sphincter-sparing technique. Options include a hand-sewn coloanal anastomosis if the tumors are >1 cm from the sphincter complex, and either partial internal anal sphincter resection for tumors <1 cm from the internal anal sphincter or complete intersphincteric resection for tumors involving the internal anal sphincter but sparing the external anal sphincters and levators [9].

For many cancers located in the distal rectum, specifically those infiltrating the levator muscles or the anal sphincter, an oncologically safe CRM and/or distal resection margin is not compatible with sphincter preservation, and an APR is therefore necessary. In a more radical version of conventional APR, the coccyx is removed en bloc with the rectum and the levators, resulting in a surgical specimen that has a cylindrical appearance; this procedure is called cylindrical or extralevator APR. Some surgeons question the need to entirely remove both levator muscles and recommend removing only the portion of the levators required to clear the tumor. The choice between standard and extralevator APR is controversial. The potential oncologic benefit of larger tissue removal needs to be weighed against the increased morbidity associated with a larger perineal defect, particularly in patients treated with neoadjuvant radiotherapy.

Optimal resection of rectal cancer according to the oncological principles of TME can be achieved by open or minimally invasive (laparoscopic or robotic) surgical techniques. Multiple trials have demonstrated the feasibility and safety of laparoscopic and robotic surgery for rectal cancer [10–12]. Transanal TME (taTME) is a more recently described minimally invasive approach for dissection of the distal rectum in patients with a narrow pelvis [13, 14]. With this technique, lymphovascular control, the entire colonic mobilization, and dissection of the upper rectum are performed using conventional transabdominal laparoscopy. The dissection of the distal rectum and mesorectum is performed transanally through an endoscopic platform. The lumen of the rectum is closed with a purse-string suture to avoid contamination, and the rectal wall is incised circumferentially distal to the tumor. The dissection is carried cephalad until the abdominal field is reached. The specimen is then removed, and the anastomosis is performed through the anus. This approach allows the surgeon to choose precisely the point for transecting the rectum while visualizing the distal edge of the tumor. Transanal TME has been associated with low conversion rates and preliminary oncologic outcomes equivalent to that of abdominal TME. Several trials are underway to assess long-term outcomes relative to laparoscopic TME. Please refer to the chapters on laparoscopic and robotic TME (Chaps. 23 and 24) for more details on operative setup and techniques of minimally invasive TME.

Multidisciplinary Management

There is increasing evidence to suggest the benefits of a multidisciplinary approach in patients with rectal cancer, involving surgical, medical, and radiation oncologists, radiologists, and pathologists [15]. Rectal cancer centers of excellence have been successfully established in several European countries over the past decade, and similar efforts in standardizing care have begun in the United States [16]. Multidisciplinary tumor (MDT) boards may change the clinical management in a non-negligible proportion of rectal cancer patients, creating a tailored plan for every individual patient [17].

Cancer outcomes are better when patients are managed according to the principles of MDT care. MDTs are associated with improved clinical decision-making, clinical outcomes, and patient experience in several cancer types, including rectal cancer. Implementation of an MDT approach to rectal cancer care in several European countries has resulted in reduced rates of local recurrence, lower rates of permanent stoma, and improved overall survival [18, 19]. We strongly encourage referral of rectal cancer patients to high-volume centers with established MDTs.

Pitfalls and Troubleshooting

Adhering to the traditional principles of following the avascular embryologic planes during dissection, proper tissue handling, ensuring adequate blood supply of the colon conduit, and avoiding tension of the anastomosis remain essential to optimizing outcomes after rectal cancer surgery. All colorectal anastomoses should undergo leak testing regardless of the donut integrity. Methods for creating adequate colon conduit length for a technically sound colorectal or coloanal anastomosis include complete mobilization of the splenic flexure and the colon mesentery, division of the inferior mesenteric vein proximally near the ligament of Treitz, and ligation of the inferior mesenteric artery proximally to the left colic artery (high ligation). In cases when, despite full mobilization of both the mesentery and the left colon, the conduit doesn't reach the pelvis, or in cases of marginal artery injury, options include performing a total colectomy and an ileorectal anastomosis or rotating the right colon 180° around the ileocolic pedicle in an effort to preserve the ileocecal valve (Deloyers procedure) or performing a retroileal anastomosis between the ascending colon and rectum [20].

Oncologic Outcomes with TME

TME has been associated with improved local control and survival rates. The local recurrence rate following TME ranges from 4% to 10%. This represents an improvement compared with local recurrence rates following the conventional blunt approach, which range from 15% to 45% with or without chemoradiation or radiation. Local recurrence and survival from selected representative studies on TME are shown in Table 22.1 [21–25]. Radiation or chemoradiation in addition to TME has further decreased local recurrence rates.

The importance of TME technique in local recurrence has been demonstrated in Sweden, Norway, and the Netherlands, where implementation of educational programs and hands-on surgical TME workshops were shown to markedly reduce local recurrence, improve survival, and reduce the permanent stoma rate (Table 22.2) [26–28].

Table 22.1 Representative studies assessing local recurrence and survival following TME surgery

Author	Country	Year	*N*	Local recurrence (%)	Five-year survival (%)
MacFarlane et al. [21]	UK	1993	135	4	78
Enker et al. [22]	Germany	1995	246	7	74
Arbman et al. [23]	Sweden	1996	128	6	68
Bjerkeset et al. [24]	Norway	1996	81	4	65
Heald et al. [25]	UK	1998	405	3	80

N, number of patients

Table 22.2 Local recurrence rates before and after the introduction of and training in TME in Northern Europe

Country	Local recurrence rate	
	Pre-TME era	Post-TME era
Norway [26]	12%	6%
Netherlands [27]	16%	9%
Stockholm [28]	14%	6%

Functional Outcomes with TME

High rates of postoperative bowel, sexual, and urinary dysfunction have been a well-known phenomenon in rectal cancer surgery, ranging between 30% and 60% [29]. Bowel dysfunction, otherwise referred to as low anterior resection syndrome (LARS), is present in up to 50–60% of patients after TME; symptoms may include incontinence, frequent bowel movements, bowel emptying difficulties, and urge, and may affect quality of life significantly. Outcomes in urologic and sexual function improved with the advent of sharp dissection and precise technique used in TME, which made the identification and preservation of the autonomic pelvic nerves an integral part of the procedure. In an early study of 42 men undergoing sphincter-preserving operations for treatment of rectal cancer, Enker demonstrated high rates of potency (86.7%) and normal ejaculation (87.9%) with the introduction of nerve-preserving TME [30]. In a comprehensive, retrospective study in both women and men, Havenga reported the sexual and urinary function of 136 patients undergoing nerve-sparing TME for cancer [31], as assessed by survey. The ability to engage in intercourse was maintained by 86% of patients younger than 60 years of age and by 67% of patients 60 years and older. Eighty-seven percent of men maintained their ability to achieve orgasm. Type of surgery (APR compared to LAR) and age greater than 60 were significantly associated with worse male sexual function. Women had similarly good results, with 85% able to experience arousal with vaginal lubrication and 91% able to achieve an orgasm. The majority of patients had few or no complaints related to urinary function. Serious urinary dysfunction such as neurogenic bladder was not encountered in this study. The importance of autonomic nerve identification and preservation during TME was also highlighted in a study by Shirouzu and colleagues, who assessed outcomes of 403 patients undergoing TME with or without nerve-sparing over a 20-year period [32]. In patients who underwent TME with nerve preservation, urinary function was preserved in over 80% of patients, erection in 79%, and ejaculation in 65%, whereas when TME was performed without nerve preservation, urinary disorders were found in over 90% and sexual dysfunction in virtually all patients, even in those younger than age 60.

Preoperative Versus Postoperative Chemoradiation

Multiple trials have established preoperative chemoradiation as a standard of care for patients with stage II and III rectal cancer. The German CAO/ARO/AIO-94 trial was the landmark study that established the superiority of preoperative chemoradiation over postoperative chemoradiation for rectal cancer [33]. In this trial, 823 patients were randomized to receive either preoperative chemoradiation or postoperative chemoradiation, along with TME and adjuvant chemotherapy with bolus fluorouracil and leucovorin. Patients in the preoperative chemoradiation arm had significantly lower 5-year rates of local relapse (6% vs. 13%, $p = 0.006$), higher rates of sphincter preservation (39% vs. 20%), and lower rates of toxicity (grade 3–4 acute toxicity, 27% vs. 40%; grade 3–4 late toxicity, 14% vs. 24%); however, there was no significant difference in overall or disease-free survival between the two arms [33, 34]. Even after a median follow-up of 11 years, patients in the preoperative chemoradiation arm had a significantly lower 10-year rate of local relapse (7% vs. 10%, $p = 0.048$) [34]. The National Surgical Adjuvant Breast and Bowel Project R-03 trial, in which patients were randomized to either preoperative or postoperative chemoradiation, provided further support for the use of preoperative chemoradiation [35]. Unlike in the German trial, the 5-year rate of disease-free survival was significantly higher (65% vs. 53%, $p = 0.011$) in patients who received chemoradiation preoperatively. The results of this trial provided general support for the preoperative approach; however, they should be interpreted cautiously, as the trial enrolled only 267 patients instead of 900 as was initially planned. Two randomized trials have compared preoperative chemoradiation and preoperative long-course radiation alone: the European Organization for Research and Treatment of Cancer (EORTC) 22,921 trial, which included 1,011 patients, and the Federation Francophone de Cancerologie Digestive (FFCD) trial, which included 762 patients [36–38]. Both trials showed that preoperative chemoradiation resulted in significantly higher rates of pathologic complete response and significantly lower rates of local recurrence, with somewhat higher toxicity.

Short-Course Radiotherapy

Preoperative short-course radiotherapy (SCRT) is used mainly in Scandinavia, the Netherlands, and the United Kingdom. It consists of a radiation schedule of 25 Gy delivered in a single week, with 5 treatments of 5 Gy each (5 × 5). SCRT offers the potential benefits of shorter duration of treatment, more efficient utilization of resources, and lower cost compared to traditional long-course chemoradiation. However, the higher dose per fraction increases the risk of delayed toxicity, and tumor regression is lower with SCRT. Two prospective randomized trials comparing SCRT with long-course chemoradiation have reported equivalent local tumor control for the two regimens, and the selection between SCRT and long-course chemoradiation is usually based on doctor and patient preference [39].

Recent results from the Stockholm III trial suggest that an 8-week interval between the end of SCRT and surgery may be more beneficial than the conventional 3- to 7-day interval [40]. In this trial, 840 patients with intermediate-risk (locally advanced) rectal cancer were randomized to preoperative radiotherapy using SCRT with either immediate (3–7 days) or delayed (4–8 weeks) surgery, or long-course conventionally fractionated radiotherapy (25 × 2 Gy) without chemotherapy and delayed surgery (4–8 weeks). The trial showed no difference in local recurrence rates, distant metastases, or recurrence-free or overall survival between the 3 arms. Postoperative mortality was the same, but postoperative morbidity (53% vs. 41%, $p = 0.001$) and surgical morbidity (36% vs. 28%, $p = 0.03$) were higher in patients who underwent SCRT with immediate surgery.

Intraoperative Radiation

Intraoperative radiotherapy (IORT) involves the delivery of a single, large dose of radiation (biologically equivalent to 2–3 times its nominal dose) intraoperatively to high-risk areas, using either electron beams or high dose-rate brachytherapy applicators. IORT allows radiation to be delivered to a small, specified area that is at highest risk of recurrence, taking advantage of direct visualization of the treated area and operative mobilization of normal structures away from the radiation field. A recent systematic review and meta-analysis of 29 studies including a total of 3,003 patients on IORT for locally advanced or recurrent colorectal cancer indicated a significant improvement in local control (odds ratio, 0.22; $p = 0.03$), disease-free survival (hazard ratio, 0.51; $p = 0.009$), and overall survival (hazard ratio, 0.33; $p = 0.001$), albeit at the expense of an increase in wound complications (odds ratio, 1.86; $p = 0.049$), but no significant difference in total complications [41]. IORT therefore appears to result in favorable perioperative and long-term outcomes and should be considered for selected patients who are at high risk of local recurrence.

Selective Omission of Radiotherapy and Neoadjuvant Chemotherapy

Certain patient subgroups have a relatively low risk of local recurrence and can potentially be treated without radiation, thereby avoiding the associated acute and late side effects.

In the multicenter MERCURY study, which evaluated the role of MRI in identifying patients with low risk of local recurrence who could be treated with surgery without radiotherapy, 33% of patients identified as having a good prognosis based on specific MRI criteria (safe CRM with tumor >1 mm from the mesorectal fascia, no extramural venous invasion, extramural spread <5 mm, and no encroachment into intersphincteric plane or levators for low-rectal tumors) were treated with surgery alone. Patients with good prognosis had a local recurrence rate of only 3%. Moreover, the 5-year rates of disease-free survival and overall survival in this group were 85% and 68%, respectively [42]. Based on the findings of the MERCURY study, good quality rectal cancer protocol MRI and appropriate interpretation of the images by highly trained radiologists can be used to select patients who can be treated with TME without radiation.

A small prospective Phase II trial conducted at Memorial Sloan Kettering Cancer Center also investigated the use of preoperative chemotherapy without radiation in patients with intermediate-risk rectal cancer (tumor located 5–12 cm from the anal verge that does not threaten the mesorectal fascia on MRI) [43]. In this trial, 32 patients with resectable, clinically staged II–III rectal cancer were treated with preoperative FOLFOX (fluorouracil, leucovorin, and oxaliplatin)/anti-VEGF and selective chemoradiotherapy, based on tumor response. The 30 patients who completed preoperative chemotherapy had tumor regression and underwent proctectomy without preoperative chemoradiotherapy. Eight (27%) had pathologic complete responses. No local recurrences were noted at 4 years, and disease-free survival was 84%. The findings of this trial suggest that preoperative chemotherapy can be a potential alternative to preoperative chemoradiation for selected patients.

To further investigate this treatment approach, the ongoing multicenter Phase II/III study CALGB PROSPECT (Preoperative Radiation or Selective Preoperative Evaluation of Chemotherapy and TME) is randomizing patients to either the standard treatment arm (chemoradiotherapy, surgery, and adjuvant FOLFOX chemotherapy) or the selective arm, with 6 cycles of FOLFOX, evaluation of response, followed by TME, with consideration for standard chemoradiotherapy if the reduction of the primary tumor is <20% on endoscopic and radiographic findings [44]. Eligible patients must have biopsy-proven adenocarcinoma with the primary tumor located 5–12 cm from the anal verge and must be candidates for sphincter-sparing surgery. The primary outcomes of the Phase II component are R0 resection rate and time to local recurrence. The primary endpoints of the Phase III component are time to local recurrence and disease-free survival. This study has accrued, and results will provide important insight into the potential for a more individualized treatment approach for rectal cancer through selective use of radiation.

Adjuvant Chemotherapy

Most patients with rectal cancer eventually experience metastatic disease. Consequently, similarly to patients with stage III colon cancer, patients with locally advanced (stage II and III) rectal cancer treated with neoadjuvant chemoradiotherapy and proctectomy are considered for postoperative adjuvant chemotherapy regardless of the histologic tumor stage identified in the final pathology specimen. Postoperative chemotherapy usually consists of fluorouracil or capecitabine plus oxaliplatin. While the use of postoperative adjuvant chemotherapy for rectal cancer lacks the unequivocal support that data from prospective randomized trial would provide, a recent meta-analysis of 21 randomized controlled trials concluded that postoperative fluorouracil-based chemotherapy is effective against locally advanced rectal cancer [45].

Initiation of adjuvant chemotherapy within 8 weeks of TME is recommended based on a meta-analysis that reported that each 4-week delay in initiation of adjuvant chemotherapy resulted in significant decreases in overall survival (hazard ratio, 1.14; 95% confidence interval 1.10–1.17) and disease-free survival (hazard ratio, 1.14; 95% confidence interval, 1.10–1.18) [46]. These data have to be interpreted with caution, as worse outcomes in patients starting chemotherapy at later times may be confounded by significant comorbidities or surgical complications, which are linked to delays in initiation of therapy following surgery and to worse overall survival. While acknowledging potential confounding by age and comorbidities, we do recommend starting chemotherapy as soon as feasible after full recovery from surgery. It is important to highlight that up to a third of eligible patients with locally advanced rectal cancer never start adjuvant chemotherapy and less than half receive the full treatment course without interruptions or delay, due to either postoperative complications, slow recovery, or treatment refusal [47]. Even at specialty cancer centers, a sizable proportion of patients (as high as 17%) do not complete postoperative chemotherapy [48].

Optimal duration of adjuvant chemotherapy after proctectomy also remains undetermined. Based on extrapolation from the MOSAIC trial, which led to the adoption of 6 months of FOLFOX as the standard of care for locally advanced colon cancer, the National Comprehensive Cancer Network guidelines currently recommend a total of 6 months of chemotherapy for rectal cancer. Accounting for the 2 months of fluoropyrimidine chemotherapy administered concurrently with radiation prior to proctectomy, this translates to approximately 4 months of adjuvant FOLFOX.

Total Neoadjuvant Therapy

In the modern era, patients with rectal cancer more commonly experience distant metastatic disease than local recurrence, with more than 25% of stage II and III rectal cancers causing metastatic disease. Although neoadjuvant chemoradiation has been shown to decrease the incidence of local recurrence, overall survival and risk of distant metastases are not impacted by chemoradiation. In an effort to prevent distant disease and increase long-term survival, the early introduction of both chemotherapy and chemoradiation prior to surgery is being investigated. Theoretical benefits include earlier protection against dissemination of micrometastatic disease, delivery of chemotherapy to the primary tumor with undisrupted vasculature, tumor downstaging, less toxicity, and better adherence to prescribed treatment.

The novel concept of total neoadjuvant therapy (TNT), in which chemoradiation and chemotherapy are administered prior to surgery, has been shown to be safe and effective [49]. A recent retrospective study conducted at Memorial Sloan Kettering analyzed records of patients treated between 2009 and 2015. Of the 811 patients identified, 320 received chemoradiation with planned adjuvant chemotherapy, and 308 received TNT (induction FOLFOX-based chemotherapy followed by chemoradiation). Patients in the TNT cohort received greater percentages of the planned chemotherapy than those in the chemoradiation with planned adjuvant chemotherapy cohort. The rate of complete response, including both pathologic complete response in patients who underwent surgery and sustained clinical complete response for at least 12 months posttreatment in patients who did not undergo surgery, was 36% in the TNT cohort compared with 21% in the chemoradiation with planned adjuvant chemotherapy cohort. These findings provide additional support for TNT as a viable treatment strategy for rectal cancer. TNT may facilitate nonoperative treatment strategies aimed at organ preservation.

Nonoperative Management

Chemoradiation can lead to pCR, and selected patients with such response can potentially avoid surgery. This nonoperative management strategy is referred to as the watch-and-wait approach. Avoiding surgery can potentially lead to better functional outcomes and better quality of life. The largest systematic study on this approach was conducted in Brazil [50]. Of 361 patients treated with chemoradiation, 122 attained clinical complete response, and 99 (27%) had sustained complete regression for at least 1 year. Clinical complete response was defined as absence of residual mass or ulcer on clinical evaluation and endoscopy, as well as no residual tumor on imaging studies. Of the 99 patients with sustained complete regression, only 5% developed endoluminal recurrences, none developed pelvic regional recurrence, and 8% developed metastatic disease. Of the 5 patients who developed endoluminal recurrences, 3 underwent salvage APR or low anterior resection, while 2 declined radical surgery and underwent local excision or brachytherapy. The 5-year rates of overall and disease-free survival were 93% and 85%, respectively. Retrospective studies conducted in the United Kingdom, the Netherlands, and the United States reported similar findings, suggesting that watch-and-wait can be a reasonable option in carefully selected and closely followed patients [51, 52]. A number of multi-institutional prospective observational studies and Phase II trials are currently testing the feasibility of incorporating nonoperative management in multimodal treatment of rectal cancer, but at the present time, nonoperative management should be considered experimental and should ideally take place in the setting of a clinical trial.

Conclusion

Decades of basic science and clinical research have resulted in a multitude of treatment options for patients with rectal cancer, providing dramatic improvement in local control and patient survival. Multidisciplinary management of rectal cancer – involving surgical, radiation, and medical oncologists; pathologists; and radiologists – has been shown to improve clinical decision-making and clinical outcomes. The ability to differentiate levels of risk for tumor recurrence and survival prognoses based on baseline tumor characteristics and response to therapy will enable future tailoring of treatment to disease biology to reduce morbidity and improve outcomes.

Acknowledgments The authors thank Arthur Gelmis, editor in the Colorectal Surgery Service at the Memorial Sloan Kettering Cancer Center, for his assistance in editing this chapter.

References

1. Extramural depth of tumor invasion at thin-section MR in patients with rectal cancer: results of the MERCURY study. Radiology. 2007;243(1):132–9.
2. Glynne-Jones R, Wyrwicz L, Tiret E, Brown G, Rodel C, Cervantes A, et al. Rectal cancer: ESMO Clinical Practice Guidelines for diagnosis, treatment and follow-up. Ann Oncol. 2017;28(suppl_4):iv22–40.

3. Callender GG, Das P, Rodriguez-Bigas MA, Skibber JM, Crane CH, Krishnan S, et al. Local excision after preoperative chemoradiation results in an equivalent outcome to total mesorectal excision in selected patients with T3 rectal cancer. Ann Surg Oncol. 2010;17(2):441–7.
4. Shin YS, Yoon YS, Lim SB, Yu CS, Kim TW, Chang HM, et al. Preoperative chemoradiotherapy followed by local excision in clinical T2N0 rectal cancer. Radiat Oncol J. 2016;34(3):177–85.
5. Nair RM, Siegel EM, Chen DT, Fulp WJ, Yeatman TJ, Malafa MP, et al. Long-term results of transanal excision after neoadjuvant chemoradiation for T2 and T3 adenocarcinomas of the rectum. J Gastrointest Surg. 2008;12(10):1797–805; discussion 805–6.
6. Garcia-Aguilar J, Renfro LA, Chow OS, Shi Q, Carrero XW, Lynn PB, et al. Organ preservation for clinical T2N0 distal rectal cancer using neoadjuvant chemoradiotherapy and local excision (ACOSOG Z6041): results of an open-label, single-arm, multi-institutional, phase 2 trial. Lancet Oncol. 2015;16(15):1537–46.
7. Maslekar S, Sharma A, Macdonald A, Gunn J, Monson JR, Hartley JE. Mesorectal grades predict recurrences after curative resection for rectal cancer. Dis Colon Rectum. 2007;50(2):168–75.
8. Nagtegaal ID, van de Velde CJ, van der Worp E, Kapiteijn E, Quirke P, van Krieken JH. Macroscopic evaluation of rectal cancer resection specimen: clinical significance of the pathologist in quality control. J Clin Oncol. 2002;20(7):1729–34.
9. Rullier E, Denost Q, Vendrely V, Rullier A, Laurent C. Low rectal cancer: classification and standardization of surgery. Dis Colon Rectum. 2013;56(5):560–7.
10. Bonjer HJ, Deijen CL, Haglind EA. Randomized trial of laparoscopic versus open surgery for rectal cancer. N Engl J Med. 2015;373(2):194.
11. Stevenson ARL, Solomon MJ, Brown CSB, Lumley JW, Hewett P, Clouston AD, et al. Disease-free survival and local recurrence after laparoscopic-assisted resection or open resection for rectal cancer: the Australasian laparoscopic cancer of the rectum randomized clinical trial. Ann Surg. 2019;269(4):596–602.
12. Jayne D, Pigazzi A, Marshall H, Croft J, Corrigan N, Copeland J, et al. Effect of robotic-assisted vs conventional laparoscopic surgery on risk of conversion to open laparotomy among patients undergoing resection for rectal cancer: the ROLARR randomized clinical trial. JAMA. 2017;318(16):1569–80.
13. Penna M, Hompes R, Arnold S, Wynn G, Austin R, Warusavitarne J, et al. Transanal total mesorectal excision: international registry results of the first 720 cases. Ann Surg. 2017;266(1):111–7.
14. Lee GC, Sylla P. Shifting paradigms in minimally invasive surgery: applications of transanal natural orifice transluminal endoscopic surgery in colorectal surgery. Clin Colon Rectal Surg. 2015;28(3):181–93.
15. Dietz DW. Multidisciplinary management of rectal cancer: the OSTRICH. J Gastrointest Surg. 2013;17(10):1863–8.
16. Monson JRT, Dietz DW, Boughey JC, You YN. Improving rectal cancer outcomes through advocacy, education, and research: the OSTRiCh Consortium and the new NAPRC. Bull Am Coll Surg. 2016;101(11):45–6.
17. Karagkounis G, Stocchi L, Lavery IC, Liska D, Gorgun E, Veniero J, et al. Multidisciplinary conference and clinical management of rectal cancer. J Am Coll Surg. 2018;226(5):874–80.
18. Khani MH, Smedh K. Centralization of rectal cancer surgery improves long-term survival. Colorectal Dis. 2010;12(9):874–9.
19. Bulow S, Harling H, Iversen LH, Ladelund S. Improved survival after rectal cancer in Denmark. Colorectal Dis. 2010;12(7 Online):e37–42.
20. Rombeau JL, Collins JP, Turnbull RB Jr. Left-sided colectomy with retroileal colorectal anastomosis. Arch Surg. 1978;113(8):1004–5.
21. MacFarlane JK, Ryall RD, Heald RJ. Mesorectal excision for rectal cancer. Lancet. 1993;341(8843):457–60.
22. Enker WE, Thaler HT, Cranor ML, Polyak T. Total mesorectal excision in the operative treatment of carcinoma of the rectum. J Am Coll Surg. 1995;181(4):335–46.

23. Arbman G, Nilsson E, Hallbook O, Sjodahl R. Local recurrence following total mesorectal excision for rectal cancer. Br J Surg. 1996;83(3):375–9.
24. Bjerkeset T, Edna TH. Rectal cancer: the influence of type of operation on local recurrence and survival. Eur J Surg. 1996;162(8):643–8.
25. Heald RJ, Moran BJ, Ryall RD, Sexton R, MacFarlane JK. Rectal cancer: the Basingstoke experience of total mesorectal excision, 1978-1997. Arch Surg. 1998;133(8):894–9.
26. Wibe A, Moller B, Norstein J, Carlsen E, Wiig JN, Heald RJ, et al. A national strategic change in treatment policy for rectal cancer – implementation of total mesorectal excision as routine treatment in Norway. A national audit. Dis Colon Rectum. 2002;45(7):857–66.
27. Kapiteijn E, Putter H, van de Velde CJ. Impact of the introduction and training of total mesorectal excision on recurrence and survival in rectal cancer in the Netherlands. Br J Surg. 2002;89(9):1142–9.
28. Martling AL, Holm T, Rutqvist LE, Moran BJ, Heald RJ, Cedemark B. Effect of a surgical training programme on outcome of rectal cancer in the County of Stockholm. Stockholm Colorectal Cancer Study Group, Basingstoke Bowel Cancer Research Project. Lancet. 2000;356(9224):93–6.
29. Camilleri-Brennan J, Steele RJ. Quality of life after treatment for rectal cancer. Br J Surg. 1998;85(8):1036–43.
30. Enker WE. Potency, cure, and local control in the operative treatment of rectal cancer. Arch Surg. 1992;127(12):1396–401; discussion 402.
31. Havenga K, Enker WE, McDermott K, Cohen AM, Minsky BD, Guillem J. Male and female sexual and urinary function after total mesorectal excision with autonomic nerve preservation for carcinoma of the rectum. J Am Coll Surg. 1996;182(6):495–502.
32. Shirouzu K, Ogata Y, Araki Y. Oncologic and functional results of total mesorectal excision and autonomic nerve-preserving operation for advanced lower rectal cancer. Dis Colon Rectum. 2004;47(9):1442–7.
33. Sauer R, Becker H, Hohenberger W, Rodel C, Wittekind C, Fietkau R, et al. Preoperative versus postoperative chemoradiotherapy for rectal cancer. N Engl J Med. 2004;351(17):1731–40.
34. Sauer R, Liersch T, Merkel S, Fietkau R, Hohenberger W, Hess C, et al. Preoperative versus postoperative chemoradiotherapy for locally advanced rectal cancer: results of the German CAO/ARO/AIO-94 randomized phase III trial after a median follow-up of 11 years. J Clin Oncol. 2012;30(16):1926–33.
35. Roh MS, Colangelo LH, O'Connell MJ, Yothers G, Deutsch M, Allegra CJ, et al. Preoperative multimodality therapy improves disease-free survival in patients with carcinoma of the rectum: NSABP R-03. J Clin Oncol. 2009;27(31):5124–30.
36. Bosset JF, Calais G, Mineur L, Maingon P, Radosevic-Jelic L, Daban A, et al. Enhanced tumorocidal effect of chemotherapy with preoperative radiotherapy for rectal cancer: preliminary results--EORTC 22921. J Clin Oncol. 2005;23(24):5620–7.
37. Bosset JF, Collette L, Calais G, Mineur L, Maingon P, Radosevic-Jelic L, et al. Chemotherapy with preoperative radiotherapy in rectal cancer. N Engl J Med. 2006;355(11):1114–23.
38. Gerard JP, Conroy T, Bonnetain F, Bouche O, Chapet O, Closon-Dejardin MT, et al. Preoperative radiotherapy with or without concurrent fluorouracil and leucovorin in T3-4 rectal cancers: results of FFCD 9203. J Clin Oncol. 2006;24(28):4620–5.
39. Ngan SY, Burmeister B, Fisher RJ, Solomon M, Goldstein D, Joseph D, et al. Randomized trial of short-course radiotherapy versus long-course chemoradiation comparing rates of local recurrence in patients with T3 rectal cancer: Trans-Tasman Radiation Oncology Group trial 01.04. J Clin Oncol. 2012;30(31):3827–33.
40. Erlandsson J, Holm T, Pettersson D, Berglund A, Cedermark B, Radu C, et al. Optimal fractionation of preoperative radiotherapy and timing to surgery for rectal cancer (Stockholm III): a multicentre, randomised, non-blinded, phase 3, non-inferiority trial. Lancet Oncol. 2017;18(3):336–46.
41. Mirnezami R, Chang GJ, Das P, Chandrakumaran K, Tekkis P, Darzi A, et al. Intraoperative radiotherapy in colorectal cancer: systematic review and meta-analysis of techniques, long-term outcomes, and complications. Surg Oncol. 2013;22(1):22–35.

42. Taylor FG, Quirke P, Heald RJ, Moran B, Blomqvist L, Swift I, et al. Preoperative high-resolution magnetic resonance imaging can identify good prognosis stage I, II, and III rectal cancer best managed by surgery alone: a prospective, multicenter, European study. Ann Surg. 2011;253(4):711–9.
43. Schrag D, Weiser MR, Goodman KA, Gonen M, Hollywood E, Cercek A, et al. Neoadjuvant chemotherapy without routine use of radiation therapy for patients with locally advanced rectal cancer: a pilot trial. J Clin Oncol. 2014;32(6):513–8.
44. Weiser MR, Fichera A, Schrag D, Boughey JC, You YN. Progress in the PROSPECT trial: precision treatment for rectal cancer? Bull Am Coll Surg. 2015;100(4):51–2.
45. Petersen SH, Harling H, Kirkeby LT, Wille-Jorgensen P, Mocellin S. Postoperative adjuvant chemotherapy in rectal cancer operated for cure. Cochrane Database Syst Rev. 2012;(3):CD004078.
46. Biagi JJ, Raphael MJ, Mackillop WJ, Kong W, King WD, Booth CM. Association between time to initiation of adjuvant chemotherapy and survival in colorectal cancer: a systematic review and meta-analysis. JAMA. 2011;305(22):2335–42.
47. Haynes AB, You YN, Hu CY, Eng C, Kopetz ES, Rodriguez-Bigas MA, et al. Postoperative chemotherapy use after neoadjuvant chemoradiotherapy for rectal cancer: Analysis of Surveillance, Epidemiology, and End Results-Medicare data, 1998-2007. Cancer. 2014;120(8):1162–70.
48. Khrizman P, Niland JC, ter Veer A, Milne D, Bullard Dunn K, Carson WE 3rd, et al. Postoperative adjuvant chemotherapy use in patients with stage II/III rectal cancer treated with neoadjuvant therapy: a national comprehensive cancer network analysis. J Clin Oncol. 2013;31(1):30–8.
49. Cercek A, Roxburgh CSD, Strombom P, Smith JJ, Temple LKF, Nash GM, et al. Adoption of total neoadjuvant therapy for locally advanced rectal cancer. JAMA Oncol. 2018;4(6):e180071.
50. Habr-Gama A, Perez RO, Proscurshim I, Campos FG, Nadalin W, Kiss D, et al. Patterns of failure and survival for nonoperative treatment of stage c0 distal rectal cancer following neoadjuvant chemoradiation therapy. J Gastrointest Surg. 2006;10(10):1319–28; discussion 28–9.
51. Smith JJ, Strombom P, Chow OS, Roxburgh CS, Lynn P, Eaton A, et al. Assessment of a watch-and-wait strategy for rectal cancer in patients with a complete response after neoadjuvant therapy. JAMA Oncol. 2019;5:e185896.
52. Renehan AG, Malcomson L, Emsley R, Gollins S, Maw A, Myint AS, et al. Watch-and-wait approach versus surgical resection after chemoradiotherapy for patients with rectal cancer (the OnCoRe project): a propensity-score matched cohort analysis. Lancet Oncol. 2016;17(2):174–83.
53. Valinluck Lao V, Fichera A. Endorectal ultrasound. In: Chang GJ, editor. Rectal cancer: modern approaches to treatment. Cham: Springer International Publishing; 2018.
54. Ferrari L, Fichera A. Neoadjuvant chemoradiation therapy and pathological complete response in rectal cancer. Gastroenterol Rep (Oxf). 2015;3(4):277–88.
55. Hakiman H, Boostrom S, Fleshman J. Total mesorectal excision with autonomic nerve preservation: "optimized surgery". In: Long WE, Reddy V, Audisio RA, editors. Modern management of cancer of the rectum. 2nd ed. Cham: Springer International Publishing; 2015

Laparoscopic Low Anterior Resection for Rectal Cancer: TME Planes and Surgery of the Upper and Mid-Rectum

23

Eric M. Haas and Amanda V. Hayman

Introduction and Rationale

Laparoscopic low anterior resection for rectal cancer is one of the more challenging minimally invasive colorectal procedures to master. The confined and narrow spaces of the pelvis often limit visualization, exposure, and access. Additionally, it is imperative to maintain proper planes of dissection to achieve a sound oncologic resection. Straying from the embryologic planes may result in a field obscured with nuisance bleeding and injury to critical structures. It is therefore essential to approach each case in a stepwise fashion with a clear understanding of the anatomical considerations as well as the precise location of the tumor.

The benefits of laparoscopy are well known and include less pain, earlier return of bowel function, shorter length of stay, and fewer wound complications. With modern techniques and newer technologies, there is rarely a case that cannot be approached using laparoscopic technique. More challenging patients including those with multiple medical morbidities, extreme obesity, or prior open abdominal procedures, often tend to benefit the most. Therefore, our initial approach is to gain access laparoscopically and assess if all or parts of the procedure can be accomplished in this fashion to limit the morbidity of a large incision.

In the absence of locally advanced disease or a threatened circumferential resection margin (CRM), upper rectal tumors, and select mid-rectal tumors, are treated like colon cancers via upfront surgical resection, avoiding the morbidity of

E. M. Haas (✉)
Division of Colon and Rectal Surgery, Houston Methodist Hospital, Department of Surgery, Houston, TX, USA
e-mail: ehaasmd@houstoncolon.com

A. V. Hayman
The Oregon Clinic, Division of Gastrointestinal and Minimally Invasive Surgery, Oregon Health and Science University, Department of Surgery, Portland, OR, USA
e-mail: ahayman@orclinic.com

P. Sylla et al. (eds.), *The SAGES Manual of Colorectal Surgery*,
https://doi.org/10.1007/978-3-030-24812-3_23

neoadjuvant chemoradiotherapy. Standard oncologic vascular pedicle ligation of the inferior mesenteric artery (IMA) is performed with regional lymphadenectomy and is referred to as tumor-specific mesorectal excision (TSME).

However, the delineation between the upper and mid-rectum and the lower rectum can be controversial. Intraoperatively, the top of the rectum can be identified by where the taenias play and the epiploic appendages peter out. Obviously, this is not applicable preoperatively. If the tumor is large enough, it can be detected by CT or MRI, thus providing reliable anatomic landmarks, such as distance from the values of Houston or the sacral promontory. An approximation of the location of the anterior reflection, and thus the delineation between the sigmoid colon and the rectum, is a line drawn between the top of the sacral promontory and the bottom of the pubic symphysis. However, in many cases, the exact intraluminal borders of the tumor are not easily seen on cross-sectional imaging. Therefore, the most important initial step for the surgeon in the workup for a newly diagnosed rectal cancer is rigid proctoscopy. This is a much more reliable assessment of "true" distance from the anal verge than flexible endoscopy, which should not be solely relied upon for surgical planning. Marking the tumor distally via tattoo may also aid in identification, intraoperatively, especially if CO_2 colonoscopy is not readily available. The surgeon should also be aware, however, that occasionally tattoo marks can obscure the anatomical visualization during the minimally invasive procedure. Proctoscopy also allows the surgeon to determine in which quadrant(s) the tumor is located, which has implication during resection about what structures would be potentially threatened (i.e., an anterior-based tumor may closely abut or involve the prostate or vagina). Further, patient habitus may influence surgical approach. An obese, muscular man may have a longer anal canal, and thus the tumor may be closer to the top of the anal sphincters (aka the "anorectal ring") making a laparoscopic approach more difficult. Proctoscopy also allows for serial assessment of response to neoadjuvant treatment, as well as to detect recurrence during surveillance.

This chapter addresses rectal cancer involving the upper and mid-rectum and, despite many similarities, leaves out the most distal rectal cancer. For the purposes of this chapter, we define the lower rectum as the distal 5 cm, the mid-rectum from 6–11 cm, and the upper rectum as above 11 cm (or above the second valve of Houston). Most studies on rectal cancer define the top of the rectum as 15 cm from the anal verge [1]. There are several important distinctions between upper and middle rectal cancers. Upper rectal cancers are typically managed with upfront surgical resection. An adequate distal resection margin and mesorectal excision can be readily achieved with a laparoscopic technique. It is important to understand the anatomical concepts of a tumor-specific mesorectal excision (TSME). To achieve a TSME, a minimum of 2 cm distal margin on the rectum is required, as well as a 5 cm distal margin of the mesorectum [2, 3]. Care is taken to avoid the tendency to cone inward and divide across the mesentery within the required margins.

Mid-rectal cancers are more often subject to neoadjuvant chemoradiation therapy if determined to be locally advanced (Stage II or III disease, i.e., T3 and/or node-positive disease). TSME is not typically feasible for most tumors of the mid-rectum due to the constraints of the narrow pelvis and bulky mesentery of the mid-rectum. In most cases, a total mesorectal excision (TME) with low pelvic colorectal anastomosis is the most technically feasible approach to surgical resection of mid-rectal cancers. Minimally invasive techniques become much more cumbersome and difficult in these cases and are addressed in the chapters on principles of rectal cancer and robotic low anterior resection (Chaps. 22 and 24).

Indications and Contraindications

A laparoscopic TSME can be considered in many, but not all, patients. Patients with certain comorbidities, such as extreme obesity or severe pulmonary dysfunction, may not tolerate prolonged Trendelenburg positioning and/or insufflation, as can be seen intraoperatively by high airway pressures or CO_2 retention. The surgeon can choose to partially mitigate these concerns by using lower insufflation pressures (such as 10–12 mmHg instead of the standard 15), but this may still be insufficient. Another option is to perform only the splenic flexure mobilization laparoscopically, which typically uses reverse Trendelenburg positioning, and then completing the pelvic dissection via a Pfannenstiel or lower midline incision. In addition to these patient factors, there are also tumor characteristics that may make a laparoscopic approach more challenging: a large, bulky tumor or presence of a colonic stent can prevent adequate retraction and visualization. Occasionally, adding another assist port can help, but not always. Additionally, presence of a perforated tumor or involved radial margins may require dissection outside the standard TME planes. This can result in a bloodier field, impeding laparoscopic visualization. Further, ensuring a negative radial margin in the setting of extreme fibrosis, such as after an intense radiation reaction, reoperative surgery, or previous perforation, can be difficult without direct tactile feedback. However, except for patient intolerance of laparoscopy, the cases listed above are relative contraindications and highly depend on the skill of the individual surgeon.

If the surgeon is able to maintain the principles of adhering to the avascular mesorectal planes of dissection, ensure proper radial and distal margins, ensure proper lymph node harvest to the base of the inferior mesenteric artery (IMA), and ensure an intact specimen, the laparoscopic approach is appropriate.

Principles and Quality Benchmarks

Ultimately, regardless of the operative approach chosen by the surgeon, a quality oncologic outcome should never be sacrificed. The same quality oncologic benchmarks for TME apply to TSME. As per the National Comprehensive Cancer Network (NCCN) guidelines and National Accreditation Program in Rectal Cancer (NAPRC) standards, an adequate lymphadenectomy is a harvest of a minimum of 12 lymph nodes. The commonly accepted distances to be considered an adequate margin are as follows: radial (>1 mm), distal (2 cm), and mesenteric (5 cm) [3]. Although the exact factors that predispose for low anterior resection syndrome (bowel dysfunction characterized by stool clustering, increased frequency, urgency, or incomplete emptying) are multifactorial, taking care to preserve the paired hypogastric nerves that run along the back of the rectum distal to the sacral promontory may mitigate this risk. Because of this risk, it is important to preoperatively assess the patient's bowel function and at all future postoperative appointments. There are many validated questionnaires that assess patient-reported outcomes regarding bowel function, including the FIQOL (fecal incontinence quality of life), the MSKCC bowel function instrument, or the EORTC QOL questionnaire for colorectal cancer surgery (QLQ-CR38). Sexual function may also be impaired postoperatively, likely due to injury to the nervi erigentes that course horizontally near the lateral rectal stalks.

Although the surgeon will not be performing a complete mesorectal excision, the same avascular presacral plane needs to be maintained while keeping the fascia propria of the mesorectum intact. Similar to the surgical principles of a TME, it is essential to not "cone in" on the mesentery when planning where to perform the rectal transection. It is also essential to harvest the lymph nodes at the base of the IMA and maintain the dissection into the retroperitoneal planes along the superior rectal artery leading to the mesorectal dissection.

Preoperative Planning, Patient Workup, and Optimization

The initial workup includes serum CEA level and CT scan of the chest, abdomen, and pelvis to rule out metastatic disease as per NCCN guidelines. Rigid proctoscopy is performed to assess clinical features of the cancer including measurement of the precise distance from the anal verge. Locoregional staging evaluation is performed with MRI using a rectal cancer staging protocol, unless MRI is medically contraindicated. Per NAPRC guidelines, endorectal ultrasound is considered an inferior staging option, due to the lack of reproducibility and inability to serially assess radial margins in a multidisciplinary fashion. [4] Based on the assessment, decision is rendered to proceed with neoadjuvant therapy followed by surgical resection versus immediate surgical resection. Each rectal cancer case should be presented for consensus recommendations in the setting of a multidisciplinary tumor conference.

Managing perioperative risks are essential. All diabetic patients must have good perioperative glucose management, as reflected by a preoperative Hba1c level. If elevated (>7.5%), aggressive comanagement with their endocrinologist is recommended. Additional modifiable risk factors such as tobacco and alcohol use should be addressed with a cessation program in the allotted time period prior to the resection. Nutritional optimization should also be addressed and maximized, and obese patients are encouraged to lose excess weight. Preoperatively, all patients undergo oral antibiotics and mechanical bowel preparation, as well as a standardized enhanced recovery protocol that includes multimodal pain regimen, early feeding, goal-directed fluid therapy to minimize IV fluids, and early mobilization. For additional details, please refer to Chaps. 7 and 8 on enhanced recovery protocols in colorectal surgery.

Although we do not routinely utilize ureteral stents, consideration of placement is important in cases that involve difficult pelvic anatomy such as a redo pelvic surgery or selected patients with T4 disease or history of perforated tumor. Lastly, if an ileostomy is planned (i.e., when performing a low pelvic anastomosis within 5 cm from the anal verge or following neoadjuvant radiation or in the setting of malnutrition or immunosuppression), patients should meet with a wound ostomy nurse preoperatively for education and stoma marking.

Room Setup and Patient Positioning

The most common laparoscopic approach is multiport surgery with the placement of four or five ports. Reduced port techniques are feasible and included below. Single-port laparoscopic surgery can be performed, but anatomical constraints of the lower pelvic anatomy result in less-than-ideal exposure and access with this approach. Another approach, which can be especially useful is the morbidly obese, is a hand-assisted technique via either a Pfannenstiel or lower midline approach. The patient is secured to safely enable steep Trendelenburg and left-side elevation throughout the procedure. This should be ensured by a preoperative "Trendelenburg test."

Intraoperative Positioning (Fig. 23.1)

- Both arms tucked
- Modified lithotomy or split leg
- 5 (or 10) mm camera port at umbilicus
- 5 mm ports in right upper quadrant (RUQ) and right lower quadrant (RLQ)
- Optional 5 mm port in left lower quadrant (LLQ) or subxiphoid

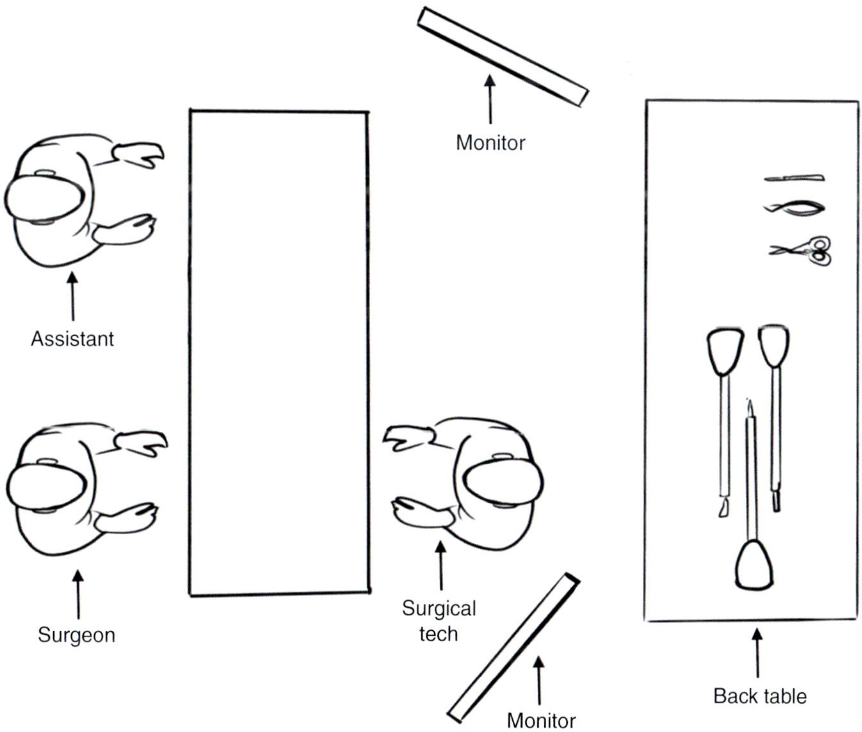

Fig. 23.1 Surgeon and room setup

- Pfannenstiel incision for extraction
- Surgeon and assist on patient's right side
- Surgical tech and sterile instrument table on patient's left side
- Monitor angled at left shoulder and left lower extremity

Port Placement (Fig. 23.2)

- If you prefer a 10 mm camera, the umbilical port will need to be upsized to a 12 mm port size. On occasion, placing the camera in another port may be required, and these ports will also need to be upsized or an additional 5 mm camera opened.
- The midline 5 mm port can usually be hidden in the upper ridge of the umbilicus; however, if the distance between the umbilicus and suprapubic region is relatively short, then the optical field of view may be limited. In these cases, placing the midline port a few centimeters superior the umbilicus is an option.
- If planning to fashion an ileostomy, the 12 mm RLQ can be placed at the lateral margin of the predetermined ileostomy site. Care should be taken not to place the

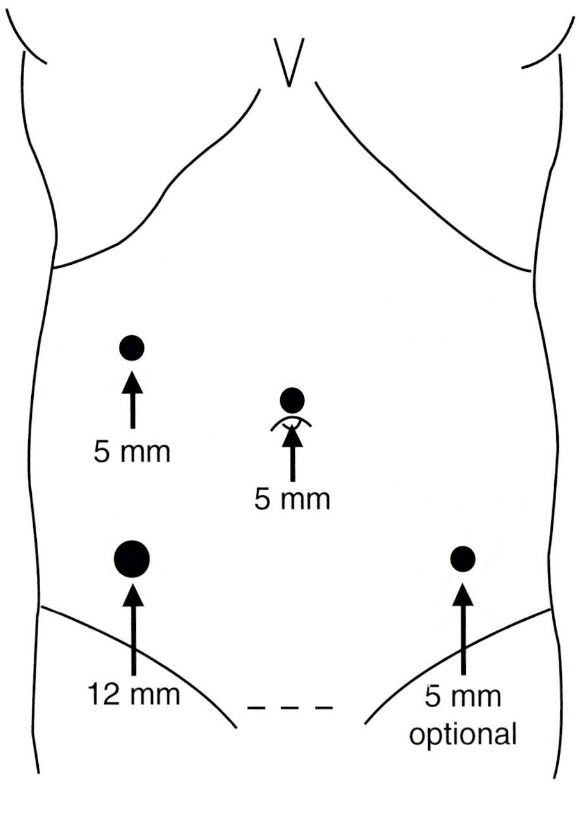

Fig. 23.2 Port placement

12 mm RLQ port adjacent to the planned ileostomy site as this may result in difficulty pouching the stoma.
- It is recommended to close the fascia on all 12 mm port sites due to hernia risk.

Other Equipment/Incisions

- *Extraction site:* Several options exist for the extraction site. We prefer a Pfannenstiel incision because it can usually also allow direct access to the anastomosis in cases in which repair of an anastomotic defect is required. It is also associated with a very low rate of hernia risk. Other extraction sites, however, can be used such as an umbilical site or the left lower quadrant. In cases in which we plan to perform an ileostomy, we use the ileostomy site as extraction site.
- *Camera*: A 5 mm 30 degree or flexible tip camera is preferred.
- *Instruments*: Atraumatic bowel graspers are required. It is recommended to have extended length graspers available.
- *Energy devices*: Monopolar energy devices include the L or J hook, spatula, or scissors with cautery. Thermal energy can include various devices designed to control vessels up to 7 mm size, such as a bipolar device or ultrasonic device.

Operative Technique and Surgical Steps

Planes of the Mesorectum

Both medial-to-lateral and lateral-to-medial approaches are utilized during the laparoscopic procedure. The procedure is preferably initiated in a medial-to-lateral fashion to identify the critical landmarks and develop the proper planes of mesenteric dissection. The medial side of the mesentery is exposed by elevating the rectosigmoid with a bowel grasper to identify the thin base near the sacral promontory. The peritoneum is carefully scored and the avascular presacral plane is dissected. Pneumodissection in the alveolar tissue signifies the correct plane between presacral fascia and the fascia propria of the rectum. The superior rectal artery (SRA) is identified and elevated to further expose the plane of dissection (Fig. 23.3). The left ureter and gonadal vessels are exposed very early in the dissection. The avascular plane is dissected further while elevating the SRA taking care not to injury the nerves in the deeper plane. Dissection continues laterally in the retroperitoneal plane toward the white line of Toldt, inferiorly to the level of the sacral promontory and superiorly toward the base of the IMA. At this level, the peritoneal plane is scored in an upside-down "U" fashion, starting at the base of the bifurcation, sweeping up as it follows the vessel's course into the pelvis, and then extending distally to where the anterior reflection terminates laterally in the pararectal gutter.

The plane between the retroperitoneal structures posteriorly and the mesorectum anteriorly is then developed. Dissection from the CO_2 insufflation again helps identify this avascular plane; after infiltrating into the tissues, they appear as white,

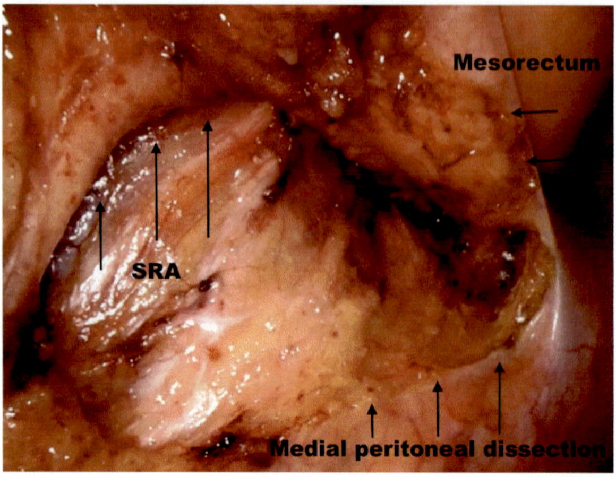

Fig. 23.3 Medial-to-lateral dissection with elevation of the superior rectal artery (SRA) and exposure of the retroperitoneal plane

crackly fibers. After sweeping over the sacral promontory from right to left, it is important to remember that the lateral retroperitoneal structures of interest, specifically the ureter, gonadal vessels, and internal iliac artery and vein, lie slightly superior to the presacral fascia. Therefore, the surgeon has to be careful to not proceed in so linear a fashion as to injure these structures. The dissection plane will be identified quite high on the edge of the mesorectum when dissecting the lateral-most area.

In order to avoid creating a tunnel when performing the above dissection, the surgeon should periodically reexamine the right peritoneal edge and continue to open up the triangle that forms between the aorta and IMA pedicle, scoring the peritoneum in a radial fashion right up to the IMA take off. The surgeon will encounter small bridging nerves in this area. These should be preserved if possible or ligated as anteriorly as possible.

In order to preserve planes and perform a meticulous dissection, many use hot scissors, L hook, or thermal energy device tip to carefully dissect between planes. The use of thermal or bipolar energy is typically not used to establish the planes of dissection and is reserved to control bleeding or division of vascular pedicles.

Once the vascular pedicle has been adequately skeletonized, and the surgeon has ensured that the left retroperitoneal structures at risk (i.e., ureter, gonadal vein) are lateral, the vessel can be divided (Fig. 23.4). Either a low (preserving the left colic (LCA) and/or sigmoid branches) or high ligation of the IMA and inferior mesenteric vein (IMV) is then performed (Table 23.1). If performing a low ligation, care is taken to dissect the mesenteric lymph nodes in the fatty tissue along the base of the IMA and draw this tissue into the resection margins so as not to leave behind draining lymph nodes (Fig. 23.5).

The surgeon then continues the mesenteric transection up to the site of planned proximal colonic division, which can be immediately performed via endoscopic stapler or via the extraction site. In the case of a particularly bulky colorectal mesentery, early bowel division can improve visualization when performing the pelvic dissection.

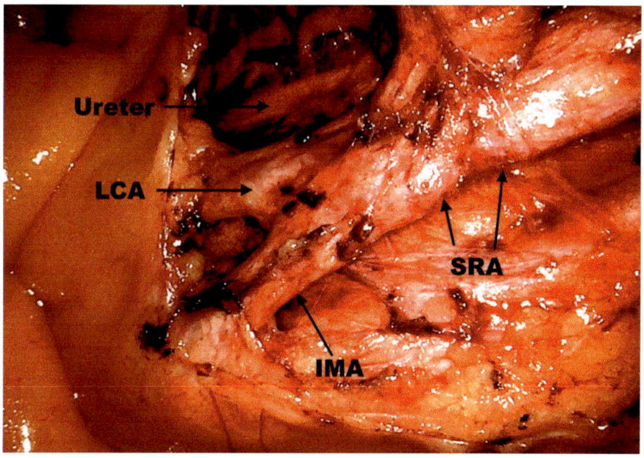

Fig. 23.4 Isolation of the inferior mesenteric artery (IMA) with dissection of the para-aortic lymph nodes

Table 23.1 Oncologic and functional outcomes of high versus low IMA ligation during LAR for rectal cancer

Matsuda et al. *GI tumors* 2017 [5]	*N* = 100, '08-'11. RCT: high vs. low ligation in LAR for rectal cancer	NS: OS, DFS (including stage III), # LN 16.7 vs. 14.9
Matsuda et al. *BJS* 2015 [6]	*N* = 100, '08-'11, TCT: high vs. low ligation in LAR for rectal caner	NS: defecatory dysfunction, FIQOL, fecal incontinence, anastomotic leak, 16% vs. 10% ($p = 0.42$)
Fujii, et al. *BJS* Open [7]	*N* = 331, '06-'12, RCT: high vs. low ligation	NS: anastomotic leak, 17.7% vs. 16.3%
Mari et al. *Ann Surg* 2018. (HIGHLOW trial) [8]	*N* = 214, '14-'16, RCT: high vs. low ligation	Low ligation: significant for better continence, fewer urinary symptoms ($p < 0.05$ @ 1 and 9 months), better QOL and sexual function NS: anastomotic leak: 8.1% vs. 6.7%

RCT randomized controlled trial, *OS* overall survival, *DFS* disease-free survival, *FIQOL* fecal incontinence quality of life, *NS* not significant, *LN* lymph nodes

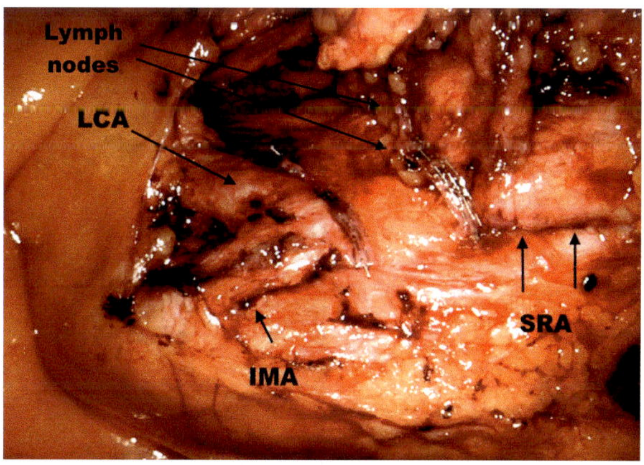

Fig. 23.5 Low IMA ligation with lymph nodes in specimen and preservation of the LCA

Splenic Flexure Mobilization

Additional length of the proximal colon may be needed to perform the anastomosis in a tension-free fashion. If so, we generally use the sub-IMV approach, either before or after IMA ligation, to accomplish this. With this technique, the patient is placed in slight reverse Trendelenburg position. The key is to carefully sweep the small intestine right lateral and cephalad to expose the ligament of Treitz. It is helpful to have the assistant retract the transverse colon cephalad to expose this area. The surgeon then identifies the IMV and incises the peritoneum in a horizontal fashion posterior to the vein along border of the ligament of Treitz. The retroperitoneal plane deep to the vein is then developed, and the vein is isolated and divided. The borders of the retroperitoneal dissection plane are the white line of Toldt along the descending colon (lateral), the inferior border of the pancreas (superior), and the origin the left colic artery (inferior). When dividing the IMV, allow for 1–2 cm cuff of vessel to avoid retraction of a bleeding vein beneath the pancreas should ligation be inadequate. We have found that the sub-IMV technique allows for easier identification of the dissection planes around the pedicle. For more details on various approaches for splenic flexure take down, please refer to Chapter 4 on splenic flexure release.

Lateral Dissection

Prior to starting the pelvic dissection, we then complete the lateral dissection. We initiate this dissection along the sigmoid colon and continue in a cranial fashion. If the sub-IMV approach has been accomplished, the peritoneal attachments will be well defined and separated from the retroperitoneal plane. The best way to accomplish the lateral dissection is to have the assistant gently retract the proximal colon medial and cephalad to expose and stretch the peritoneal refection. The surgeon uses an atraumatic instrument to push the colon medially for counter-traction (it is important to guide trainees with this technique as their instincts are often to traumatically grasp the mesentery), putting the peritoneal attachments on tension (Fig. 23.6). This

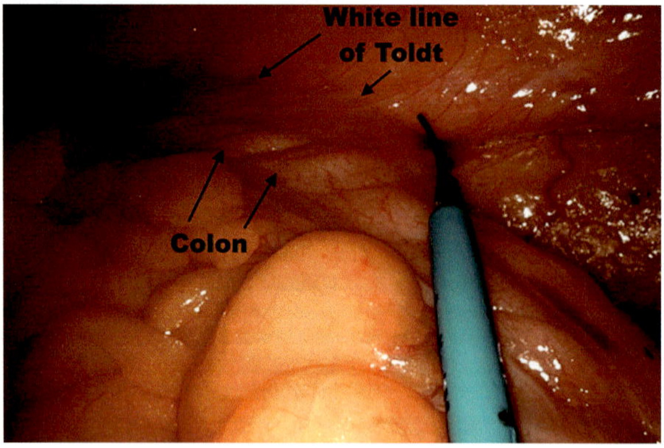

Fig. 23.6 The colon is retracted to stretch the peritoneal reflection for lateral to medial dissection along the white line of Toldt

will allow for efficient division of these attachments all the way up to the splenic flexure, staying just medial to Gerota's fascia.

One helpful tip is that the peritoneum over the lateral retroperitoneal structures appears slightly pink, as opposed to the peritoneum over the colon mesentery which appears slightly yellow. In order to maintain the correct plane, it is advised to score 1 mm on the yellow fat to avoid stripping the peritoneum off the side wall.

This technique is continued proximally around the splenic flexure, staying close to the colon, to enter the lesser sac. As we approach the splenocolic ligament, we often switch from hot scissors to a thermal energy device such as a bipolar device or harmonic scalpel to minimize thermal spread and achieve adequate hemostasis. Dissection is continued until entry into the lesser sac is achieved, usually marked by visualization of the posterior wall of the stomach. If the colon is closely adhered to the spleen or exposure is otherwise limited, we will change our approach and attack it proximally. The assistant retracts the mid-transverse colon omentum cephalad, while the surgeon pulls inferiorly on the transverse colon tenia. The omentum is then dissected off the colon until the lesser sac is opened. This dissection plane is carried distally until it meets the descending colon plane. Typically, there will be a few more attachments anterior to Gerota's fascia that will need to be ligated.

Lastly, we return our attention to the rectosigmoid colon and release the lateral attachments at the intersigmoid fold, taking care to avoid injury to the left gonadal vein and left ureter. Continue the peritoneal release as distally as possible by retracting the rectum medially and cephalad to expose the left pararectal gutter (Fig. 23.7). We score the peritoneum up and over the lateral edge of sacral promontory, being careful to stay just medial to the peritoneal edge. We perform the contralateral peritoneal release on the right during the IMA pedicle ligation (Fig. 23.8). Remember from embryology that the colon was a midline structure. Especially for low colorectal anastomoses, splenic flexure mobilization is not complete until the colon is able to be fully mobilized to the midline.

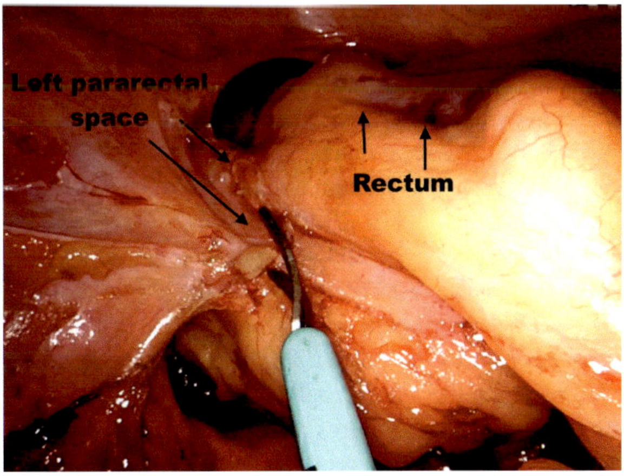

Fig. 23.7 The rectum is retracted medially to expose the left pararectal gutter

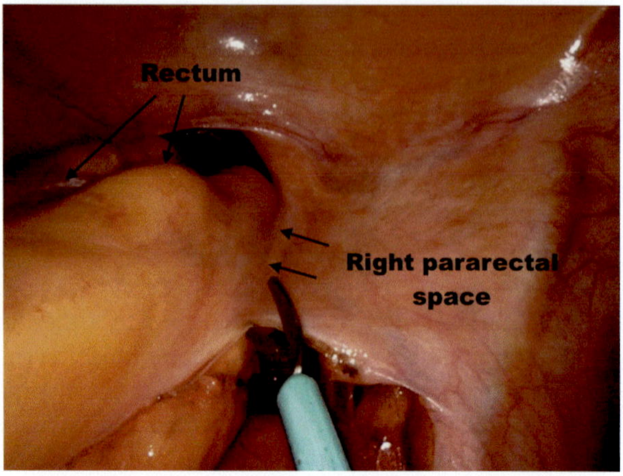

Fig. 23.8 Exposure and release of the right pararectal peritoneal attachments

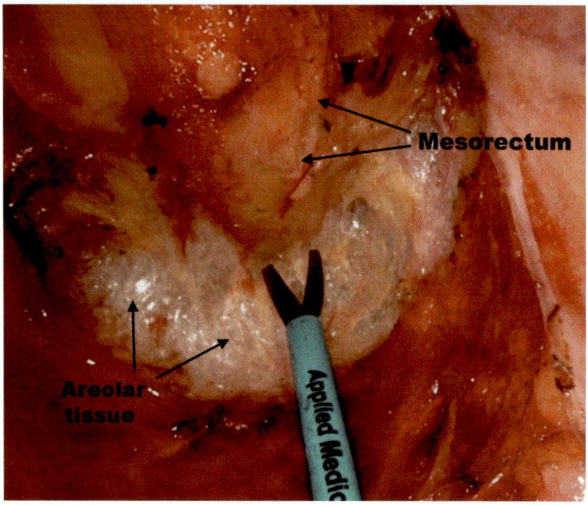

Fig. 23.9 Dissection in the avascular presacral plane

Pelvic Dissection

Dissection continues in the presacral mesorectal plane from the sacral promontory toward the retrosacral fascia. Care is taken to maintain the correct dissection plane identified by the avascular alveolar tissue while keeping the investing fascia of mesorectum intact (Fig. 23.9). The surgeon scores the peritoneum where the blood pools along the right and left pararectal gutters, until the anterior reflection is reached. With the assistant grasping the sigmoid, the surgeon then lifts the rectum with a blunt instrument and dissects in the posterior plane up and over the sacral promontory into the pelvis. The lateral stalks of the rectum are divided with hot cautery. Next, the anterior reflection of the rectum is scored and the plane between the anterior pelvic strictures (seminal vesicles in a man and vagina in a woman) and the anterior wall of the rectum is developed until the rectum has been adequately mobilized based on the location of the tumor. In the case of an upper rectal tumor, at least 2 centimeters of distal margin and 5 centimeters of mesenteric margin are required. A tangential resection across the mesorectum is performed with the aid of thermal energy device to control the mesenteric vessels. Care is taken to keep the investing fascia of the mesorectum intact and to avoid the tendency to cone into the mesenteric envelope.

Dividing the Rectum

During specimen division, the surgeon must decide whether to divide the mesentery or the bowel lumen first. Typically, the mesentery is initially divided. This is performed in a tangential fashion using thermal energy device with care taken not to injure the rectal wall. A reticulating linear stapler is placed though the 12 mm RLQ port, and the rectal wall is stapled and divided. It is important to compress the bowel wall in a linear fashion, and use of a second staple cartridge load is often necessary. In cases of a particularly bulky mesorectum and/or narrow male pelvis, dividing the bowel first can be helpful. A tunnel beneath the bowel wall is carefully created by developing a plane between the bowel wall and the mesentery. The reticulating linear stapler slides into this plane, and the bowel is then divided in one or two loads. The mesorectum is now readily exposed for division.

Alternatively, one can widen the Pfannestiel extraction incision and perform division of the bowel and mesentery under direct nonlaparoscopic access. This should be reserved for large bulky tumor or otherwise unfavorable anatomy.

The most important aspect of this portion of the case is to maintain adequate distal and circumferential resection margins. A proper distal margin of at least 2 cm can be ensured by concomitant intraoperative endoscopic visualization of the tumor. Again, it is important to achieve a 5 cm mesenteric margin due to the vagaries of local lymph node drainage (Fig. 23.10).

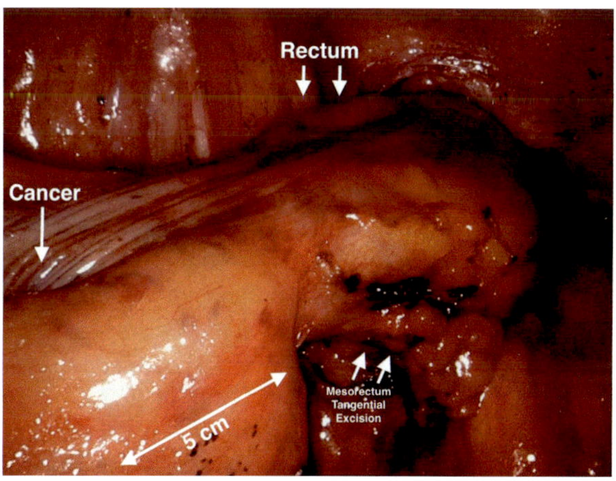

Fig. 23.10 Tumor-specific mesorectal excision for showing 5 cm mesenteric margin

Specimen Extraction and Creating the Anastomosis

We utilize a small Pfannenstiel incision for our extraction site to minimize pain, hernia rate, and improve cosmesis. Generally, we also place and secure the anvil of the circular stapler into the proximal end of colon via this site. The assistant then places the circular stapler through the rectum and opens the stapler just anterior to the rectal staple line. The anvil is then attached to the head of the stapler, which is closed and then actuated. The patient is then taken out of Trendelenburg and the pelvis filled with saline, submerging the anastomosis. The assistant advances a flexible or rigid endoscope past the anastomosis under direct visualization to assess for anastomotic integrity and hemostasis while insufflating. The operating surgeon assesses for any bubbling from the anastomosis, indicating a potential leak. Generally, for upper and mid-rectal tumors, we do not perform a diverting loop ileostomy unless there are poor prognostic features of healing, most commonly in the background of a radiated field.

Pitfalls and Troubleshooting

When to Convert

Typically, the most difficult portion of the case is the pelvic dissection, especially when operating in a postradiated or postoperative field or in the presence of a bulky, locally advanced, or previously perforated tumor. In these cases, we still commence the procedure with a minimally invasive approach performing the splenic flexure, sub-IMV dissection and colon mobilization laparoscopically, then performing the remainder of the pelvic dissection and specimen extraction through the Pfannenstiel extraction incision. Although for novices, laparoscopic dissection and exposure of challenging anatomy or splenic flexure takedown may be daunting and result in early conversion to open surgery, with experience this approach will become more routine. However, as with difficult low pelvic dissections, although conversion to open may allow for more effective retraction and counter-traction, visualization is often sacrificed, due to the loss of magnification and high-definition imaging supplied by modern laparoscopes. Therefore, in order to minimize the morbidity of an open incision, whenever possible, we attempt to keep our incisions subumbilical even when we need to convert.

Another tool that aids in anatomic identification is preoperative cystoscopy and ureteral catheter placement by urology. If preoperative ureteral catheters are utilized, intraoperative identification can be accomplished laparoscopically by injecting 25 mg of indocyanine green in 10 mL of saline via a Luer lock attachment into each catheter and performing intraoperative fluorescence imaging utilizing Spy or, if using the robot, FireFly technology. This will allow the ureters to light up green throughout the duration of the case (Fig. 23.11a, b). However, if these tools are insufficient to allow safe visualization, or if at any point the surgeon is concerned about safely proceeding with the procedure, the surgeon should consider conversion to an open or, when possible, a hand-assisted approach.

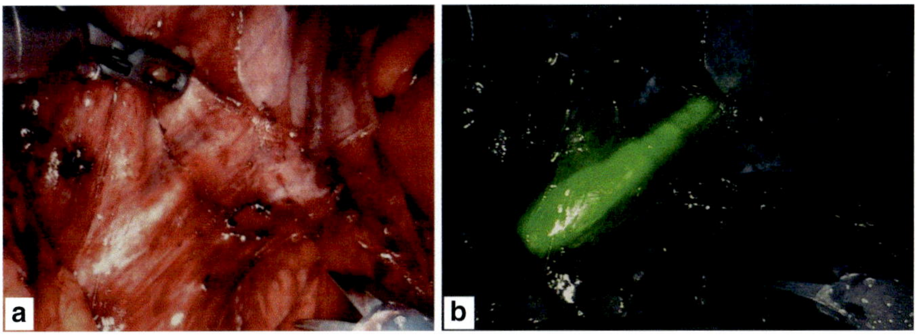

Fig. 23.11 (**a**, **b**) Intraoperative localization of the left ureter using Firefly fluorescence and ICG injection into the left ureteral stent. (Courtesy of Josh Wallet, MD)

The laparoscopic surgeon should be constantly vigilant about avoiding intraoperative injury to major vascular structures (IMA, iliac vessels, pelvic side wall vessels, and presacral venous plexus) or adjacent organs (small intestine, spleen, bladder). One tip is to alert the operating room staff prior to a critical portion of the procedure (IMA ligation, splenic flexure takedown) and ensure that any potential equipment needed in the event of an unintended injury is immediately available. In the event of IMA stump bleed, a large plastic clip or looped laparoscopic ligature may be helpful in controlling bleeding. Hollow organ injury (bladder, small intestine) can be repaired, either definitely or for temporary control, via laparoscopic suturing with an absorbable suture. Although a detailed discussion about managing intraoperative splenic bleeding is beyond the scope of this chapter, briefly, the laparoscopic surgeon must be aware that any undue traction on the splenocolic ligament can result in splenic bleeding. If just a subcapsular tear, a useful tool for managing this can be intraoperative placement of an absorbable hemostatic knit mesh, along with extended pressure.

Outcomes

Every prospective proctectomy patient should be asked about any baseline bowel, sexual, or urinary dysfunction. They should be counseled about the risk of surgery including low anterior resection syndrome (LARS), incontinence, impotence, bladder dysfunction, and others especially in those who will undergo neoadjuvant radiation therapy.

There are debates about the risk versus benefit ratio of high versus low ligation of the IMA during LAR; one must balance oncologic outcomes (i.e., overall land disease-free survival) with functional outcomes (defecatory, urinary, and sexual function). Some purists insist that it is essential to perform a full lymphadenectomy for LAR completed for malignancy, up to just after the takeoff of the IMA from the aorta and cephalad to the aortic bifurcation. However, other surgeons have argued that this adds unnecessary risk of injury to the autonomic nerves, specifically the superior hypogastric plexus that runs anterior to the aortic bifurcation, with increased risk of defecatory and urinary dysfunction, compromised blood supply, thus increasing the risk of anastomotic leak. If, indeed, there is regional lymph node involvement between the takeoff of the left colic artery and the IMA, this may be a marker for more distant tumor spread up the paraaortic chain and thus represent occult metastatic (M1) disease. Most studies comparing oncologic outcomes following high versus low IMA ligation during LAR for cancer did not report any significant difference in oncologic outcomes but did highlight functional differences favoring low ligation (Table 23.1) [5–8]. Our approach is to carefully examine the cross-sectional imaging prior to resection to assess for any lymph node involvement near the bifurcation and to perform selective high ligation.

A more important question of whether laparoscopic LAR is oncologically equivalent to open low anterior resection. Multiple well-publicized trials have had conflicting results, as summarized in Table 23.2 [2, 3, 9]. Three multinational and multi-institutional randomized trials, evaluated outcomes of laparoscopic versus open TME for rectal cancer performed by expert laparoscopic colon and rectal surgeons. Because of the early timeline of follow-up, long-term oncologic results (i.e., overall and disease-free survival) were not yet available. Consequentially, a proxy measure of oncologic efficacy was used to compare the pathologic results via a composite score of negative margins (circumferential radial and distal) and

Table 23.2 Results of randomized controlled trials of laparoscopic versus open total mesorectal excision for rectal cancer

Fleshman et al. *JAMA* 2015. (ACOSOG Z6051 trial) [2]	$N = 486$, '08-'13, RCT: lap vs. open TME for stage II/III rectal CA	Successful resection (neg CRM/distal margin, complete/near complete TME), 81.7% vs. 86.9% (p 0.41 for noninferiority)[a]
Stevenson et al. *JAMA* 2015. (ALACART trial) [3]	$N = 475$, '10-'14 RCT: lap vs. open TME for stage I–III rectal CA	Successful resection (neg CRM/distal margin, TME completeness), 82% vs. 89% ($p = 0.38$ for noninferiority)[a]
Jeong et al. *Lancet Oncol* 2010. (COREAN trial) [9]	$N = 340$, '06-'09. RCT: lap vs. open TME for stage II/III rectal CA	NS: involvement of CRM, TME specimen, #LNs harvested
Jeong et al. *Lancet Oncol* 2014 [11]	$N = 340$, '06'09. RCT: lap vs. open TME for stage II/III rectal CA (COREAN trial f/u: 3YS)	NS: 3Y DFS (79.2% vs 72.5%), $p < 0.0001$ for noninferiority[a]
Fleshman et al. *Ann Surg* 2019 [10]	$N = 486$, '08-'13, RCT: lap vs. open TME for stage II/III rectal CA (ACOSOG Z6051 trial f/u: median 48 months)	NS: 2Y DFS (79.5% vs 83.2%), locoregional (4.6% vs. 4.5%) or distant (14.6% vs. 16.7%) recurrence

CRM circumferential resection margin, *TME* total mesorectal excision, *DFS* disease-free survival, *LN* lymph nodes

[a]Establishing "noninferiority" of laparoscopic versus open approach was the end point chosen by the authors of these trials. Therefore, a nonsignificant p-value ($p \geq 0.05$) suggests that there are insufficient data to conclude that laparoscopy was "not *not* inferior" to an open approach. Conversely, significant p-value (<0.05) would suggest that laparoscopy was not inferior to an open approach

completeness of the TME specimen. The burden of proof was to determine that a laparoscopic approach was noninferior to open TME, which could not be demonstrated in two of the three major trials [2, 3]. Although results of long-term survival are eagerly awaited, the most recent publications on short-term oncologic outcomes including disease-free survival rates from two of the trials suggests oncologic equivalence [10, 11].

Conclusions

Laparoscopic low anterior resection with a mesenteric-specific tumor resection allows for functionally acceptable outcome while preserving minimizing morbidity. However, performing these procedures safely requires a thorough understanding of the relevant anatomic landmarks, knowledge about intraoperative pitfalls and how to avoid them, and are best performed by surgeons experienced in minimally invasive techniques. Although early randomized trial results suggest probable oncologic equivalence, ongoing controversy about the oncologic inferiority of minimally invasive TME and potential ramifications on long-term survival should be approached with thoughtful consideration by all rectal cancer surgeons when deciding on surgical approach and individualized based on patient and tumor factors.

References

1. Taylor F, Quirke P, Heald R, Moran B, Blomqvist L, Swift I, et al. Preoperative high-resolution magnetic resonance imaging can identify good prognosis stage I, II, and III rectal cancer best managed by surgery alone. Ann Surg. 2011;253(4):711–9.
2. Fleshman J, Branda M, Sargent DJ, Boller AM, George V, Abbas M, et al. Effect of laparoscopic-assisted resection vs open resection of stage II or III rectal cancer on pathologic outcomes: the ACOSOG Z6051 randomized clinical trial. JAMA. 2015;314(13):1346–55.
3. Stevenson ARL, Solomon MJ, Lumley JW, Hewett P, Clouston AD, Gebski VJ, et al. Effect of laparoscopic-assisted resection of open resection on pathological outcomes in rectal cancer: the ALACART trial. JAMA. 2015;314(13):1356–63.
4. https://www.Facs.org/Quality-Programs/Cancer/Naprc/Standards.
5. Matsuda K, Yokoyama S, Hotta T, Hakifuji K, Watanabe T, Tamura K, et al. Oncological outcomes following rectal cancer surgery with high or low ligation of the inferior mesenteric artery. Gastrointest Tumors. 2017;4(1–2):45–52.
6. Matsuda K, Hotta T, Takifuji K, Yokoyama S, Oku Y, Watanabe T, et al. Randomized clinical trial of defaecatory function after anterior resection for rectal cancer with high versus low ligation of the inferior mesenteric artery. Br J Surg. 2015;102(5):501–8.
7. Fujii S, Ishibe A, Ota M, Watanabe K, Watanabe J, Kunisaki C, et al. Randomized clinical trial of high versus low inferior mesenteric artery ligation during anterior resection for rectal cancer. BJS Open. 2018;2(4):195–202.
8. Mari GM, Crippa J, Cocozza E, Berselli M, Livraghi L, Carzaniga P, et al. Low ligation of inferior mesenteric artery in laparoscopic anterior resection for rectal cancer reduces genitourinary dysfunction. Ann Surg. 2018; https://doi.org/10.1097/SLA.0000000000002947. [Epub ahead of print]
9. Jeong SY, Park JW, Nam BH, Kim S, Kang SB, Lim SB, et al. Open versus laparoscopic surgery for mid-rectal or low-rectal cancer after neoadjuvant chemoradiotherapy (COREAN

trial): short-term outcomes of an open-label randomised controlled trial. Lancet Oncol. 2010;11(7):637–45.
10. Fleshman J, Branda ME, Sargent DJ, Boller AM, George VV, Abbas MA, et al. Disease-free survival and local recurrence for laparoscopic resection compared with open reseciton fo stage II to III rectal cancer: follow-up results of the ACOSOG Z6051 randomized controlled trial. Ann Surg. 2019;269(4):589–95.
11. Jeong SY, Park JW, Nam BH, Kim S, Kang SB, Lim SB, et al. Open versus laparoscopic surgery for mid-rectal or low-rectal cancer after neoadjuvant chemoradiotherapy (COREAN trial): survival outcomes of an open-label, noninferiority, randomized controlled trial. Lancet Oncol. 2014;15(7):767–74.

Robotic Low Anterior Resection: Unique Considerations and Optimal Setup

24

Slawomir Marecik, John J. Park, and Kunal Kochar

Introduction and Rationale

The objective of robotic assistance has always been to facilitate completion of complex laparoscopic procedures [1–7], which is particularly crucial during total mesorectal excision (TME). No randomized study has yet demonstrated the superiority of the robotic technique over laparoscopy for rectal cancer resections, but surgeons have consistently reported advantages of the robotic approach with respect to the ease of dissection, control of the operating field, and the ergonomics during these demanding cases [1, 2].

At the end of 2018, there are more than 40 companies actively developing new surgical robots. At least two of these companies offer integrated transabdominal platforms pending FDA approval. The cost of these emerging technologies remains the main point of contention and will need to be addressed [8, 9].

When examining robotics from a purely technical standpoint, and in the context of pelvic dissection, there are several inherent features of the robotic system that make it more advantageous to use when compared with laparoscopic, transanal minimally invasive, and open techniques. First, the robotic platform allows the

S. Marecik (✉) · K. Kochar
Advocate Lutheran General Hospital, Division of Colorectal Surgery, Park Ridge, IL, USA

University of Illinois at Chicago, Chicago, IL, USA
e-mail: smarecik@uic.edu

J. J. Park
Advocate Lutheran General Hospital, Division of Colorectal Surgery, Park Ridge, IL, USA

Chicago Medical School, Chicago, IL, USA

P. Sylla et al. (eds.), *The SAGES Manual of Colorectal Surgery*,
https://doi.org/10.1007/978-3-030-24812-3_24

primary surgeon to control the camera in a very stable way, allowing for constant operator-friendly adjustments, as well as "freezing" of the entire operating field. This, together with simultaneous control of three working articulating wrist instruments (often supported by two additional instruments controlled by the bedside assistant), gives the primary surgeon the ability to completely control the operating field. This is essential when working with obese patients, bulky tumors, or narrow pelvic confines.

While other chapters will detail the principles of rectal cancer management as well as the technique of laparoscopic LAR, this will review robotic techniques for low anterior resection with special emphasis on optimal robotic setup and best practices.

Indications and Contraindications of Approach

There are currently no strict guidelines with regard to which patients with rectal cancer are appropriate candidates for robotic low anterior resection (rLAR). As a general principle, however, candidates for a laparoscopic approach can also be operated with robotic assistance. Patients with previous abdominal surgeries should be carefully selected. The most difficult cases to include mid and low rectal cancers, bulky tumors, high body mass index (BMI), male patients, and abdominoperineal resections may be easier with the robotic approach. Surgeons still early along their robotic learning curve should not proceed with these complex cases without assistance by a proctor or an experienced co-surgeon. Conversion rates have been used as surrogate parameter for failure to pursue a minimally invasive approach [3].

Principles and Quality Benchmarks

The main objective of any emerging surgical technique is to perform a safe and controlled operation to the benefit of the patient. The robotic surgeon should have sufficient laparoscopic and open experience to complete the procedure [10, 11]. Good clinical judgment is crucial to determine the appropriate technique (laparoscopic, robotic, transanal, or open) for a particular patient while considering value-based outcomes [8].

The main principle of rectal dissection for cancer is the universal concept of total (or tumor-specific) mesorectal excision [12], i.e., to resect the necessary mesorectum with an intact mesorectal fascia (>90% of cases), low rate of positive circumferential and distal resection margins (<5%), and a low anastomotic leak rate (<5%) [3, 4, 13]. Total mesorectal excision (TME) requires an adequate knowledge of the pelvic anatomy and specialized training in this technique in order to perform an oncological, technically safe operation with good functional outcomes. When the anatomical landmarks are difficult to identify, the surgeon should look for the roundness and symmetry of the mesorectal compartment.

rLAR can be performed as a pure robotic technique or as hybrid approach (with traditional laparoscopy) [14, 15]. The latter is recommended at the beginning of the learning curve, in order to keep the procedures as short and easy as possible. A stepwise approach, i.e., adding robotically performed parts of the procedure with increasing robotic experience, will eventually enable the surgeon to convert to a fully robotic procedure (if appropriate) while considering each individual surgeon's learning curve [14, 16].

The fourth-generation system (da Vinci Xi®) from Intuitive Surgical® (Sunnyvale, CA, USA) is more versatile and allows a wider reach of the arms with less chance for external collisions. This makes it more suitable for multi-quadrant surgeries such as TME, without the need to redock. Conversely, the da Vinci Si® (or X) system will require redocking of the robot in order to complete the left colon mobilization and perform the TME.

Preoperative Planning, Patient Workup, and Optimization

Newly diagnosed rectal cancer patient should undergo a standardized staging workup, per the National Accreditation Program for Rectal Cancer [17]. The results of pathology; computer tomography of the chest, abdomen, and pelvis; as well as magnetic resonance (MRI of the pelvis, rectal cancer protocol with standardized synoptic reporting) and blood tests (CBC, CMP, CEA) are then presented to the multidisciplinary tumor board to determine if any neoadjuvant therapy is recommended. Digital rectal examination and flexible and/or rigid sigmoidoscopy are performed by the surgeon her/himself in order to localize the tumor and assess its relationship to the anal sphincters. Video documentation of the tumor (pre and post-neoadjuvant treatment) can be particularly helpful as it allows the surgeon to recall specific details just before surgery. This is especially important when assessing for tumor downstaging and when surgery is delayed by weeks or months after sigmoidoscopy.

When a plan for immediate or future LAR is made, the patient undergoes medical optimization. The first part involves smoking and alcohol cessation, weight loss as needed, nutrition optimization, and prehabilitation. Patients are extensively educated with respect to what to expect perioperatively as part of standard enhanced recovery protocols. For more information on specific protocols, refer to Chaps. 7 and 8 on enhanced recovery in colorectal surgery.

Most patients with tumors in the mid and lower rectum, particularly after neoadjuvant chemoradiation, are considered for a protective diverting ileostomy, based on the low level of the anticipated colorectal anastomosis. Some experienced surgeons are more selective in that decision. Preoperative stoma marking should be routinely performed by an enterostomal therapist.

Operative Setup

Positioning

The patient is placed in the modified lithotomy position with the thighs at level with the abdomen. If available, an anti-sliding pad is used (e.g., The Pink Pad®, Xodus Medical, New Kensington, PA, USA) with both arms tucked along the torso in a neutral position. Care is taken to provide full access to the perineum, taking into consideration the possibility of cephalad and caudal patient sliding during steep Trendelenburg positioning. Bony prominences and potential nerve entrapment sides should be secured with a protective padding to avoid neuropathy [18]. The most common sites of potential nerve injury are the cervical portion of the brachial plexus, the ulnar nerve at the epicondylar groove (elbow), the median nerve at the wrist, and the peroneal nerve at the fibular head. The patient is strapped to the table at the chest, with a towel between the chest and the strap so respiratory movement is not compromised. The shoulder brackets are then secured to avoid compression on the brachial plexus. Before draping the patient, the bed is tilted to the extreme positions to observe any possible patient sliding. The anesthesia equipment is moved as far cephalad as possible to prevent contamination during robotic arm setup and instrument exchange. The minimum amount of necessary table tilt is used throughout the procedure.

Robotic Cart Position (Fig. 24.1)

For LAR using the Si system, the cart is placed by the left hip and along the left leg while straddling the left lower corner of the operating room base. Occasionally, the Si (or X) system can be placed between the legs (provides excellent robotic arm distribution for pelvic dissection). However, this position precludes easy access to the perineum.

When using the Xi system, the cart can be brought from either side with the exception of the right upper quadrant, which is reserved for the bedside assistant. A rotating boom of the Xi system allows the arms to be directed toward the left abdomen and pelvis.

Port Placement

Standard principles of safe port placement should be respected. These include ensuring the appropriate distance between the ports and depth of port insertion. In cases of insufficient instrument reach, which may be encountered during deep pelvic dissection, the ports and the robotic arms may need to be pushed deeper beyond the black line marked on the port's cannula. Additionally, attention should be given

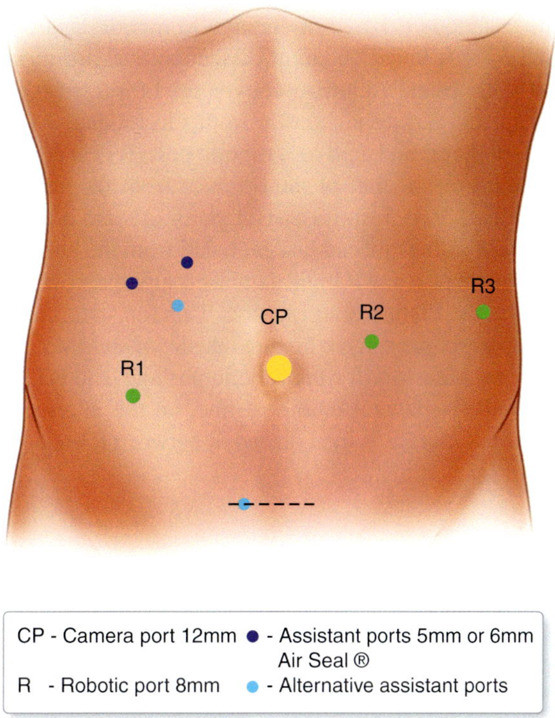

Fig. 24.1 Port setup for Si (and X) system. R1-robotic dissecting instrument, CP-12 mm camera port (8 mm in X system), R2-micro-retracting bipolar grasper, R3-macro-retracting grasper; assistant ports (5 mm or 6 mm AirSeal®, Conmed System, Utica, NY, USA)

to the position of the robotic base (Si or X system) or the center of the rotating boom (Xi system) in relation to the ports. The shorter distance between the ports and the abovementioned central parts of the robotic system can result in cramming of the external arms, with the possibility of external arm collision. The longer distance would result in decreased reach of the instruments. During the learning curve, it is recommended that the robotic ports be placed in the most optimal location with no regard for a future ileostomy site, or even the extraction site. With time and experience, the ileostomy site and the extraction incision can be incorporated into the port placement.

There are many possible ways to achieve successful port placement. There are, however, differences between the Si and Xi systems in terms of port setup. Overall, the Xi system provides a wider reach of the arms with less chance for external collisions. The Si (or X) system will typically require redocking of the robot in order to complete the left colon mobilization and perform the TME. The techniques for a completely rLAR with the Si (or X) system have been described; however, the authors suggest using them only after obtaining sufficient experience with the simpler techniques [14, 15, 19].

Robotic LAR with the Si System

The technique is based on the hybrid robotic-laparoscopic technique. The robot is used for left lower quadrant dissection, inferior mesenteric artery (IMA) control, and TME. Standard laparoscopy is used for inferior mesenteric vein (IMV) control and splenic flexure takedown. In this technique, a 12 mm camera port is placed at the umbilicus, and an 8 mm robotic port (R1) is placed in the right lower quadrant, one third to one half of the distance from the anterior superior iliac spine to the umbilicus. Two 5 mm assistant ports (a1 and a2) are inserted in the right upper quadrant with a1 placed just cephalad from the horizontal umbilical line in between the camera port and R1 and a2 placed suprapubic on the line of the future extraction port via the Pfannenstiel incision. This four-port configuration should be sufficient for laparoscopic splenic flexure takedown and IMV control. Two additional robotic ports are necessary for the robotic portion. The R3 is an 8 mm robotic port placed above the horizontal umbilical line, on the intersection with the anterior axillary line. An 8 mm R2 is then placed in between R3 and the camera port (Fig. 24.2).

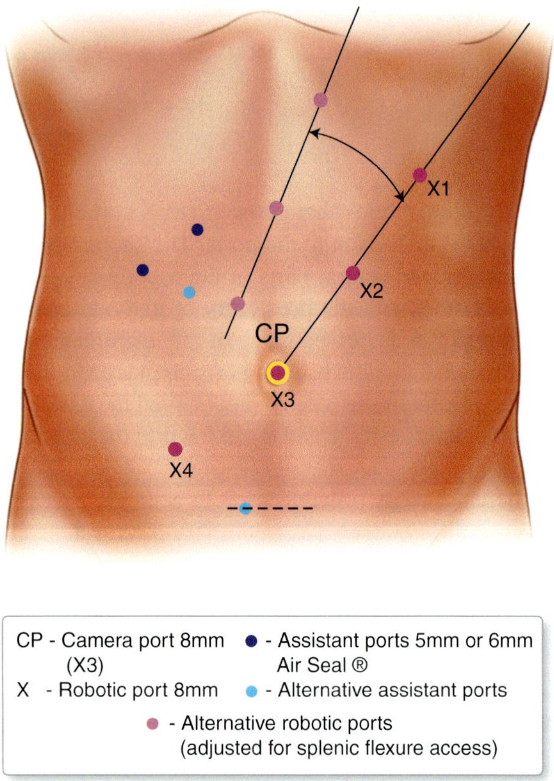

Fig. 24.2 Port setup for Xi system. X1-macro-retracting grasper for pelvic dissection, X2-micro-retracting bipolar grasper for pelvic dissection, X3–8 mm camera port, X4-robotic dissecting instrument; assistant ports (5 mm, 6 mm AirSeal®, Conmed System, Utica, NY, USA)

During the robotic part of the procedure, R1 is used for a monopolar cautery hook or hot shears, which are assigned to the right hand of the operator. The R2 port accommodates a bipolar grasper-type instrument, and R3 is used for a Cadiere-type (no cautery) grasper. Both R2 and R3 ports are assigned to the left hand of the operator. The R3 instrument is primarily responsible for stationary retraction (macroretraction) of the rectosigmoid during posterior rectal mobilization. It is also used to retract anterior pelvic structures during anterior rectal mobilization. The left hand of the assistant (a1) controls a grasper and helps with macro- and microretraction, while the right assistant hand (a2) is supplied with a suction irrigator in order to actively evacuate the plume and fluid from the pelvis and to assist with retraction and exposure. Zero-degree or 30-degree down camera is used for most of the procedure.

Robotic LAR with This Xi System

The Xi system differentiates from the Si system by its central rotating boom and a reverse numbering of the arms from the left to right. The 8 mm Xi camera can be placed in any robotic port. The ports are placed in an almost linear configuration from the right lower quadrant (one third to one half of the distance between the anterior superior iliac spine and the umbilicus) to the left upper quadrant mid-costal region (Fig. 24.3). Subsequently, the 8 mm camera port (X3) and two additional robotic ports (X2 and X1) are placed on that line, evenly distributed. Frequently, the camera port (X3) corresponds with the umbilicus, which is the preferred site for the camera. The line for the port positions can be modified by pivoting it around the X4 port (which is constant). A more vertical port placement line brings the X1 closer to the midline and allows for more comfortable dissection around the splenic flexure and the left colon. A rotation of the port placement line in a more horizontal direction allows for more comfortable pelvic dissection and with better reach of the X1 and X2 instruments into the deep pelvis. The assistant port configuration includes two ports in the right upper quadrant or one port in that location and the other one in the suprapubic location. Alternatively, the entire robotic port line, including the X4 port, may be moved in parallel toward the right upper quadrant.

The assignment of the arms for the pelvic dissection is essentially the same as in the Si technique, but for the splenic flexure mobilization, the instruments can be rearranged, including the 8 mm camera, which can be placed in any robotic port. If the assistant port is chosen to be placed in the suprapubic location, the right hand of the assistant will have to be inserted between the robotic arm of the right lower quadrant (R1 or X4) and the camera arm. This maneuver is not usually problematic; however, the assistant should be alert for any sudden swings of the nearby robotic arms.

Once the rectal mobilization is complete, a robotic stapler is typically introduced via the right lower quadrant port (R1 or X4), after upsizing of that port with a 12 mm designated stapler port.

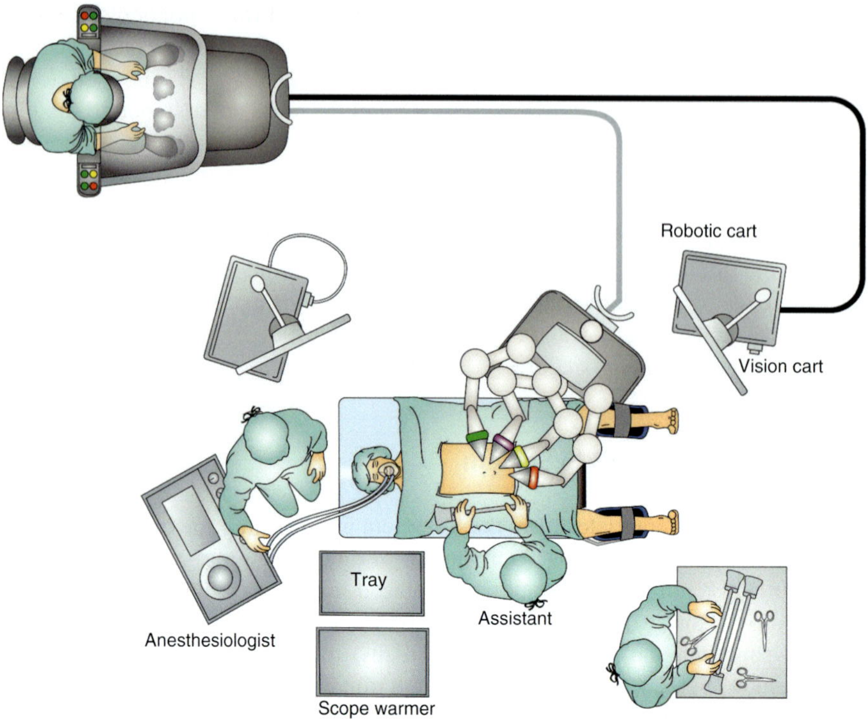

Fig. 24.3 Robotic cart positioning

The X system utilizes the Xi system ports and instruments, but the port placement can be chosen between Si and Xi.

Extraction Site

The preferred extraction site is a Pfannenstiel incision for cosmetic reasons and an extremely low hernia formation rate [20]. Alternatively, the specimen can be extracted through the ileostomy site. In this case, the incision would likely have to be enlarged at the skin and fascial levels for the larger specimens. This could increase the risk of stomal prolapse and/or parastomal hernia. Select patients can undergo transanal or transvaginal specimen extraction, particularly when hand-sewn anastomosis follows the pull-through procedure [21].

Operative Technique: Surgical Steps

After safely establishing the pneumoperitoneum, diagnostic laparoscopy is carried out to confirm the appropriateness of the planned resection, including plans for splenic flexure release and use of a hybrid or fully robotic technique.

Exposure of the base of the left colon mesentery and the sacral promontory is obtained by adjusting the table tilt and sweeping of the small bowel to the right and upper abdomen. All necessary ports are then placed, the robot docked, and the instruments inserted under direct vision.

A decision is made regarding where to initiate the dissection and the sequence of dissection. Most surgeons prefer a medial to lateral approach for mesenteric dissection. However, the surgeon should be familiar with the lateral to medial approach if exposure of the base of the mesentery is complicated by severe visceral obesity or inability to sweep away small bowel loops, uncertainty regarding the anatomy, aneurysmal aorta, suspiciously enlarged lymph nodes, or extensive scarring or inflammation. The medial to lateral approach can be initiated by incising below the IMV, above or below the IMA, or at the level of the sacral promontory. Likewise, the splenic flexure can be mobilized using a lateral to medial, supra-mesocolic or infra-mesocolic approach.

Mesenteric Dissection and IMA Ligation

When starting the dissection below the IMV or above the IMA, the peritoneal incision should be initiated between the vein and a distinct autonomic (sympathetic) nerve running along the left side of the aortic surface. This nerve, which serves as a very helpful anatomical landmark, eventually joins the (peri) IMA nerve plexus. A proper initial incision guarantees easiest access to the correct plane within lamellar Toldt's fascia, between the retroperitoneal and the mesocolic fascia [22]. Squiggly vessels of Toldt's fascia, left on the mesocolic side of the dissection, indicate that the dissection was carried out too deep. Small oozing from these vessels can eventually stain the dissection plane. A proper (non-bloody) dissection plane should keep the squiggly vessels on the retroperitoneal side.

When the dissection is initiated below the IMA, it is more difficult to find the proper plane (Toldt's fascia). This almost always leads to dissection in the deeper plane, below the retroperitoneal fascia. The main reason for this difficulty is the presence of a distinct autonomic nerve layer in front of the aorta, in addition to often seen fibrosis, inflammation, and sometimes lymphadenopathy between the IMA and the aorta. The main consequence of too deep of a dissection is oozing from the small vessels and potential injury to the ureter and the gonadal vessels.

For the reasons stated above, the dissection is frequently initiated at the level of the sacral promontory. This is done by retracting the rectosigmoid, with the far-left instrument stretching the peritoneum at the base of the rectosigmoid. Hot dissection also helps in plane identification between the mesentery and the prehypogastric nerve fascia (pHGNF). The latter is a fascial layer covering the superior hypogastric plexus (below the aortic bifurcation), both hypogastric nerves, and the sacral splanchnic nerves (SSN) deeper in the pelvis (Fig. 24.4) [23]. The pHGNF must be kept intact in order to minimize injury to these important autonomic nerves.

Dissection is continued cephalad along and above the nerves and pHGNF layer, toward the root of the IMA, avoiding further lateral dissection. A helpful maneuver

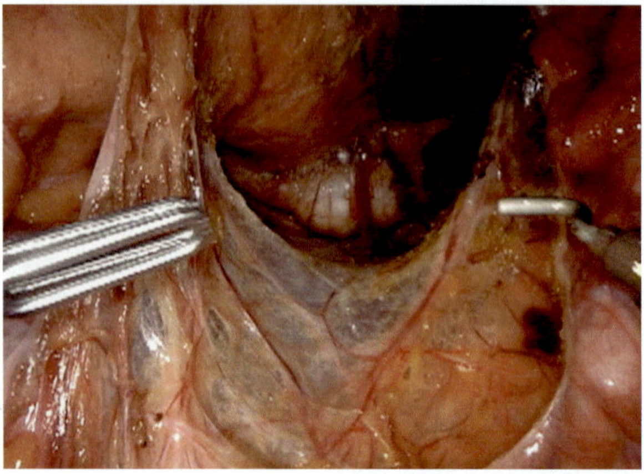

Fig. 24.4 Prehypogastric nerve fascia (pHGNF) covering the superior hypogastric plexus and both hypogastric nerves. The fascia was incised between both diverging nerves, and the plane of dissection was changed, leaving the pHGNF attached to the mesorectum

at this point involves moving the dissection above the IMA. This helps to establish a proper layer of easily identifiable Toldt's fascia above (cephalad from) the IMA. In addition, "connecting the dots" between the planes above and below (cephalad and caudal of) the IMA helps prevent violation of the retroperitoneal fascia along the entire length of dissection. Thus, if the retroperitoneal fascia remains intact in a bloodless operating field, the left ureter and gonadal vessels will also be left intact below the fascia, and a search for the ureter by dissection through the retroperitoneal fascia will not be necessary. Conversely, if the operating field becomes bloody and/or the retroperitoneal fascia is violated, the ureter must be clearly identified.

Dissection continues at the root of the IMA, where it is circumferentially dissected, isolated, and then divided. Several methods can be used, including the laparoscopic or robotic clip applier (most cost effective), a robotic vessel sealer, a vascular stapler, or a laparoscopic bipolar energy device. The dissection is then carried from the medial to the lateral aspect by dissecting between the retroperitoneal and mesocolic fascia. One of the robotic arms, usually the far-left one, provides a macroretraction to the detached mesenteric base and should be continually adjusted to provide adequate tension during medial to lateral dissection. The dissection is extended onto the white line of Toldt. Any difficulty encountered during medial to lateral dissection, such as difficulties identifying the correct plane or the left ureter, can be circumnavigated by changing the dissection to the lateral to medial approach. When the lateral to medial dissection is performed, the far-left robotic arm is applied laterally to the white line of Toldt. The other retracting arm provides the medial microretraction on the bowel and mesentery.

Splenic Flexure Release

The various strategies for laparoscopic splenic flexure release (SFR) are described in the Masters chapter (Chap. 4) on laparoscopic SFR, tips and tricks. Robotic surgeons should be familiar with the lateral to medial, supra-mesocolic or infra-mesocolic approach, in case difficulties arise and an alternative approach is needed.

Several techniques of splenic flexure mobilization have been described for both the Si and Xi systems [14, 15, 24]. While it is possible to mobilize the flexure and perform the TME with one robotic setup, the Si system techniques are generally more demanding. They frequently require arm repositioning and/or system redocking and may be achieved easier with the hybrid (laparoscopic) approach. On the other hand, the design of the Xi system allows for less external arm collisions and better reach. When combined with integrated table motion and appropriate port placement, it allows for more effective one port setup for splenic flexure mobilization as well as for rectal dissection. Also as mentioned, the in-line port setup must be done in a more vertical fashion, thus opening a more effective angle for the splenic flexure. Alternatively, a completely horizontal, mid-abdominal robotic port placement can effectively serve the splenic flexure and pelvis, following boom rotation and instrument exchange.

Rectal Mobilization

This part of the dissection is fairly standardized and very reproducible with repetitive movements, particularly when compared with splenic flexure mobilization. The objective of successful TME is to perform a gradual release of the mesorectum (posterior, anterior, and both lateral) using effective and atraumatic retraction of the mesorectal specimen.

Posterior Dissection

The rectum is mobilized posteriorly to the level of the lower sacrum. During the upper part of the dissection, care should be taken to preserve the pHGNF (the innermost layer of the presacral (Waldeyer's fascia). The pHGNF covers the superior hypogastric plexus, the right and left hypogastric nerves, and a significant portion of the sacral splanchnic nerves), all of which are important as safety landmarks and are essential for both sexual and urinary function (Fig. 24.5). Additionally, because the

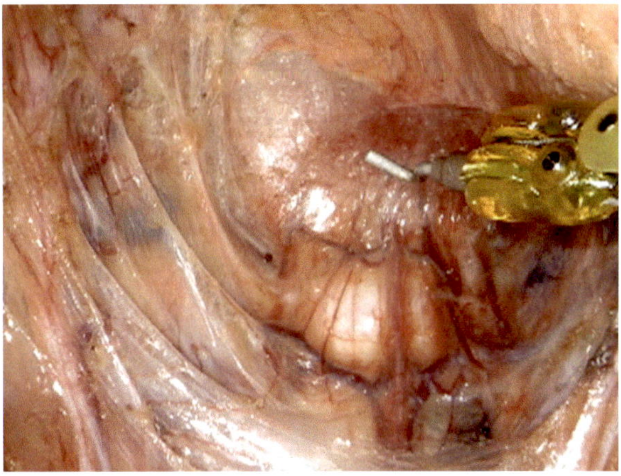

Fig. 24.5 Sacral splanchnic nerves (SSN) originating from the pelvic sympathetic trunks and converging in the pelvic plexus (seen in the left upper corner); pHGNF lifted with the mesorectum

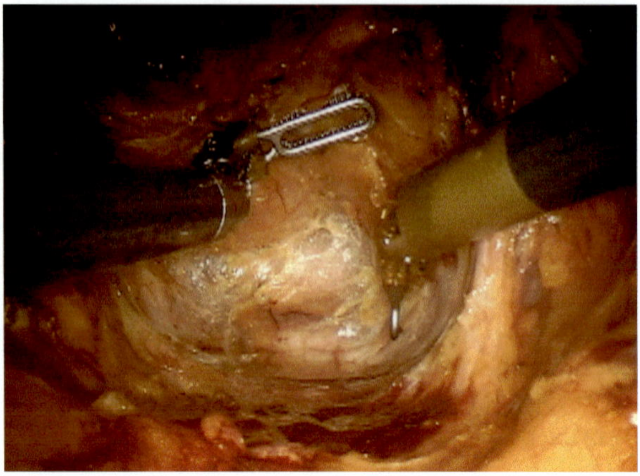

Fig. 24.6 Retraction of the mesorectum during posterior dissection, left hand grasper with 90-degree wrist angulation

posterior avascular plane can be easily identified, it is often advantageous to continue this plane of dissection around the rectum, mobilizing the mesorectum from the right and left lateral pelvic compartments. In order to provide the best exposure, the far-left robotic arm with Cadiere forceps is used to provide a macroretraction to the rectum in the cephalad and anterior direction. The medial left robotic arm with the fenestrated bipolar grasper is then used to provide a gentle microretraction on the mesorectum, close to the area of hook/scissors dissection (performed with the right arm). In experienced hands, using the wrist of the instrument at a 90-degree angle to the shaft, the macro-retracting arm can frequently lift and support the mesorectum without actually grasping it (Fig. 24.6). Posterior TME dissection proceeds either between the mesorectal fascia and the pHGNF (with reduced risk of injury to the nerves) or between the pHGNF and the nerves, which exposes the nerves but may extend the posterior resection margin in cases where the mesorectal fascia is threatened by tumor. It is the authors' preference to preserve the pHGNF until a clear divergence of the two hypogastric nerves can be seen toward both pelvic sidewalls. At that point, the pHGNF is routinely incised, and dissection falls into the plane between the pHGNF and the sacral splanchnic nerves (Fig. 24.4).

Another implication of precise and bloodless surgery is the ability to visualize anatomical landmarks to guide the dissection. This is important in the case of unclear anatomy due to inflammation, tumor, previous radiation, or previous dissection. While it is rare to visualize SSN during open surgery, they are easily identified during robotic surgery and should be preserved (Fig. 24.5).

It is also important to point out that many general surgery and colorectal textbooks describe Waldeyer's fascia as a structure penetrating the mesorectum and spreading between the sacrum and the rectal tube. It is often referred to as "rectosacral" or "retrosacral." In fact, the presacral Waldeyer's fascia has two components, with a more posterior one covering the presacral vessels and a more superficial one covering the hypogastric and sacral splanchnic nerves. The name of the latter layer is the pHGNF (prehypogastric nerve fascia). Waldeyer's fascia spreads onto the lateral aspects of the mesorectal compartment, where it ultimately embeds the pelvic (inferior hypogastric) plexi (Fig. 24.7).

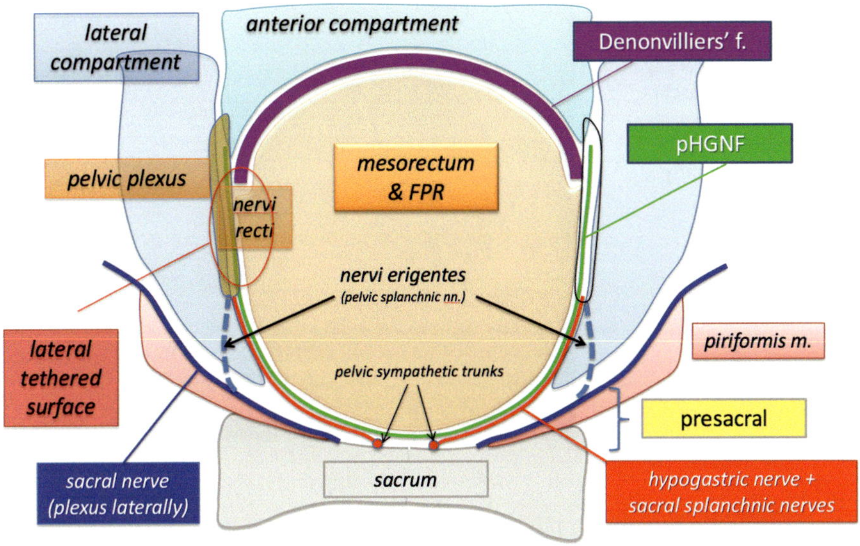

Fig. 24.7 Pelvic fasciae and nerve structures. (Used with permission of Wolters Kluwer from Marecik et al. [25])

Fig. 24.8 Dissection through the left lateral tethered surface; left hypogastric nerve converging with the sacral splanchnic nerves to form left pelvic plexus; mesorectum – bottom/right

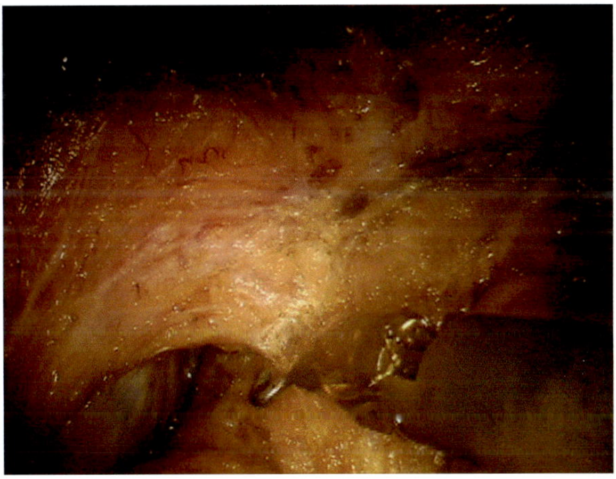

Lateral Dissection

The area of the lateral rectal attachments (stalks) is referred to by authors as "lateral tethered surface" and not "lateral ligament." These are often taken down by cautery and sharp dissection (Fig. 24.8). When most of the lateral mobilization is completed as a continuum of the posterior dissection around the rectum, this part of the dissection is relatively easy, particularly if the line of anterior dissection has been previously marked (Fig. 24.9). Care should be taken,

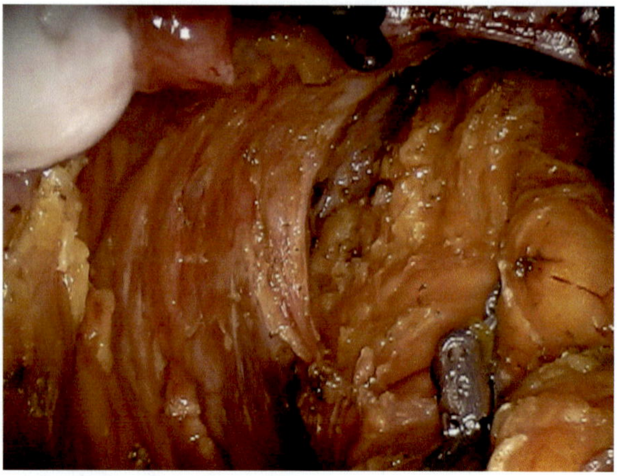

Fig. 24.9 Dissection through the left lateral tethered surface; left edge of Denonvilliers' fascia still attached to the mesorectum; left pelvic plexus visible laterally

however, not to injure the lateral pelvic plexi. This is where the sympathetic hypogastric nerves and sacral splanchnic nerves converge with the parasympathetic sacral pelvic nerves (known as *nervi erigentes*, located in the posterior aspect of the lateral compartment) (Fig. 24.7) [25]. The left lateral dissection is performed with the far-left instrument retracting the lateral wall, the medial left instrument pushing the mesorectum to the right, and the right-hand instrument crossing the medial left instrument for dissection. The right lateral dissection is performed with the far-left instrument retracting the mesorectum (macroretraction to the left), while the medial left instrument pushes the right anterior Denonvilliers' fascia (DF), or the lateral wall, while positioned in front of or behind the right-hand dissecting instrument.

Anterior Dissection

The rectovaginal/rectovesical peritoneal fold is incised to expose the DF, and the rectum is mobilized from the vagina/prostate. The key to avoiding potential bleeding from the fine vascular plexus that surrounds the seminal vesicles or posterior vaginal wall (venous sinuses) is to maintain the plane of dissection just posterior to DF, unless the tumor is threatening it. This also helps to avoid injury to the neurovascular bundles of the prostate (and vagina). These are covered by the lower portion of DF just above the pubococcygeus levator muscle in the anterolateral portion of the mesorectal compartment (Fig. 24.10). The fixed macroretraction provided by the far-left robotic arm on the bladder/prostate/vagina facilitates surgical access and visualization during anterior rectal dissection, while the micro-retracting arm pushes the mesorectum posteriorly (downward) (Fig. 24.11a, b). Of note, during a clean TME technique, the lateral edges of the trapezoid-shaped DF can be seen covering the anterior half portion of the pelvic plexus (Fig. 24.12).

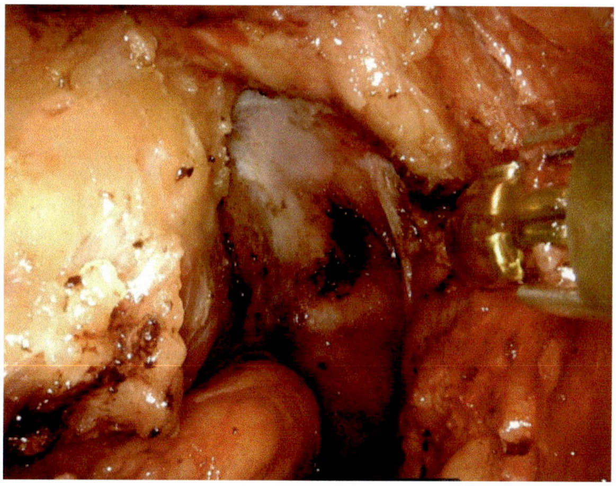

Fig. 24.10 Right anterior dissection at the level of the pubococcygeus levator muscle; mesorectum on the left, right neurovascular prostatic bundle ("erigent pillar") above the cautery hook, covered by Denonvilliers' fascia

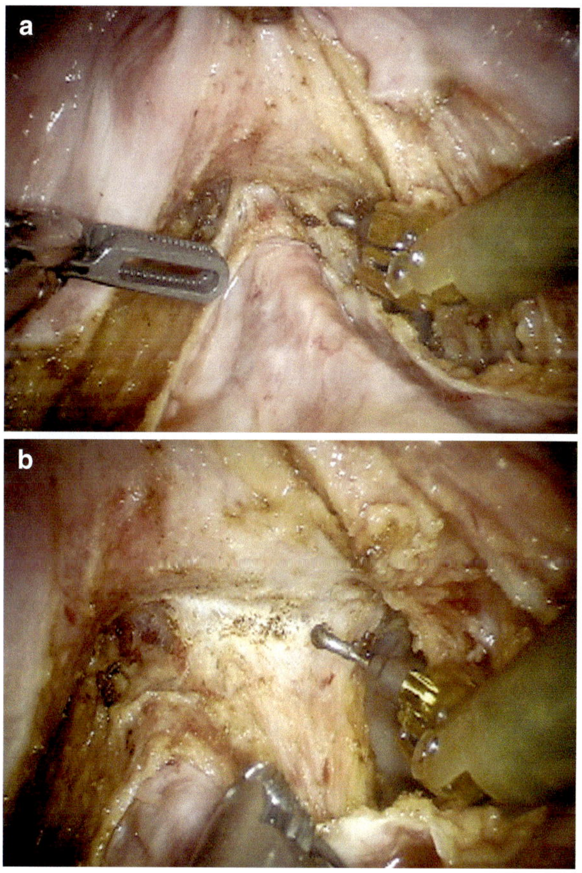

Fig. 24.11 (**a**) Anterior dissection, the macro-retracting arm (top) is retracting the anterior pelvic structures (cephalad and anterior direction). (**b**) The micro-retracting arm (left) pushing on the mesorectum downwards

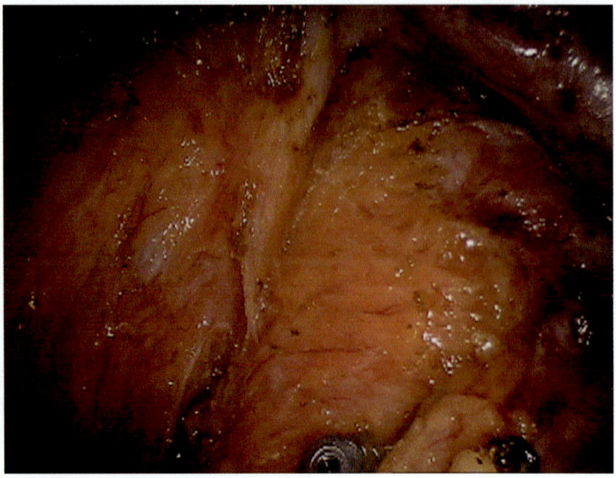

Fig. 24.12 Left edge of Denonvilliers' fascia; mesorectum on the right side, pelvic plexus visible laterally

Pelvic Floor Dissection

This part of the dissection can be challenging because it is the most distal part of the TME. Occasionally, the robotic ports need to be pushed in beyond the recommended black mark on the cannula, in order to obtain adequate reach in tall patients. It is also possible for the instrument wrists to start losing their responsiveness at times. This requires resetting by simple removal and reinsertion. The exposure can also be challenging in very obese patients with a narrow and muscular pelvis, as well as in thin patients with a stretchy rectum and levators with their fascia. Finally, for low rectal cancers, there is a narrow margin for error because of the converging pelvic space and lack of mesorectal fat coverage.

The anterior mobilization is often easier during deep pelvic floor dissection due to the shorter distance to reach the levators. Here, a small segment of the pubococcygeus muscle can be exposed posteriorly next to the base of the arcuate DF (Fig. 24.10). In fact, it is also easy to reach the levators in the lateral aspects, right at the lateral edge of DF and medial to the pelvic plexus. This is where the domes of the iliococcygeus muscles are located.

Medial dissection of the dome-like portion of the levators can be more difficult due to the depth of dissection. In addition, the endopelvic fascia (levators' fascia in this case) becomes quite stretchy and often difficult to dissect from the stretchy mesorectal fascia. Similarly, the posterior dissection of the pelvic floor, which starts below the posterior impressions of the piriformis muscle (S4/5 level), with a flat and tendinous coccygeus muscle, will lead deeper into the levator "funnel," along the levators' raphe, and toward the anorectal junction. These nuances, together with the fact that posterior dissection requires significantly more work than anterior dissection, may lead to difficulty in determining at what level to stop the dissection for adequate distal margin below the tumor. As a result, deep pelvic dissection may require a 30-degree-up camera angulation.

Distal Mesorectal Clearance, Rectal Transection, and Anastomosis

Once the mesorectum is adequately mobilized, the distal transection site is prepared. If the goal is to perform an ultralow anterior resection with a staple line on or close to the anorectal junction, a circumferential clearance of the mesorectum or thickened mesorectal fascia is usually simple due to the minimal amount of mesorectal tissue at that level. For the more proximal stapler application, the mesorectum must be transected first. It is helpful to perform an intraoperative flexible sigmoidoscopy to confirm a tumor-specific transection site or, alternatively, one can rely on India ink marking. Mesenteric transection can be easily performed using a cautery hook. It is best to start in the right anterior aspect, where the rectal wall is subsequently exposed. The dissection is gradually moved toward the posterior midline, exposing more circumference of the rectal wall. The process is repeated on the left side, establishing the rendezvous in the posterior midline. Large and bulky mesorectum can be challenging, and care should be taken to transect the mesorectum on the same level during the left- and right-sided division. Care should also be taken to avoid the "spiral apple peel" effect, with unequally transected left and right side. Depending on the level of transection, the macro-retracting far-left arm may need to support the anterior pelvic structures for adequate exposure or to retract the specimen. The assistant's instruments can be very helpful in supporting the exposure or the specimen during this part of procedure.

Once the distal transection site is prepared, a linear and articulating robotic stapler can be applied. The robotic stapler has smart clamp technology which makes it more comfortable and easier to control than the laparoscopic instrument. It is typically inserted through the right-hand port; however, the port itself needs to be first upgraded to a 12 mm cannula. During the stapling process, the far-left robotic arm provides a macroretraction to the anterior pelvic structures. Meanwhile, the medial left arm stretches and flattens the rectum for stapler application. The stapler can be supplied with blue or green cartridges and is available in 30 mm, 45 mm, and 60 mm length. On average, at least two stapler applications are necessary for successful rectal transection. The smart clamp technology allows for initial tissue compression, active feedback, and stapler reapplication during this process, in order to optimize the amount of tissue in the stapler jaws to the height of closing staples.

The proximal mesenteric transection in the sigmoid or descending colon can be performed using a robotic or laparoscopic vessel sealer. The stapler is used to transect the bowel. Alternatively, the colon with a resected rectum can be exteriorized for extracorporeal division and anvil application, including the transanal route. A suprapubic horizontal incision and the ileostomy site are preferred extraction sites. With experience, an intracorporal purse-string suture application and anvil insertion can be performed after the staple line from the proximal colonic end is removed. The anastomosis is performed in a standard fashion, with two left robotic arms retracting the anterolateral walls of the mesorectal compartment, providing excellent exposure. A double-stapled anastomosis can also be performed in the laparoscopic technique once the robot is undocked. It is not recommended to perform a robotic double purse-string (single stapled) technique until proficiency with the robotic system is gained [21, 26]. Each completed anastomosis is inspected with a sigmoidoscope to watch for signs of intraluminal bleeding. An air-water leak test is also performed.

Pitfalls and Troubleshooting

The da Vinci surgical robot system is a mechanical and highly sophisticated computer system. As such, there is potential for malfunction or failure. Fortunately, general system failures are rare, provided that proper maintenance and its software updates have been carried out [10, 27].

The system has a user-friendly communication system to help with routine setup and the docking process. The Xi system offers a self-optimizing robotic boom and arm positioning, but it is important to note that strict reliance on that self-optimization is not always beneficial. The surgeon should know how to adjust the arms and the boom, how to position the robotic cart, and how to distribute the arms in the most ergonomic fashion. When setting up and docking the robotic cart, the assistant should be provided with a comfortable place to stand or sit by the bedside, without assuming any contorted positions or being placed near swinging robotic arms. Finally, it is important that the console surgeon be actively engaged in port and instrument placement during the setup. This is to ensure full understanding of the limitations of reach and instrument collisions, should they arise. Strict reliance on the assistant without constructive feedback will not allow the team to evolve efficiently.

Port setup is also crucial and can be a major factor for progress in the procedure. If any restrictions or persistent collisions arise during instrument manipulation, the layout should be assessed and, if necessary, more ports be added in better locations. Likewise, the robotic cart needs to be positioned correctly. If it is placed too close to the field, cramming of the arms and instruments will occur. If it is placed too far away, the instruments will not have the full range of motion. The blue mark on the Si system shows the optimal distance range between the robotic cart and the field. This can be adjusted, depending on the body habitus of the patient and the distance between ports.

Once the arms are docked with the ports, the elbows of the arms should be spread sufficiently to allow for clearance and avoidance of collisions. If the ports are placed too far from the pelvis, the instruments may not reach the pelvic floor or may get hung up on the pelvic brim, limiting the access to the posterior (presacral) aspect of the mesorectal compartment. Similarly, if the instruments intended to dissect in the deep pelvis are placed too far laterally (too close to the anterior superior iliac spine), access to the ipsilateral pelvic sidewall will be limited as well. In case of insufficient reach to the pelvic floor, advancing the robotic ports beyond the recommended black mark on the robotic port cannula is suggested.

Proficient camera operation is one of the primary determinants of fluidity and rhythm of the case. Proper visualization is not only important for the operator but also helps to orient the assistant, whose instrument frequently retracts and protects the operating field outside of the active camera view. For this reason, frequent zooming out and pan viewing of the field must be performed. During TME in the deep pelvis, there is a natural tendency to inadvertently "spiral" the camera (rotate the horizon), especially during anterolateral dissection. This results in improper recognition of anatomical landmarks. It is true that experienced robotic surgeons are known to perform up to four times more camera (and instrument) adjustments than novice surgeons while still demonstrating the economy of movements [27]. What should be avoided is dissection on the outskirts of the active view. Instead, the camera should have the working instruments in center view at all times.

Similar to constant camera adjustment is constant instrument adjustment with the clutching mechanisms [27]. The surgeon's hands should rest comfortably on the support and never be positioned "in the air." This guarantees precision of movements and control of the operating field. Thus, by controlling three working instruments, the camera, and "conducting" the position of the assistant's instruments, the surgeon is in full control of the entire case. It is imperative for the operator to subconsciously know the spatial position of all instruments at any given time. Without this awareness, the instruments tend to clash internally and get damaged, but there is also an increased risk of collateral tissue damage if the instruments are not seen.

The part of the instrument most susceptible to damage is the plastic wrist cover of the monopolar cautery hook, which should always be checked when removed from the patient body. The internal and external collisions can lead to loss of instrument wrist responsiveness. This requires resetting by simple removal and reinsertion. This malfunction can sometimes be observed during dissection around the very distal rectum. Frequently, less experienced surgeons do not recognize the full ability of the wrist articulation and use this sophisticated system in the traditional laparoscopic-like fashion. The skill of proficient utilization of the wrist articulation is especially crucial during right pelvic sidewall dissection with the right-hand instrument (hook or scissors) placed in the right lower quadrant. This often requires cocking the wrist toward the right side (Fig. 24.13). Additional unique articulation

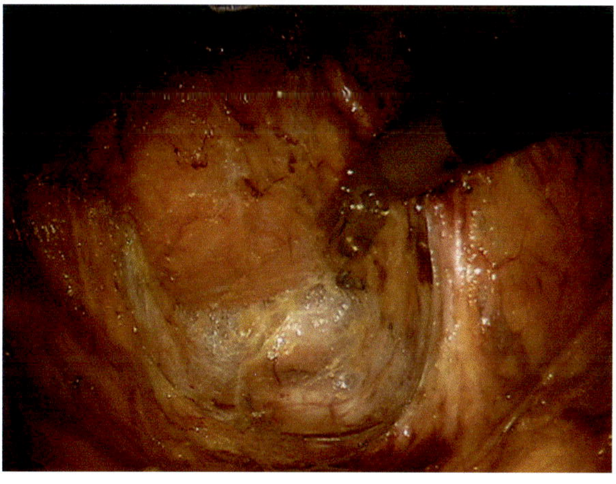

Fig. 24.13 Cocking of the right-hand dissecting instrument during the right-side pelvic dissection

techniques are used for atraumatic retraction (L-shaping of the closed graspers), including lifting of the mesorectum and resting it on the instrument shaft without grabbing any tissue during posterior dissection (Fig. 24.6). Essentially, all techniques of robotic TME rely on two robotic instruments to provide micro- and macroretraction and one dissecting monopolar cautery instrument. While the most lateral retracting instrument is typically used for macroretraction, one has to remember that switching roles of the retracting instruments can sometimes improve the retraction. There is also a possibility, particularly during difficult and long cases, to confuse the pedals of the monopolar and bipolar cautery, resulting in burning of the specimen or, even worse, applying the heat to the grasper that is retracting the walls of the mesorectal compartment.

The newest Xi system comes with a built-in electrocautery generator unit which has different cautery settings than commonly used external units. As of now, the former may have a slightly inferior performance than the latter. Some operative adjustments may be necessary, and the settings increased to higher values than expected from traditional units.

Multiple problems can arise from inadequate communication between the console surgeon and the bedside assistant. Closed-loop communication in a standardized fashion is mandatory to confirm receipt and implementation of mutual instructions. Noise, insufficient microphone volume, or lack of team concentration can set off intraoperative disasters. Unexperienced bedside assistants may be unable to dock the robot efficiently or may injure tissues (most commonly small bowel) during instrument exchanges. In the newest Xi version, protective visual mechanisms (hazard bars) allow one to visualize the path of the inserted instruments, even when they are outside of the active visual field. It is recommended that instruments always be inserted under the camera's vision. Typically, the assistant's instruments are 5 or 6 mm in size, and occasionally they will collide with the robotic instruments or arms, rendering them ineffective. If such problems arise, a liberal new port insertion in the optimal location is recommended. Additionally, because of the design of the robotic arms, the instrument insertion or replacement requires more clearance over the sterile field toward the anesthesia stand. Therefore, the anesthesia screen and the poles must be moved more cephalad in order to avoid instrument contamination.

It is important to remember that newer, integrated motion tables, designed for use with the Xi system, will likely not have as extreme of a right-sided tilt when combined with simultaneous extreme Trendelenburg positioning seen in most traditional tables. Because of this, a more methodical small bowel positioning, or even different approach (lateral to medial), might be required to gain access to the base of the left colon mesentery. Finally, when the console operator leaves the console and returns to resume the case, care must be taken to safely insert the fingers in the manipulators before the surgeon's head rests on the support with the system activation sensors. This will help to avoid inadvertent movement of the instruments which could be holding or retracting crucial anatomical structures.

Common Errors and Intraoperative Difficulties

The most common errors specific to robotic cases result from inadequate retraction and visualization of anatomic landmarks, failure to recognize visual cues of tissue tension without a haptic interface, use of excessive or mistaken instrument energy application, loss of visualization of the instruments, or unrecognized collision of the instruments (Box 24.1).

Box 24.1 Most Common Errors Specific to Robotic Cases

- Improper retraction or clearance of small bowel and redundant sigmoid from the pelvis
- Initial incision into the mesentery of the rectosigmoid (more common in obese patients) or below the pHGNF, thus endangering the autonomic nerves
- Traumatic macroretraction of the rectosigmoid with break of the peritoneum or mesentery and bowel deserolization
- Dissection below the retroperitoneal fascia (very common), thus exposing the ureter and gonadal vessels
- Too deep dissection through the layers of Toldt's fascia (nuisance error resulting in bleeding from the squiggly vessels of Toldt's fascia)
- Inadequate clearance of the fibrotic trunk of IMA and not addressing vessel calcification
- Inadequate lymphadenectomy at the IMA root
- Transection of IMV distal to splenic flexure tributary (not close enough to the origin at the inferior pancreatic border)
- Disruption of splenic flexure vascular arcades (venous outflow is more common)
- Devascularization of omentum, with special emphasis to posterior omental leaflet attached to the cephalad surface of the transverse mesocolon
- Pulling on the omentum, resulting in splenic decapsulation, or rupture and bleeding
- Stripping of the peritoneal or retroperitoneal layer of the sigmoid fossa
- Stripping the retroperitoneal areolar layer (fascia) of the left common iliac vessels and psoas muscle (leading to a false pelvic dissection plane)
- Injury to the superior hypogastric plexus or the hypogastric nerves due to unrecognized dissection below the pHGNF
- Presacral dissection below or through the sacral splanchnic nerve (SSN) layer and too close to presacral vessels
- Lateral dissection below and outside of the SSN layer (exposing the internal iliac vein and injuring the pelvic plexus, where the nerves converge)
- Lateral dissection beyond the lateral edge of Denonvilliers' fascia (exposing the anterior portion of the pelvic plexus) (Figs. 24.8 and 24.11)

- Unrecognized dissection in front of Denonvilliers' fascia (safe and intentional anterior dissection can be championed with experience)
- Lateral dissection into the mesorectum, leaving the mesorectum of the lateral tethered surface remaining
- Breach of the mesorectal fascia
- Unintentional breach of Denonvilliers' fascia during retraction or dissection, with resulted sagging of seminal vesicles resulting in oozing
- Anterolateral dissection beyond the distal portion of Denonvilliers' fascia, resulting in bleeding from the neurovascular prostatic bundles
- Anterior and anterolateral dissection too close to sinuses of the posterior vaginal wall
- Inadequate distal rectal mobilization
- Improper mesorectal transection ("spiral apple peel") below the tumor, resulting in too close distal margin or transection line (more common in large specimens)
- Improper stapler application (green cartridges are likely more adequate for thick rectal tissue) with insecure staple line after multiple stapler firings, ischemic dog ears, and large amount of loose foreign body (free floating staples)
- Devascularization of colonic conduit (indocyanine green angiography may be helpful in suspected cases)
- Proximal purse-string application incorporating a diverticulum into the circular staple line
- Tension on the anastomosis
- Insecure anastomosis with failed pressure-bubble test
- Not protecting the high-risk anastomosis with a proximal diversion

Management of Intraoperative Complications and Conversion

Most intraoperative complications during a robotic low anterior resection are similar to those seen during traditional laparoscopic or open procedures. The lack of haptic feedback is outweighed by the steady view, instrument articulation, and tireless retraction. The ability to take visual cues of tissue or suture tension in lieu of haptic feedback develops with experience.

In the simplest cases of non-life-threatening bleeding, compression of the bleeding structure can be sufficient. The robotic platform allows the field, including the compressing instrument, to "freeze." This allows for self-hemostasis or preparation for the hemostatic maneuver (evacuation of blood and irrigation, application of vessel sealer or suture-ligature). In cases of more severe and potentially life-threatening bleeding, all robotic graspers should release any tissue, the robot be undocked, and a rapid laparotomy be performed.

Suturing is easier with the robot and can be easily employed to repair a bowel injury. The left ureter injury can be avoided if the retroperitoneal fascia is kept intact, and the dissection is performed in the bloodless fashion. In all other cases, a methodical, limited exposure of the ureter is required. Ureteral stents are helpful during complicated redo surgeries, but routine stent placement is not recommended. Lack of control of the powerful instruments in the pelvis can lead to violation of the presacral Waldeyer's fascia, with injury to the presacral venous plexus or, less likely, sacral artery (median or lateral). Small injuries can be controlled with robotic arm compression of the bleeding structure for 5–15 minutes; however, more severe injuries may require conversion and specialized hemostatic techniques.

The most common reason for conversion during low anterior resection is the inability to progress due to unclear anatomy as a result of extensive pelvic pathology. Unclear anatomy can even be encountered when preoperative imaging appears to be clear. It helps in these situations to look for two features of a complete mesorectal compartment – roundness and symmetry – which are universally present. They can be appreciated with appropriate exposure and deliberate slowing (or stopping) of the dissection to zoom out and in for reorientation.

Conversions have historically been associated with negative perioperative, functional, and oncologic outcomes [28, 29]. It remains prudent to reevaluate the various options and rather convert in a difficult situation than to proceed with excessive case prolongation and suboptimal outcome [9, 30].

Prerequisite Skills and Learning Curves

Advanced laparoscopic skills and adequate case volumes are keys to performing safe low anterior resection of the rectum [11]. The learning curve for robotic low anterior resection is estimated to be approximately 30–40 cases to achieve primary technical competence and around 70 cases to achieve proficiency [31, 32]. Many of the necessary robotic skills can be acquired with the help of virtual reality simulators and cadavers [16, 24, 33]. In order to keep operative times as short as possible, a stepwise transition from hybrid to complete robotic procedures may be prudent.

Outcomes

Since the landmark paper by Pigazzi and colleagues in 2006, demonstrating the feasibility of rLAR, many case series and several nonrandomized, retrospective, and prospective comparative studies of robotic and laparoscopic technique followed [1, 2, 6, 7, 11]. Until now, only two randomized controlled trial were performed. The ROLARR trial compared robotic and laparoscopic techniques, while the ACOSOG study compared a robotic subgroup with laparoscopic and open cohorts [3, 4]. In addition, several meta-analyses were conducted comparing robotic and laparoscopic techniques and others comparing all three techniques [34, 35].

Altogether, robotic surgery was shown to be safe and feasible but had longer operative times when compared to the laparoscopic technique. Oncologic superiority of the robotic technique could not be demonstrated. Nonrandomized studies and meta-analyses frequently pointed toward lower conversion rates in the robotic technique [34, 35]. The pivotal ROLARR study (2017) suggested lower conversions and lower positive circumferential resection margins with the robotic technique but failed to reach statistical significance [3]. Additionally, the study found no difference in operative and postoperative complication rates, or functional genitourinary outcomes, in contrast to several nonrandomized studies that had suggested a potential respective advantage of the robotic technique [36–39].

Conclusions

Since its inception, the robotic technique for low anterior resection has continued to undergo a constant evolution. Currently, it remains one of the many available tools in the surgical armamentarium for surgeons treating rectal cancer. Further studies are necessary to the optimal role of this technology.

References

1. Pigazzi A, Ellenhorn JD, Ballantyne GH, Paz IB. Robotic-assisted laparoscopic low anterior resection with total mesorectal excision for rectal cancer. Surg Endosc. 2006;20(10):1521–5.
2. Park JS, Choi GS, Lim KH, Jang YS, Jun SH. Robotic-assisted versus laparoscopic surgery for low rectal cancer: case-matched analysis of short-term outcomes. Ann Surg Oncol. 2010;17(12):3195–202.
3. Jayne D, Pigazzi A, Marshall H, Croft J, Corrigan N, Copeland J, et al. Effect of robotic-assisted vs conventional laparoscopic surgery on risk of conversion to open laparotomy among patients undergoing resection for rectal cancer: The ROLARR Randomized Clinical Trial. JAMA. 2017;318(16):1569–80.
4. Fleshman J, Branda ME, Sargent DJ, Boller AM, George VV, Abbas MA, et al. Disease-free survival and local recurrence for laparoscopic resection compared with open resection of stage II to III rectal cancer: follow-up results of the ACOSOG Z6051 Randomized Controlled Trial. Ann Surg. 2019;269(4):589–95.
5. Khan JS, Banerjee AK, Kim SH, Rockall TA, Jayne DG. Robotic rectal surgery has advantages over laparoscopic surgery in selected patients and centres. Colorectal Dis. 2018;20(10):845–53.
6. Lee L, de Lacy B, Gomez Ruiz M, Liberman AS, Albert MR, Monson JRT, et al. A multicenter matched comparison of transanal and robotic total mesorectal excision for mid and low-rectal adenocarcinoma. Ann Surg. 2018; https://doi.org/10.1097/SLA.0000000000002862. [Epub ahead of print].
7. Rouanet P, Bertrand MM, Jarlier M, Mourregot A, Traore D, Taoum C, et al. Robotic versus laparoscopic total mesorectal excision for sphincter-saving surgery: Results of a single-center series of 400 consecutive patients and perspectives. Ann Surg Oncol. 2018;25(12):3572–9.
8. Zelhart M, Kaiser AM. Robotic versus laparoscopic versus open colorectal surgery: towards defining criteria to the right choice. Surg Endosc. 2018;32(1):24–38.
9. Marecik S, Park JJ. Editorial. Promising times in rectal cancer treatment. Curr Med Res Pract. 2017;7:39–40.
10. Agcaoglu O, Aliyev S, Taskin HE, Chalikonda S, Walsh M, Costedio MM, et al. Malfunction and failure of robotic systems during general surgical procedures. Surg Endosc. 2012;26(12):3580–3.
11. Odermatt M, Ahmed J, Panteleimonitis S, Khan J, Parvaiz A. Prior experience in laparoscopic rectal surgery can minimise the learning curve for robotic rectal resections: a cumulative sum analysis. Surg Endosc. 2017;31(10):4067–76.

12. Heald RJ, Husband EM, Ryall RD. The mesorectum in rectal cancer surgery--the clue to pelvic recurrence? Br J Surg. 1982;69(10):613–6.
13. Stevenson AR, Solomon MJ, Lumley JW, Hewett P, Clouston AD, Gebski VJ, et al. Effect of laparoscopic-assisted resection vs open resection on pathological outcomes in rectal cancer: The ALaCaRT Randomized Clinical Trial. JAMA. 2015;314(13):1356–63.
14. Ahmed J, Siddiqi N, Khan L, Kuzu A, Parvaiz A. Standardized technique for single-docking robotic rectal surgery. Colorectal Dis. 2016;18(10):O380–4.
15. Toh JWT, Kim SH. Port positioning and docking for single-stage totally robotic dissection for rectal cancer surgery with the Si and Xi Da Vinci Surgical System. J Robot Surg. 2018;12(3):545–8.
16. Petz W, Spinoglio G, Choi GS, Parvaiz A, Santiago C, Marecik S, et al. Structured training and competence assessment in colorectal robotic surgery. Results of a consensus experts round table. Int J Med Robot. 2016;12(4):634–41.
17. Commission on Cancer. National accreditation program for rectal cancer standards manual. https://www.facs.org/quality-programs/cancer/naprc/standards. 2017.
18. Velchuru VR, Domajnko B, deSouza A, Marecik S, Prasad LM, Park JJ, et al. Obesity increases the risk of postoperative peripheral neuropathy after minimally invasive colon and rectal surgery. Dis Colon Rectum. 2014;57(2):187–93.
19. Popeskou SG, Panteleimonitis S, Figueiredo N, Qureshi T, Parvaiz A. Robotic vascular ligation, medial to lateral dissection and splenic flexure mobilization for rectal cancer – a video vignette. Colorectal Dis. 2018;20(2):165–6.
20. DeSouza A, Domajnko B, Park J, Marecik S, Prasad L, Abcarian H. Incisional hernia, midline versus low transverse incision: what is the ideal incision for specimen extraction and hand-assisted laparoscopy? Surg Endosc. 2011;25(4):1031–6.
21. Choi GS, Park IJ, Kang BM, Lim KH, Jun SH. A novel approach of robotic-assisted anterior resection with transanal or transvaginal retrieval of the specimen for colorectal cancer. Surg Endosc. 2009;23(12):2831–5.
22. Culligan K, Walsh S, Dunne C, Walsh M, Ryan S, Quondamatteo F, et al. The mesocolon: a histological and electron microscopic characterization of the mesenteric attachment of the colon prior to and after surgical mobilization. Ann Surg. 2014;260(6):1048–56.
23. Kinugasa Y, Murakami G, Suzuki D, Sugihara K. Histological identification of fascial structures posterolateral to the rectum. Br J Surg. 2007;94(5):620–6.
24. Bertrand MM, Colombo PE, Mourregot A, Traore D, Carrère S, Quénet F, et al. Standardized single docking, four arms and fully robotic proctectomy for rectal cancer: the key points are the ports and arms placement. J Robot Surg. 2016;10(2):171–4.
25. Marecik SJ, Pai A, Sheikh T, Park JJ, Prasad LM. Transanal total mesorectal excision: save the nerves and Urethra. Dis Colon Rectum. 2016;59(7):e410–4.
26. Prasad LM, deSouza AL, Marecik SJ, Park JJ, Abcarian H. Robotic pursestring technique in low anterior resection. Dis Colon Rectum. 2010;53(2):230–4.
27. Raza SJ, Froghi S, Chowriappa A, Ahmed K, Field E, Stegemann AP, et al. Construct validation of the key components of Fundamental Skills of Robotic Surgery (FSRS) curriculum--a multi-institution prospective study. J Surg Educ. 2014;71(3):316–24.
28. Tam MS, Kaoutzanis C, Mullard AJ, Regenbogen SE, Franz MG, Hendren S, et al. A population-based study comparing laparoscopic and robotic outcomes in colorectal surgery. Surg Endosc. 2016;30(2):455–63.
29. Yamamoto S, Fukunaga M, Miyajima N, Okuda J, Konishi F, Watanabe M, et al. Impact of conversion on surgical outcomes after laparoscopic operation for rectal carcinoma: a retrospective study of 1,073 patients. J Am Coll Surg. 2009;208(3):383–9.
30. Melich G, Hong YK, Kim J, Hur H, Baik SH, Kim NK, et al. Simultaneous development of laparoscopy and robotics provides acceptable perioperative outcomes and shows robotics to have a faster learning curve and to be overall faster in rectal cancer surgery: analysis of novice MIS surgeon learning curves. Surg Endosc. 2015;29(3):558–68.
31. Kim HJ, Choi GS, Park JS, Park SY. Multidimensional analysis of the learning curve for robotic total mesorectal excision for rectal cancer: lessons from a single surgeon's experience. Dis Colon Rectum. 2014;57(9):1066–74.

32. Jiménez-Rodríguez RM, Rubio-Dorado-Manzanares M, Díaz-Pavón JM, Reyes-Díaz ML, Vazquez-Monchul JM, Garcia-Cabrera AM, et al. Learning curve in robotic rectal cancer surgery: current state of affairs. Int J Colorectal Dis. 2016;31(12):1807–15.
33. Melich G, Pai A, Shoela R, Kochar K, Patel S, Park J, et al. Rectal dissection simulator for da Vinci Surgery: details of simulator manufacturing with evidence of construct, face, and content validity. Dis Colon Rectum. 2018;61(4):514–9.
34. Ohtani H, Maeda K, Nomura S, Shinto O, Mizuyama Y, Nakagawa H, et al. Meta-analysis of robot-assisted versus laparoscopic surgery for rectal cancer. In Vivo. 2018;32(3):611–23.
35. Prete FP, Pezzolla A, Prete F, Testini M, Marzaioli R, Patriti A, et al. Robotic versus laparoscopic minimally invasive surgery for rectal cancer: a systematic review and meta-analysis of randomized controlled trials. Ann Surg. 2018;267(6):1034–46.
36. Kim HJ, Choi GS, Park JS, Park SY, Yang CS, Lee HJ, et al. The impact of robotic surgery on quality of life, urinary and sexual function following total mesorectal excision for rectal cancer: a propensity score-matched analysis with laparoscopic surgery. Colorectal Dis. 2018;20(5):O103–13.
37. Kim JY, Kim NK, Lee KY, Hur H, Min BS, Kim JH. A comparative study of voiding and sexual function after total mesorectal excision with autonomic nerve preservation for rectal cancer: laparoscopic versus robotic surgery. Ann Surg Oncol. 2012;19(8):2485–93.
38. Panteleimonitis S, Ahmed J, Harper M, Parvaiz A. Critical analysis of the literature investigating urogenital function preservation following robotic rectal cancer surgery. World J Gastrointest Surg. 2016;8(11):744–54.
39. Panteleimonitis S, Ahmed J, Ramachandra M, Farooq M, Harper M, Parvaiz A. Urogenital function in robotic vs laparoscopic rectal cancer surgery: a comparative study. Int J Colorectal Dis. 2017;32(2):241–8.

Part V

Emergencies and Troubleshooting

Unexpected Findings During Laparoscopic Colectomy for Cancer: Techniques and Strategies

25

Eric G. Weiss and Giovanna da Silva

Introduction

Laparoscopic colectomy for colon cancer is widely accepted and perhaps the procedure of choice for the majority of patients with colon cancer. Despite sophisticated preoperative imaging that typically includes a CT scan of the chest, abdomen, and pelvis, as recommended by the National Comprehensive Cancer Network (NCCN) Guidelines and most surgeons' practices, unexpected intraoperative findings are sometimes encountered. This chapter focuses on eight findings that may be encountered during the performance of laparoscopic surgery for colon cancer and how to manage these unexpected findings so that patient outcome is optimized.

Identification of the Primary Tumor or Lack Thereof

Of primary importance in laparoscopic surgery for colon cancer are identification of the cancerous segment and its removal in an oncologically appropriate manner. Although this seems basic and routine, in the early learning curve of laparoscopic colon cancer management, wrong segments were removed for a variety of reasons. Surgeons often embarked on laparoscopic surgery to remove segments based solely on colonoscopic reports rather than intraoperative confirmation. This leads to the realization that preoperative marking using tattoo techniques was extremely important owing to the fact that, with the loss of tactile sensation associated with

E. G. Weiss (✉) · G. da Silva
Department of Colorectal Surgery, Cleveland Clinic Florida, Weston, FL, USA
e-mail: weisse@ccf.org; dasilvag@ccf.org

P. Sylla et al. (eds.), *The SAGES Manual of Colorectal Surgery*,
https://doi.org/10.1007/978-3-030-24812-3_25

laparoscopic surgery, the surgeon is more highly reliant on other methods of identifying tumors intraoperatively or preoperatively. Thus the importance of reviewing the preoperative imaging, even when a report does not explicitly state that there is a mass or tumor identified in a segment, cannot be overstated. Subtle findings, particularly with the surgeon's familiarity with the colonoscopy report, their own physical examination, and, possibly, their own endoscopy (colonoscopy or flexible sigmoidoscopy) depending on the situation, will often allow for confirmation of a tumor location. If a PET/CT has been ordered, unless the tumor is mucinous, the location of the tumor is typically PET-avid and will reappear, thus adding a corroborating study in addition to the colonoscopy. In cases of rectal or rectosigmoid tumors, flexible endoscopy is notoriously inaccurate in identifying the specific level of the tumor in relation to the anal verge or dentate line. Thus, in these cases, it behooves all surgeons to perform preoperative rigid proctoscopy or flexible sigmoidoscopy in the office or endoscopy suite to ensure that the tumor is a colonic rather than a rectal lesion. This is important both to ensure removal of the appropriate bowel segment and, in the case of rectal cancer, to consider alternative therapeutic options based on local staging such as neoadjuvant chemoradiotherapy, a diverting stoma, chemotherapy, etc. Other scenarios in which preoperative imaging can be useful is obtaining a water-soluble contrast enema study (WSCE) in the case of incomplete colonoscopy due to obstruction or partial obstruction. This will provide information regarding the areas not visualized by colonoscopy as well as a "hard copy, road map" as to the location of the tumor.

At the time of the initial colonoscopy, the endoscopist should consider marking a tumor with tattoos [1]. Although until recently there was no standard method of tattooing for localization of tumors during laparoscopic colectomy, several principles should be adhered to. Tattooing should always be placed distal to the tumor so that removal of the tattoo within the segment ensures removal of the tumor. Tattooing should be placed in multiple quadrants of the bowel wall to facilitate visualization of the tattooing. If only one or two tattoos are placed and they happen to be in the mesenteric surface, they will at times be difficult if not impossible to visualize. Therefore placing tattoos in three or four quadrants should be routinely performed. Reviewing the colonoscopy report is sometimes helpful, but the specifics of marking are often omitted, and the reports only confirm that marking/tattooing was performed. In these cases, discussion with the endoscopist can be useful. Furthermore, in cases where an endoscopist frequently refers patients, it is helpful to discuss the specifics of marking/tattooing in advance, which will often preclude the need for repeat colonoscopy and further marking/tattooing or intraoperative maneuvers to identify the correct segment with its associated tumor (Fig. 25.1).

At the onset of a laparoscopic procedure, an initial diagnostic laparoscopy should be performed. This entails a general inspection of the peritoneal cavity, liver, and pelvis to look for identifying characteristics of an underlying colonic tumor such as an obvious mass, adherence of omentum to the colon, puckering of the serosa, serosal involvement by the tumor, and visualization of the tattoo markings. If none of the characteristics of a colonic tumor are present and tattooing is

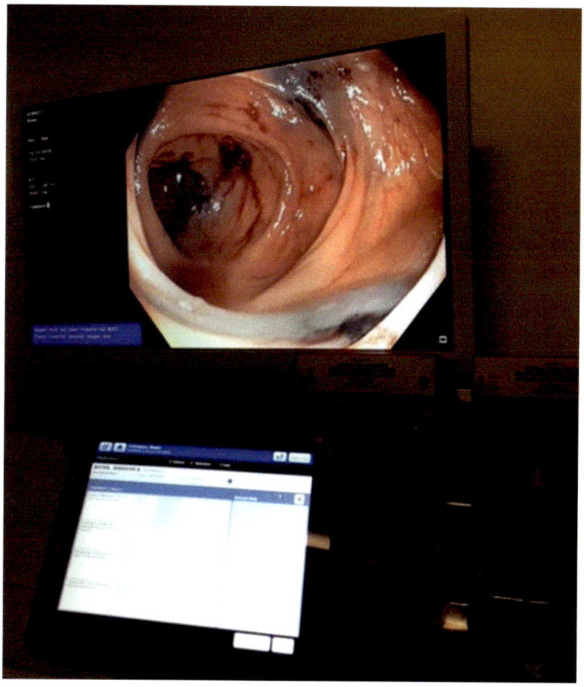

Fig. 25.1 Preoperative tattooing

not visualized, one needs to consider why the tattoos are not visualized. Is the surgeon looking in the wrong location? Just because a colonoscopy report states a tumor is in the sigmoid, it does not mean that it could not be in the descending, splenic flexure, transverse colon, and at times even more proximal. Flipping the omentum up over the transverse colon should be undertaken as sometimes this maneuver will allow visualization of the tattoos/markings. Lastly, mobilizing the flexure(s) will sometimes allow visualization if tattoos are on the mesenteric surface or blocked by folded or adhesed areas. Another approach is to place a hand port through the expected extraction site to restore tactile sensation and help to identify the tumor and its associated segment.

If all of the above maneuvers are unsuccessful, intraoperative colonoscopy should be performed. For most laparoscopic colorectal procedures, patients should be initially positioned in lithotomy, allowing access to the anus for such potential needs as intraoperative colonoscopy. If this has not already been done, repositioning will be required. Ideally, intraoperative colonoscopy should be performed using CO_2 endoscopy equipment [2]. If unavailable, clamping the terminal ileum will prevent insufflation of the small bowel with room air, which will limit working space and make completion of the surgery more difficult. Once the tumor is identified, placing a tattoo intraoperatively, placing a suture at the site of the tumor, and marking with endoclips are all viable options to preserve identification of the tumor once the colonoscopy has been completed. With all of the tools available both preoperatively and intraoperatively, a "blind colectomy" – without the ability to identify the correct segment prior to excision – should never be performed.

Invasion of Other Organs

Despite preoperative, routine, and high-quality CT scans of the chest, abdomen, and pelvis, more advanced disease does sometimes present intraoperatively. Thus on initial diagnostic laparoscopy, assessment for adherence to or involvement of the tumor to other structures should be undertaken. Structures that a primary colon cancer may be adherent to or invading into would include the abdominal wall, omentum, small bowel, duodenum, stomach, retroperitoneum, bladder, and female reproductive organs including the fallopian tubes, ovaries, uterus, and/or vagina. Other structures may be less frequently involved. Regardless, intraoperative assessment as to the resectability of these structures en bloc with the primary tumor needs to be undertaken. In addition, a decision needs to be made as to whether the procedure should be continued as a laparoscopic approach or converted to an open procedure [3]. Involvement of other specialists, if available, may also be required depending on the expertise of the operating surgeon and the organ(s) involved.

One of "the out of the OR" considerations is the potential lack of informed consent for the additional surgery that may be necessary. Speaking to family members may be of some benefit; however, from a medicolegal standpoint, unless a family member has healthcare power of attorney on behalf of the patient, consent may not be binding or legal. Regardless, doing what is in the patient's best interest should take precedence and should guide decisions.

The best decision may sometimes be to abort the procedure. However, this is advisable only if an initial diagnostic laparoscopy has been performed. If the procedure has advanced (mobilization, vascular division, etc.) in an effort to recognize any secondary involvement of structures, aborting the procedure is not an option.

If the decision is made to proceed with en bloc resection, the operative team should take a "time-out" to discuss the new operation and the steps required and the need for other teams or services, if required. This will then allow the OR staff, the operative team(s), and potential additional services to be called and prepared.

Synchronous Masses/Tumors

Synchronous tumors or cancers are relatively rare, occurring in less than 1–2% of patients with colon cancer, and are usually intraoperatively identified rather than preoperatively during colonoscopy. Although there is a small "miss rate" on colonoscopy, more typically a synchronous tumor would be proximal to a partially or obstructing tumor that was not traversed at the time of colonoscopy, thereby leaving a segment(s) of the colon that was not endoscopically evaluated. In cases where a complete colonoscopy cannot be performed, a preoperative WSCE is recommended. Not only does WSCE confirm the location of the primary tumor, it can also assess areas that were not endoscopically evaluated. In cases where a second tumor is noted preoperatively, an extended resection or, less commonly, two segmental resections should be performed [4, 5].

If the synchronous tumor is noted intraoperatively, similar options are available to the surgeon and patient. Synchronous tumors should raise the suspicion of hereditary nonpolyposis colorectal cancer (HNPCC) in the appropriately aged patient. Depending on the location of the first and second tumors, the options remain as above: extended resection such as an extended right colectomy, subtotal colectomy, or total colectomy with ileorectal anastomosis. Even in cases of total abdominal colectomy with ileorectal anastomosis, functional outcomes are good with an average of 24-hour bowel function of two to four bowel movements per day.

Meckel's Diverticulum

Meckel's diverticulum occurs in 2% of the population as per the "rule of 2s": a location of 2 feet from the ileocecal valve and ectopic gastric tissue within the diverticulum predisposing to GI bleeding in 2% of cases. Incidentally finding a Meckel's diverticulum is rarely an indication for surgical excision unless bleeding, perforation, diverticulitis, and obstructions have occurred prior to the incidental identification [6]. However, if a decision is made to excise a Meckel's diverticulum, it is generally safe and well tolerated.

Peritoneal Carcinomatosis

Patients with peritoneal carcinomatosis (PC) typically have other sites of metastasis. However, PC may be the only site in up to 25%, and in 10% it is diagnosed at the time of surgery [7]. The presence of PC implies a poorer prognosis to the patient. Traditionally, management of PC has included a combination of systemic therapy and cytoreductive surgery (CRS) followed by intraoperative hyperthermic intraperitoneal chemotherapy (HIPEC) with mitomycin-C or oxaliplatin (Fig. 25.2). Recently, a French randomized phase III multicenter trial has questioned the addition of HIPEC in these patients showing no difference in survival and an increased incidence of severe complications when compared to CRS alone [8]. Nevertheless, several studies have shown that CRS/HIPEC confers increased median 5-year survival of approximately 30% after R0/R1 resection, depending on the extent of disease and the completeness of CRS [7, 9].

Up-front knowledge of the presence of PC allows the surgeon to prepare for CRS, which entails removal of all visible disease, omentum/parietal peritoneum followed by HIPEC, which is time-consuming and demands structure with special equipment and drugs. More importantly, advance knowledge provides an opportunity for a thorough preoperative discussion with the patient regarding the prognosis, benefits, and morbidity related to the procedure. CT scan is still considered the best imaging modality to detect PC. The presence of nodular or plaque-like soft tissue

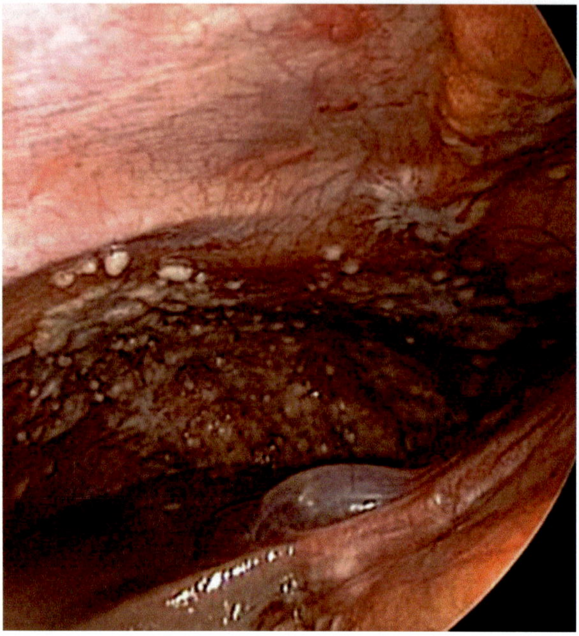

Fig. 25.2 Peritoneal carcinomatosis. (Courtesy of Patricia Sylla, MD)

masses and thickening of the mesentery in association with ascites are suggestive of the diagnosis. Unfortunately, CT scan accuracy is approximately 65% with low sensitivity for implants less than 1 cm. This results in often missed or underestimated PC on preoperative imaging [10].

When the surgeon encounters unexpected PC, the first step is to evaluate the extent of the disease. The peritoneal cancer index (PCI) is one of the most commonly used tools to evaluate the extent of disease. The PCI scores the lesion size from 0 to 3 (0 no tumor, 1 implants ≤5 mm, 2 >5–50 mm, or 3 >50 mm) in 13 abdominopelvic regions, for a score range from 0 to 39 (13 × 3). Patients who are physically fit and have limited (PCI < 20) and potentially completely resectable and/or ablatable disease with no extra-abdominal metastasis are candidates for the procedure [8]. In these cases, a surgeon experienced with CRS/HIPEC should be called in for evaluation and/or the extent of the disease well documented with photos or video. While colectomy has been performed in these scenarios, few studies have suggested worse outcomes with CRS/HIPEC preceded by nondefinitive surgical intervention due to violation of the planes and adherence of cancer cells in traumatized tissue [11]. A better option might be to perform biopsies and, at a later date, colectomy with concomitant CRS/HIPEC. Similarly, if the patient has multiple liver metastasis, CRS should not be attempted. The implants should be biopsied and the primary tumor left in place. If the patient is symptomatic, however, the tumor might be resected and/or a stoma constructed or a gastrostomy tube placed, as indicated. In all situations, the case should be discussed in a multidisciplinary team, and the patient is referred for combination treatment with systemic chemotherapy, CRS, and HIPEC.

Liver Metastasis

Liver metastasis is present in approximately 25% of patients diagnosed with colorectal cancer. CT scan is the imaging modality of choice for patients undergoing colectomy for colon cancer. As with PC, the diagnosis of liver metastasis alters the patient's treatment and prognosis. High-quality preoperative imaging is crucial as it demonstrates the number, size, and distribution of the metastasis and the volume of the remaining liver, which is important to determine the resectability of the lesions(s) and best treatment approach.

When the surgeon encounters lesions during laparoscopic exploration that are suggestive of metastasis not detected preoperatively, the decision to proceed with colectomy depends on the number/burden of the liver by the lesion(s) and the patient's symptoms. If the lesions are multiple and occupy a significant portion of the liver, biopsy of the most assessable lesion might be performed using an energy device and sent for frozen biopsy, if available. If the patient is asymptomatic, the surgeon may forego colectomy, whereas resection should be performed in the presence of symptoms such as obstruction or bleeding. If only few lesions are noted, the surgeon may proceed with colectomy. In all cases, high-quality imaging +/− biopsy should be obtained postoperatively for further treatment planning. In addition, the patient should be referred to chemotherapy and hepatobiliary surgery, and the case should be discussed in a multidisciplinary tumor board.

Ovarian Mass

The differential diagnosis for ovarian mass includes functional cyst, endometrioma, and benign or malignant neoplasm. The incidence of malignant ovarian tumors increases with age. Approximately 5 30% of ovarian tumors originate from other sites and 3–8% are from the colon. Whereas the appearance of a benign cyst filled with clear fluid is reassuring, the findings of a large, irregular, solid, multiloculated, or fixed mass are concerning. The approach to ovarian mass includes a diagnostic or staging phase and an operative phase. The diagnostic phase entails washing for cytologic examination and thorough inspection of all pelvic organs, peritoneal surfaces, the upper abdomen, the diaphragm, and the liver, in order to rule out macroscopic evidence of malignancy. Surgical treatment of known ovarian tumors may include debulking with removal of all visible disease and a staging procedure with hysterectomy, bilateral salpingo-oophorectomy, omentectomy, peritoneal biopsies, and bilateral pelvic and para-aortic lymphadenectomy [12]. This might be followed by intraperitoneal or systemic chemotherapy. Metastatic ovarian tumor may be managed with unilateral or bilateral oophorectomy. Careful preoperative evaluation should identify women who have suspicious adnexal masses, and the patient is referred to a gynecologic oncologic surgeon for possible oophorectomy and immediate staging by laparoscopy or laparotomy at the time of colon resection.

If an incidental isolated ovarian mass is found during colectomy for colon cancer, the surgeon may proceed as planned with colectomy, and gynecologic oncology consult should be obtained, if available. If the mass is suspicious and the patient is postmenopausal, after consent is obtained from the next of kin, the specialist may perform oophorectomy with care to avoid rupture and sent for frozen biopsy. If malignancy is confirmed, immediate full staging including peritoneal washings, total abdominal hysterectomy with bilateral salpingo-oophorectomy, omentectomy, peritoneal biopsies, and pelvic and para-aortic lymphadenectomy might be performed, or in a second surgery [13]. This staging procedure can be performed by laparotomy or laparoscopy in experienced hands. If frozen biopsy is not available or the patient's wishes are unknown, the ovary may be sent for permanent pathology and a second surgery performed at a later date by a specialist after discussion with the patient. Tumor markers can be sent intraoperatively or in the postoperative period.

In a premenopausal patient, reproductive and hormonal issues render the scenario more complex. A gynecologic oncology surgeon is called in for evaluation and/or the findings documented and photos taken. Oophorectomy should be performed at a later date after proper discussion and counseling relative to the patient's reproductive wishes and expected hormonal changes. In cases when a benign-looking cyst is incidentally found, management should be postponed and the patient referred to a specialist.

Malrotation

Intestinal malrotation is a rare congenital disorder that results from incomplete rotation and fixation during fetal development. It is usually diagnosed in the first month of life and is extremely rare in adults. Presentation may be acute or chronic, with symptoms of obstruction with abdominal pain and vomiting. Although preoperative CT scan is usually obtained in patients undergoing colectomy for colon cancer, the diagnosis of malrotation is often missed. Findings of reversed relation of superior mesenteric artery and superior mesenteric vein with the vein to the right of the artery, a duodenojejunal junction lying on the right without crossing over to the left (corkscrew sign), a whirled appearance of the vasculature entering the volvulus (whirlpool sign), small bowel loops in the right upper abdomen, lack of visualization of the cecum in the right lower abdomen, and dilatation of small bowel are suggestive of malrotation (Fig. 25.3a, b). The best imaging modality is upper gastrointestinal series, which may show the duodenojejunal flexure to the right of the

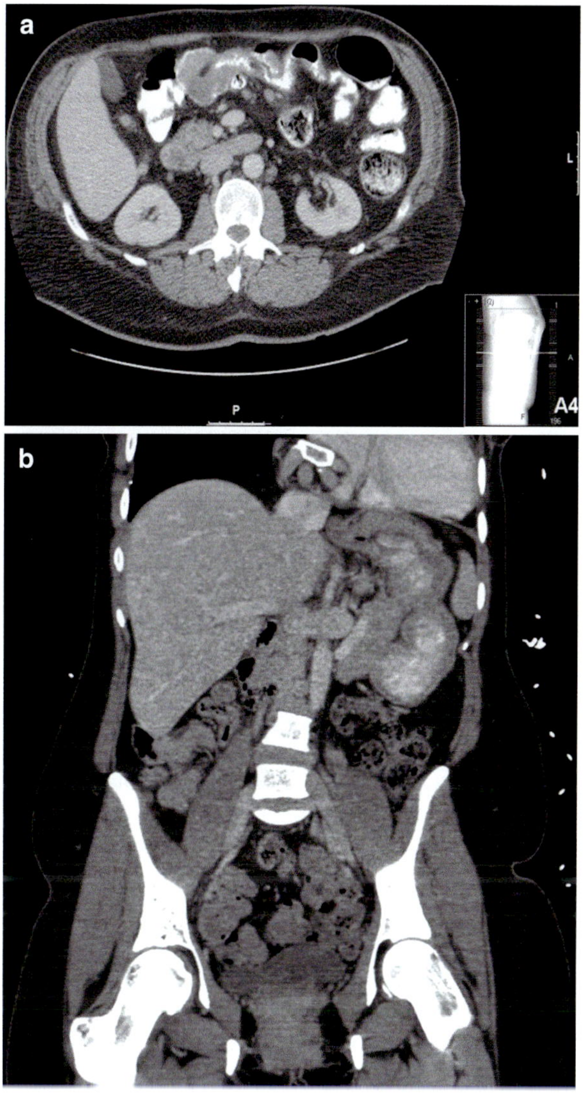

Fig. 25.3 (**a**) CT scan showing superior mesenteric artery dorsal to superior mesenteric vein. (**a** Source: From Donaire et al. [14]. Copyright © 2013 Michael Donaire et al. Used under the Creative Commons Attribution License 3.0, which permits unrestricted use, distribution, and reproduction in any medium, provided the original work is properly cited.). (**b**) Duodenum does not cross the midline

abdomen. Upon entering the abdominal cavity, the surgeon may encounter the small bowel to the right of the abdomen (Fig. 25.4). Lysis of adhesions should be carried on until the bowel is mobilized off the right abdomen. The colon might be difficult to visualize as it may be dislodged to the left. One should not hesitate to convert to open surgery to properly identify the anatomy. Care should be taken with division of the blood supply.

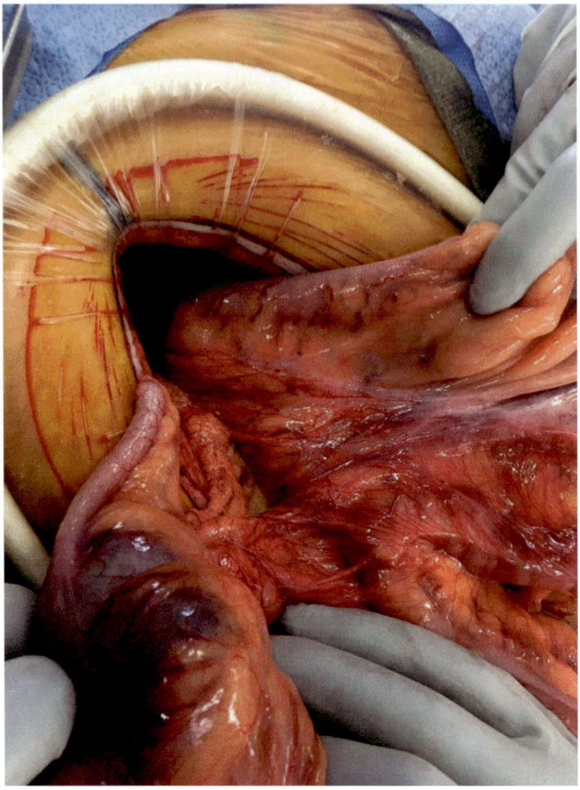

Fig. 25.4 Intestinal malrotation: cecum to the left and sigmoid to the right

Conclusion

Unexpected intraoperative findings are minimized by thorough and high-quality preoperative evaluation and imaging. The decision-making process is based on the knowledge of how to proceed when these findings are known prior to surgery; morbidity of additional treatment; natural history of the disease; surgeon's experience, resources, and skills; availability of the next of kin; the pathologist for frozen biopsy in some cases; and, above all, the patient's best interest.

References

1. Letarte F, Webb M, Raval M, Karimuddin A, Brown CJ, Phang PT. Tattooing or not? A review of current practice and outcomes for laparoscopic colonic resection following endoscopy at a tertiary care centre. Can J Surg. 2017;60(6):394–8.
2. Nakajima K, Lee SW, Sonoda T, Milsom JW. Intraoperative carbon dioxide colonoscopy: a safe insufflation alternative for locating colonic lesions during laparoscopic surgery. Surg Endosc. 2005;19(3):321–5.

3. Kumamoto T, Toda S, Matoba S, Moriyama J, Hanaoka Y, Tomizawa K, et al. Short- and long-term outcomes of laparoscopic multivisceral resection for clinically suspected T4 colon cancer. World J Surg. 2017;41(8):2153–9.
4. Kim KY, Hwang DW, Park YK, Lee HS. A single surgeon's experience with 54 consecutive cases of multivisceral resection for locally advanced primary colorectal cancer: can the laparoscopic approach be performed safely? Surg Endosc. 2012;26(2):493–500.
5. Kim MS, Park YJ. Detection and treatment of synchronous lesions in colorectal cancer: the clinical implication of perioperative colonoscopy. World J Gastroenterol. 2007;13(30):4108–11.
6. Alexander A, Farish-Williford H, Hashmi M. Recognizing and treating Meckel diverticulum. JAAPA. 2015;28(9):1–2.
7. Ihemelandu CU, Shen P, Stewart JH, Votanopoulos K, Levine EA. Management of peritoneal carcinomatosis from colorectal cancer. Semin Oncol. 2011;38(4):568–75.
8. Quenet F, Elias D, Roca L,Goere D, Ghouti L, Pocard M, et al. A UNICANCER phase III trial of hyperthermic intra-peritoneal chemotherapy (HIPEC) for colorectal peritoneal carcinomatosis (PC): PRODIGE 7. Abstract LBA3503. Oral presentation ASCO meeting 2018.
9. Esquivel J. Cytoreductive surgery and hyperthermic intraperitoneal chemotherapy for colorectal cancer: survival outcomes and patient selection. J Gastrointest Oncol. 2016;7(1):72–8.
10. Esquivel J, Chua TC, Stojadinovic A, Melero JT, Levine EA, Gutman M, et al. Accuracy and clinical relevance of computed tomography scan interpretation of peritoneal cancer index in colorectal cancer peritoneal carcinomatosis: a multi-institutional study. J Surg Oncol. 2010;102:565–70.
11. Paul BK, Ihemelandu C, Sugarbaker PH. Prior surgical score: an analysis of the prognostic significance of an initial nondefinitive surgical intervention in patients with peritoneal carcinomatosis of a colorectal origin undergoing cytoreductive surgery and perioperative intraperitoneal chemotherapy. Dis Colon Rectum. 2018;61:347–54.
12. Kline RC, Bazzett-Matabele LB. Adnexal masses and malignancies of importance to the colorectal surgeon. Clin Colon Rectal Surg. 2010;23(2):63–71.
13. Dias DS, Bueloni-Dias FN, Delmanto A, Tonon ÂF, Tayfour NM, Traiman P, et al. Clinical management of incidental findings on pelvic adnexal masses. Rev Assoc Med Bras. 2015;61(5):469–73.
14. Donaire M, Mariadason J, Stephens D, Pillarisetty S, Wallack MK. Carcinoma of the colon in an adult with intestinal malrotation. Case Rep Surg. 2013;2013:525081.

The Role of Laparoscopy in the Management of Bowel Obstruction

26

Angela H. Kuhnen

Introduction and Rationale

Traditionally, laparotomy has been the approach of choice for small bowel obstruction even though laparoscopy may offer improved outcomes. Despite early adoption of laparoscopy for evaluation and treatment of a wide variety of abdominal pathology, acceptance of laparoscopy as an adequate approach to small bowel obstruction occurred late in the history of laparoscopy. Laparoscopic release of a single adhesive band was first described in 1991 by Bastug [1]. An estimated 300,000 patients are hospitalized and/or undergo surgery annually for adhesion-related SBO. Approximately 85% of small bowel obstructions in the Western world are caused by adhesions [2]. The overall risk of developing an adhesive SBO after abdominal surgery is approximately 5% historically, and after major abdominal surgery, the risk increases to between 15% and 42%. In a meta-analysis of over 440,000 patients who underwent abdominal surgery, the highest incidence of SBO occurred after open adnexal surgery or ileal pouch-anal anastomosis. With many procedures, laparoscopy resulted in fewer adhesions than an open approach, though this has not clearly translated to a lower incidence of SBO in colorectal surgery [3].

Although laparoscopic surgery is associated with early recovery, reduced length of hospital stay, and decreased morbidity compared with open surgery, the laparoscopic approach for treatment of small bowel obstruction has been slow to become established as the optimal approach, but laparoscopy is now considered an acceptable approach for cases of SBO in which it was previously felt to be contraindicated.

A. H. Kuhnen (✉)
Division of Colon and Rectal Surgery, Lahey Hospital and Medical Center, Burlington, MA, USA
e-mail: Angela.h.kuhnen@lahey.org

P. Sylla et al. (eds.), *The SAGES Manual of Colorectal Surgery*,
https://doi.org/10.1007/978-3-030-24812-3_26

Indications and Contraindications of Laparoscopy in SBO

The cause of a bowel obstruction frequently determines whether a laparoscopic approach is possible. Most commonly adhesions are the source of obstruction, but other causes including hernia (both internal hernias and abdominal wall defects), tumor, bezoar, intussusception, acute appendicitis, and terminal ileitis may be implicated. Preoperative imaging studies often point to a cause and assist with planning of the operative approach (Figs. 26.1a, b and 26.2a–c). Laparoscopy offers the advantage of a diagnostic opportunity in cases where preoperative imaging is ambiguous. Several predictors of successful laparoscopic lysis of adhesions have been reported, as well as relative contraindications to a laparoscopic approach (Table 26.1).

Principles and Quality Benchmarks

Principles of surgery for small bowel obstruction include identification of the cause of obstruction, relief of the obstruction, resection of nonviable bowel, and avoidance of inadvertent enterotomy. Laparoscopy can be a valuable tool in

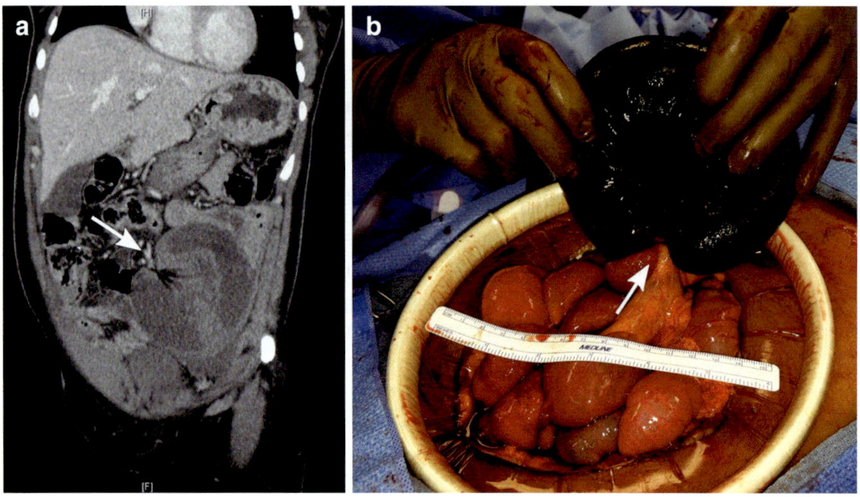

Fig. 26.1 (**a**, **b**) Abdominal CT scan images and operative findings in a woman with an adhesive closed loop small bowel obstruction after low-anterior resection for rectal cancer. Given the CT findings and peritonitis on exam, the patient was felt to be a poor candidate for laparoscopic exploration and underwent laparotomy and small bowel resection. **a** shows a coronal image with a class C-shaped closed loop obstruction with thickening and hypoenhancement of the bowel wall as well as edema and lack of perfusion in the associated mesentery. The arrow points to the location of both proximal and distal obstruction. **b** shows findings on exploratory laparotomy, with internal hernia through a short adhesive band causing closed loop obstruction and ischemia of a loop of small intestine

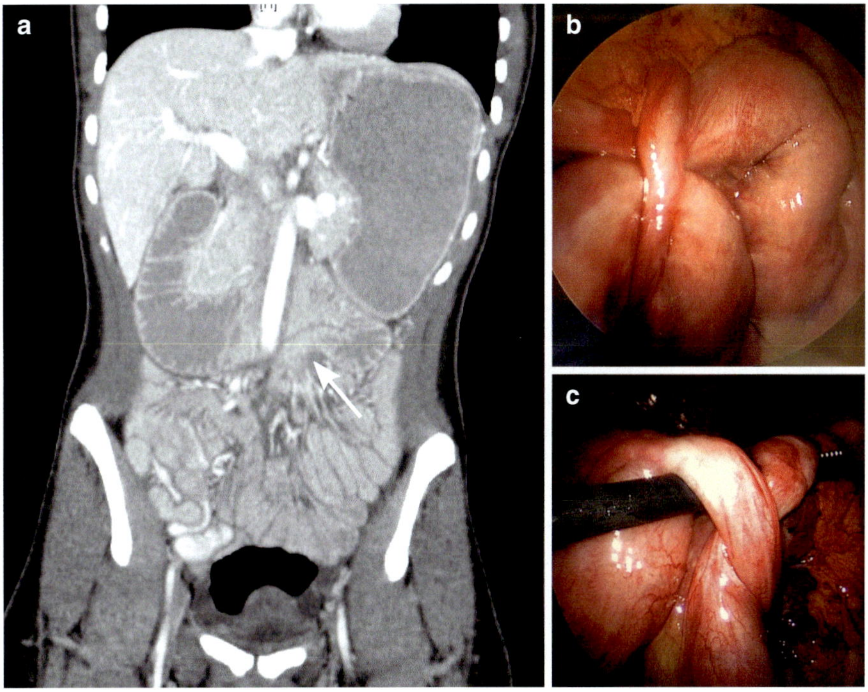

Fig. 26.2 (**a**–**c**) Abdominal CT scan images and operative findings in a woman with adhesive small bowel obstruction of the proximal jejunum after laparoscopic total proctocolectomy and ileal pouch-anal anastomosis for familial adenomatous polyposis. Given the proximal point of obstruction and prior laparoscopic approach, the patient was felt to be a good candidate for laparoscopic exploration and lysis of adhesions, which successfully resolved her obstruction. **a** shows a coronal image with dilated stomach, duodenum, and proximal jejunum. The arrow points to the point of obstruction from the adhesive band. Note the distal decompressed loops of small intestine in the pelvis. **b** and **c** show laparoscopic findings, with a broad adhesive band compressing the proximal jejunum

Table 26.1 Predictors for success and contraindications to laparoscopy for small bowel obstruction

Predictors of successful laparoscopic lysis of adhesions	Contraindications to laparoscopic approach for SBO
Two or fewer prior abdominal operations Previous upper abdominal incision Appendectomy as only prior operation Transition point outside of the pelvis Bowel dilation less than 4 cm Partial bowel obstruction Surgeon training in advanced laparoscopic techniques	Massive abdominal distension that prevents safe entry into the peritoneal space and limits working space Peritonitis with the need for bowel resection Hemodynamic instability Inability to tolerate pneumoperitoneum due to comorbid disease

accomplishing these goals, but conversion to open surgery should be undertaken without delay if any of these goals cannot be accomplished via laparoscopic approach.

Preoperative Planning, Patient Workup, and Optimization

Initial evaluation of the patient should address early stabilization with nasogastric decompression, fluid resuscitation, and correction of electrolyte abnormalities. Nasogastric decompression should be performed prior to induction of general anesthesia to minimize risk of aspiration.

Early attention to the urgency of surgery is critical in avoiding complications of strangulated bowel. Severe pain, incarcerated hernia, overlying skin changes, significant leukocytosis, free peritoneal fluid or air, or suggestion of compromised perfusion on imaging warrants consideration of emergent surgery. It is important to remember that with a closed loop obstruction, fluid-filled loops are often not seen on abdominal x-ray. If a patient is felt to be stable without impending strangulation, observation with nasogastric decompression is appropriate, but if an obstructed patient does not improve in 24–48 hours, the abdomen should be explored.

The skill level and experience of the surgeon are important in operative planning, both in terms of technical skill and ability to judge if and when it is appropriate to convert to laparotomy. Absolute contraindications for laparoscopy include pulmonary or cardiac status that cannot tolerate abdominal insufflation. Relative contraindications include diffuse abdominal distension, which risks bowel injury both during initial access to the abdomen and in dissection and visualization of the anatomy due to limited exposure. A history of previous abdominal surgery is a relative contraindication to a laparoscopic approach, with prior laparotomy or prior diffuse peritonitis yielding lower probability of success than a prior laparoscopic operation.

Operative Setup and Technique

The patient should be positioned on the operating room table with the entire abdomen exposed and sterilized. The patient's torso and all extremities should be secured to the operating table such that the table can be tilted in different directions for best visualization. In cases where intraoperative lower endoscopy may be useful (e.g., SBO after ileal pouch-anal anastomosis), a split-leg table or lithotomy position should be considered.

Pneumoperitoneum can be established using either Hasson technique or Veress needle depending on surgeon's preference, but ideally initial access should be gained away from prior surgical sites. Initial use of an optical viewing trocar can facilitate safe peritoneal entry as it allows direct visualization of the layers of the abdominal wall. Insertion of subsequent trocars under direct laparoscopic visualization is critical. Surgeons should not shy away from using several additional 5 mm trocars in order to improve access and exposure. Using a 5 mm rather than 10 mm 30 degree scope allows for frequent change in camera port position during the case. This is particularly helpful in keeping the camera in line with the surgeon's instruments when running the bowel from distal to proximal. Using a pair of atraumatic laparoscopic forceps, the surgeon follows the loops of bowel, attempting to find a transition point between distended and collapsed bowel. Careful attention to gentle manipulation of the bowel, especially dilated segments, is critical to avoid creating enterotomies. Adhesive bands are lysed with sharp laparoscopic scissors, and blunt dissection of adhesions is minimized in order to avoid tearing of tissue in planes out of direct view. As in reoperative surgery, the use of energy, either monopolar cautery or bipolar energy, should be minimized in order to avoid the risk of inadvertent burn injury and delayed enterotomy. Endo peanuts can be particularly helpful during blunt dissection of soft adhesions. Hemostasis can be achieved with suction and sponges.

Laparoscopy is a very good option to evaluate bowel obstruction in the virgin abdomen, as it allows for diagnosis and, if tumor or other reasons for minilaparotomy are found, helps optimize incision placement.

Pitfalls and Troubleshooting

The decision to convert to open surgery should be made expediently if any of the goals of surgery for SBO cannot be accomplished (identification of the cause of obstruction, relief of the obstruction, resection of nonviable bowel, and avoidance of inadvertent enterotomy). Frequently laparoscopy provides improved visualization over open surgery, but with obstruction, dilated bowel may preclude adequate visualization. Changing camera ports, adding working ports, and tilting the operating table may allow for identification of the transition point. Often after prior open surgery, adhesions to the prior abdominal incision can be divided via lateral laparoscopic ports, and laparoscopic approach is successful.

Ideally, all adhesions should be lysed to allow for running of the entire small bowel. It is necessary, however, to balance the advantage of complete visualization with the risk of bowel injury and causing bleeding by dividing further adhesions. The surgeon should maintain a low threshold for conversion if severely distended bowel or matted adhesions are present, especially in the deep pelvis. If enterotomy with minor contamination occurs and the bowel is minimally distended and otherwise healthy, laparoscopic repair can be considered, but unfortunately these conditions are rarely met, and at least minilaparotomy is typically advisable after iatrogenic bowel injury.

If the cause of obstruction is corrected but question of bowel strangulation exists, the loop of bowel should be observed for at least 5 minutes in the operating room. Return of normal color and peristalsis suggests viability, but with uncertainty the loop of bowel should be resected or at minimum the patient should be closely observed after surgery with a low threshold for second-look laparoscopy. If nonviable bowel is identified, resection should be performed through at least a minilaparotomy to minimize peritoneal contamination.

Laparoscopy can be a safe and effective first-line approach to small bowel obstruction, but maintaining a low threshold to convert to laparotomy is imperative for patient safety.

Outcomes

Logic would suggest that a laparoscopic approach for adhesive small bowel obstruction would confer the same benefits to patients as laparoscopy for other conditions, but the data are not so clear. An important consideration is that the retrospective, nonrandomized nature of nearly all publications on surgery for adhesive SBO heavily biases open surgery toward patients with more comorbidities or worse clinical presentation. As a result, outcomes will tend to favor laparoscopy despite attempts to mediate these confounders with multivariate analysis and case matching. However, it is unlikely that a randomized controlled trial large enough to provide useful results will ever be completed, and so best analysis of the available data is important. Several single institution retrospective reviews, some of which utilize propensity score matching, have been published on the topic. In addition, several authors have pooled analyses of case-matched control or comparative studies, and nationwide databases have been queried on the topic.

Adhesive SBO is approached laparoscopically in about one third of cases [4, 5] with conversion to laparotomy in 25–39% of these [2, 4, 5]. The number of prior operations did not correlate with need for conversion to open surgery in all studies, but a documented history of dense adhesions was associated with a higher rate of conversion to open surgery. In addition, emergency operations resulted in twice the rate of conversion to laparotomy [6]. The most commonly cited reasons for conversion are dense adhesions (29–70%), ischemic bowel with need for resection (16–24%), iatrogenic injury (10–16%), and inadequate exposure (9–16%) [2, 4, 5]. Enterotomy rates ranged from 6.6 to 25% [2, 4, 6] (Table 26.2). It is unclear whether laparoscopic or open surgery poses a higher risk for enterotomy, with conflicting results showing higher rates of enterotomy in open surgery [4], some showing higher rates in laparoscopy [7], and some equivocal [8]. Importantly, Dindo and colleagues found in their review of a prospective Swiss nationwide database of

Table 26.2 Outcomes in laparoscopy for small bowel obstruction

Reasons for conversion to open surgery during laparoscopic approach to small bowel obstruction	Incidence
Dense adhesions	29–70%
Ischemic bowel, need for resection	16–24%
Iatrogenic injury	10–16%
Inadequate exposure	9–16%
Laparoscopic approach to small bowel obstruction is associated with:	
Enterotomy rates of 6.6–25%	
Reduced rates of mortality, morbidity, pneumonia, length of stay compared to open approach	
Possibly increased long-term incidence of reoperation for recurrent obstruction compared to open approach	

laparoscopic approach for SBO that reactive conversions forced by intra-abdominal complications almost doubled the morbidity rate compared to early preemptive conversions [6].

Laparoscopic surgery for adhesive SBO has been associated with a significant reduction in mortality [2, 8], morbidity [2, 4, 8–10], rates of pneumonia [8], and length of stay [4, 5, 8–11] (Table 26.2). Most [4, 9] but not all [8] studies showed early return of bowel function with laparoscopy compared to open surgery. No difference has been found between laparoscopy and laparotomy in need for early return to the OR [8, 9, 11].

With introduction and wider adoption of laparoscopy for intestinal surgery, comfort levels with more challenging cases have risen. Pei et al. used the ACS NSQIP database to evaluate trends in use of laparoscopy for SBO and found that the proportion of SBO cases treated laparoscopically increased by 1.6% per year from 17.2% in 2006 to 28.7% in 2013 [10]. Behman and colleagues showed a threefold increase in laparoscopic approach over a 10-year period, from 4.3% to 14.3% in 2014 [7]. In a separate study, patient outcomes did not differ when the operating surgeon was fellowship-trained in minimally invasive surgery [5].

One argument for the use of laparoscopy is the attractive logic that long-term recurrence of adhesive small bowel obstruction might be less if the index obstruction is treated laparoscopically, resulting in fewer future adhesions. Yao and colleagues [9] followed 156 patients for 3 years after laparoscopic and open adhesiolysis and evaluated incidence of recurrent obstructive symptoms and reoperation for obstruction. Laparoscopy yielded good short-term outcomes including early return of bowel function, reduced incidence of complications, and shorter hospital stay. At 1 and 3 years postoperatively, etiology of previous SBO, surgical approach (laparoscopic vs. open), and postoperative clinical course had no impact on recurrence of obstructive symptoms. At 1 and 3 years, however, the incidence of reoperation for recurrence was significantly higher in the laparoscopically treated group (7.7% vs. 0%), though only four patients in total required reoperation (Table 26.2). Overall the authors were unable to show a long-term benefit of laparoscopy over open surgery, especially in terms of recurrent symptoms. The authors speculate that in laparoscopy, insufficient exposure of the entire small bowel can contribute to recurrence.

Conclusions

Relative to the open approach, laparoscopic management of small bowel obstruction is feasible in selected patients with reduced morbidity and mortality among surgeons experienced in laparoscopy but with a significant conversion rate. It is important to keep in mind that a low threshold for conversion may decrease postoperative morbidity. Laparoscopy may reduce the risk of adhesions compared to laparotomy, though further long-term studies are needed to determine whether laparoscopic treatment of adhesive SBO can help reduce the risk of recurrent episodes of SBO.

References

1. Bastug DF, Trammell SW, Boland JP, Mantz EP, Tiley EH. Laparoscopic adhesiolysis for small bowel obstruction. Surg Laparosc Endosc. 1991;1(4):259–62.
2. O'Connor DB, Winter DC. The role of laparoscopy in the management of acute small-bowel obstruction: a review of over 2,000 cases. Surg Endosc. 2012;26(1):12–7.
3. Foster NM, McGory ML, Zingmond DS, Ko CY. Small bowel obstruction: a population-based appraisal. J Am Coll Surg. 2006;203(2):170–6.
4. Byrne J, Saleh F, Ambrosini L, Quereshy F, Jackson TD, Okrainec A. Laparoscopic versus open surgical management of adhesive small bowel obstruction: a comparison of outcomes. Surg Endosc. 2015;29(9):2525–32.
5. Davies SW, Gillen JR, Guidry CA, Newhook TE, Pope NH, Hranjec T, et al. A comparative analysis between laparoscopic and open adhesiolysis at a tertiary care center. Am Surg. 2014;80(3):261–9.
6. Dindo D, Schafer M, Muller MK, Clavien PA, Hahnloser D. Laparoscopy for small bowel obstruction: the reason for conversion matters. Surg Endosc. 2010;24(4):792–7.
7. Behman R, Nathens AB, Byrne JP, Mason S, Look Hong N, Karanicolas PJ. Laparoscopic surgery for adhesive small bowel obstruction is associated with a higher risk of bowel injury: a population-based analysis of 8584 patients. Ann Surg. 2017;266(3):489–98.
8. Wiggins T, Markar SR, Harris A. Laparoscopic adhesiolysis for acute small bowel obstruction: systematic review and pooled analysis. Surg Endosc. 2015;29(12):3432–42.
9. Yao S, Tanaka E, Matsui Y, Ikeda A, Murakami T, Okumoto T, et al. Does laparoscopic adhesiolysis decrease the risk of recurrent symptoms in small bowel obstruction? A propensity score-matched analysis. Surg Endosc. 2017;31(12):5348–55.
10. Pei KY, Asuzu D, Davis KA. Will laparoscopic lysis of adhesions become the standard of care? Evaluating trends and outcomes in laparoscopic management of small-bowel obstruction using the American College of Surgeons National Surgical Quality Improvement Project Database. Surg Endosc. 2017;31(5):2180–6.
11. Patel R, Borad NP, Merchant AM. Comparison of outcomes following laparoscopic and open treatment of emergent small bowel obstruction: an 11-year analysis of ACS NSQIP. Surg Endosc. 2018;32(12):4900–11.

Large Bowel Obstruction: When Should Colon Stenting Be Considered as First-Line Strategy?

27

George Melich, Elena Vikis, and Alberto Arezzo

Introduction and Rationale

Introduced in the 1990s [1, 2] and found to be a lower cost alternative to emergency surgery (ES) for symptomatic obstructing left-sided colon cancer [3], the role of self-expanding metal stents (SEMS) has continued to evolve. There are two types of colonic stents available on the market, covered and uncovered stents. While no differences in technical and clinical success rates or complication rates have been found between the stents, covered stents have significantly higher rates of tumor ingrowth but lower migration rates [4, 5]. Correct stent insertion is mostly dependent on the location of the stenosis and length of the stent, which may be difficult to advance through the loops of the sigmoid tract (mainly if >10 cm long). Stent diameter also influences the rate of migration, as stents <24 mm in diameter are associated with higher migration rates [6, 7, 8]. As SEMS tend to shorten after deployment, it is advisable to cover at least 2 cm on each side of the obstruction to guarantee long-lasting efficacy [9].

The indications for stent placement in patients with malignant colonic obstruction include:

- Palliation of surgically incurable colorectal cancer
- Stenting as a bridge to surgery to avoid an emergent, two-step procedure and to allow for optimization of medical status and for preoperative staging including colonoscopy
- Management of some patients with extracolonic pelvic tumors (e.g., ovarian cancer)

G. Melich (✉) · E. Vikis
Royal Columbian Hospital, Department of General Surgery, New Westminster, BC, Canada

University of British Columbia, Department of General Surgery, New Westminster, BC, Canada

A. Arezzo
Department of Surgical Sciences, University of Torino, Torino, Italy

P. Sylla et al. (eds.), *The SAGES Manual of Colorectal Surgery*,
https://doi.org/10.1007/978-3-030-24812-3_27

This chapter will review indications and contraindications for colonic stents placement in large-bowel obstruction, based on available data regarding technical success/failure, risk for early and delayed perforation, and oncologic outcomes relative to emergency surgery based on recurrence rates and 5-year survival rates.

Indications for SEMS

While first-line use of SEMS for palliation of obstructing left-sided colon cancer in the face of significant comorbidity is widely accepted [10–13], its role in colonic stent decompression as a bridge to elective surgery (SBTS) remains controversial. This is reflected by conflicting international guidelines that are summarized in Table 27.1.

The 2013 American Society for Gastrointestinal Endoscopy (ASGE) guidelines state colonic SEMS may also be used as "bridge to surgery" for patients with malignant obstruction who are surgical candidates [10]. These were followed by the 2014 update of the European Society of Gastrointestinal Endoscopy (ESGE) guidelines [11]. Heavily influenced by outcomes from the halted STENT-In 2 trial [14], the largest multicenter randomized controlled trial (RCT) published at the time, the guidelines strongly recommended against colonic SEMS placement as a standard treatment for symptomatic left-sided malignant obstruction. Nonetheless, several critics of the STENT-In 2 study questioned the SEMS skills and experience of some of the centers, due to the low clinical and endoscopic success rate reported [15]. Though not a recommended first-line treatment for all patients with potentially curable left-sided obstructing colon cancer, the ESGE still conceded that SEMS placement may be considered as an alternative to emergency surgery in those who have an increased risk of postoperative mortality, e.g., ASA > III and/or age > 70 years (weak recommendation, low quality evidence) [11].

More recent guidelines are no less at odds. In 2016, the Eastern Association for the Surgery of Trauma (EAST) conditionally recommended colonic stenting (if available) as the initial therapy for malignant colonic obstruction after finding stent use being associated with decreased mortality and decreased rates for emergency procedures, including reoperations [11], based on a meta-analysis of results from six RCTs [16–20]. These conclusions are supported by findings from the subsequent 2016 ESCO trial, the largest RCT published to date [21]. Here the findings indicate that the two treatment strategies (stent bridge to elective surgery and emergency surgery) are equivalent. No difference in oncologic outcome was found at a median follow-up of 36 months. The significantly lower stoma rate noted in the SBTS group argues in favor of the stent bridge to elective surgery procedure when performed in expert hands.

The 2017 consensus conference of the World Society of Emergency Surgery (WSES) states SEMS as a bridge to elective surgery offers a better short-term outcome than direct emergency surgery with significantly lower stoma rates [21, 22]. However, SEMS could not with certainty be recommended as the treatment of choice in the management of obstructing left-sided colon cancer, because evidence

Table 27.1 Main recommendations on the use of stents of the most recent international guidelines

	Prophylactic colonic stent placement	Stent bridge to elective surgery	Stent as palliation of malignant colonic obstruction
ASGE, 2013		"Colonic SEMS may also be used as a 'bridge to surgery' for patients with malignant obstruction who are surgical candidates"	
ESGE, 2014	Not recommended. Colonic stenting should be reserved for patients with clinical symptoms and imaging evidence of malignant large-bowel obstruction, without signs of perforation	Not recommended, unless increased risk of postoperative mortality, i.e., American Society of Anesthesiologists (ASA) physical status RIII and/or age >70 years (weak recommendation, low quality evidence)	SEMS placement is recommended as the preferred treatment for palliation of malignant colonic obstruction except in patients treated or considered for treatment with antiangiogenic drugs (e.g., bevacizumab)
EAST, 2016		We conditionally recommend endoscopic, colonic stenting (if available) as the initial therapy for colonic obstruction	
WSES, 2017		*SEMS as bridge to elective surgery offers a better short-term outcome than direct emergency surgery. The complications are comparable, but the stoma rate is significantly smaller. Long-term outcomes appear comparable, but evidence remains suboptimal; further studies are necessary. For these reasons, SEMS as BTS cannot be considered the treatment of choice in the management of OLCC, while it may represent a valid option in selected cases and in tertiary referral hospitals*	*In facilities with capability for stent placement, SEMS should be preferred to colostomy for palliation of OLCC since it is associated with similar mortality/morbidity rates and shorter hospital stay. Alternative treatments to SEMS should be considered in patients eligible to a bevacizumab-based therapy. Involvement of the oncologist in the decision is strongly recommended*

Data from Refs. [10, 11, 16-20, 21-26]

ASGE American Society for Gastrointestinal Endoscopy, *ESGE* European Society for Gastrointestinal Endoscopy, *EAST* Eastern Association for the Surgery of Trauma, *WSES* World Society of Emergency Surgery, *SEMS* self-expanding metal stents, *OLCC* obstructing left colon carcinoma, *BTS* bridge to elective surgery

remained suboptimal for long-term outcomes [23]. Further studies were deemed necessary to alleviate concerns that SEMS insertion may promote tumor progression and metastasis. A 2015 meta-analysis by Erichsen and coauthors reports a comparable 5-year survival of 49% among patients with SEMS vs 40% who underwent urgent resection. However, the same study also reports a 5-year recurrence risk of

39% after SEMS placement compared with 30% after urgent resection [24]. More recently, a 2017 meta-analysis of randomized trials and observational studies found SBTS had similar long-term oncologic outcomes to ES, leading the authors to conclude that it should be considered the best treatment option for left-sided malignant colonic obstructions in centers with appropriate experience [25]. A similar meta-analysis considering only RCTs showed that SBTS was associated with lower short-term overall morbidity and lower rates of temporary and permanent stoma [9]. The authors concluded that depending on multiple factors such as local expertise and clinical status, including level of obstruction and level of certainty of diagnosis, SBTS does offer some advantages with less risk than ES for left-sided malignant colonic obstruction in the short-term. Patients' characteristics and main findings of the meta-analysis of only RCTs are summarized in Tables 27.2 and 27.3.

Although the evidence quality is low, because of the potential complications associated with SEMS, prophylactic stenting in the case of asymptomatic left-sided colon cancer cannot be recommended outside clinical trials [11]. Results of the CREST study are awaited to eventually reconsider this conclusion [26].

Contraindications for SEMS

Absolute contraindications to colorectal stenting include documented perforation on imaging, concomitant small bowel obstruction, and very distal rectal lesions where stent placement poses a high risk of tenesmus and, when within 2 cm of the anal verge, incontinence [27, 28]. In addition, stents are not recommended if bevacizumab-based chemotherapy is intended, due to increased risk of perforation [28–30].

Relative contraindications include peritoneal carcinomatosis due to increased risk of perforation, uncorrectable coagulopathy, and extensive bleeding [31].

Principles and Quality Benchmarks

Most commercial SEMS are manufactured from the flexible nickel-titanium alloy Nitinol and may be covered with polyurethane, polyethylene, or silicone, which makes them resistant to tumor invasion and tissue ingrowth but more prone to migration [27, 28, 30, 32].

Stent placement may be radiologic, endoscopic, or, as we prefer, a combination of both. The combined approach not only enables precise placement of the stent by facilitating guidewire delivery, particularly in tortuous colons and angulated or tight stenoses, but endoscopy permits biopsy when a pathologic diagnosis has yet to be made and decreases patient and operator exposure to radiation compared with fluoroscopy alone [33].

Stent length is selected by allowing an additional 2 cm to extend proximally and distally past the lesion while ensuring the expanded stent fully abuts the bowel wall to prevent migration.

Table 27.2 Characteristics of included studies and principal outcomes

Author	Year	Country	Type of publication	Recruitment	Type of surgery	Stent type	Time from SEMS to surgery	Significant difference	No significant difference	Notes
Cheung [16]	2009	China	Single center; RCT	Jan 2002/ May 2005	SBTS and lap Versus ES open	Wallstent	<2 weeks	Blood loss, pain, wound infection, anastomotic leak rates, stoma rate	–	–
Alcántara [18]	2011	Spain	Single center; RCT	Feb 2004/ Dec 2006	SBTS and lap versus open ES	N/A	<10 days	Blood loss, permanent stoma pain, postoperative complications	–	Trial included 2 SBTS groups, operated at 3 or at 10 days, these showing higher 1-stage treatment and lower conversion rate
Cui [38]	2011	China	Single center: RCT	–	SBTS and open versus open ES with IOCL	Wallstent	5–7 days	Overall morbidity and anastomotic leak	SSI, hospital stay, mortality	Trial stopped as emergency surgery group had significantly increased rate of anastomotic leak
Van Hooft [14]	2011	Netherlands	Multicenter; RCT	Mar 2007/ Aug 2009	SBTS and open surgery versus open ES	Wallstent/ Wallflex	<4 weeks	Initial stoma rates	Mean global health status, mortality, morbidity, stoma rates	Trial stopped as SBTS group had increased absolute risk of 30-day morbidity on interim analysis

(continued)

Table 27.2 (continued)

Author	Year	Country	Type of publication	Recruitment	Type of surgery	Stent type	Time from SEMS to surgery	Significant difference	No significant difference	Notes
Pirlet [20]	2011	France	Multicenter; RCT	Dec 2002/ Oct 2006	SBTS and open surgery versus open ES	Bard	N/A	–	Stoma, colonic resection, in-hospital mortality, surgical and medical morbidity rates	Trial stopped owing to 3 colonic perforations during stent placement and high rate of technical failure of stent placement (16 of 30)
Ho [19]	2012	Singapore	Single center; RCT	Oct 2004/ Feb 2008	SBTS and surgery versus ES	Wallflex	1–2 weeks	Shorter hospital stay	Stoma, overall complications, mortality	12 IOCL and 7 STC in ES group
Ghazal [17]	2013	Egypt	Single center RCT	Jan 2009/ May 2012	SBTS and surgery versus subtotal colectomy	N/A	<10 days	Postoperative complications, bowel movements	–	30 TACIR in ES group
Arezzo [21]	2017	Italy; Spain	Multicenter; RCT	Mar 2008/ Nov 2015	SBTS and surgery versus ES	Wallflex/ Hanaro	<4 weeks	Initial stoma rates (pro SBTS), hospital stay (pro ES)	Morbidity, mortality, blood transfusion, relapse, OS, and PFS curves	13% misdiagnosis at CT

Cui et al. [38]

RCT randomized controlled trial, *SBTS* stent bridge to surgery, *ES* emergency surgery, *SSI* surgical site infection, *IOCL* intra-operative colonic lavage, *TACIR* total abdominal colectomy and ileorectal anastomosis, *SEMS* self-expandable metallic stents, *CT* computed tomography, *OS* overall survival, *PFS* progression-free survival

Table 27.3 Characteristics of patients

Author	No. of randomized patients	Group	No. of analyzed patients	M/F	Mean age in years (SD or range)	BMI Kg/m^2 (SD or range)	ASA score (I/II/III/IV)	POSSUM score	Mean follow-up in months (SD or range)
Cheung (2009) [16]	50	SBTS	24	14/10	64.5 (39–68)	23.8 (17.5–27.2)	–	–	65 (18–139)
		ES	24	12/12	68.5 (27–86)	24 (17.4–30.3)	–	–	32 (4–118)
Alcántara (2011) [18]	28	SBTS	15	5/10	71.9 (8.96)	–	–/5/8/2	17.13	*37.6 (16.08)*[a]
		ES	13	7/6	71.15 (9)	–	–/1/9/3	19.15	
Cui (2011) [38]	49	SBTS	29	16/13	64	22.3	–	–	–
		ES	20	9/11	67.5	23.7	–	–	
Van Hooft (2011) [14]	98	SBTS	47	24/23	70.4 (11.9)	–	16/24/6/0	–	6
		ES	51	27/24	71.4 (9.7)	–	17/27/6/0	–	
Pirlet (2011) [20]	67	SBTS	30	16/14	70.4 (10.3)	24.2 (5.1)	–	24.2 (7.6)	–
		ES	30	13/17	74.7 (11.3)	23.3 (4.2)	–	21 (5.2)	
Ho (2012) [19]	40	SBTS	20	13/7	68 (51–85)	–	–	–	–
		ES	19	9/10	65 (49–84)	–	–	–	
Ghazal (2013) [17]	60	SBTS	30	12/18	52 (37–68)	–	–	–	18 (6–40)
		ES	30	11/19	51 (35–66)	–	–	–	
Arezzo (2017) [21]	144	SBTS	56	28/28	72 (43–90)	24.8 (19.5–40.2)	12/27/14/3	–	36 (16–38)
		ES	59	32/27	71 (44–94)	24.5 (18–35)	11/28/16/4	–	
Total	**536**	**SBTS**	**251**	**128/123**					
		ES	**246**	**120/126**					

Cui et al. [38]

SBTS stent bridge to surgery, *ES* emergency surgery, *BMI* body-mass index, *ASA* American Society of Anesthesiologists, *SD* standard deviation, *POSSUM* physiological and operative severity score for the enumeration of mortality and morbidity

[a]Mean + SD

Although there is no agreement on how long the stent should or could be kept in place depending on the different applications, it is generally recommended to await a minimum of 5 days before proceeding to elective surgery if the stent was meant as a bridge to surgery. Some centers prefer to discharge patients and readmit them after a minimum of 2 weeks before subsequent surgery. A full bowel preparation is questionable after SEMS placement but generally not performed for concerns regarding possible stent migration. No evidence is provided in the literature to provide specific guidance in any of these topics.

Subsequent surgery is ideally carried out as a single procedure, but patients with multiple comorbidities (i.e., distant metastases) may require staged surgery, i.e., first colorectal resection followed by systemic chemotherapy, after which liver-directed operation is performed.

Preoperative Planning, Patient Workup, and Optimization

Complete blood count and, in cases where a bleeding diathesis is known or suspected, INR and PTT are ordered. If applicable, abnormalities are corrected. CT scans of the chest, abdomen, and pelvis are performed to localize the tumor, to assess for metastatic spread, and to identify contraindications to stent placement.

Prior to stent placement, patients can usually undergo a simple water enema.

Technique

Once the lesion is visualized endoscopically, a 5 Fr catheter threaded with a hydrophilic guidewire is passed via the endoscope's 3.7 mm working channel beyond the lesion. Threading is further facilitated via radiological guidance using static X-rays or fluoroscopy (Fig. 27.1) [34]. Angulated strictures may require initial traversal either with a J-wire or with the use of a sphincterotome as cannula. The guidewire is retrieved, and water-soluble contrast is injected through the catheter to delineate the lesion and confirm required stent length under radiological guidance, if this is not clear by just observation of air contrast. A super stiff guidewire replaces the hydrophilic one (Fig. 27.2), the catheter is removed, and the compressed SEMS delivery system is passed over the guidewire into position (Fig. 27.3) and expanded under both fluoroscopic and endoscopic visualization (Fig. 27.4). Patency is confirmed by water-soluble contrast which also ensures the absence of leaks. Additional dilation via balloon is not performed to avoid perforation. X-rays are taken the day of the procedure and the day after to confirm appropriate placement, non-migration, and rule out asymptomatic perforation.

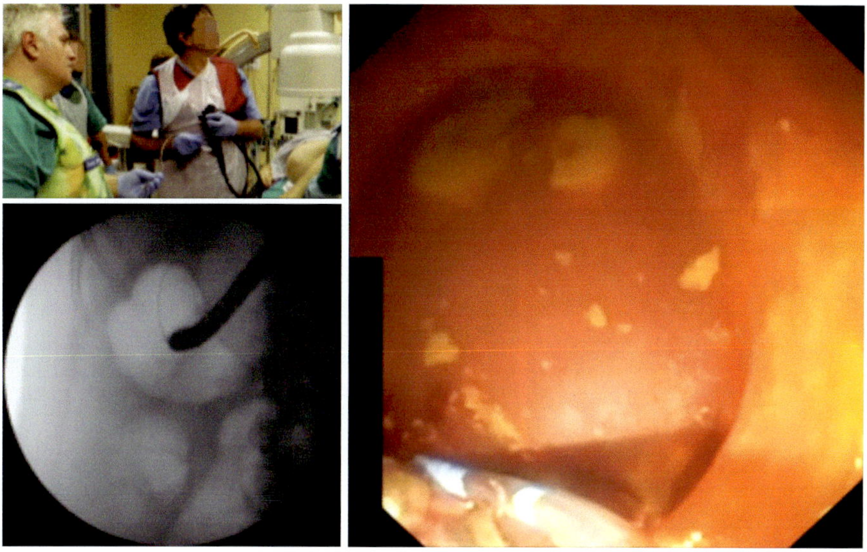

Fig. 27.1 Insertion of the J-wire under endoscopic and fluoroscopic guidance

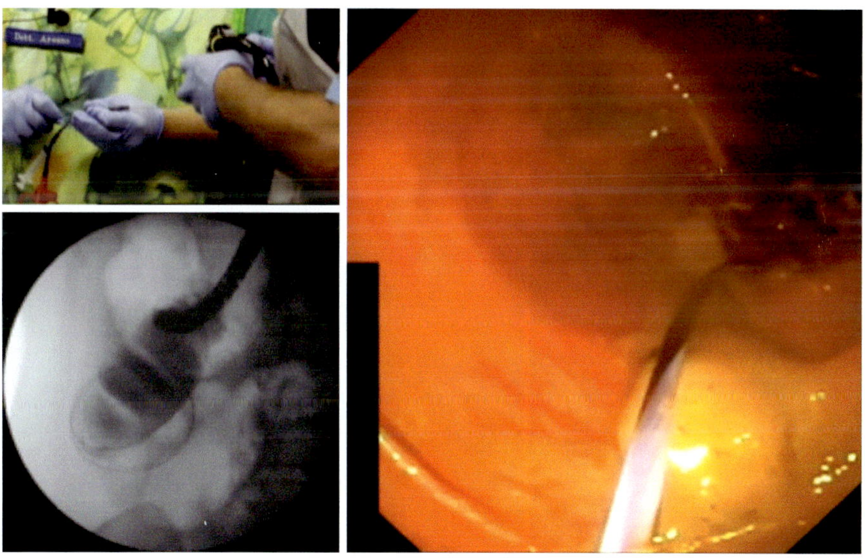

Fig. 27.2 Advancement of the super-stiff wire

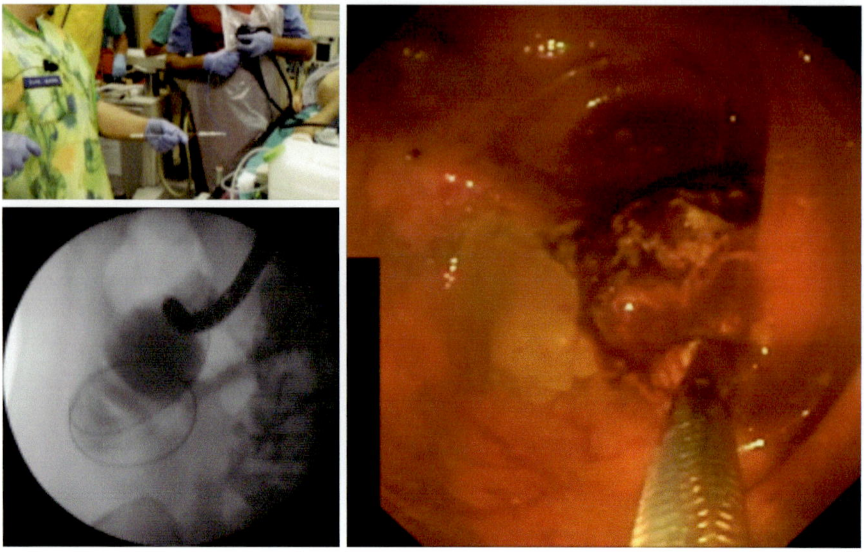

Fig. 27.3 Advancement of the SEMS delivery system

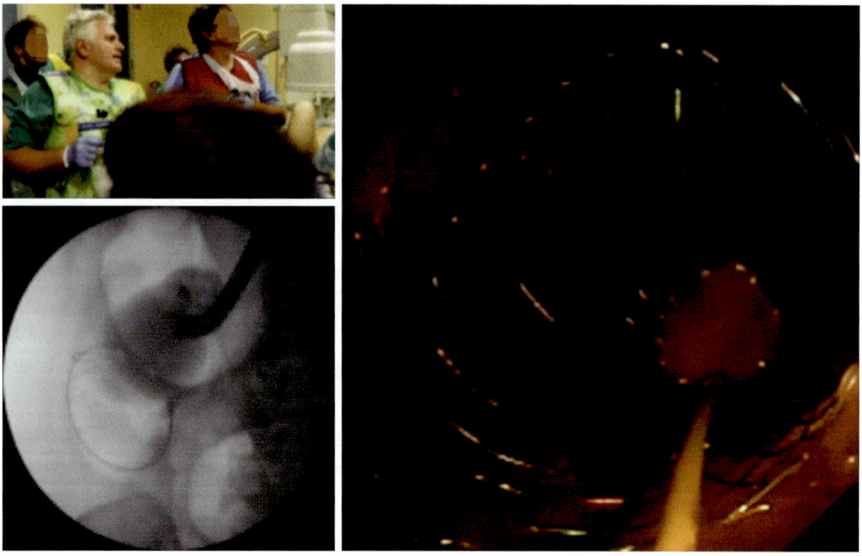

Fig. 27.4 Stent deployment

Pitfalls and Troubleshooting

Complications of SEMS include perforation, migration, obstruction, and bleeding. Immediate perforation typically occurs during guidewire or catheter advancement, while delayed perforation is associated with stent quality and high angulation strictures at the rectosigmoid junction [27, 31, 35, 36].

Partial migration or foreshortened stent length may be managed with placing a second overlapping stent. For re-obstruction, stent-in-stent deployment must be balanced against the increased risk of surgical failure with the placement of additional stents.

Bleeding is usually due to a friable tumor or mucosal injury and is typically self-limited.

Emergency surgery is required in cases of perforation, incorrect or unsalvageable stent placement, and unrelieved obstructive symptoms.

Learning Curve

Initial proctoring by a skilled operator is strongly recommended with the learning curve for colorectal stent insertion being reported as about 30 procedures for an experienced endoscopist [37]. We now know that one of the weaknesses of the Stent-In 2 trial study that significantly influenced subsequent statements and guidelines was the variation in operator experience with stenting in the participating centers, which could partly explain the high rate of perforations as compared with the published literature. As a result, in order to minimize the risk of perforation, surgeons in the Netherlands must prove sufficient expertise before they can perform colonic stenting. The general consensus is that larger trials are mandatory and that stent placement should only be performed in centers where experienced endoscopists are available.

Outcomes

Tables 27.2 and 27.3 summarize the findings of all randomized trials pertaining to SBTS vs ES. The meta-analysis of RCTs investigated overall mortality and morbidity rates within 60 days as primary outcomes. The overall mortality rate was 9.6% in the SBTS group and 9.9% in the ES group (RR = 0.98, 95% CI 0.53–1.82, $p = 0.955$). The overall morbidity rate was 33.9% in the SBTS group and 51.2% in the ES group (RR = 0.59, 95% CI 0.38–0.93, $p = 0.023$). Among secondary outcomes, the temporary stoma rate was 33.9% in the SBTS group and 51.4% in the ES group ($p < 0.001$); the permanent stoma rate was 22.2% in the SBTS group and 35.2% in the ES group ($p = 0.003$); the primary anastomosis success rate was 70.0% in the SBTS group and 54.1% in the ES group ($p = 0.043$).

Major concern has been raised regarding oncologic outcomes after SBTS and the increased risk of disease spread, particularly of liver metastases. The same meta-analysis showed that tumor recurrence rate was reported in four of the eight studies, with a median follow-up period ranging from 18 to 65 months; the rate was 40.5% in the SBTS group and 26.6% in the ES group, with an overall RR of 1.80 (95% CI 0.91–3.54, $p = 0.09$; $I^2 = 61.1\%$). Data about overall survival and progression-free survival as well as quality of life and cost analysis were insufficient for inferential analysis.

Conclusions

First-line use of colonic stenting is universally recognized for the palliation of symptomatic left-sided obstruction due to colon cancer when patient comorbidity is high. Its role in symptomatic, potentially curable obstructing left-sided colon cancer is less defined, and we await the 5-year oncologic outcomes from the ESCO trial [21] to provide further clarity. Prophylactic stenting in asymptomatic left-sided colon cancer is not recommended.

References

1. Rupp KD, Dohmoto M, Meffert R, Holzgreve A, Hohlbach G. Cancer of the rectum- palliative endoscopic treatment. Eur J Surg Oncol. 1995;21(6):644–7.
2. Tejero E, Mainar A, Fernández L, Tobío R, De Gregorio MA. New procedure for the treatment of colorectal neoplastic obstructions. Dis Colon Rectum. 1994;37(11):1158–9.
3. Flor-Lorente B, Báguena G, Frasson M, García-Granero A, Cervantes A, Sanchiz V, et al. Self-expanding metallic stent as a bridge to surgery in the treatment of left colon cancer obstruction: Cost-benefit analysis and oncologic results. Cir Esp. 2017;95(3):143–51.
4. Zhang Y, Shi J, Shi B, Song CY, Xie WF, Chen YX. Comparison of efficacy between uncovered and covered self-expanding metallic stents in malignant large bowel obstruction: a systematic review and meta-analysis. Colorectal Dis. 2012;14(7):e367–74.
5. Yang Z, Wu Q, Wang F, Ye X, Qi X, Fan D. A systematic review and meta-analysis of randomized trials and prospective studies comparing covered and bare self-expandable metal stents for the treatment of malignant obstruction in the digestive tract. Int J Med Sci. 2013;10(7):825–35.
6. Small AJ, Coelho-Prabhu N, Baron TH. Endoscopic placement of self-expandable metal stents for malignant colonic obstruction: long-term outcomes and complication factors. Gastrointest Endosc. 2010;71(3):560–72.
7. Kim BC, Han KS, Hong CW, Sohn DK, Park JW, Park SC, et al. Clinical outcomes of palliative self-expanding metallic stents in patients with malignant colorectal obstruction. J Dig Dis. 2012;13(5):258–66.
8. Im JP, Kim SG, Kang HW, Kim JS, Jung HC, Song IS. Clinical outcomes and patency of self-expanding metal stents in patients with malignant colorectal obstruction: a prospective single center study. Int J Colorectal Dis. 2008;23(8):789–94.
9. Baron TH, Wong Kee Song LM, Repici A. Role of self-expandable stents for patients with colon cancer (with videos). Gastrointest Endosc. 2012 Mar;75(3):653–62.
10. ASGE Standards of Practice Committee, Fisher DA, Shergill AK, Early DS, Acosta RD, Chandrasekhara V, et al. Role of endoscopy in the staging and management of colorectal cancer. Gastrointest Endosc. 2013;78(1):8–12. Erratum in: Gastrointest Endosc. 2013;78(3):559.

11. van Hooft JE, van Halsema EE, Vanbiervliet G, Beets-Tan RGH, DeWitt JM, Donnellan F. Self-expandable metal stents for obstructing colonic and extracolonic cancer: European Society of Gastrointestinal Endoscopy (ESGE) Clinical Guideline. Gastrointest Endosc. 2014;80(5):747–61.
12. Ferrada P, Patel MB, Poylin V, Bruns BR, Leichtle SW, Wydo S, et al. Surgery or stenting for colonic obstruction: a practice management guideline from the Eastern Association for the Surgery of Trauma. J Trauma Acute Care Surg. 2016;80(4):659–64.
13. Pisano M, Zorcolo L, Merli C, Cimbanassi S, Poiasina E, Ceresoli M, et al. 2017 WSES guidelines on colon and rectal cancer emergencies: obstruction and perforation. World J Emerg Surg. 2018;13:36.
14. van Hooft JE, Bemelman WA, Oldenburg B, Marinelli AW, Lutke Holzik MF, Grubben MJ, et al. Colonic stenting versus emergency surgery for acute left-sided malignant colonic obstruction: a multicentre randomised trial. Lancet Oncol. 2011;12(4):344–52.
15. Arezzo A, Passera R, Lo Secco G, Verra M, Bonino MA, Targarona E, et al. Stent as bridge to surgery for left-sided malignant colonic obstruction reduces adverse events and stoma rate compared with emergency surgery: results of a systematic review and meta-analysis of randomized controlled trials. Gastrointest Endosc. 2017;86(3):416–26.
16. Cheung HY, Chung CC, Tsang WW, Wong JC, Yau KK, Li MK. Endolaparoscopic approach vs conventional open surgery in the treatment of obstructing left-sided colon cancer: a randomized controlled trial. Arch Surg. 2009;144(12):1127–32.
17. Ghazal AH, El-Shazly WG, Bessa SS, El-Riwini MT, Hussein AM. Colonic endolumenal stenting devices and elective surgery versus emergency subtotal/total colectomy in the management of malignant obstructed left colon carcinoma. J Gastrointest Surg. 2013;17(6):1123–9.
18. Alcántara M, Serra-Aracil X, Falcó J, Mora L, Bombardó J, Navarro S. Prospective, controlled, randomized study of intraoperative colonic lavage versus stent placement in obstructive left-sided colonic cancer. World J Surg. 2011;35(8):1904–10.
19. Ho KS, Quah HM, Lim JF, Tang CL, Eu KW. Endoscopic stenting and elective surgery versus emergency surgery for left-sided malignant colonic obstruction: a prospective randomized trial. Int J Colorectal Dis. 2012;27(3):355–62.
20. Pirlet IA, Slim K, Kwiatkowski F, Michot F, Millat BL. Emergency preoperative stenting versus surgery for acute left-sided malignant colonic obstruction: a multicenter randomized controlled trial. Surg Endosc. 2011;25(6):1814–21.
21. Arezzo A, Balague C, Targarona E, Borghi F, Giraudo G, Ghezzo L, et al. Colonic stenting as a bridge to surgery versus emergency surgery for malignant colonic obstruction: results of a multicentre randomised controlled trial (ESCO trial). Surg Endosc. 2017;31(8):3297–305.
22. Allievi N, Ceresoli M, Fugazzola P, Montori G, Coccolini F, Ansaloni L. Endoscopic stenting as bridge to surgery versus emergency resection for left-sided malignant colorectal obstruction: an updated meta analysis. Int J Surg Oncol. 2017;2017:2863272.
23. Ribeiro IB, Bernardo WM, Martins BDC, de Moura DTH, Baba ER, Josino IR, et al. Colonic stent versus emergency surgery as treatment of malignant colonic obstruction in the palliative setting: a systematic review and meta-analysis. Endosc Int Open. 2018;6(5):E558–67. Erratum in: Endosc Int Open. 2018;6(5):C1.
24. Erichsen R, Horváth-Puhó E, Jacobsen JB, Nilsson T, Baron JA, Sørensen HT. Long-term mortality and recurrence after colorectal cancer surgery with preoperative stenting: a Danish nationwide cohort study. Endoscopy. 2015;47(6):517–24.
25. Ceresoli M, Allievi N, Coccolini F, Montori G, Fugazzola P, Pisano M, et al. Long-term oncologic outcomes of stent as a bridge to surgery versus emergency surgery in malignant left side colonic obstructions: a meta-analysis. J Gastrointest Oncol. 2017;8(5):867–76.
26. Hill J, Kay C, Morton D, Magill L, Handley K, Gray RG. CREST Trial Collaborative Group: CREST: Randomised phase III study of stenting as a bridge to surgery in obstructing colorectal cancer-results of the UK ColoRectal Endoscopic Stenting Trial (CREST). J Clin Oncol. 2016;34(Suppl):abstr 3507.
27. Repici A, de Paula Pessoa Ferreira D. Expandable metal stents for malignant colorectal strictures. Gastrointest Endosc Clin N Am. 2011;21(3):511–33.

28. Manes G, de Bellis M, Fuccio L, Repici A, Masci E, Ardizzone S, et al. Endoscopic palliation in patients with incurable malignant colorectal obstruction by means of self-expanding metal stent: analysis of results and predictors of outcomes in a large multicenter series. Arch Surg. 2011;146(10):1157–62.
29. Cennamo V, Fuccio L, Mutri V, Minardi ME, Eusebi LH, Ceroni L, et al. Does stent placement for advanced colon cancer increase the risk of perforation during bevacizumab-based therapy? Clin Gastroenterol Hepatol. 2009;7(11):1174–6.
30. Small AJ, Coelho-Prabhu N, Baron TH. Endoscopic placement of self-expandable metal stents for malignant colonic obstruction: long-term outcomes and complication factors. Gastrointest Endosc. 2010;71(3):560–72.
31. Yoon JY, Jung YS, Hong SP, Kim TI, Kim WH, Cheon JH. Clinical outcomes and risk factors for technical and clinical failures of self-expandable metal stent insertion for malignant colorectal obstruction. Gastrointest Endosc. 2011;74(4):858–68.
32. Branger F, Thibaudeau E, Mucci-Hennekinne S, Métivier-Cesbron E, Vychnevskaia K, Hamy A, et al. Management of acute malignant large-bowel obstruction with self-expanding metal stent. Int J Colorectal Dis. 2010;25(12):1481–5.
33. de Gregorio MA, Mainar A, Rodriguez J, Alfonso ER, Tejero E, Herrera M, et al. Colon stenting: a review. Semin Intervent Radiol. 2004;21(3):205–16.
34. Melich G, Pai A, Balachandran B, Marecik SJ, Prasad LM, Park JJ. Endoscopic control of enterocutaneous fistula by dual intussuscepting stent technique. Surg Endosc. 2016;30(9):4150–1.
35. Kim BC, Han KS, Hong CW, Sohn DK, Park JW, Park SC, et al. Clinical outcomes of palliative self-expanding metallic stents in patients with malignant colorectal obstruction. J Dig Dis. 2012;13(5):258–66.
36. Lee YJ, Yoon JY, Park JJ, Park SJ, Kim JH, Youn YH, et al. Clinical outcomes and factors related to colonic perforations in patients receiving self-expandable metal stent insertion for malignant colorectal obstruction. Gastrointest Endosc. 2018;87(6):1548–57.
37. Lee JH, Yoon JY, Park SJ, Hong SP, Kim TI, Kim WH, et al. The learning curve for colorectal stent insertion for the treatment of malignant colorectal obstruction. Gut Liver. 2012;6(3):328–33.
38. Cui J, Zhang JL, Wang S, Sun ZQ, Jiang XL. A preliminary study of stenting followed by laparoscopic surgery for obstructing left-sided colon cancer [Article in Chinese]. Zhonghua Wei Chang Wai Ke Za Zhi. 2011;14(1):40–3.

28 Minimally Invasive Management of Complicated Sigmoid Diverticulitis in the Emergency Setting: Patient Selection, Prerequisite Skills, and Operative Strategies

Ron G. Landmann and Todd D. Francone

Introduction and Rationale

Complicated diverticulitis is defined as diverticulitis with associated abscess, phlegmon, fistula, obstruction, bleeding, or perforation with purulent or fecal peritonitis [1]. National guidelines for the management of diverticular disease continue to evolve with the pendulum swung in full force toward a more conservative approach, individualized for both complicated and uncomplicated diverticulitis. These guidelines have also been modified to include minimally invasive surgery as a safe and effective modality for diverticular disease. This is mainly in part related to the increased utilization of robotic and laparoscopic approaches for not only benign disease but also malignant processes.

As with the decision to operate, the technique should be tailored to the individual. No matter the choice of technique, open or minimally invasive, surgery for complicated diverticulitis comes with inherent challenges due to perforation, sepsis, abscess, fistula, and peritonitis. Surgical options vary between the historically conservative Hartmann's procedure (HP) with segmental colectomy and end colostomy, segmental resection with primary anastomosis (PRA) with or without fecal diversion, and, the least invasive approach, laparoscopic peritoneal lavage (LL).

Safe and effective management of complicated diverticulitis requires a personalized approach to the patient based on the clinical presentation, diagnostic imaging,

R. G. Landmann
Section of Colon and Rectal Surgery, Department of Surgical Oncology, Inflammatory Bowel Disease Center, Baptist-MD Anderson Cancer Center, Jacksonville, FL, USA

T. D. Francone (✉)
Newton/Wellesley Hospital, Newton, MA, USA

Massachusetts General Hospital, Boston, MA, USA

Tufts Medical University, Boston, MA, USA
e-mail: tfrancone@partners.org

P. Sylla et al. (eds.), *The SAGES Manual of Colorectal Surgery*,
https://doi.org/10.1007/978-3-030-24812-3_28

Box 28.1 Hinchey Classification

- *Stage Ia:* phlegmon
- *Stage Ib:* diverticulitis with pericolic or mesenteric abscess
- *Stage II:* diverticulitis with walled off pelvic abscess
- *Stage III:* diverticulitis with generalized purulent peritonitis
- *Stage IV:* diverticulitis with generalized fecal peritonitis

Data from Refs. [2–6]

Box 28.2 Indications for Surgery with Complicated Diverticulitis

1. Hemodynamic instability
2. Failure to respond to medical therapy (i.e., percutaneous drainage of abscess and IV antibiotics)
3. Fistula disease (colovesicular, colovaginal, colocutaneous)
4. Large bowel obstruction with impending perforation
5. Gastrointestinal hemorrhage.

and underlying disease presentation such as the presence of purulent (Hinchey III) or feculent (Hinchey IV) peritonitis (Box 28.1). For these reasons, it is essential to be familiar with various approaches (i.e., medial-to-lateral, lateral-to-medial, superior to inferior, etc.) resulting in optimal exposure as well as safer, quicker, and a more reproducible dissection in an otherwise hostile surgical environment. This chapter aims to provide insight into the considerations required and techniques available to safely perform minimally invasive surgery for complicated diverticulitis.

Indications and Contraindications

The management of patients with peritonitis from perforated diverticulitis is challenging. Patient presentation may vary from hemodynamically stable to critically ill and labile. Accordingly, rapid and accurate diagnosis and evaluation is essential to facilitate selection of an appropriate surgical strategy. Indications for surgery in patients with complicated diverticulitis include the presence of diffuse peritonitis such as in patients with Hinchey III or IV disease, failure to respond to medical therapy such as with percutaneous drainage or IV antibiotics, or the development of complex disease such as a fistula to the vagina or bladder (Box 28.2). As one would expect, bowel resection in the setting of acute inflammation can be quite problematic and potentially detrimental to the patient with increased risk of injury to other critical structures. As such, nonoperative management, such as percutaneous drainage and intravenous antibiotic therapy, should always be considered and favored in patients who are not critically ill. A study by Dharmaarjan and coauthors demonstrated that 93% of patients with remote air on CT scan were able to be managed effectively nonoperatively with almost 50% of patients eventually undergoing an elective minimally invasive resection highlighting the importance of correlating clinical assessment with diagnostic imaging [7].

The decision to perform minimally invasive surgery in the setting of complicated diverticulitis should be based not only on the physiologic state and comorbidities of the patient but also the experience of the operating surgeon and surgical team. In the hemodynamically stable patient, laparoscopy offers both diagnostic and therapeutic utility, including drainage of abscesses, lavage, or bowel resection. The decision to proceed in a minimally invasive fashion or convert to an open approach is multifactorial. Factors such as poor exposure, difficult anatomy, and patient intolerance related to cardiopulmonary status or failure to make progress highlight the importance of an experienced surgeon to recognize when the benefit of a minimally invasive approach is dwarfed by the risk to patient safety.

Although an open approach does not necessarily resolve all the difficulties encountered during those complex cases, it may allow certain advantages such as increased exposure and the ability to palpate structures as well as the use of blunt dissection. In the setting of purulent or feculent peritonitis, aggressive abdominal irrigation may also be facilitated. Those familiar with hand-assist laparoscopy may be able to avoid conversion to an open procedure as this technique utilizes the advantages of both minimally invasive and open techniques. Whatever the approach, the surgeon and the operating room staff should frequently reevaluate the intraoperative conditions to ensure there is appropriate prioritizing of patients' safety and that procedures are progressing in a safe and effective manner.

Principles and Quality Benchmarks

The goals of treating patients with complicated diverticulitis remain simple: (1) stabilize the patient and (2) control the sepsis. Once achieved, definitive management can be determined. In the critically ill patient with physiologic compromise, MIS should be avoided, and damage control techniques may need to be employed. The principles of damage control surgery in non-trauma care include abbreviated surgery to control contamination in the abdomen, simultaneous resuscitation, and definitive surgical management at a later stage after restoration of hemodynamic stability. The staged management of damage control has been shown to minimize the physiological impact of shock, allowing definitive reconstruction under more favorable conditions. In the setting of perforated diverticular disease, the patient may be taken to the operating room for exploratory laparotomy where the segment of perforated diverticular disease is resected with minimal dissection or simply diverted. Diversion can be achieved with either a diverting loop sigmoid colostomy, transverse colostomy, or "blow hole" [8]. The abdomen is thoroughly washed with irrigation, and the patient is transferred to the ICU for further resuscitation with plans for more definitive care once stable [9].

There is minimal benefit to "damage control" techniques in the setting of hemodynamic stability. Less critical patients may be considered for a minimally invasive approach although the principles of concurrent physiologic resuscitation and sepsis control remain relevant. The source of sepsis should be identified and controlled either by diversion or resection. Resection is often feasible; however, the surgeon should avoid extensive dissection along the retroperitoneum and avoid mobilizing the splenic flexure if possible. This may not be possible in certain situations, especially in the morbidly obese when a diverting colostomy can be difficult to create in the setting of a thick abdominal wall. Once the sepsis is controlled, primary definitive care may occur at the time of the initial operation. If resection is performed, the potential for restoring intestinal continuity should be considered. Alternative management to resection in patients with mainly Hinchey III disease includes laparoscopic lavage and is discussed later in the chapter in detail.

Preoperative Planning, Patient Workup, and Optimization

In the emergency setting, extensive preoperative workup and planning are often precluded by the need for urgent operative intervention. In the critically ill patient, operative intervention may be required before further diagnostic imaging such as a CT scan can be performed; however, preoperative optimization, either in the emergency department or surgical intensive care unit with IV fluid resuscitation, IV antibiotics, as well as potentially afterload reduction or inotropic support may reduce intraoperative events and improve postoperative outcomes. Additionally, improved hemodynamic status may allow opportunity for further diagnostic imaging including CT scan to further narrow the differential diagnosis and etiology.

Physiologic state notwithstanding, clinical assessment should at minimum include a detailed medical history including prior operative interventions as well as an appropriate physical exam and laboratory workup. Past medical history includes prior endoscopic evaluation such as colonoscopy. This is particularly important in patients who present with perforation secondary to large bowel obstruction raising the possibility of a neoplastic etiology in the absence of a prior endoscopic evaluation. Hemodynamic stability often affords more time for a detailed clinical history and physical exam habitually supplemented by a CT scan of the abdomen and pelvis. Identification of free air or fluid throughout the abdomen may give further clues to the classification of the presenting diverticular disease with categorization into Hinchey I–IV (Box 28.1) and as such dictate further management. In the absence of free fluid or diffuse air throughout the abdomen, nonoperative management should be considered as the preferred pathway. Failure to respond to medical management should trigger conversion to an operative approach. Patients with presumed Hinchey III diverticular disease may be considered for laparoscopic lavage with the understanding that delineation between Hinchey III and IV can be challenging and may require conversion to a bowel resection either by laparoscopy or open. Other preoperative considerations may include ureteral stents depending on availability at the time of surgery.

Routine mechanical bowel preparation should be performed if possible, for left-sided resections, and is recommended in the elective setting in conjunction with oral antibiotics as per enhanced recovery protocols [10]. Elective resection with primary anastomosis without bowel preparation has been shown to be safe and feasible; however, if fecal diversion is deemed necessary, then an on-table lavage should be performed to reduce the fecal load proximal to the new anastomosis. Fecal diversion will have minimal benefit if the colon distal to the diverting ostomy is full of stool. On-table lavage has been shown to be safe but can be time-consuming and expose the patient to unnecessary risk with increased fecal contamination, bowel handlining, and ileus [11]. The authors do not generally perform nor advocate for on-table lavage.

It also is worth noting that all patients undergoing emergent operation for presumed diverticular disease receive preoperative stoma marking and teaching. It is well documented that a well-sited stoma and pre-counseling have been associated with improved postoperative outcomes and higher quality of lie scores [12]. Often a Wound Ostomy Care Nurse (WOCN) is not available; therefore, it is up to the surgeon to discuss the possibility of a stoma, provide adequate education, and appropriately mark potential sites. Both the right and left sides of the abdomen should be marked for potential stomas in preparation for either Hartmann's procedure or segmental resection with primary anastomosis and loop ileostomy creation. Stoma creation without considerations of certain factors such as prior scars, belt lines, and abdominal crease can result in a poorly functioning stoma no matter how well it is fashioned.

Operative Strategy

Operative strategy will be dictated by multiple factors including but not limited to the physiologic state of the patient, medical comorbidities, prior surgical history, diagnostic imaging suggesting feculent or purulent peritonitis, timing of presentation, as well as the experience of the surgeon and surgical staff. Consideration of these factors among others should aid the surgeon in devising a strategic operative plan for the patient, in particular whether to approach the patient using a minimally invasive approach. Furthermore, any patient planed for a minimally invasive approach should be prepared the possibility of conversion to an open procedure.

When operating in an emergent hostile abdomen, it is essential to be familiar with various approaches for dissection of the bowel and its mesentery (i.e., medial-to-lateral, lateral-to-medial, superior to inferior, etc) in order to optimize exposure, perform a safer and quicker dissection, and minimize the risk of injury and postoperative morbidity. This is undoubtedly facilitated by a fundamental understanding of the surgical anatomy, allowing the surgeon to identify key anatomic landmarks such as the bladder and ureters prior to proceeding with planned resection while being prepared to perform additional diagnostic evaluations and therapeutic interventions as needed.

Surgical options can range from sigmoid resection with end colostomy, well known as a Hartmann's procedure (HP), sigmoid resection with primary anastomosis (PRA) with or without temporary fecal diversion, or laparoscopic lavage (LL). Recent systematic reviews and meta-analyses have reported comparable complication rates for those undergoing PRA and HP suggesting that PRA is safe and feasible in the setting of generalized peritonitis (Hinchey III and IV). Results have been less favorable for laparoscopic lavage with data suggesting no clear benefit to lavage when compared to PRA or HP [13, 14]. In a recent meta-analysis by Schmidt and coauthors, mortality rates were similar between HP and PRA (RR 2.03 (95% CI 0.79–5.25); $p = 0.14$) but showed higher stoma reversal rates for those patients undergoing PRA (RR 0.73 (95% CI 0.58–0.98); $p = 0.008$). In addition, the meta-analysis showed no significant benefit of laparoscopic lavage when compared to resection, with similar mortality (RR 1.07 (95% CI 0.65–1.76); $p = 0.79$) and morbidity rates (RR 0.86 (95% CI 0.69–1.08); $p = 0.20$), respectively [14].

Diagnostic laparoscopy is first performed to inspect the abdominal and pelvic cavity to evaluate for any altered anatomy and discern for feculent peritonitis not previously identified on preoperative staging and imaging. For the most part, the decision to convert from minimally invasive to open should occur early in the operative intervention with studies demonstrating improved patient outcomes with proactive conversion rather than reactive [15]. The decision to restore intestinal continuity at the time of emergency resection rather than diverting with an end colostomy can be challenging. The surgeon has to consider multiple factors including the patient's condition, the condition of the bowel and the amount of fecal load proximal to the anastomosis, the risk of morbidity and mortality based on comorbidities, as well as the potential for long-term impact on the patient's quality of life. Primary anastomosis with or without mechanical bowel preparation has been shown to be safe and feasible. If the fecal load above the new anastomosis is considerable, then on-table lavage should be considered.

Operative Setup

The following patient setup can be utilized for any procedure (resection, lavage, or fecal diversion). Patient positioning and port placement may need to be adjusted based on the patient's prior surgical history, body habitus, and pathology.

Patient Positioning

Patients are positioned on gel pads or bean bags with safety straps or tape to minimize patient slipping and movement during extremes of positioning (Trendelenburg and reverse-Trendelenburg, right or left-side tilt). Furthermore, all patients are placed in modified lithotomy (legs in slight hip flexion) or split-leg position with both arms tucked at the sides (Fig. 28.1). Positioning in this manner affords the

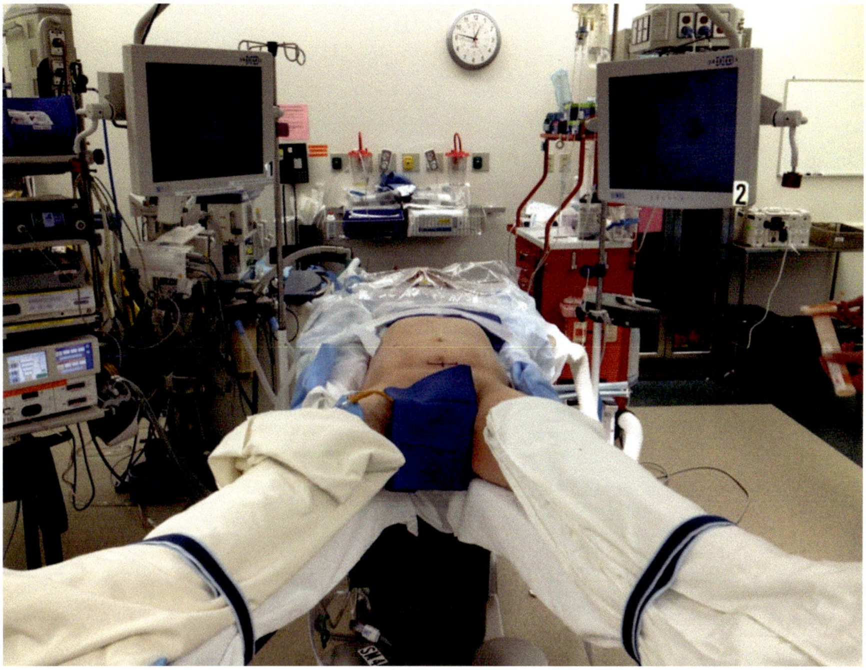

Fig. 28.1 Patient setup. Patient is placed in the split-leg position for all cases

surgeons numerous advantages including (1) insertion of a stapling device and (2) exposure to the anus/rectum for intraoperative colonoscopy if needed. This can be particularly useful to help rule out a tumor that may not have been appreciated on preoperative workup, as well as to assess the anastomosis endoscopically for integrity and adequate perfusion (3) operator positioning between the legs during more complex procedures.

Port Placement

Appropriate port placement is critical in facilitating exposure and anatomic definition. For a left or sigmoid colectomy, a total of four "working" ports are utilized (12 mm umbilical, 12 mm right lower quadrant (RLQ), 5 mm right upper quadrant (RUQ), 5 mm left lower quadrant (LLQ)) (Fig. 28.2a). An open cut-down technique (Hasson technique) is used to place a supra-umbilical port and then utilized for introduction of the 10 mm laparoscope. This allows for initial exploration. The RLQ trocar is used for the endoscopic stapler. The LLQ port is often helpful for assistance with retraction and possible drain placement. For a hand-assist approach, access to the peritoneal cavity is achieved by making a 6–8 cm Pfannenstiel incision (Fig. 28.2b); however, in cases that have high probability of conversions to an open

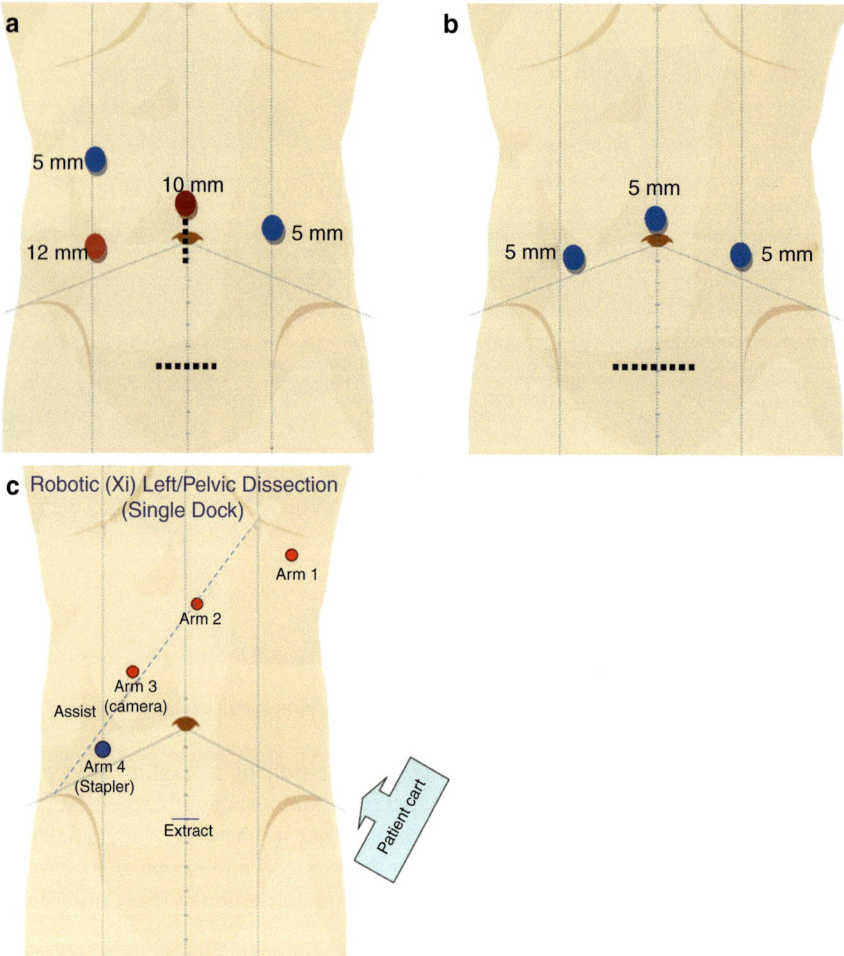

Fig. 28.2 (**a–c**) Port setup. (**a**) Depicts a laparoscopic four-port technique. Abdominal access is typically achieved via the Hasson technique, and a 10 mm port is placed. The two ports in the right upper and lower quadrant are utilized as working ports. The 4th port is placed on the left side of the abdomen and is typically used for additional retraction. This port maybe excluded as one gains more experience. Extraction can vary with surgeon preference. The diagram depicts the extraction site (dotted line) in the two most common locations. (**b**) Hand-port port placement. (**c**) Port placement for Xi Robotic approach with supra-pubic extraction site

procedure, a lower midline incision may be used as it can be easily extended cephalad if conversion to an open procedure is warranted. For elective procedures with complex disease such as colovesicular or colovaginal fistulas, robotic surgery techniques may be utilized. Port placement for an elective left colectomy is demonstrated in Fig. 28.2c.

Diagnostic Laparoscopy

The patient is placed in Trendelenburg position with the left side tilted up, which assists in displacing the small intestine into the upper abdomen. Prior to any mobilization or resection, inspect the abdominal and pelvic cavity to rule out feculent peritonitis and localize abscesses or phlegmons and evaluate their relationship to the sigmoid colon. It is also appropriate to take this opportunity to visualize the pelvis including the relationship of the inflammatory sigmoid mass to the bladder, left pelvic sidewall and retroperitoneum, ovaries, adjacent colon and small bowel loops, and anterior peritoneal reflection. The small bowel should also be thoroughly inspected to assess the degree of peritonitis and the likelihood that a minimally invasive approach is feasible.

Identification of Pathology

The pathology is often identified during diagnostic laparoscopy at which point adjustments to the preoperative surgical plan may be required. In the setting of perforated diverticulitis, the extent of peritonitis will dictate whether minimally invasive approach is feasible. The identification of feculent peritonitis is often difficult to control with minimally invasive techniques, even hand-assist, and is typically associated with conversion to an open procedure. Patients with purulent peritonitis (Hinchey III) may only require laparoscopic lavage.

Those who present with large bowel obstruction may be difficult to resect due to chronic inflammation such that fecal diversion may be the safest option. In this circumstance the entire large and small bowel should be inspected to rule bowel compromise which may present as large serosal tears or even frank perforation. If there is a concern for malignancy, then an intraoperative colonoscopy is warranted if feasible and temporary fecal diversion may be in the patient's best interest. Subsequently, the patient may undergo appropriate staging, allow inflammation to settle, and subsequently undergo an appropriate oncologic resection in the future. Pathology located in the proximal sigmoid colon or distal descending colon may necessitate mobilization of the splenic flexure for appropriate tension-free anastomosis or fecal diversion.

Minimally Invasive Resectional Approach

Critical Steps of Resection

Best Approach

In the elective setting, a medial-to-lateral approach is the author's preferred approach. However, in the setting of a perforation, the anatomy of the left lower quadrant, pelvis, and retroperitoneum is often distorted. The retroperitoneum at the

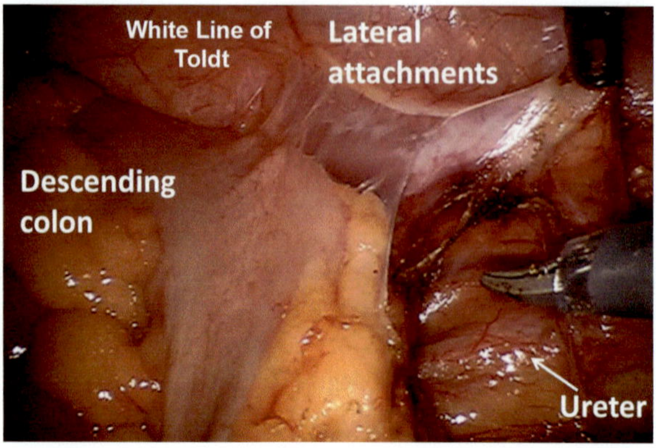

Fig. 28.3 When dividing the lateral attachments, dissection is carried from the pelvis toward the splenic flexure

site of the perforation is often inflamed such that critical retroperitoneal structures can be challenging to identify or kept out of harm's way. A phlegmon may involve loops of small bowel or densely adhere the colon to the pelvic sidewall. For this reason, a lateral-to-medial mobilization is most useful and safe especially in the setting of benign disease where regional lymph node harvest is not of importance (Fig. 28.3). The colon mesentery needs only to be mobilized enough for resection leaving much of the colonic mesentery in place overlying the retroperitoneum and avoiding injury to critical structures such as the left ureter. The dissection should be started above the pathology typically along the proximal descending colon where the planes are less inflamed. The correct plane is followed as the dissection is extended toward the pelvis.

Identifying the Vascular Anatomy

The inferior mesenteric artery (IMA) is typically preserved during an emergent operation. The takeoff of the IMA occurs roughly at the level of L3 vertebrae. The IMA and its branches are the vascular supply to the hindgut structures including the distal transverse, descending, and sigmoid colon, as well as the rectum. Leaving the IMA intact preserves blood flow to the proximal colon and rectal stump while also avoiding the retroperitoneum and circumventing the potential risk of injury to underlying structures.

Identification of the Left Ureter

Given the left ureter's close proximity to the rectosigmoid and left pelvic sidewall, it is often at risk for becoming secondarily involved from diverticular inflammation. Therefore, it is particularly vulnerable to injury during emergent surgery for complicated sigmoid diverticulitis. It lies under the parietal peritoneum along the pelvic sidewall and rests on the anterior surface of the psoas muscle (Fig. 28.4a, b). The right and left ureters generally both follow a straight path from the renal pelvis to the pelvic brim and then cross over the iliac vessels to enter the pelvic brim. The right ureter classically traverses the external iliac artery, whereas the left ureter lies slightly more medial and typically crosses the common iliac artery. The ureters then

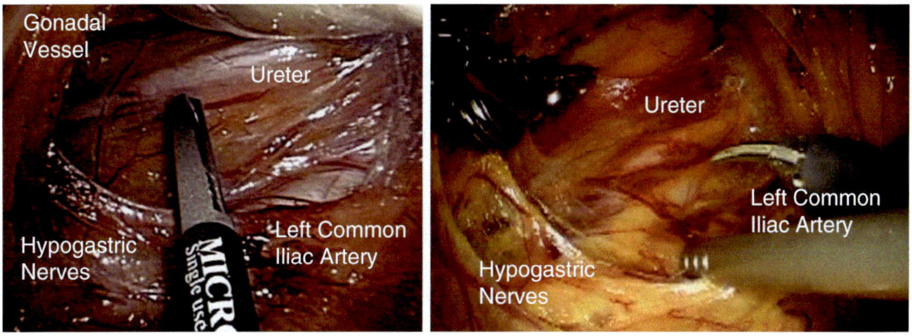

Fig. 28.4 (**a**, **b**) Pelvic anatomy highlighting the ureter, gonadal vessels, sacral promontory, hypogastric nerves, and avascular alveolar space between fascia propria and presacral fascia

run posterior and inferior along the lateral pelvic sidewall before entering the posterolateral surface of the bladder to form the trigone. If possible, avoiding extensive mobilization in a lateral-to-medial fashion should avoid injury to the ureter and other underlying retroperitoneal structures such as the left gonadal vessels and the hypogastric nerve plexus.

If the underlying disease and circumstances dictate a more extensive retroperitoneal dissection, the ureter must be visualized and dissected out to avoid inadvertent injury. In cases where the ureter is not easily identified, it is prudent to alter the approach and mobilization to ensure that it is visualized prior to mesentery or bowel transection. In certain cases, the ureter may have been mobilized medially and placed on stretch with the mobilized left colon mesentery. Alternatively, it may be involved in a phlegmon and require dissection to free it. The latter cases require a different approach to dissect the colon mesentery safely away from the left ureter to avoid transection. In the non-emergent setting, preoperative ureteral catheters/stents placement can be particularly helpful to aide in laparoscopic palpation of the ureters. Though these stents do not reduce the risk for transection or injury, they do permit for earlier identification of these events and facilitate prompt repair.

Splenic Flexure Mobilization (If Needed)

Splenic flexure mobilization is typically not required when performing an HP unless the patient is morbidly obese and with a thick abdominal wall or PRA is planned. Splenic flexure mobilization is generally performed using a combination of approaches. A lateral-to-medial approach is our preferred approach in the emergency setting. The patient is placed in reverse Trendelenburg position with the table inclined toward the right. Laterally, the peritoneal attachments to the abdominal sidewall and spleen are carefully divided while being mindful not to injure the splenic capsule (Fig. 28.5). Often, there will be close and dense adhesions of the colon to the spleen. The hand-assist technique can also be advantageous in this scenario. The lesser sac can be entered and used to direct the dissection around the splenic flexure and safely mobilize left colon (Fig. 28.6). Dissection continues separating the attachments of the splenic flexure and its mesentery away from the spleen and pancreas.

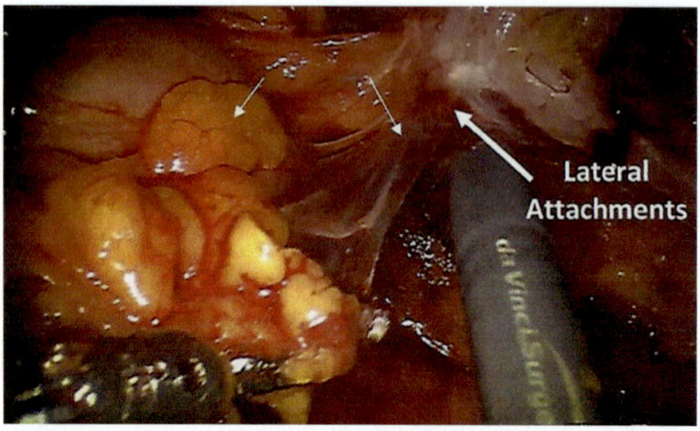

Fig. 28.5 The attachments to the sidewall and spleen are carefully divided while being mindful not to injure the splenic capsule

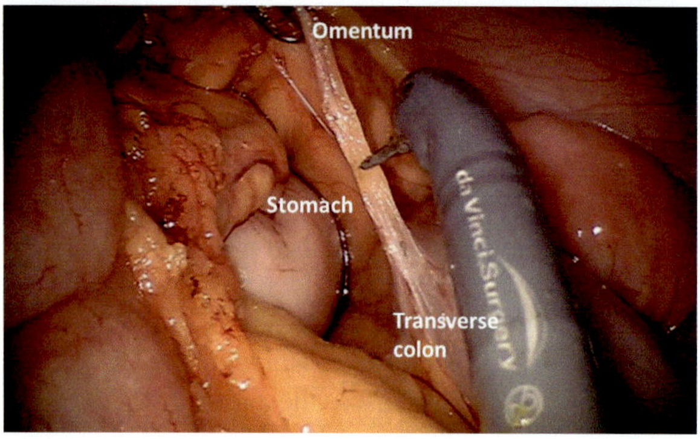

Fig. 28.6 The lesser sac is identified by visualization of the posterior wall of the stomach. Often, congenital fusion attachments must be divided to enter the correct space. Entry into the lesser sac often facilitates complete mobilization of the splenic flexure

Resecting the Source of Sepsis

Once the colon is adequately mobilized and the left ureter identified and protected, bowel resection is carried out. In the setting of a large perforation, the proximal and distal colon should be divided laparoscopically to control contamination. The mesentery is then divided using an energy device or stapler. Staying close to the colon will avoid injury to the underlying structures of the retroperitoneum. In the setting of a phlegmon or perforation, tissues are often friable, necrotic, and ischemic with little bleeding. The mesentery is divided caudally until the site of distal transection is reached.

Distal Colon Transection

A critical step in any left or sigmoid resection is identification of a distal transection point. The colon should be soft and viable. If planning a Hartmann's procedure, then a lengthier rectal stump can be utilized. The superior hemorrhoidal arteries can be left intact ensuring the retroperitoneum is undisturbed facilitating possible reversal of the colostomy in the future.

When planning a primary anastomosis, division is generally performed at the level of the proximal rectum, past the splaying of the tenia coli on the anti-mesenteric surface. For diverticular disease, this minimizes recurrence by transection distal to

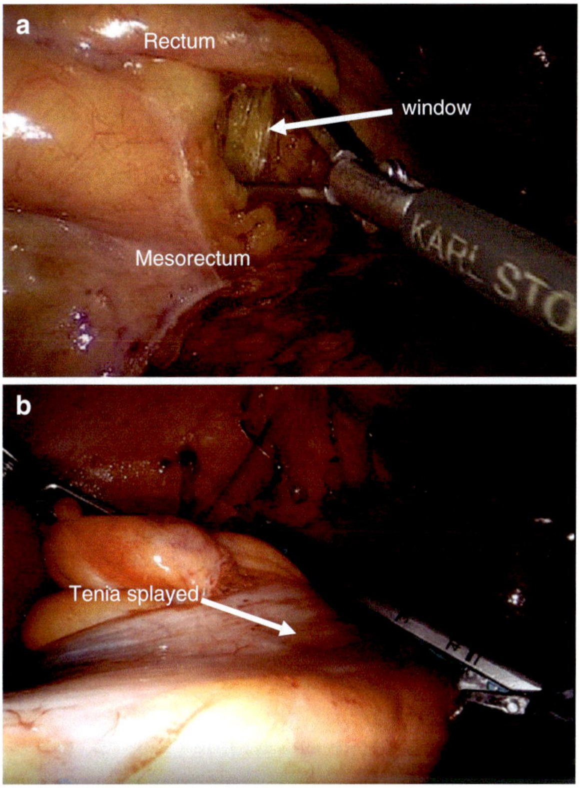

Fig. 28.7 (**a**) Once the site of distal transection has been identified, the mesorectum is divided by creating a window between the posterior wall of the rectum and the mesorectal fat. (**b**) The upper rectum is divided with an endoscopic stapler. Multiple loads may be required; careful attention should be taken to avoid a staggered staple line

the high-pressure zone encountered in the rectosigmoid colon. The upper rectum is isolated by creation of a window between the posterior wall of the rectum and mesentery at the proposed transection site (Fig. 28.7a). Once the bare rectum is appropriately dissected and exposed, division is generally performed with an endoscopic stapling device through the RLQ port (Fig. 28.7b). The appropriate stapling load should be chosen based on the thickness and integrity of the tissue to be divided. It may be required to use additional loads of the stapler in some cases.

Integrity and airtightness of the rectal stump staple line may be tested at this point. The stump is submerged under sterile solution, and gentle insufflation per anus is performed. This can be done with a variety of modalities including rigid proctoscopy, flexible sigmoidoscopy, or bulb syringe insufflation. The former two allow for visualization of the mucosa and staple line. Direct laparoscopic visualization during rectal insufflation should confirm appropriate distension of the stump without air leak (visualized bubbles). If air leak is encountered at this point, two options are available. The first is to introduce the spike of the end-to-end anastomotic circular stapler through the defect. The second option is to resect an additional distal margin incorporating the prior staple line. Air testing may then be repeated.

Extraction and Proximal Colon Transection

Prior to extraction, the distal end of the colon is held with a locking grasper and placed under the location of the anticipated extraction site. Potential extraction sites include extension of the periumbilical incision, creation of a Pfannenstiel incision, or extension of the RLQ incision. When performing a minimally invasive HP, the specimen can be extracted through the marked colostomy site. In a patient who has had prior abdominal operations, using a prior incision may be appropriate. Cosmetically, a Pfannenstiel incision may be preferable and may minimize hernia rates [16]. The incision size will vary between 3 and 6 cm but ultimately is determined by the size of the pathology. Once the abdominal wall is opened appropriately and the peritoneal cavity entered, a wound protector is inserted to protect the skin and soft tissue from contamination during externalization and creation of anastomosis.

Through the wound protector, the distal stapled end of the colon and the proximal mobilized colon and mesentery are extracorporealized. The proximal dissection point is predicated upon a number of factors including inflammation, edema, induration, and perfusion. Appropriate maintenance of vascular supply must be assured to minimize risk of ischemia of the anastomosis. Sharp transection of the marginal artery with resultant pulsatile flow from the proximal end is one method to verify and document appropriate healthy vascular tissue. In the elective setting, newer methods including fluorescence imaging may also be utilized to identify well-perfused tissue prior to transection.

Anastomosis and Intraoperative Leak Testing

A double-stapled technique is often employed during a left or sigmoid colectomy. An end-to-end anastomotic (EEA) stapler height is chosen based on tissue thickness and compliance. Common staple heights range between 3.5 and 4.8 mm staples with optimal closure of 1.5–2 mm in height, respectively. When dealing with the rectum, inflamed or not, the authors typically prefer the latter, green loads. The diameter of the stapler will also vary between 21 and 33 mm and may be selected based on the diameter of the proximal and distal bowel as well as the compliance of the patient's anal tone. Testing of the anastomosis is essential with recent data suggesting the ability to reduce the incidence of missed anastomotic leak [17]. The bowel proximal to the anastomosis is clamped, and an air leak test is performed as described above. Flexible sigmoidoscopy is preferred by the authors as it allows superior visualization of the mucosa and staple line as well as quick resolution of CO_2. If an air leak is encountered, several options exist including direct repair of the anastomotic leak point(s) with or without fecal diversion, takedown and creation of a new anastomosis, or creation of an end colostomy. Choosing the appropriate surgical management of a positive air leak test is dependent on multiple factors and is beyond the scope of this chapter.

Given that risks for anastomotic leak are multifactorial, the absence of a "positive" leak test does not preclude later occurrence of an anastomotic leak. Other factors should be considered when deciding whether to divert including the severity of immunosuppression, worsening hemodynamic instability, difficult dissection or anatomy resulting in increased tension on the anastomosis, malnutrition, and obesity. Routine prophylactic drain placement is not recommended as it was not shown to reduce surgical site infection or anastomotic leaks [18]. Drains should be used selectively in the setting of residual purulent collections or phlegmons or gross feculent spillage.

Considerations During Laparoscopic Hartmann's Procedure

In certain cases, anatomic, physiologic, or disease processes preclude safe or appropriate anastomosis. In those cases, as above, the distal colon or proximal rectum should be transected and divided using an endoscopic stapling device. If there is any potential for future anastomosis, it is helpful to add tags at the staple line using permanent monofilament suture to ease future identification of the rectal stump. When mobilizing the proximal sigmoid and descending colon, all attempts should be made to minimize excess dissection and mobilization more than is necessary to bring out a tension-free colostomy. This will aide in future Hartmann's reversal. Similarly, it may be prudent to have localizing ureteral stents placed at the time of Hartmann's reversal. For more details, please refer to Chap. 20 on Key Steps During Hartmann's Procedures to Facilitate Minimally Invasive Hartman's Reversal.

Pitfalls and Troubleshooting

Fistula/Phlegmon in Diverticular Disease

In the case of fistulas between the colon and other intraperitoneal structures or processes involving phlegmonous collections, care should be taken to minimize concomitant injury/resection (Fig. 28.8a). In general, the authors prefer to place preoperative ureteral catheters (or stents) to help in identification of these structures during dissection. Oftentimes, a combination of lateral-to-medial and medial-to-lateral dissection is required. Initiating the dissection with a medial-to-lateral mobilization close to the takeoff of the IMA may help gain access to the retroperitoneal surface and space between the colon and its mesentery and the sidewall due to decreased acute on chronic inflammatory processes in the central mesentery. This will then help in identification of the ureter and other structures more easily than a primary lateral-to-medial dissection. Dissection may then proceed laterally with anterior retraction of the colon and mesentery. In some cases, it may be helpful to initiate the dissection proximally along the descending colon at an area of decreased inflammatory reaction and proceed caudally. Similarly, rectal mobilization with retrograde dissection can also be a helpful adjunct in mobilizing the colon from the pelvic sidewall and ureter. In certain cases, this dissection and separation of the colon to the sidewall and ureter may require manual disruption with a finger-fracture technique. If significant inflammation and/or abscess are encountered (Fig. 28.8b), in certain cases, anastomosis may be precluded or protected with the use of a diverting loop ileostomy.

Colovesical fistulas may be dissected free without the need for repair. If a small or no bladder defect is visualized, catheter drainage for a few days [8–10] with

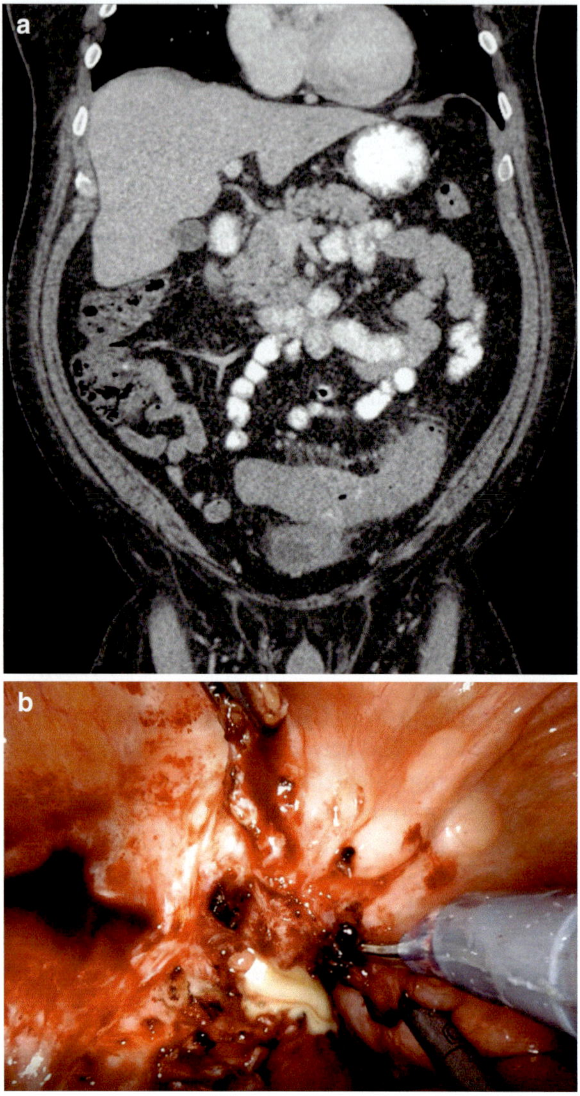

Fig. 28.8 (**a**) CT scan demonstrating a colovesicular fistula secondary to diverticular disease. (**b**) Separating the colon from the bladder reveals a small pericolic abscess

removal predicated upon a negative retrograde cystogram is advised. If a larger bladder defect is uncovered, a two-layer closure of the bladder is advised. Takedown of colovaginal fistulas frequently requires closure of the vaginal defect. Smaller defects may generally heal spontaneously once the inciting phlegmon or fistula has been removed. In these instances, the defect may function as a drain. Larger defects can be closed in a single-layer fashion with an absorbable suture.

In the setting of a prior fistula (colovesical or colovaginal), the anastomosis should be distal to and away from the previously dissected process. Furthermore, a pedicle of healthy and well-vascularized mobilized omentum should be interposed and secured between the anastomosis and the anterior fistula defect to prevent future contamination and fistulous communication with the new anastomosis.

If small bowel is noted to be fistulized with the diseased colon, after takedown of the fistula, either primary repair or small bowel resection is usually indicated. The decision is predicated upon overall condition of the small bowel and size of the fistula.

Obese Patients

Obesity presents a challenge to the surgeon, specifically due to increased mesenteric adiposity and patient weight. To prevent falls and slippage during extremes of positioning required in these cases, extra care must be taken to tape and securely strap the patient to the bed (Fig. 28.9). Obesity can create challenges in identification of landmarks and typical planes that would otherwise be easily accessed (i.e., space over the sacral promontory, around the takeoff of the IMA, retroperitoneal reflections). Additionally, the additional weight of the colon and mesentery may make appropriate retraction and visualization difficult. In these instances, liberal use of additional ports with retracting devices and/or hand assistance may be utilized. It is helpful to differentiate between visceral mesenteric fat and retroperitoneal fat during dissection. Basic knowledge of the typical anatomy and landmarks as well as

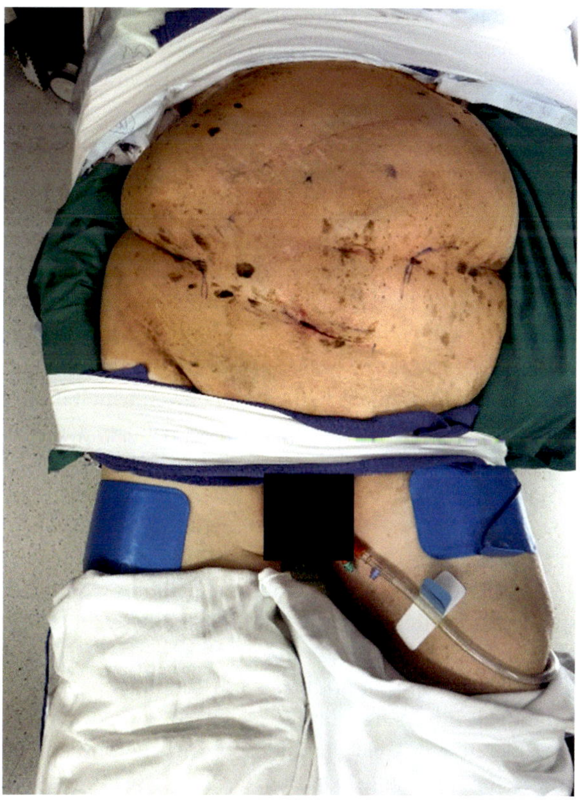

Fig. 28.9 Obesity provides additional challenges with patient positioning, intraoperative exposure, and postoperative fluid management

prior experience in non-obese patient will help the surgeon safely progress during dissection. If the anatomy is not clear or safety becomes a concern, conversion to an open procedure is advised.

Minimally Invasive Non-resectional Approach

Laparoscopic Peritoneal Lavage

Over the past several years, several studies have investigated alternative minimally invasive approaches to mitigate the morbidity of resectional approaches (i.e., Hartmann's procedure) in the setting of Hinchey III diverticulitis. Colectomy and stoma can have profound long-term sequelae, including prolonged ICU stay and permanent stoma. LL has been advocated as an alternative to resectional approaches in carefully selected patients with Hinchey III disease.

Operative Setup

Port Placement

Appropriate port placement is critical in facilitating exposure and anatomic definition. Though no resection is intended, it may be advisable to place the ports accordingly in case colectomy becomes necessary. The authors have advocated a modified 3-"working"-port technique: 5/10 mm umbilical, 5 mm RLQ, and 5 mm RUQ trocars (Fig. 28.2a with omission of the LLQ trocar). The surgeon should be prepared to place an additional LLQ working port for help with manipulation and retraction and also be prepared to upsize the RLQ port to a 10/12 mm port in case of the need to convert to a resectional approach.

Diagnostic Laparoscopy and Identification of Pathology

The decision to proceed with laparoscopic lavage is made early with the presence of frank stool indicating the need for resection. At this stage, gentle retraction of the small bowel should be performed away from the disease process. Care is utilized to avoid inadvertent injury to the small bowel, which if encountered should be promptly repaired or resected. Once the diseased segment and/or abscess is isolated away from the remainder of the abdominal and pelvic contents, suction followed by copious irrigation should be performed. There is no consensus on how much irrigation should be utilized; however, enough volume of sterile fluid should be utilized to minimize the bacterial burden in the peritoneal cavity. Careful inspection of the colon is then performed to identify any additional pathology. In the majority of cases, no demonstrable perforation will be found. In rare cases, a small isolated perforation may be observed and subsequently oversewn. If a large colonic defect is encountered, lavage with oversewing will not be successful, and conversion to a resection procedure is warranted. If a malignancy is suspected, resection is then mandated. Availability of intraoperative flexible sigmoidoscopy is a helpful adjunct to diagnose any malignant process or ongoing perforation. Once lavage is completed, a drain is left in place.

Postoperative Management

Most of patients should then be placed on broad-spectrum antibiotics to treat purulent peritonitis and class IV/infected wounds. Resumption of an oral diet may be instituted if no significant small bowel dilatation was noted (indicative of an impending ileus/obstruction). If successful, most patients will demonstrate a prompt improvement and normalization of their leukocytosis, resolution of abdominal distension, and an ability to tolerate a low-residue diet with return of bowel function. Once all parameters have been achieved on an acceptable pain management regimen, patients can then be discharged with follow-up. If no colonoscopy has been documented within the past 2 years, a full colonoscopy is imperative generally performed to exclude malignancy or other pathology 6 weeks after discharge.

Pitfalls and Troubleshooting

Any operative intervention in the setting of Hinchey III diverticular disease is complex and fraught with risks of further complications. The surgeon must have a strong grasp of the anatomy and experience managing unexpected intraoperative as well as complications. When evaluating the peritoneal cavity, if anatomic landmarks cannot be clearly identified and dissection safely performed, conversion to an open resectional procedure should be contemplated early in the interest of patients' safety.

If the patient's condition fails to improve postoperatively (elevated WBC, prolonged ileus), then the source of persistent intra-abdominal sepsis must be evaluated. If the patient becomes hemodynamically unstable with worsening leukocytosis and/or signs of ongoing sepsis or peritonitis, urgent reoperation is indicated, which may need to be performed open if a minimally invasive approach is not feasible. In the absence of hemodynamic compromise, a CT may be performed 3–4 days postoperatively to evaluate for undrained abscesses which may be drained percutaneously. Management would then proceed as if the patient had Hinchey II disease. If continued disseminated intra-abdominal fluid is noted, there should be a high index of suspicion for continued uncontrolled perforation. Patients may demonstrate ongoing signs of sepsis or a systemic inflammatory response (SIRS). Though additional imaging could be performed (CT or water soluble contrast enema), the general consensus is that patients with ongoing sepsis following LL should undergo resectional therapy (either resection with primary anastomosis and diversion or Hartmann's procedure).

Many cases of LL have been reported as complicated by small bowel fistulas from the laparoscopic attempt at separating and mobilizing the small bowel away from the inflammatory mass. Partial- or full-thickness enterotomy may not have been appreciated at the time of initial lavage. If encountered, primary repair and/or bowel resection should be performed and might require conversion and/or sigmoid resection as well. It is common to see delayed fistulization from the small bowel to another segment of small bowel or colon on follow-up. In these situations, interval resection is necessary. If the patient is otherwise asymptomatic, these procedures can be delayed by at least 6–8 weeks following initial LL and in some instances by 6 months or more.

When performing lavage, it is rarely indicated to mobilize the colon from the left pelvic sidewall. If this becomes necessary, it is imperative that pelvic sidewall structures (i.e., ureter and gonadal vessels) be appropriately identified and preserved. Failure to identify anatomic landmarks during minimally invasive approach is an indication to convert to an open procedure and proceed with a resectional approach as described above.

Outcomes

Resection

Patient with perforated diverticulitis and peritonitis should be considered for early operative intervention to control sepsis. Emergency surgery for perforated diverticulitis is associated with increased morbidity and mortality compared to elective surgery [2]. That being said, studies suggest that the laparoscopic approach for sigmoid resection with or without a stoma decreases overall complications compared to open resections in the emergency setting and should be considered in patients with perforated diverticulitis who are otherwise hemodynamically stable [3, 4, 19].

The optimal treatment strategy for perforated diverticulitis remains controversial. In Hinchey III diverticulitis, sigmoid resection with PRA and proximal diversion has been demonstrated to have similar mortality, lower mobility, and a lower stoma rate at 12 months compared to HP [5, 20–23]. A recent systematic review and meta-analysis demonstrated significantly lower overall mortality in patients with PRA compared with patients with HP [OR (95% CI) = 0.38 (0.24, 0.60), $p < 0.0001$]. Organ/space surgical site infection, reoperation, and ostomy non-reversal rates were significantly lower in PRA [21]. HP remains to the preferred operation in hemodynamically unstable patients with perforated diverticulitis and is associated with acceptable mortality and morbidity.

Laparoscopic Lavage

Numerous groups have performed randomized studies investigating lavage and comparing this modality to HP and resection with PRA and diverting ileostomy. See Tables 28.1 and 28.2. There are three major randomized trials investigating LL for diverticulitis: LOLA/LADIES [24], DILALA [27], and SCANDIV [25].

Acuna and coauthors recently published a Current Status guideline report reviewing six studies, incorporating 626 patients who underwent surgery for perforated diverticulitis. Though early reoperation rates and postoperative mortality were similar in the lavage vs sigmoidectomy group, major complications (Clavien-Dindo > IIIa) were significantly higher after LL group, RR = 1.68 (95% CI, 1.1–2.56) ($p = 0.02$). Similarly, early reoperation rates were slightly higher in the laparoscopic lavage group, RR = 1.93 (95% CI, 1.71–5.22) ($p = 0.20$), as was postoperative

Table 28.1 Primary outcomes of laparoscopic lavage compared to resection – including long-term updates

Study	Author	Year	*N*	Comparisons	Morbidity rates, RR (95% CI)	Reoperation rates, RR (95% CI)	Mortality, RR (95% CI)	Others
LADIES-LOLA	Vennix [24]	2015	90	LL vs PRA ± DLI vs HP	39% vs 13% ($p = 0.043$) RR 1.83 (95% CI 0.97–3.44) Discontinued early due to increased morbidity	20% vs 7% RR 2.74 (0.79–9.45)	9 vs 14% ($p = 0.43$) 1.83 (0.17–19.41)	
SCANDIV	Schultz [25]	2015	199	LL vs HP or PRA ± DLI	31% vs 26% ($p = 0.53$) RR 1.80 (0.90–3.59)	20% vs 6% ($p = 0.01$) RR 3.78 (1.11–12.84)	14% vs 21% ($p = 0.67$) 0.63 (0.11–3.66)	
SCANDIV	Schultz [26]	2017	199	LL vs HP or PRA ± DLI	34% vs 27% ($p = 32\%$) Deep sepsis: 32% vs 13% ($p = 0.006$)	27% vs 10% ($p = 0.01$)		Stoma 14% vs 42% ($p < 0.001$)
DILALA	Angenete [27]	2016	83	LL vs HP	NS RR 1.23 (0.47–3.19)	13% vs 17% ($p = 0.63$) 0.77 (0.26–2.29)	8% vs 0% 6.47 (0.35–121.17)	Lower operating time ($p < 0.0001$)
DILALA	Thornell [28]	2016	83	LL vs HP	NS	28% vs 63% ($p = 0.004$)	NS	
DILALA	Gerhman [29]	2016	83	LL vs HP				Lower cost −8983€, −19,794€/expected life years
	Angenete [30]	2017	358	LL vs HP or PRA ± I		Reduced OR 0.54 (95% CI, 0.38–0.76)		
DILALA	Kohl [31]	2018	83	LL vs HP		42% vs 68%0.55 (0.36–0.84) $p = 0.012$		Long-term stoma rates: 7% vs 22%
	Shaikh [32]	2017	372	LL vs HP or PRA ± DLI	OR 1.87 (95% CI, 0.68–5.12) ($p = 0.23$)			Increased deep space abscess, OR 4.12 (95% CI, 1.89–8.98) ($p = 0.0004$) Increased risk of percutaneous drainage, OR 5.41 (95% CI, 1.62–18.12) ($p = 0.006$)

LL laparoscopic peritoneal lavage, *HP* Hartmann's procedure, *PRA* primary resection and anastomosis, *DLI* diverting loop ileostomy, *NS* non-significant, *OR* Odd's ratio, *CI* confidence interval, *RR* relative risk

Table 28.2 Long-term secondary outcomes of laparoscopic lavage compared to resection at 12 months

Measures	Trials	Risk ratio (95% CI)	Favoring	*P*
Major postoperative complication	LOLA, SCANDIV [24, 25]	1.27 (0.89–1.80)	Resection	0.19
Reoperations, including stoma reversal, at 12 months	DILALA, LOLA, SCANDIV	0.67 (0.45–1.02)	Lavage	0.06
Mortality at 12 months	LOLA, DILALA, SCANDIV	0.89 (0.49–1.61)	Lavage	0.70
Patients with stoma at 12 months	DILALA, SCANDIV, LOLA	0.43 (0.22–0.83)	Lavage	0.01

mortality, RR = 1.33 (95% CI, 0.37–4.74) ($p = 0.66$). All three above measured outcomes favored resection over laparoscopic lavage [33].

When evaluating patients undergoing primary sigmoidectomy with PRA and stoma to patients undergoing Hartmann's procedure, similar complication rates (RR = 0.88 (95% CI, 0.49–1.55)) and postoperatively mortality were noted (RR = 0.58 (95% CI, 0.20–1.70)). However, those patients that underwent PRA were more likely to be stoma-free at 1 year compared to those undergoing Hartmann's procedure (RR = 1.40 (95% CI, 1.18–1.67)) and experience fewer major complications related to stoma reversal (RR = 0.26 (95% CI, 0.07–0.89)).

Acuna also performed a meta-analysis attempting to evaluate quality of life and comparing laparoscopic lavage group with the resection group. Due to significant differences in survey instrumentations and variable time points, no appropriate differences nor conclusions could be drawn. Overall, the DILALA trial found similarly poor quality of life at discharge among both groups. The LOLA trial similarly found no differences overall. Lastly, the SCANDIV trial found no significant differences in any of the quality of life measures at 90 days [33].

Beyer-Berjot published a meta-analysis evaluating surgical outcomes following emergency surgery for acute diverticulitis which included LL, open or laparoscopic sigmoidectomy with PRA with or without ostomy. This comprehensive review included 5 guideline papers, 4 meta-analysis, 14 systematic reviews, and 5 randomized controlled trials. Laparoscopic lavage was associated with an increased rate of deep space infections and abscess and a higher rate of unplanned reoperations. When comparing Hartmann's procedure to resection with PRA, the latter had an improved stoma-free rate and improved quality of life [13].

Penna similarly reviewed clinical outcomes between LL and colonic resection for Hinchey III diverticulitis. Based on their analysis, the former had higher rates of intra-abdominal abscesses (RR = 2.85 (95% CI 1.52–5.34), $p = 0.001$), peritonitis (RR = 7.80 (95% CI 2.12–28.69), $p = 0.002$), and increased long-term emergency reoperations (RR = 3.32 (95% CI 1.73–6.38), $p < 0.001$). After stoma reversal, 23% had a stoma after 1 year in the resection group, compared to 7.2% in the lavage group. Of note, 36% of the lavage group eventually underwent elective sigmoid resection [34].

Kohl presented long-term results of the DILALA trial comparing LL to HP. At 2 years, there was a statistically significant increase in the number of reoperations in the Hartmann's group; however, reasons for these secondary operations were similar among the two groups and likely related to the index operation [31].

Though initially advocated as a significant adjunct to minimize morbidity in patients with perforated Hinchey III diverticulitis, an abundance of data from multiple large prospective trials demonstrates that LL is associated with increased major complication rate, increased short-term re-operative rate, and permanent stoma rate when compared to primary resection. In summary, resection with primary anastomosis and diverting ileostomy should be the preferred approach in the management of Hinchey III disease.

In conclusion, when possible, we currently recommend percutaneous drainage of diverticular abscesses which, when successful, can be followed by observation vs definitive resection on an elective basis. In the setting of Hinchey III perforated diverticulitis with purulent peritonitis, the current guidelines and data suggest resection of the diseased sigmoid colon with primary colorectal anastomosis and diverting loop ileostomy in patients that are otherwise stable for an operation is superior to LL and HP. HP remains a viable safe alternative in patients hemodynamically unstable or unfit for creation of an anastomosis. This treatment paradigm results in a significantly lower rate of permanent stoma with lower or equivalent long-term morbidity and mortality when compared to LL (or selective HP). Lavage may be considered in selected Hinchey III patients by surgeons with appropriate expertise and the ability to closely watch for and manage complications. The lower stoma rate should be weighed against the higher risk of postoperative complications and re-intervention encountered after LL.

Conclusions

Emergent laparoscopic colectomy with or without fecal diversion is feasible and safe in carefully selected patients. Current data do not support the routine use of laparoscopic peritoneal lavage for Hinchey III (or IV) diverticulitis. The optimal resectional strategy (open or laparoscopic HP, PRA with or without ileostomy) is determined by multiple factors including surgical experience, patient clinical presentation, and intraoperative findings with consideration of short-term and long-term outcomes and impact on quality of life. The surgical team should frequently reevaluate the intraoperative conditions to ensure the patient's safety is maximized. It is essential to be familiar with various approaches (i.e., medial-to-lateral, lateral-to-medial, superior to inferior, etc.) resulting in optimal exposure as well as safer, quicker, and a more reproducible dissection. This is undoubtedly facilitated by a fundamental understanding of the surgical anatomy, allowing the surgeon the ability to proceed in a safe manner and allow for additional diagnostic and therapeutic maneuvering while maximizing patient quality of life and simultaneously reducing morbidity.

References

1. Abraha I, Binda GA, Montedori A, Arezzo A, Cirocchi R. Laparoscopic versus open resection for sigmoid diverticulitis. Cochrane Database Syst Rev. 2017;(11):CD009277.
2. Alves A, Panis Y, Mantion G, Slim K, Kwiatkowski F, Vicaut E. The AFC score: validation of a 4-item predicting score of postoperative mortality after colorectal resection for cancer or diverticulitis: results of a prospective multicenter study in 1049 patients. Ann Surg. 2007;246(1):91–6.
3. Vennix S, Boersema GS, Buskens CJ, Menon AG, Tanis PJ, Lange JF, et al. Emergency laparoscopic sigmoidectomy for perforated diverticulitis with generalized peritonitis: a systematic review. Dig Surg. 2016;33(1):1–7.
4. Vennix S, Lips DJ, Di Saverio S, van Wagensveld BA, Brokelman WJ, Gerhards MF, et al. Acute laparoscopic and open sigmoidectomy for perforated diverticulitis: a propensity score-matched cohort. Surg Endosc. 2016;30(9):3889–96.
5. Biondo S, Lopez Borao J, Millan M, Kreisler E, Jaurrieta E. Current status of the treatment of acute colonic diverticulitis: a systematic review. Color Dis. 2012;14(1):e1–e11.
6. Hinchey EJ, Schaal PG, Richards GK. Treatment of perforated diverticular disease of the colon. Adv Surg. 1978;12:85–109.
7. Dharmarajan S, Hunt SR, Birnbaum EH, Fleshman JW, Mutch MG. The efficacy of nonoperative management of acute complicated diverticulitis. Dis Colon Rectum. 2011;54(6):663–71.
8. Remzi FH, Oncel M, Hull TL, Strong SA, Lavery IC, Fazio VW. Current indications for blow-hole colostomy:ileostomy procedure. A single center experience. Int J Color Dis. 2003;18(4):361–4.
9. Weber DG, Bendinelli C, Balogh ZJ. Damage control surgery for abdominal emergencies. Br J Surg. 2014;101(1):e109–18.
10. Greco M, Capretti G, Beretta L, Gemma M, Pecorelli N, Braga M. Enhanced recovery program in colorectal surgery: a meta-analysis of randomized controlled trials. World J Surg. 2014;38(6):1531–41.
11. Awotar GK, Guan G, Sun W, Yu H, Zhu M, Cui X, et al. Reviewing the management of obstructive left colon cancer: assessing the feasibility of the one-stage resection and anastomosis after intraoperative colonic irrigation. Clin Colorectal Cancer. 2017;16(2):e89–e103.
12. Person B, Ifargan R, Lachter J, Duek SD, Kluger Y, Assalia A. The impact of preoperative stoma site marking on the incidence of complications, quality of life, and patient's independence. Dis Colon Rectum. 2012;55(7):783–7.
13. Beyer-Berjot L, Maggiori L, Loiseau D, De Korwin JD, Bongiovanni JP, Lesprit P, et al. Emergency surgery in acute diverticulitis: a systematic review. Dis Colon Rectum. 2019; https://doi.org/10.1097/DCR.0000000000001327. [Epub ahead of print].
14. Schmidt S, Ismail T, Puhan MA, Soll C, Breitenstein S. Meta-analysis of surgical strategies in perforated left colonic diverticulitis with generalized peritonitis. Langenbeck's Arch Surg. 2018;403(4):425–33.
15. Belizon A, Sardinha CT, Sher ME. Converted laparoscopic colectomy: what are the consequences? Surg Endosc. 2006;20(6):947–51.
16. DeSouza A, Domajnko B, Park J, Marecik S, Prasad L, Abcarian H. Incisional hernia, midline versus low transverse incision: what is the ideal incision for specimen extraction and hand-assisted laparoscopy? Surg Endosc. 2011;25(4):1031–6.
17. Ricciardi R, Roberts PL, Marcello PW, Hall JF, Read TE, Schoetz DJ. Anastomotic leak testing after colorectal resection: what are the data? Arch Surg. 2009;144(5):407–11; discussion 11–2.
18. Reiffel AJ, Barie PS, Spector JA. A multi-disciplinary review of the potential association between closed-suction drains and surgical site infection. Surg Infect. 2013;14(3):244–69.
19. Turley RS, Barbas AS, Lidsky ME, Mantyh CR, Migaly J, Scarborough JE. Laparoscopic versus open Hartmann procedure for the emergency treatment of diverticulitis: a propensity-matched analysis. Dis Colon Rectum. 2013;56(1):72–82.

20. Cirocchi R, Trastulli S, Desiderio J, Listorti C, Boselli C, Parisi A, et al. Treatment of Hinchey stage III-IV diverticulitis: a systematic review and meta-analysis. Int J Color Dis. 2013;28(4):447–57.
21. Gachabayov M, Oberkofler CE, Tuech JJ, Hahnloser D, Bergamaschi R. Resection with primary anastomosis vs nonrestorative resection for perforated diverticulitis with peritonitis: a systematic review and meta-analysis. Color Dis. 2018;20(9):753–70.
22. Oberkofler CE, Rickenbacher A, Raptis DA, Lehmann K, Villiger P, Buchli C, et al. A multicenter randomized clinical trial of primary anastomosis or Hartmann's procedure for perforated left colonic diverticulitis with purulent or fecal peritonitis. Ann Surg. 2012;256(5):819–26; discussion 26–7.
23. Toro A, Mannino M, Reale G, Cappello G, Di Carlo I. Primary anastomosis vs Hartmann procedure in acute complicated diverticulitis. Evolution over the last twenty years. Chirurgia (Bucur). 2012;107(5):598–604.
24. Vennix S, Musters GD, Mulder IM, Swank HA, Consten EC, Belgers EH, et al. Laparoscopic peritoneal lavage or sigmoidectomy for perforated diverticulitis with purulent peritonitis: a multicenter, parallel-group, randomized, open-label trial. Lancet. 2015;386(10000):1269–77.
25. Schultz JK, Yaqub S, Wallon C, Blecic L, Forsmo HM, Folkesson J, et al. Laparoscopic lavage vs primary resection for acute perforated diverticulitis: the SCANDIV randomized clinical trial. JAMA. 2015;314(13):1364–75.
26. Schultz JK, Wallon C, Blecic L, Forsmo HM, Folkesson J, Buchwald P, et al. One-year results of the SCANDIV randomized clinical trial of laparoscopic lavage versus primary resection for acute perforated diverticulitis. Br J Surg. 2017;104(10):1382–92.
27. Angenete E, Thornell A, Burcharth J, Pommergaard HC, Skullman S, Bisgaard T, et al. Laparoscopic lavage is feasible and safe for the treatment of perforated diverticulitis with purulent peritonitis: the first results from the randomized controlled trial DILALA. Ann Surg. 2016;263(1):117–22.
28. Thornell A, Angenete E, Gonzales E, Heath J, Jess P, Lackberg Z, et al. Treatment of acute diverticulitis laparoscopic lavage vs. resection (DILALA): study protocol for a randomized controlled trial. Trials. 2011;12:186.
29. Gehrman J, Angenete E, Bjorholt I, Bock D, Rosenberg J, Haglind E. Health economic analysis of laparoscopic lavage versus Hartmann's procedure for diverticulitis in the randomized DILALA trial. Br J Surg. 2016;103(11):1539–47.
30. Angenete E, Bock D, Rosenberg J, Haglind E. Laparoscopic lavage is superior to colon resection for perforated purulent diverticulitis-a meta-analysis. Int J Color Dis. 2017;32(2):163–9.
31. Kohl A, Rosenberg J, Bock D, Bisgaard T, Skullman S, Thornell A, et al. Two-year results of the randomized clinical trial DILALA comparing laparoscopic lavage with resection as treatment for perforated diverticulitis. Br J Surg. 2018;105(9):1128–34.
32. Shaikh FM, Stewart PM, Walsh SR, Davies RJ. Laparoscopic peritoneal lavage or surgical resection for acute perforated sigmoid diverticulitis: a systematic review and meta-analysis. Int J Surg. 2017;38:130–7.
33. Acuna SA, Wood T, Chesney TR, Dossa F, Wexner SD, Quereshy FA, et al. Operative strategies for perforated diverticulitis: a systematic review and meta-analysis. Dis Colon Rectum. 2018;61(12):1442–53.
34. Penna M, Markar SR, Mackenzie H, Hompes R, Cunningham C. Laparoscopic lavage versus primary resection for acute perforated diverticulitis: review and meta-analysis. Ann Surg. 2018;267(2):252–8.

Minimizing Colorectal Anastomotic Leaks: Best Practices to Assess the Integrity and Perfusion of Left-Sided Anastomoses

29

Mehraneh D. Jafari and Alessio Pigazzi

Introduction and Rationale

Anastomotic leak can be a serious complication of colon and rectal resections. Although all the factors contributing to anastomotic leak are not well understood, leaks are commonly caused by a combination of patient factors such as malnutrition, obesity, smoking, and diabetes or technical factors including excessive tension on the anastomosis, inadequate perfusion, or other errors in their construction. Leaks from right-sided (ileocolic) anastomoses are uncommon, with less than 2% reported in a meta-analysis of seven series [1]. Rates for left-sided (colorectal) anastomoses vary depending on the distance of the anastomosis relative to the anal verge and range from 5 to 18%, even among high-volume surgeons [2–5].

The sequelae of leaks can range from subclinical leaks that require no interventions to life-threatening sepsis requiring emergency surgery. Randomized trial data report mortality of 1.3–6.7% in patients with anastomotic leaks, with higher rates in anastomoses closer to the anal verge [4, 6]. Mortality after right-sided colon resections are less than 0.5%, corresponding to the lower leak rates [1].

Intraoperative examination of the anastomosis with air leak testing and rigid or flexible endoscopy should be used to evaluate for the mechanical integrity and perfusion of the anastomosis. Bowel perfusion with fluorescence angiography may be used as an adjunct to further delineate and identify areas of compromised perfusion. Endoscopy can also aid in correcting technical errors and help perform anastomotic revision intraoperatively, possibly reducing the rate of postoperative leak.

M. D. Jafari · A. Pigazzi (✉)
University of California, Irvine, Colon and Rectal Surgery, Orange, CA, USA
e-mail: apigazzi@uci.edu

P. Sylla et al. (eds.), *The SAGES Manual of Colorectal Surgery*,
https://doi.org/10.1007/978-3-030-24812-3_29

Indications for Endoscopic Evaluation

In our view, all left-sided colorectal anastomoses should be evaluated with intraoperative endoscopy. Though no randomized trial of flexible endoscopy versus air leak testing without visualization has been performed, data from large case series support evaluation with direct visualization over air leak testing alone. A single-institution review of 415 consecutive laparoscopic left-sided colorectal resections identified abnormalities on 17 (4.1%) of cases, 15 of which also had an air leak. These anastomoses were resected and refashioned, and none subsequently leaked [7]. However, a negative air leak testing does not necessarily eliminate the risk of a postoperative leak. Grading with visual inspection of the anastomoses can potentially predict leaks, allowing for intraoperative revision and lower risk of anastomotic leak. Areas of ischemia or congestion at the anastomosis warrant intraoperative revision [8]. Evaluation with fluorescent imaging that highlights the vasculature, and thus perfusion to the anastomosis, can help identify and/or confirm areas of suspected bowel ischemia, allowing for correction and reducing the risk of postoperative leakage [9]. Endoscopic evaluation carries almost no risk if properly performed and does not significantly prolong operative time. This modality is recommended for evaluation of all left-sided colorectal anastomoses.

Principles and Quality Benchmarks for Endoscopic Evaluation

When evaluating a colorectal anastomosis, surgeons should evaluate for the integrity of the anastomosis with insufflation, evaluate the perfusion of the colon and rectum at the anastomosis, and evaluate for any brisk bleeding which can be controlled.

The integrity of the anastomosis can be performed by visualization of the anastomosis with simultaneous CO_2 (or air if CO_2 is unavailable) insufflation and proximal bowel occlusion via either open or laparoscopic techniques. This combination will allow the surgeon to visualize any defect and potentially repair via suture ligation or, in cases of large defects, revise the anastomosis entirely. Any obvious defects at the anastomosis, with or without air leak, warrant immediate revision. Flexible sigmoidoscopy offers excellent visualization, but rigid proctoscopy can also be performed. We highly encourage every surgeon who performs high-risk anastomosis to perform an endoscopic evaluation with care to fully visualize the anastomosis.

One technique we developed at the University of California, Irvine, involves examination and grading of the distal and proximal mucosa at the staple line. This novel technique allows the surgeon to objectively evaluate the perfusion at the index operation (Table 29.1 and Fig. 29.1a–c) [8]. Grade 1 anastomoses have no signs of ischemia or congestion and have a low risk of leak. Grade 2 anastomoses have ischemia or congestion involving less than 30% of either the colon or rectal mucosa. These anastomoses have a higher risk of leak, and intraoperative revision or diversion should be considered. Grade 3 anastomoses have more than 30%

Table 29.1 Endoscopic mucosal grading system for colorectal anastomoses

	Anastomosis appearance on endoscopy		
	Grade 1: No ischemia or congestion	Grade 2: <30% ischemia or congestion	Grade 3: >30% ischemia or congestion
Patients	92	10	4
Leaks (%)	9 (9.4%)	4 (40%)	–
Odds ratio of leak (95% CI)	Ref	4.09 (1.21–13.6)	–

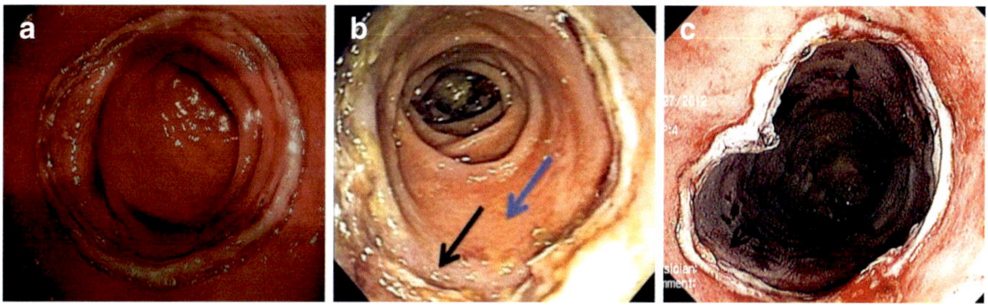

Fig. 29.1 (**a**) Grade 1 anastomosis. No areas of ischemia or congestion are noted, and the entire circumference is visible. (**b**) Grade 2 anastomosis. Less than 30% of the circumference (arrows) appears congested. (**c**) Grade 3 anastomosis. Greater than 30% of the colonic mucosa appears ischemic. All 4 Grade 3 anastomoses were revised to Grade 1 with no subsequent leaks

ischemia on either side or any ischemia on both sides of the staple line. They have a high risk of leak and should always be revised. Re-evaluation with endoscopy after revision is warranted. Please refer to Chap. 30 on salvage of the failed anastomosis for additional details on how to manage colonic ischemia.

Techniques for Assessing Tension and Perfusion During Colorectal Anastomosis Creation

A tension-free, well-perfused anastomosis is the key to reducing the risk of anastomotic leak, especially in pelvic anastomoses. Excessive tension can compromise perfusion, but overzealous division of the mesocolon will also cause ischemia. With this in mind, complete mobilization of the left side of the colon, including the splenic flexure, and division of the inferior mesenteric vein and artery (IMV and IMA) are encouraged for low anterior resections. Division of the gastrocolic ligament to the mid transverse colon and separation of the mesocolic attachment to the pancreatic tail will also provide additional colon length. After mobilization, the left colonic conduit should easily descend down toward the rectal stump without any tension. The mesocolon is often the site of persistent tension even after mobilization of these attachments, and division of the azygous portion of inferior mesenteric vein superior to the ligament of Treitz can provide additional length. Please refer to Chap. 4 on laparoscopic splenic flexure release for additional details on surgical techniques.

Perfusion of the colon can be assessed through direct visual inspection of the serosa and evaluation of blood flow after sharp division of the colon. Any concerns should prompt identification of a better perfused area for division. Further mobilization of retroperitoneal, gastrocolic, and lateral attachments may be required to avoid tension on the anastomosis. Care should be given to avoid injury of the marginal artery to avoid ischemia of the colonic conduit.

Various fluorescent dyes have been developed for assessment of bowel perfusion. The most commonly used of these is indocyanine green (ICG). This is a nontoxic, stable dye that has been used for a half century in ophthalmology for retinal angiography [10]. It is readily excreted in bile and does not stain the tissues. Allergy to the dye is extremely rare. Angiography with this dye requires specialized light sources and cameras that can capture the near-infrared spectrum, which are present on some robotic and laparoscopic camera systems. 3.75–7.5 mg of ICG dye is injected intravenously and imaging performed approximately 2–3 minutes afterward. The dye washes out after 3–5 minutes; thus, close communication with the anesthesiologist and surgeon is critical. Repeated injections can be performed if necessary. Ideally, visualization should be performed prior to division of the colon to identify a transection point between well-perfused and ischemic bowel. The proximal rectal pouch can also be evaluated simultaneously as the dye perfuses the entire bowel vasculature. Well-perfused bowel will fluoresce green or blue, and a sharp cutoff of malperfused distal bowel should be noted (Fig. 29.2). With rigid proctoscopy, fluorescent perfusion of the mucosa after anastomosis can also be visualized; however, this option is not currently available with flexible endoscopes. This technique can be used in conjunction with, but not in lieu of, direct visual inspection of the bowel's blood supply. Using both ICG imaging techniques, leak rates of only 1.4% were achieved in a phase II multicenter trial [11].

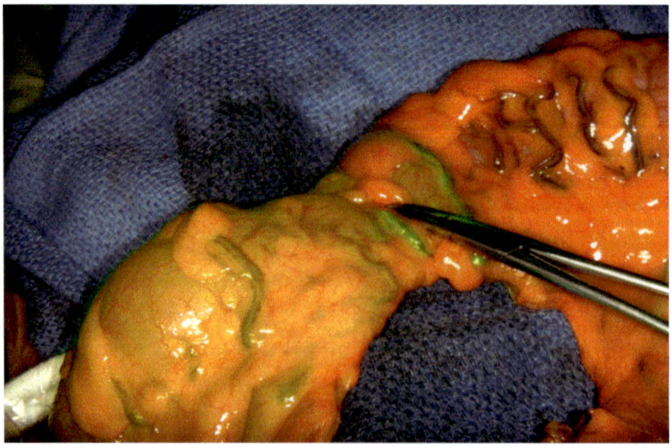

Fig. 29.2 Intraoperative ICG perfusion imaging. Green fluorescence highlights the proximal, perfused bowel. Clamp delineates the transition between perfused and unperfused bowel

Techniques for Intraoperative Endoscopy

The patient should undergo bowel preparation with oral laxatives and rectal enemas prior to the day of operation, and rectal irrigation should be performed at the start of the procedure to ensure adequate evacuation of residual rectal contents. The patient should remain in a modified lithotomy position and Trendelenburg after creation of the anastomosis. With the anastomosis under direct visualization from the abdomen, a flexible colonoscope is inserted via the anus. If a laparoscopic approach is used, the extraction incision should be temporarily closed with a wound retractor (Fig. 29.3), and the abdomen should be re-insufflated. If an open approach is used, the extraction site should be large enough to provide adequate visualization of the anastomosis. The colon proximal to the anastomosis is gently occluded with a blunt grasper by an assistant. The pelvis should be irrigated of clots, and any organs obscuring the anastomosis should be retracted away. Irrigation (water) is instilled into the pelvis to submerge the anastomosis. Any residual bubbles from instilling irrigation should be suctioned away. The rectum is then insufflated with CO_2 or air. The colonoscope or proctoscope is gently advanced to the anastomosis and beyond. Any air leak noted within the pelvis should warrant investigation of the anastomosis. If positive air leak continues after suctioning, consider repair of the anastomosis under direct visualization at the exact location of the air leak. This can be performed transabdominally with interrupted absorbable sutures to close the defect. Visualization of the defect during repair can ease accurate placement of sutures. If the anastomosis is very low, suture repair of the defect may need to be performed transanally. In either case, careful inspection via a colonoscope or proctoscope should be performed and air leak testing repeated after repair to confirm resolution of leak. If the leak persists or is associated with a large or posterior defect, revision of the entire anastomosis with either stapled or hand-sewn techniques may be required. In the setting of a small air leak that cannot be identified, in a patient who has undergone a full bowel preparation, fecal diversion with a loop ileostomy can be considered, in conjunction with placement of reinforcing sutures at the anastomosis, but only after endoscopic and/or perfusion assessment has confirmed adequate perfusion.

As the endoscope is slowly pulled back, the colon mucosa proximal to the anastomosis is inspected for any changes in perfusion. Once the entire anastomosis is in

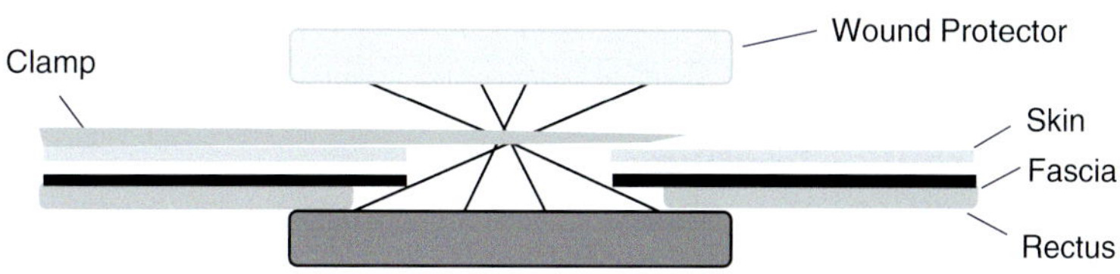

Fig. 29.3 Technique for re-insufflating abdomen by occluding the specimen extraction site. A flexible wound protector inserted into the specimen extraction site can be twisted and clamped flush with the incision to maintain pneumoperitoneum during the anastomosis creation and inspection

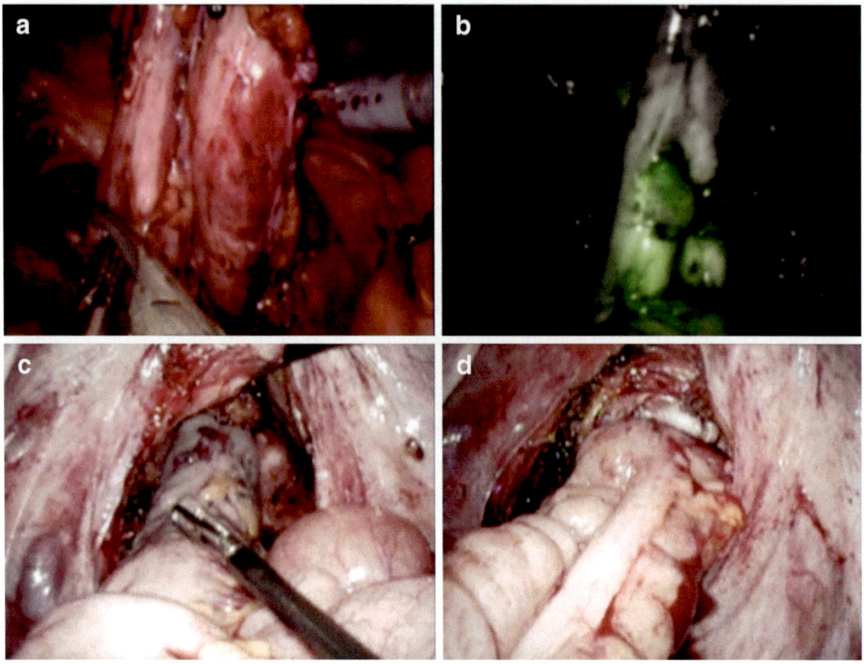

Fig. 29.4 (**a**–**d**) Intraoperative evaluation of a high-risk low rectal anastomosis with laparoscopic techniques for revision. Colon is shown prior to transection in white light (**a**) and with ICG fluorescence imaging (**b**). The distal colon appears ischemic after the initial anastomosis is performed (**c**) and well perfused after complete revision of the anastomosis with viable bowel (**d**)

view, any clots and debris are gently irrigated away with the endoscope flush. Signs of ischemia or congestion are noted, and the approximate extent around the circumference of the anastomosis is determined (Fig. 29.1a–c). If the area is small (UCI Grade 2), suture reinforcement may be adequate. If a UCI Grade 3 anastomosis is noted, takedown and revision of anastomosis with possible diversion must be considered (Fig. 29.4a–d). The remainder of the rectal remnant is inspected as the endoscope is removed. Retroflexion should not be performed to avoid undue tension on the anastomosis. The rectum should be desufflated with suction. If any brisk arterial bleeding is encountered, endoscopic clips can be utilized to control bleeding. If clips are not available, the area should be visualized intraabdominally, and suture ligation should be attempted.

Pitfalls and Troubleshooting

Evaluation of the anastomosis with intraoperative and endoscopic assessment is a straightforward technique that is readily applicable in elective colon resections. The surgeon should be familiar with basic endoscopy techniques. The major pitfall with endoscopic evaluation is incomplete or inaccurate assessment of the anastomosis. Assessment of the degree of ischemia requires experience, but simple grading systems such as the one provided in this chapter are useful benchmarks. Determining the need for revision must be tailored for each patient's situation, with the understanding that immediate revision in a non-inflamed and non-contaminated field will be technically easier than revision in the setting of a clinically significant leak.

Incomplete assessment of the anastomosis is technically preventable by ensuring sufficient exposure to allow for careful inspection of the entire circumference of the anastomosis. It is essential to irrigate any clots or stool and ensure sufficient insufflation so that mucosal folds do not obscure the anastomosis. Therefore, we recommend rectal irrigation prior to anastomosis. Proximal occlusion of the colon will help retain gas within the rectum, and a well-made anastomosis will not leak with normal levels of insufflation. Flexible, rather than rigid, endoscopy greatly facilitates evaluation of the anastomosis by multiple observers in the operating room and allows for endoscopic intervention. Ensuring that the anastomosis is well exposed from the abdomen, and the bladder and uterus are retracted off the rectum, will also improve visualization.

Outcomes

Many methods for evaluating anastomotic leaks have been described in the literature. Gross assessment of the anastomosis without endoscopic evaluation is neither sensitive nor specific for predicting leaks [12]. A meta-analysis of 20 studies evaluating air leak testing with out endoscopy found no significant decrease in postoperative leaks, even if diverting ostomies were created after repair of the anastomosis (OR 0.61, 95% CI 0.32–1.18, $p = 0.15$) [13]. The overall leak rate across all studies was 11.2%, consistent with ranges of 10–15% in randomized colorectal surgery trials [3, 4]. These findings highlight the importance of direct endoscopic inspection of left-sided colorectal anastomoses.

Large series examining the use of intraoperative endoscopy in evaluating anastomoses demonstrated significant reductions in leak rates when compared to patients who had not undergone endoscopy. A series of 215 rectal cancer patients matched for demographics, AJCC stage, and tumor location demonstrated a 4.2% leak rate after endoscopy vs. 12.1% with air leak testing alone ($p = 0.004$) [14]. Of note, only 1 of the 26 patients with postoperative leaks after air leak testing alone had had a positive air leak test. A series of 415 consecutive patients who underwent intraoperative endoscopy reported a 4.1% rate of abnormalities requiring revision. No postoperative leaks occurred in these patients [7]. The overall leak rate in this series was 2.1%, much lower than the 13% rate reported in a recent Cochrane review of the literature [15]. However, neither group reported a systemic method of evaluating the integrity of the anastomosis.

A simple classification scheme has been developed at our institution to grade the quality of colorectal anastomoses (Table 29.1) [8]. This is the only reported systemic method of grading colorectal anastomoses with intraoperative endoscopy.

Table 29.2 Evaluation of anastomoses with ICG

Study	Series type and comparison	*n*	% Left-sided anastomosis	Leak rate	Change in operation due to ICG imaging *n* (%)
Jafari [11]	ICG series	139	100%	2 (1.4%)	9 (6.5%)
Ris [18]	ICG series	30	6 (20%)	0 (0%)	3 (10%)
Boni [19]	ICG series	42	100%	0 (0%)	2 (4.7%)
	Matched cases	38	100%	2 (5.3%)	–
Kudszus [17]	ICG group	201	NA	7 (3.4%)*	28 (13.9%)
	Matched cases	201	NA	15 (7.5%)	–
Protyniak [20]	ICG group	76	47 (61.8%)	0 (0%)	4 (5.2%)
Foppa [21]	ICG group	160	NA	NA	4 (2.5%)
Kawada [22]	ICG group	68	28 (41.1%)	3 (4.5%)	18 (26.5%)
Kim [23]	ICG group	123	100%	1 (0.8%)*	13 (10.6%)
	Matched cases	313	100%	17 (5.4%)	–
Kin [24]	ICG group	173	17 (9.8%)	13 (7.5%)	8 (4.6%)
	Matched cases	173	17 (9.8%)	11 (6.4%)	–
Hellan [25]	ICG group	40	27 (67.5%)	2 (5.0%)	16 (40%)
Boni [26]	ICG group	107	22 (21%)	1 (0.9%)	4 (3.7%)

NA not available
*$p < 0.05$

Using this scheme, 106 consecutive patients were evaluated intraoperatively, and significant differences in leak rates were noted between Grade 1 and 2 anastomoses (OR of leak 4.09, 95% CI 1.21–13.63, $p = 0.023$). There were no significant differences in patient demographics, indication for resection or operative approach. The majority of anastomoses were Grade 1 (86.7%), and these had a leak rate of 9.8% (9/96). Five of these patients had a symptomatic leak requiring intervention. Grade 2 anastomoses had a significantly higher leak rate of 40% (4/10), and two patients required intervention. Four patients had Grade 3 anastomoses initially, and all underwent immediate revision to a Grade 1 anastomosis. This study highlights the usefulness of a grading system to guide intraoperative decision-making.

The use of ICG for evaluating bowel perfusion during colorectal operations has gained traction in recent years as newer models of minimally invasive camera systems have included the necessary optics. A recent meta-analysis of five case-control series demonstrated a significant reduction in postoperative leaks with the use of ICG imaging (OR 0.34, 95% CI 0.160.74, $p = 0.006$) [16]. The majority of the benefit was noted in resections for cancer (1.1% with ICG vs. 6.1% without, $p = 0.02$). A series of 402 patients with matched controls demonstrated a lower leak rate and fewer reoperations with ICG use (3.1% vs. 7.7%, $p = 0.04$) [17]. In a prospective trial of ICG in laparoscopic left-sided colorectal operations, operative plans were informed by perfusion assessment in 8% of cases, and the anastomotic leak rate was 1.2% [11]. ICG is a simple to use, low-risk method of perfusion assessment that can provide important information to guide intraoperative planning and reduce postoperative complications from leaks. See Table 29.2.

Conclusion

Anastomotic leaks from colorectal anastomoses dramatically increase the morbidity and mortality of colorectal operations. However, the risk of this complication can be minimized with close attention to the quality of the anastomoses. Minimizing tension, optimizing perfusion, and evaluating the newly created anastomosis are essential to ensure its integrity. Endoscopic visualization and bowel perfusion assessment with fluorescent dyes are simple techniques that can be readily incorporated into any colorectal operation.

Acknowledgments The authors are indebted to Abhineet Uppal, MD, for his invaluable contributions to this chapter.

References

1. Cirocchi R, Trastulli S, Farinella E, Guarino S, Desiderio J, Boselli C, et al. Intracorporeal versus extracorporeal anastomosis during laparoscopic right hemicolectomy – systematic review and meta-analysis. Surg Oncol. 2013;22(1):1–13.
2. Chadi SA, Fingerhut A, Berho M, DeMeester SR, Fleshman JW, Hyman NH, et al. Emerging trends in the etiology, prevention, and treatment of gastrointestinal anastomotic leakage. J Gastrointest Surg: Off J Soc Surg Alimentary Tract. 2016;20(12):2035–51.
3. Fingerhut A, Hay JM, Elhadad A, Lacaine F, Flamant Y. Supraperitoneal colorectal anastomosis: hand-sewn versus circular staples--a controlled clinical trial. French Associations for Surgical Research. Surgery. 1995;118(3):479–85.
4. Fingerhut A, Elhadad A, Hay JM, Lacaine F, Flamant Y. Infraperitoneal colorectal anastomosis: hand-sewn versus circular staples. A controlled clinical trial. French Associations for Surgical Research. Surgery. 1994;116(3):484–90.
5. Hyman NHOT, Cataldo P, Burns EH, Shackford SR. Anastomotic leaks after bowel resection: what does peer review teach us about the relationship to postoperative mortality? J Am Coll Surg. 2009;208(1):48–52.
6. Fingerhut AHJ, Elhadad A, Lacaine F, Flamant Y. Supraperitoneal colorectal anastomosis: hand-sewn versus circular staples--a controlled clinical trial. French Associations for Surgical Research. Surgery. 1995;118(3):479–85.
7. Kamal T, Pai A, Velchuru VR, Zawadzki M, Park JJ, Marecik SJ, et al. Should anastomotic assessment with flexible sigmoidoscopy be routine following laparoscopic restorative left colorectal resection? Colorectal Dis: Off J Assoc Coloproctol Great Br Ireland. 2015;17(2):160–4.
8. Sujatha-Bhaskar S, Jafari MD, Hanna M, Koh CY, Inaba CS, Mills SD, et al. An endoscopic mucosal grading system is predictive of leak in stapled rectal anastomoses. Surg Endosc. 2018;32(4):1769–75.
9. Chen CW, Chen MJ, Yeh YS, Tsai HL, Chang YT, Wang JY. Intraoperative anastomotic dye test significantly decreases incidence of anastomotic leaks in patients undergoing resection for rectal cancer. Tech Coloproctol. 2013;17(5):579–83.
10. Alander JT, Kaartinen I, Laakso A, Patila T, Spillmann T, Tuchin VV, et al. A review of indocyanine green fluorescent imaging in surgery. Int J Biomed Imaging. 2012;2012:940585.
11. Jafari MD, Wexner SD, Martz JE, McLemore EC, Margolin DA, Sherwinter DA, et al. Perfusion assessment in laparoscopic left-sided/anterior resection (PILLAR II): a multi-institutional study. J Am Coll Surg. 2015;220(1):82–92 e1.

12. Karliczek A, Harlaar NJ, Zeebregts CJ, Wiggers T, Baas PC, van Dam GM. Surgeons lack predictive accuracy for anastomotic leakage in gastrointestinal surgery. Int J Color Dis. 2009;24(5):569–76.
13. Wu Z, van de Haar RC, Sparreboom CL, Boersema GS, Li Z, Ji J, et al. Is the intraoperative air leak test effective in the prevention of colorectal anastomotic leakage? A systematic review and meta-analysis. Int J Color Dis. 2016;31(8):1409–17.
14. Yang SY, Han J, Han YD, Cho MS, Hur H, Lee KY, et al. Intraoperative colonoscopy for the assessment and prevention of anastomotic leakage in low anterior resection for rectal cancer. Int J Color Dis. 2017;32(5):709–14.
15. Neutzling CB, Lustosa SA, Proenca IM, da Silva EM, Matos D. Stapled versus handsewn methods for colorectal anastomosis surgery. Cochrane Database Syst Rev. 2012;(2):CD003144.
16. Blanco-Colino R, Espin-Basany E. Intraoperative use of ICG fluorescence imaging to reduce the risk of anastomotic leakage in colorectal surgery: a systematic review and meta-analysis. Tech Coloproctol. 2018;22(1):15–23.
17. Kudszus S, Roesel C, Schachtrupp A, Hoer JJ. Intraoperative laser fluorescence angiography in colorectal surgery: a noninvasive analysis to reduce the rate of anastomotic leakage. Langenbeck's Arch Surg. 2010;395(8):1025–30.
18. Ris F, Hompes R, Cunningham C, et al. Near-infrared (NIR) perfusion angiography in minimally invasive colorectal surgery. Surg Endosc. 2014;28:2221–6.
19. Boni L, Fingerhut A, Marzorati A, Rausei S, Dionigi G, Cassinotti E. Indocyanine green fluorescence angiography during laparoscopic low anterior resection: results of a case-matched study. Surg Endosc. 2017;31:1836–40.
20. Protyniak B, Dinallo AM, Boyan WP Jr, Dressner RM, Arvanitis ML. Intraoperative indocyanine green fluorescence angiography: an objective evaluation of anastomotic perfusion in colorectal surgery. Am Surg. 2015;81:580–4.
21. Foppa C, et al. Indocyanine green fluorescent dye during bowel surgery: are the blood supply "guessing days" over? Tech Coloproctol. 2014;18(8):753–8.
22. Kawada K, et al. Evaluation of intestinal perfusion by ICG fluorescence imaging in laparoscopic colorectal surgery with DST anastomosis. Surg Endoscopy. 2017;31(3):1061–9.
23. Kim JC, Lee JL, Yoon YS, Alotaibi AM, Kim J. Utility of indocyanine-green fluorescent imaging during robot-assisted sphincter-saving surgery on rectal cancer patients. Int J Med Robotics Comput Assist Surg. 2016;12:710–7.
24. Kin C, Vo H, Welton L, Welton M. Equivocal effect of intraoperative fluorescence angiography on colorectal anastomotic leaks. Dis Colon Rectum. 2015;58(6):582–7. https://doi.org/10.1097/DCR.0000000000000320.
25. Hellan M, Spinoglio G, Pigazzi A, Lagares-Garcia JA. The influence of fluorescence imaging on the location of bowel transection during robotic left-sided colorectal surgery. Surg Endosc. 2014;28(5):1695–702. https://doi.org/10.1007/s00464-013-3377-6.
26. Boni L, David G, Dionigi G, Rausei S, Cassinotti E, Fingerhut A. Indocyanine green-enhanced fluorescence to assess bowel perfusion during laparoscopic colorectal resection. Surg Endosc. 2016;30(7):2736–42. https://doi.org/10.1007/s00464-015-4540-z.

Intraoperative Air Leak, Colonic Ischemia, or Tension: How to Salvage the Failed Anastomosis

30

Virginia Oliva Shaffer and Elisabeth C. McLemore

Introduction and Rationale

Dietz and Debus note that in the recorded period prior to 1882, there were 100 different suture techniques for treatment of gut wounds [1]. Between 1844 and 1908, there were approximately 60 different suture techniques described by Senn in his classic review [2]. The importance of serosa apposition was introduced by Lembert in 1826, and additional advances in asepsis by Lord Joseph Lister further advanced the field of surgery [1]. In 1887, Halsted using animal studies laid the foundation for the importance of the submucosa in an anastomosis [3]. It was not until the late nineteenth century that the principles of intestinal anastomoses became standardized.

Risk Factors for Anastomotic Leaks

Although intestinal resection and anastomoses have been standardized, anastomotic leaks (AL) continue to plague gastrointestinal surgeons. Rates of anastomotic leak range from 3% to 30% depending on the patient population and the criteria used to define anastomotic leak [4–7]. A myriad of factors both technical and patient-specific have been implicated as contributing to AL. Among many others, risk factors include excessive tension on the anastomosis, poor tissue

V. O. Shaffer (✉)
Emory University School of Medicine, Department of Surgery, Emory University Hospital, Atlanta, GA, USA
e-mail: Virginia.o.shaffer@emory.edu

E. C. McLemore
Kaiser Permanente Los Angeles Medical Center, Department of Surgery, Los Angeles, CA, USA
e-mail: Elisabeth.c.mclemore@kp.org

P. Sylla et al. (eds.), *The SAGES Manual of Colorectal Surgery*,
https://doi.org/10.1007/978-3-030-24812-3_30

perfusion, smoking, immunosuppressive medications, and radiation. Obesity and male gender have also been associated with increased risk of AL [8]. Additional factors such as gut microbiome are emerging as possible culprits in anastomotic leakage [9].

With respect to anastomotic technique, anastomoses are created in two main ways – handsewn or stapled. The first mechanical stapling devices were described in 1908 by Professor Humer Hultl and delivered two double rows of fine wire steel staples. The USSR began experimenting and developing stapling devices in the 1940s and by 1952 had a series of instruments meant for vascular surgery. In the USA, gastrointestinal staplers appeared in 1967.

With the advent of laparoscopy, the adoption of staplers grew [10]. With the increased popularity of gastrointestinal staplers, a controversy has emerged as to whether a stapled or a handsewn anastomosis has a greater risk of leaking. A recent Cochrane review found insufficient evidence that a stapled anastomosis was superior to handsewn, but there are no randomized clinical trials in the last decade comparing the two techniques [11]. However, a Cochrane review specifically examining ileocolonic anastomoses in Crohn's disease found stapled functional end-to-end ileocolic anastomoses to be associated with fewer leaks than handsewn anastomoses [12]. A recent large cohort study of 1414 patients undergoing right colectomy for cancer demonstrated a twofold increased risk of anastomotic leak in the stapled relative to handsewn anastomotic group [13]. Based on conflicting data, it is difficult to make a definitive conclusion about the superiority of one technique over another with respect to risk of anastomotic leakage.

Definitions of Anastomotic Leaks

The American College of Surgeons National Surgical Quality Improvement Project (NSQIP) defines AL as "a leak of endoluminal contents though an anastomosis… The presence of infection/abscess thought to be related to an anastomosis even if the leak cannot be definitively identified as visualization in an operation or contrast extravasation…still considered a leak if indicated by the surgeon" [14]. There are over 20 definitions of AL in the literature which makes comparison of leak rates across studies very difficult (Table 30.1) [15]. Minor disruptions are usually <1 cm or <1/3 the circumference of the lumen. Anything larger is categorized as a major disruption [16]. In general, leaks that occur within 7 days after surgery are considered "early," and those occurring after 7 days are considered "late." The different timing of these leaks affects their treatment. Operative intervention is generally preferred for early leaks, whether it be with resection of anastomosis or with a proximal diverting stoma. Patients with late-onset leaks may have already been discharged from the hospital and require readmission for symptoms of abdominal pain, fevers, ileus, or failure to thrive. A CT scan in these situations is typically helpful in making the diagnosis. Several large series report a majority of late leaks

Table 30.1 Different definitions of anastomotic leak based on diagnostic test and timing of leak

References	Operation	Study design	Sample size	No. of leaks	Definition	Test	Timing
Ambrosetti et al. [71]	CR	Cohort	199	5 (3)	No	WS contrast	Routinely on day 9–11
Biondo et al. [72]	CR	Cohort	63	3 (5)	No	Unspecified contrast	When suspected
Bokey et al. [73]	C/CR	Cohort	1846	79 (4)	Yes	WS contrast, abdominal reoperation	When suspected
Bouillot et al. [74]	C	Cohort	50	1 (2)	No	Unspecified radiography	Unclear
Burke et al. [75]	CR	RCT	186	7 (4)	Yes	WS contrast	Routinely on day 7 in first half of study, then changed to when leak suspected
Cornwell et al. [76]	C	Cohort	56	3 (5)	Yes	Surgical re-exploration, CT, or WS contrast	Variable
De Wever et al. [77]	CR	Cohort	16	5 (31)	No	Endoscopy and unspecified radiological test	3–4 months
Debus et al. [78]	CR	Cohort	77	6 (8)	No	Barium contrast	When suspected
Deen and Smart [79]	C	Cohort	53	2 (4)	Yes	Unspecified radiography	When suspected
Dehni et al. [80]	CR	Cohort	258	31 (12)	Yes	WS contrast, imaging, or reoperation	Routine contrast study 8–10 weeks before stoma
Docherty et al. [81]	CR	RCT	652	38 (6)	Yes	WS contrast, reoperation	Routine on day 4–14
Fingerhut et al. [82]	CR	RCT	159	10 (6)	Yes	WS contrast, sinography	Routine contrast study on day 7
Fingerhut et al. [83]	CR	RCT	113	17 (15)	Yes	WS contrast, sinography, reoperation	Routine contrast study on day 7
Hallbook et al. [84]	CR	RCT	97	9 (9)	Yes	Digital and endoscopic examination, contrast, reoperation, CT closure	Routine contrast study before stoma closure

(continued)

Table 30.1 (continued)

References	Operation	Study design	Sample size	No. of leaks	Definition	Test	Timing
Hansen et al. [85]	CR	Cohort	615	9 (1)	Yes	Unspecified radiography	When suspected
Hida et al. [86]	CR	RCT	43	2 (5)	No	WS contrast	Routinely at 2 months
Iversen et al. [87]	CR	Cohort	161	17 (11)	No	WS contrast	When suspected
Junger et al. [88]					Yes	LPS concentration	LPS level assessed daily
Karanjia et al. [89]	CR	Cohort	219	38 (17)	Yes	WS contrast	When suspected
Kessler et al. [90]	CR	MRCT	621	88 (14)	Yes	Unspecified radiological tests, methylene blue test	When suspected
Kockerling et al. [91]	CR	MRCT	949	46 (5)	No	Unspecified	Unspecified
Kracht et al. [92]	C	MRCT	440	31 (7)	Yes	WS contrast, reoperation	Routine contrast on day 8–10
Mann et al. [93]	CR	Cohort	370	11 (3)	Yes	WS contrast	When suspected
Merad et al. [94]	CR	RCT	705	53 (8)	Yes	WS contrast, reoperation	Routine contrast on day 8
Merad et al. [95]	CR	RCT	494	32 (6)	Yes	WS contrast, reoperation	Routine contrast on day 7
Miller et al. [96, 97]	CR	Cohort	103	6 (6)	Yes	WS contrast	Routine contrast on day 10
Moore et al. [98]	CR	Cohort	300	34 (11)	No	Unspecified radiological examination, reoperation (clinically significant)	Routine before stoma closure
Norris et al. [99]	L	Cohort	156	6 (4)	No	Unspecified imaging or reoperation	When suspected
Pakkastie et al. [100]	CR	RCT	38	15 (39)	Yes	WS contrast	Routine contrast on day 7–10
Petersen et al. [101]	CR	Cohort	467	41 (9)	Yes	WS contrast	When suspected
Redmond et al. [102]	CR	Cohort	111	13 (12)	Yes	WS contrast	Routine contrast on day 10–12
Sagar et al. [103]	CR	RCT	100	12 (12)	Yes	WS contrast	Routine contrast on day 5–7

Table 30.1 (continued)

References	Operation	Study design	Sample size	No. of leaks	Definition	Test	Timing
Santos et al. [104]	CR	RCT	149	11 (7)	Yes	Unspecified radiological examination	When suspected
Slim et al. [105]	Lap. CR	Cohort	65	6 (9)	Yes	WS contrast, reoperation for peritonitis	When suspected
Stewart et al. [106]	CR	RCT	88	1 (1)	Yes	Unspecified	Unspecified
Tagart [107]	CR	Cohort	220	79 (36)	No	Limited barium contrast	Routine contrast on day 14
Thompson et al. [108]	CR	Cohort	535	18 (3)	No	None	Unspecified (not done routinely)
Watson et al. [109]	C/CR	Cohort	477	9 (2)	No	WS contrast	When suspected
Wheeler and Gilbert [110]	CR	Cohort	102	7 (7)	No	WS contrast	Routine contrast on day 8

Used with permission of John Wiley and Sons from Bruce et al. [15]
Values in parentheses are percentages
C colonic resection, *CR* colorectal surgery, *CT* computed tomography, *L* laparotomy (for Crohn's disease), *Lap* laparoscopic, *LPS* lipopolysaccharide, *MRCT* multi-randomized clinical trial, *RCT* randomized clinical trial, *WS* water soluble

being able to be managed nonoperatively with antibiotics with or without radiologic drainage [17, 18]. The treatment ultimately hinges on the clinical picture and stability of the patient.

Studies have also noted that there may be differences between early and late AL [19] and that risk factors may be different [7]. A recent large cohort study found that early leaks were associated with male gender, rectal cancer, higher BMI, laparoscopic surgery, emergency surgery, and lack of proximal fecal diversion. Late-onset leaks were associated with male gender, ASA class greater than 3, Charlson Comorbidity Index greater than 2, advanced tumor stage, and extensive additional resection required [7].

Impact of Anastomotic Leaks

Postoperative anastomotic leaks are associated with significant morbidity, longer lengths of hospital stay, and overall worse oncological outcomes [20–23]. Up to 68% of patients live with a permanent stoma following anastomotic leakage [24, 25]. A NSQIP study of over 13,000 patients undergoing colectomy and anastomosis found that AL was associated with an increased 30-day mortality rate [6.8% vs 1.6% p <0.001] and longer lengths of hospital stay (13 vs 5 days) and was 37 times more likely to require reoperation [20]. A review of 13 studies with a total of 12,202 patients in rectal cancer found that patients with anastomotic leak had twice the odds of local recurrence. A review of seven studies on outcomes of patients undergoing resection for rectal cancer found no significant impact of AL on distant recurrence rates but did find an increased risk of cancer-specific mortality [21].

AL also has detrimental effects on bowel function and quality of life (QOL) in patient undergoing low rectal anastomoses for cancer. One year postoperatively, patients who suffered from AL had worse physical and mental SF-36 scores, more frequent daytime and nighttime bowel movements, and worse control of solid stool as compared to patients without AL [26]. A study examining the effect of pelvis sepsis on function following ileal pouch-anal anastomosis (IPAA) found that patients with pelvic sepsis had worse function and QOL [27]. A different study in over 800 patients who underwent restorative proctocolectomy found that AL did not adversely affect long-term outcomes or QOL but did increase the risk of pouch loss and ileostomy creation [28]. In addition to overall worse clinical outcomes, AL is quite costly. A study evaluating gastrointestinal leak in the NSQIP database found a mean cost of $16,085.39 vs $56,349.12 in non-leak vs leak patients [29]. Anastomotic leak has also been found to be the complication with the largest impact on 30-day end-organ dysfunction and the third largest impact on mortality after elective colorectal surgery. It also contributed the most to reoperation and readmission [30].

Principles and Quality Benchmarks

Intraoperative Testing of Colorectal Anastomoses

Intraoperative air testing of intestinal anastomosis was introduced to mitigate potential adverse outcomes [31]. Most commonly, after the anastomosis is complete, the pelvis is filled with sterile water or saline and the proximal bowel occluded. Air is insufflated through the anus through either a rigid, flexible, or bulb irrigator. When a rigid or flexible endoscope is used, the anastomosis can be directly visualized for integrity and hemostasis. If bubbles are noted, the anastomosis is not airtight. Some surgeons go a step further and perform an additional betadine-tinged saline infusion to look for extravasation [32]. Different methods for anastomotic leak testing are described in Table 30.2.

A study evaluating the selective or routine use of intraoperative endoscopy in elective laparoscopic surgery showed a trend toward more overall anastomotic complications in the selective group vs routine use group [33]. Proponents of intraoperative leak testing estimate this may identify leaks in as many as 25% of anastomoses [31, 34]. Some studies indicate a lower rate of clinically diagnosed anastomotic leaks in the air leak-tested patients when compared to controls, and several studies have shown value and efficacy with this practice [31, 35–38]. A recent study of 777 laparoscopic left-sided colon resections with primary anastomosis and no proximal diversion demonstrated a lower anastomotic leak rate in intraoperatively air leak-tested anastomoses [39]. Sasaki and colleagues reviewed 148 consecutive cases of

Table 30.2 Methods of intraoperative testing in recent studies

Authors	Year	Method of testing
Vignali et al. [111]	2000	Air insufflation into the rectum with anastomosis under saline irrigation
Schmidt et al. [112]	2003	Air insufflation into the rectum using endoscope with anastomosis under saline irrigation
Ishihara et al. [113]	2008	Air insufflation into the rectum with anastomosis under saline irrigation
Lanthaler et al. [114]	2008	Air insufflation into the rectum with anastomosis under saline irrigation
Ricciardi et al. [36]	2009	Air insufflation through a proctoscope or flexible endoscope with the anastomosis under irrigation of saline
Li et al. [33]	2009	Air insufflation into the rectum using endoscope with anastomosis under saline irrigation
Shamiyeh et al. [115]	2012	400 cc air insufflation into the rectum using a syringe with the anastomosis under saline irrigation
Ivanov et al. [116]	2011	Air insufflation into the rectum using a sigmoidoscope with the anastomosis under saline irrigation
Lieto et al. [117]	2011	Air insufflation into the rectum using endoscope with anastomosis under saline irrigation
Xiao et al. [118]	2011	Air insufflation into the rectum using a rectoscope with anastomosis under irrigation of saline
Kamal et al. [119]	2015	Air insufflation into the rectum using a sigmoidoscope with the anastomosis under saline irrigation

left-sided anastomoses and found 7 to yield a positive intraoperative leak test; they reconstructed the anastomosis and performed proximal diversion. They had no anastomotic leaks in this cohort [40].

Management of Positive Intraoperative Leak Test

If a positive air leak test is found, there are several options, including suture repair, reanastomosis, diversion, or a combination of techniques. Kamal and colleagues reviewed 415 consecutive cases of hand-assisted laparoscopic colorectal resection and had 15 patients with a positive leak test. Fourteen underwent takedown and reanastomosis with no proximal diversion with no subsequent clinical leak. Based on this, they recommend formal takedown and reconstruction of the anastomosis [38]. Davies and colleagues studied 33 patients with postoperative gastrografin (water soluble) contrast enemas. In their cohort, six patients had positive air leaks which were suture repaired only. Two of the six had radiographic leaks on postoperative day 8 (POD8), and one of the two also developed a clinical leak [41]. A recent study looked at patients that had a positive air leak test and divided patients into those receiving a suture repair alone vs suture repair with diversion or reconstruction of the anastomosis. This study of non-inferiority found 9% clinically significant leak rate in the suture repair alone group vs 0% in the diverted or reanastomosis group. The study was not able to conclude that suture repair alone was non-inferior to diversion or reanastomosis after an intraoperative positive leak

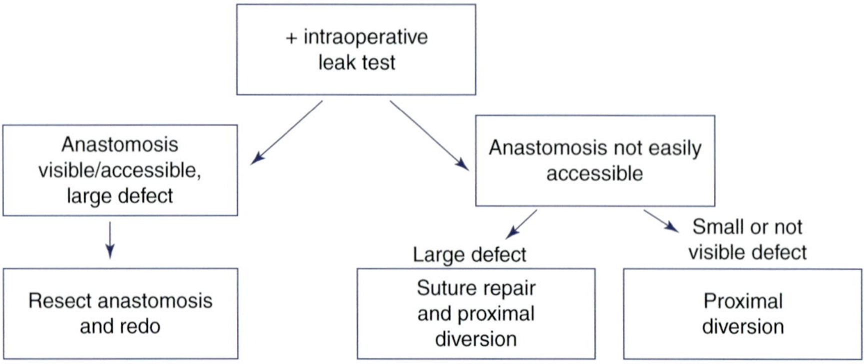

Fig. 30.1 Proposed algorithm for positive intraoperative leak test

test [25]. There is literature describing the management of postoperative leak by proximal diversion alone without repair of anastomosis as safe and non-inferior to resection [42–44]. Extrapolating these data, one might conclude that if because of location of air leak, one is unable to suture repair it or reconstruct it, it may be safe to proximally divert with a loop ileostomy (Fig. 30.1). Proximal diversion, however, does not eliminate the need for additional surgery, hospitalization, and the risk of complications. Leahy and colleagues [19] studied the rate of anastomotic leak even after diversion and found that 34 of 245 patients experienced anastomotic leak with 8 of those occurring after stoma closure. In this study, there was no difference in the proportion of positive leaks intraoperatively in patients with and without subsequent clinical leak.

Strategies to Reduce Mechanical Contributions to Leaks

Splenic Flexure Release

Factors that influence a successful outcome after colorectal anastomosis include a tension-free anastomosis, intact macro- and microcirculation of the retained colon and rectum, as well as appropriate perioperative abdominal and pelvic sepsis and wound prophylaxis [45]. In the setting of any bowel anastomosis, achieving a tension-free anastomosis is of utmost importance. Patient body habitus and anatomic variants in colonic redundancy and vascular anatomy contribute to the broad range in the variable length that can be achieved after splenic flexure mobilization and inferior mesenteric vein ligation. In both the cadaveric and in vivo laparoscopic setting, the longest length achieved is when splenic flexure mobilization is combined with high ligation of the inferior mesenteric vein [46, 47].

In a recent systematic review and meta-analysis on the safety and use of splenic mobilization, splenic flexure mobilization was associated with longer operative time, especially when performing TME for rectal cancer [48]. In addition, splenic flexure mobilization was found to be associated with a higher leak rate in the studies with both benign and malignant indications, as well as the subgroup which included only rectal cancer resections [48]. Rather than a cause and effect, splenic flexure mobilization is a surrogate marker for low colorectal or coloanal anastomosis. Splenic flexure mobilization to the level of the midbody of the pancreas combined with high ligation of the inferior mesenteric vein (IMV) is typically required to facilitate colonic conduit mobilization and reach into the pelvis to create an anastomosis within 4–5 cm from the anal verge. Please refer to Chap. 4 on laparoscopic splenic flexure release for more technical details.

Colonic Conduit Ischemia

Intraoperative colonic ischemia in the retained descending colon (colonic conduit) planed for use and restoration of bowel continuity with low pelvic colorectal or coloanal anastomosis can occur for a variety of reasons during open or minimally invasive colorectal surgery (Fig. 30.2a, b). Venous congestion can result in colonic conduit ischemia if the IMV is ligated inadvertently during high ligation of the inferior mesenteric artery (IMA). Disruption of collateral arterial blood flow to the retained descending colon conduit during mesocolic transection up to the level of

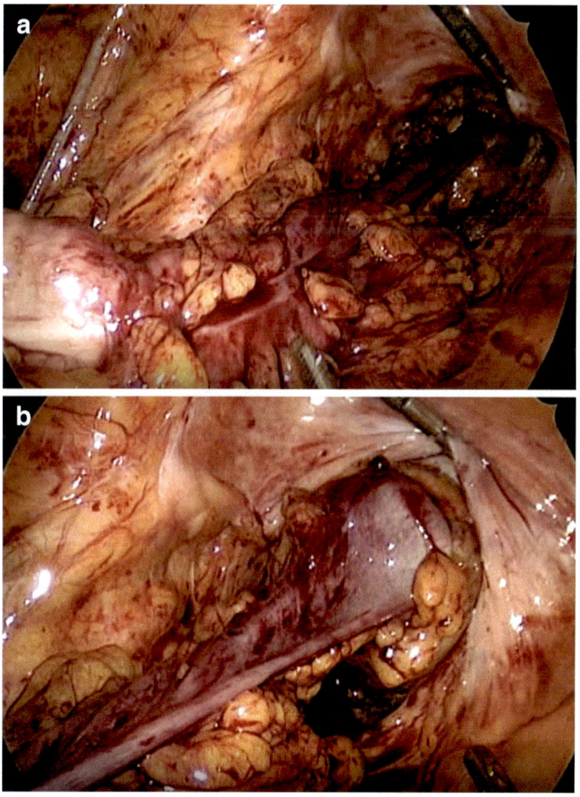

Fig. 30.2 (**a**, **b**) Left colonic conduit ischemia recognized following stapled colorectal anastomosis during laparoscopic low anterior resection. The discoloration of the left colon does not improve following multiple maneuvers to reduce tension on the anastomosis. (Both: Courtesy of Patricia Sylla, MD)

the colon can occur secondary to tension on the retained left colic, arc of Riolan, or marginal artery of Drummond resulting in spasm and/or arterial thrombosis. Colonic ischemia can also occur in patients with altered mesocolic vascular anatomy due to embryologic developmental variations and/or prior rectosigmoid surgery. (See Fig. 4.3 in Chap. 4 in this volume.) There is also potential for ischemia during specimen extraction completed either abdominally or transanally.

During mesocolic dissection and high ligation of the IMA for left-sided colon or rectal cancer, two technical errors can be made. The first is inadvertent ligation of the inferior mesenteric vein during high ligation of the IMA, and the second is disruption of collateral arterial blood flow during the mesenteric dissection. The IMV drains into the splenic vein, and high ligation of the inferior mesenteric vein is typically performed in cases in which low pelvic colorectal or coloanal anastomosis is required. A high ligation of the IMV is typically performed just to the left of the fourth portion of the duodenum at the level of the ligament of Treitz or duodenojejunal flexure (Fig. 30.3). However, the IMV can travel in close approximation to the IMA, and inadvertent ligation of the IMV during high ligation of the IMA can result in colonic ischemia due to venous congestion. Patients with central obesity and/or increased mesocolic adiposity are at risk for inadvertent ligation of the IMV during high ligation of the IMA as the IMV may be obscured or difficult to identify due to increased mesocolic adiposity.

In cases in which a high ligation of the IMV is planned for reconstructive purposes, it may be prudent to perform a high ligation of the IMV as the first step during the mesocolic dissection for distal sigmoid or rectal cancer. The IMV is typically less challenging to identify at the level of the ligament of Treitz, even in patients with increased mesocolic adiposity. After high ligation of the IMV, the mesocolic dissection caudal to the IMA can proceed in a bloodless plane.

This inframesocolic approach for splenic flexure takedown can be utilized even in cases in which a high ligation of the IMV is not required as a colonic conduit lengthening maneuver. Please refer to Chap. 4 on laparoscopic splenic flexure release for more

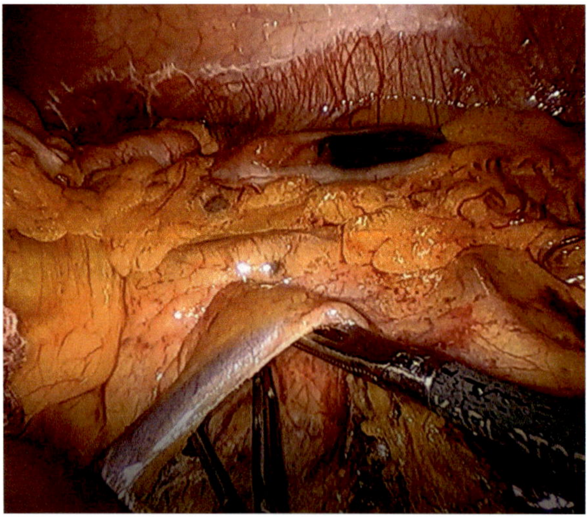

Fig. 30.3 Dissection of the inferior mesenteric vein during laparoscopic left colectomy. The tumor is located in the mid-left colon and was tattooed preoperatively. (Courtesy of Patricia Sylla, MD)

details regarding this approach. The IMV can be identified at the level of the ligament of Treitz but not divided. Inframesocolic dissection can be carried down to the level of the IMA and then high ligation of the IMA performed after identification and separation from the IMV. Anatomic variations in blood supply should be kept under consideration during the mesocolic dissection in order to avoid inadvertent devascularization of the colon conduit. The blood supply to the splenic flexure can be distributed through the superior mesenteric artery (SMA), the IMA, or both. The feeder vessels originating from these arteries can be the left colic artery, left branch of the middle colic, an accessory middle colic artery, a combination of these arteries, or no direct feeder vessel [49]. Collateral arterial blood flow disruption after high ligation of the IMA during mesocolic dissection up to the level of the colon can be a cause of colonic ischemia. Disruption of collateral arterial blood flow to the retained descending colon conduit during mesocolic transection up to the level of the colon can occur secondary to tension on the retained left colic, arc of Riolan, or marginal artery of Drummond resulting in spasm and/or arterial thrombosis. (See Fig. 4.3 in Chap. 4 in this volume.)

There are several techniques that the surgeon can adopt to avoid arterial tension and thrombosis during sigmoid and rectal resection. The first is to identify the collateral arterial flow and avoid transecting the mesentery too proximally. Direct visualization of a proximal feeding vessel supplying the conduit may be possible. More recently, fluorescence angiography has been used to help in assessing intestinal perfusion. Intravenous injection of indocyanine green (ICG) dye followed by the use of near-infrared light to assess bowel perfusion is safe and may decrease the risk anastomotic leaks by aiding the surgeons better identify ischemic segments (Figs. 30.4a, b and 30.5a, b) [50–52]. The second technique is to avoid tension on the mesentery

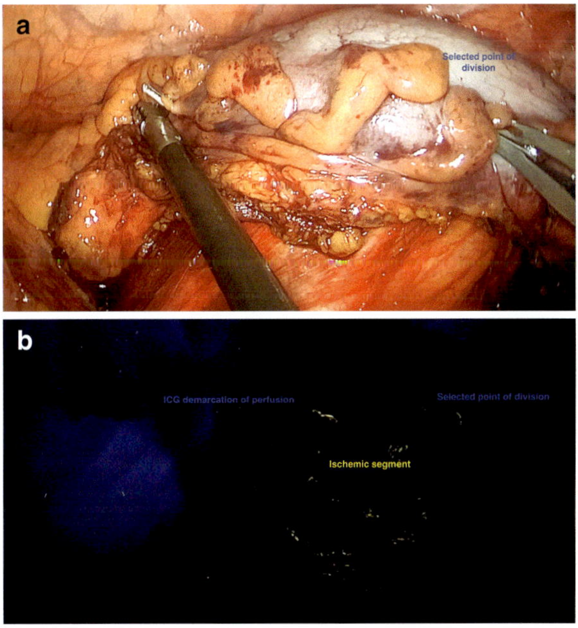

Fig. 30.4 (**a**, **b**) Perfusion assessment of the bowel during low anterior resection using ICG fluorescence angiography. (**a**) Demarcation of the bowel is assessed laparoscopically with white light. (**b**) Following ICG intravenous injection, perfusion reassessment using near-infrared light confirms the level of vascular demarcation. (Both: Courtesy of Antonio Caceydo, MD)

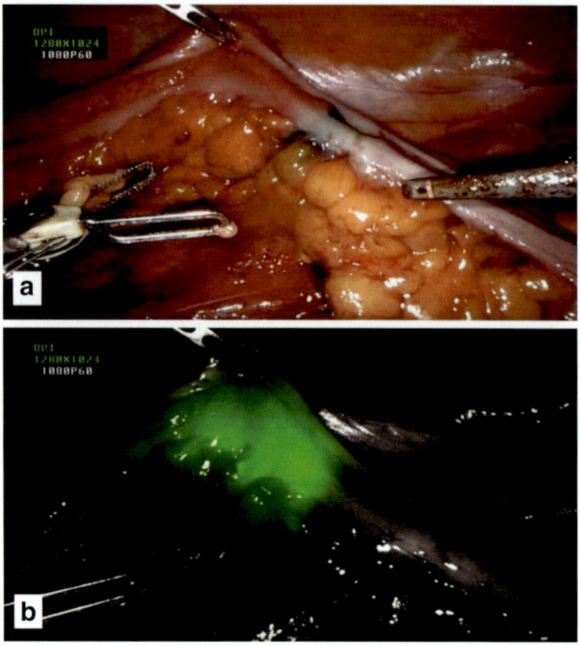

Fig. 30.5 (**a**, **b**) Perfusion assessment during robotic LAR using ICG fluorescence angiography. (**a**) Vascular demarcation is assessed with white light. (**b**) Following ICG intravenous injection, perfusion is reassessed using near-infrared light and confirms the point of vascular demarcation. (Both: Courtesy of Daniel Popowich, MD)

during mesocolic transection, either by performing the transection intracorporeally or further mobilizing the colon and its mesentery in order to reduce the tension on the vascular pedicles during extracorporeal extraction. When the mesentery performed extracorporeally, undue tension may result in spasm and tearing of the left colic, arc of Riolan, or marginal artery of Drummond leading to arterial colonic ischemia.

Special consideration should be made in cases in which transanal extraction of the specimen and conduit is planned. Even if the mesocolic transection is performed intracorporeally prior to transanal specimen extraction, the weight of the specimen can inadvertently pull on the proximal mesocolon and lead to spasm and/or arterial trauma resulting in arterial colonic ischemia. Care should be taken to maintain hold of the specimen after transanal extraction and not allow the weight of the specimen to pull on the retained colonic conduit prior to distal bowel transection. The specimen should be held at all times and not allowed to lay unsupported through the extraction site.

Options for Anastomotic Reconstruction

In the event of colonic conduit ischemia, the first step is to discuss this finding with your anesthesiology team. Vasopressors should be discontinued if the patient's hemodynamic status can be maintained with alternative agents, and normothermia should be achieved. Intravenous fluid warming devices as well as warm intraabdominal irrigation can facilitate increasing the patient's body temperature if the patient is hypothermic. In addition, temporary cessation of pneumoperitoneum and taking the patient out of steep Trendelenburg or reverse Trendelenburg position can be performed to improve mean systemic filling pressure, venous return, and microcirculation associated with pneumoperitoneum [53]. Releasing any tension on the mesentery is another important maneuver. If the tension was placed during transanal extraction, the conduit should be returned intraabdominally to see if this improves blood flow. Additionally, the mesentery should be assessed for avulsion of any blood vessels that may be contributing to the ischemia.

If colonic ischemia persists despite all the above maneuvers, alternative reconstructive options vs conversion to permanent colostomy need to be considered depending on the extent of the colonic ischemia. If this possibility was not discussed with the patient prior to surgery, the surgeon is encouraged to discuss the findings with the patient's family or emergency contact and obtain emergent informed consent for either conversion to permanent colostomy or attempt to alternative reconstructive options. In addition, the surgeon is encouraged to consult a surgical colleague to assist with decision-making for the remainder of the case. Alternative low pelvic reconstructive options utilize the right colon for low pelvic reconstruction and anastomotic options. In some cases, the transverse colon can be salvaged as well [54]. While laparoscopic approaches have been described for alternative low pelvic reconstruction [55–57], an open approach may be in the patient's best interest to facilitate reducing operative time and potentially preserving a longer segment of the colon if feasible. The anatomy becomes significantly altered and is typically easier to visualize rather than described (Fig. 30.6 AB).

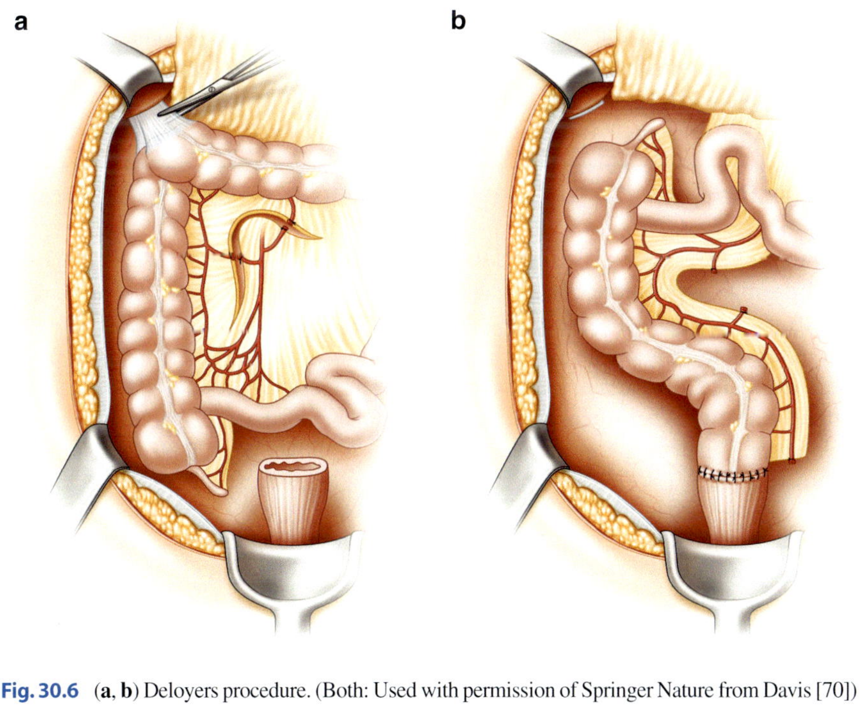

Fig. 30.6 (**a**, **b**) Deloyers procedure. (Both: Used with permission of Springer Nature from Davis [70])

Deloyers procedure was first described in 1964 and utilizes a right colon to low pelvic rectal anastomosis as a salvage technique for low colorectal or coloanal anastomosis in the setting of ischemic left conduit. In the Deloyers procedure, the right and middle colic arteries are ligated, and the right colon is inverted, so a right colon to rectal anastomosis is created [58–60]. The left and transverse colon are frequently removed secondary to ischemia during this approach. The right colon can be used either in an isoperistaltic or antiperistaltic fashion, essentially whichever conduit has less tension and better reach into the pelvis. An appendectomy is performed as well to avoid future appendicitis and delay in diagnosis or inability to treat due to the altered anatomic location of the retained appendix. The terminal ileum is relocated to the hepatic flexure in cases in which an antiperistaltic right colorectal anastomosis is created. Another option similar to the Deloyers procedure is a cecum to rectal anastomosis [61, 62]. A modification of the Deloyers technique involves maintaining the orientation of the vascular pedicle but involves two anastomosis – an antiperistaltic colorectal anastomosis and an ileocolonic anastomosis [63]. Surgeons have also described a retroileal transverse colon to rectum anastomosis. A passage is created in an avascular plane in the transverse ileal mesentery to allow the proximal transverse colon through to anastomose to the rectum [64]. If none of these techniques are successful, an option for a subtotal colectomy with an ileorectal anastomosis is a possibility. In extreme cases, a delayed coloanal anastomosis, Turnbull-Cutait [65, 66], may be attempted. In this technique, the colon is exteriorized through the anus and transected. A segment of the colon is left exteriorized through the anus and affixed to the skin with sutures. A small venting hole is created in the exteriorized colon with plans to return to the OR several days later. At the second stage, the colon is transected at the level of the anal verge, and a handsewn coloanal anastomosis is performed [65, 66]. Surgeons have found this technique to be a valuable option in difficult situations [67–69].

Conclusion

There are many factors associated with creating a viable and intact anastomosis. Intraoperative anastomotic interrogation with endoscopic evaluation for air leak as well as mucosal perfusion is recommended for all low pelvic anastomosis. Colonic ischemia and tension on the anastomosis are technical factors that can contribute to anastomotic leak. Ischemia, tension, and anastomotic integrity should be evaluated intraoperatively. When identified, the anastomosis can be salvaged with various techniques including proximal colonic mobilization and anastomotic reconstruction.

References

1. Dietz UA, Debus ES. Intestinal anastomoses prior to 1882; a legacy of ingenuity, persistence, and research form a foundation for modern gastrointestinal surgery. World J Surg. 2005;29(3):396–401.

2. Classic articles in colonic and rectal surgery. Nicholas Senn 1844–1908. Enterorrhaphy; its history, technique and present status. Dis Colon Rectum. 1985;28(1):59–68.
3. Classic articles in colonic and rectal surgery. William Stewart Halsted 1852–1922. Circular suture of the intestine–an experimental study. Dis Colon Rectum. 1984;27(12):838–41.
4. Snijders HS, Wouters MW, van Leersum NJ, Kolfschoten NE, Henneman D, de Vries AC, et al. Meta-analysis of the risk for anastomotic leakage, the postoperative mortality caused by leakage in relation to the overall postoperative mortality. Eur J Surg Oncol. 2012;38(11):1013–9.
5. Peel AL, Taylor EW. Proposed definitions for the audit of postoperative infection: a discussion paper. Surgical infection study group. Ann R Coll Surg Engl. 1991;73(6):385–8.
6. Chambers WM, Mortensen NJ. Postoperative leakage and abscess formation after colorectal surgery. Best Pract Res Clin Gastroenterol. 2004;18(5):865–80.
7. Sparreboom CL, van Groningen JT, Lingsma HF, Wouters MWJM, Menon AG, Kleinrensink GJ, et al. Different risk factors for early and late colorectal anastomotic leakage in a Nationwide audit. Dis Colon Rectum. 2018;61(11):1258–66.
8. Pellino G, Frasson M, García-Granero A, Granero-Castro P, Ramos Rodríguez JL, Flor-Lorente B, et al. Predictors of complications and mortality following left colectomy with primary stapled anastomosis for cancer: results of a multicentric study with 1111 patients. Color Dis. 2018;20(11):986–95.
9. Gaines S, Shao C, Hyman N, Alverdy JC. Gut microbiome influences on anastomotic leak and recurrence rates following colorectal cancer surgery. Br J Surg. 2018;105(2):e131–41.
10. Schiappa J, Van Hee R. From ants to staples: history and ideas concerning suturing techniques. Acta Chir Belg. 2012;112(5):395–402.
11. Neutzling CB, Lustosa SA, Proenca IM, da Silva EM, Matos D. Stapled versus handsewn methods for colorectal anastomosis surgery. Cochrane Database Syst Rev. 2012;(2):CD003144.
12. Choy PY, Bissett IP, Docherty JG, Parry BR, Merrie AE. Stapled versus handsewn methods for ileocolic anastomoses. Cochrane Database Syst Rev. 2011;(9):CD004320.
13. Nordholm-Carstensen A, Schnack Rasmussen M, Krarup PM. Increased leak rates following stapled versus Handsewn ileocolic anastomosis in patients with right-sided Colon Cancer: a Nationwide cohort study. Dis Colon Rectum. 2019;62(5):542–8.
14. Users guide for the 2017 ACS NSQIP Procedure Target Participant Use Data File. American College of Surgeons National Quality Improvement Project.
15. Bruce J, Krukowski ZH, Al-Khairy G, Russell EM, Park KG. Systematic review of the definition and measurement of anastomotic leak after gastrointestinal surgery. Br J Surg. 2001;88(9):1157–68.
16. Falcone RE, Wanamaker SR, Santanello SA, Carey LC. Colorectal trauma: primary repair or anastomosis with intracolonic bypass vs. ostomy. Dis Colon Rectum. 1992;35(10):957–63.
17. Hyman N, Manchester TL, Osler T, Burns B, Cataldo PA. Anastomotic leaks after intestinal anastomosis: it's later than you think. Ann Surg. 2007;245(2):254–8.
18. Blumetti J, Chaudhry V, Cintron JR, Park JJ, Marecik S, Harrison JL, Prasad LM, et al. Management of anastomotic leak: lessons learned from a large colon and rectal surgery training program. World J Surg. 2014;38(4):985–91.
19. Leahy J, Schoetz D, Marcello P, Read T, Hall J, Roberts P, et al. What is the risk of clinical anastomotic leak in the diverted colorectal anastomosis? J Gastrointest Surg. 2014;18(10):1812–6.
20. Midura EF, Hanseman D, Davis BR, Atkinson SJ, Abbott DE, Shah SA, et al. Risk factors and consequences of anastomotic leak after colectomy: a national analysis. Dis Colon Rectum. 2015;58(3):333–8.
21. Mirnezami A, Mirnezami R, Chandrakumaran K, Sasapu K, Sagar P, Finan P. Increased local recurrence and reduced survival from colorectal cancer following anastomotic leak: systematic review and meta-analysis. Ann Surg. 2011;253(5):890–9.
22. Lu ZR, Rajendran N, Lynch AC, Heriot AG, Warrier SK. Anastomotic leaks after restorative resections for rectal cancer compromise cancer outcomes and survival. Dis Colon Rectum. 2016;59(3):236–44.

23. Hammond J, Lim S, Wan Y, Gao X, Patkar A. The burden of gastrointestinal anastomotic leaks: an evaluation of clinical and economic outcomes. J Gastrointest Surg. 2014;18(6):1176–85.
24. Francone TD, Saleem A, Read TA, Roberts PL, Marcello PW, Schoetz DJ, et al. Ultimate fate of the leaking intestinal anastomosis: does leak mean permanent stoma? J Gastrointest Surg. 2010;14(6):987–92.
25. Mitchem JB, Stafford C, Francone TD, Roberts PL, Schoetz DJ, Marcello PW, et al. What is the optimal management of an intra-operative air leak in a colorectal anastomosis? Color Dis. 2018;20(2):O39–45.
26. Ashburn JH, Stocchi L, Kiran RP, Dietz DW, Remzi FH. Consequences of anastomotic leak after restorative proctectomy for cancer: effect on long-term function and quality of life. Dis Colon Rectum. 2013;56(3):275–80.
27. Kiely JM, Fazio VW, Remzi FH, Shen B, Kiran RP. Pelvic sepsis after IPAA adversely affects function of the pouch and quality of life. Dis Colon Rectum. 2012;55(4):387–92.
28. Chessin DB, Gorfine SR, Bub DS, Royston A, Wong D, Bauer JJ. Septic complications after restorative proctocolectomy do not impair functional outcome: long-term follow-up from a specialty center. Dis Colon Rectum. 2008;51(9):1312–7.
29. Turrentine FE, Denlinger CE, Simpson VB, Garwood RA, Guerlain S, Agrawal A, et al. Morbidity, mortality, cost, and survival estimates of gastrointestinal anastomotic leaks. J Am Coll Surg. 2015;220(2):195–206.
30. Scarborough JE, Schumacher J, Kent KC, Heise CP, Greenberg CC. Associations of specific postoperative complications with outcomes after elective colon resection: a procedure-targeted approach toward surgical quality improvement. JAMA Surg. 2017;152(2):e164681.
31. Beard JD, Nicholson ML, Sayers RD, Lloyd D, Everson NW. Intraoperative air testing of colorectal anastomoses: a prospective, randomized trial. Br J Surg. 1990;77(10):1095–7.
32. Kingham TP, Pachter HL. Colonic anastomotic leak: risk factors, diagnosis, and treatment. J Am Coll Surg. 2009;208(2):269–78.
33. Li VK, Wexner SD, Pulido N, Wang H, Jin HY, Weiss EG, et al. Use of routine intraoperative endoscopy in elective laparoscopic colorectal surgery: can it further avoid anastomotic failure? Surg Endosc. 2009;23(11):2459–65.
34. Thomas MS, Margolin DA. Management of colorectal anastomotic leak. Clin Colon Rectal Surg. 2016;29(2):138–44.
35. Kwon S, Morris A, Billingham R, Frankhouse J, Horvath K, Johnson M, et al. Routine leak testing in colorectal surgery in the surgical care and outcomes assessment program. Arch Surg. 2012;147(4):345–51.
36. Ricciardi R, Roberts PL, Marcello PW, Hall JF, Read TE, Schoetz DJ. Anastomotic leak testing after colorectal resection: what are the data? Arch Surg. 2009;144(5):407–11; discussion 411–2
37. Khan AA, Wheeler JM, Cunningham C, George B, Kettlewell M, Mortensen NJ. The management and outcome of anastomotic leaks in colorectal surgery. Color Dis. 2008;10(6):587–92.
38. Kamal T, Pai A, Velchuru VR, Zawadzki M, Park JJ, Marecik SJ, et al. Should anastomotic assessment with flexible sigmoidoscopy be routine following laparoscopic restorative left colorectal resection? Color Dis. 2015;17(2):160–4.
39. Allaix ME, Lena A, Degiuli M, Arezzo A, Passera R, Mistrangelo M, et al. Intraoperative air leak test reduces the rate of postoperative anastomotic leak: analysis of 777 laparoscopic left-sided colon resections. Surg Endosc. 2019;33(5):1592–9.
40. Sasaki K, Ishihara S, Nozawa H, Kawai K, Hata K, Kiyomatsu T, et al. Successful management of a positive air leak test during laparoscopic colorectal surgery. Dig Surg. 2018;35(3):266–70.
41. Davies AH, Bartolo DC, Richards AE, Johnson CD, McC Mortensen NJ. Intra-operative air testing: an audit on rectal anastomosis. Ann R Coll Surg Engl. 1988;70(6):345–7.
42. Stafford C, Francone TD, Marcello PW, Roberts PL, Ricciardi R. Is diversion with ileostomy non-inferior to hartmann resection for left-sided colorectal anastomotic leak? J Gastrointest Surg. 2018;22(3):503–7.

43. Fraccalvieri D, Biondo S, Saez J, Millan M, Kreisler E, Golda T, et al. Management of colorectal anastomotic leakage: differences between salvage and anastomotic takedown. Am J Surg. 2012;204(5):671–6.
44. Krarup PM, Jorgensen LN, Harling H, Danish Colorectal Cancer Group. Management of anastomotic leakage in a nationwide cohort of colonic cancer patients. J Am Coll Surg. 2014;218(5):940–9.
45. Tagart RE. Colorectal anastomosis: factors influencing success. J R Soc Med. 1981;74(2):111–8.
46. Thum-umnuaysuk S, Boonyapibal A, Geng YY, Pattana-Arun J. Lengthening of the colon for low rectal anastomosis in a cadaveric study: how much can we gain? Tech Coloproctol. 2013;17(4):377–81.
47. Kye BH, Kim HJ, Kim HS, Kim JG, Cho HM. How much colonic redundancy could be obtained by splenic flexure mobilization in laparoscopic anterior or low anterior resection? Int J Med Sci. 2014;11(9):857–62.
48. Nowakowski M, Małczak P, Mizera M, Rubinkiewicz M, Lasek A, Wierdak M, et al. The safety of selective use of splenic flexure mobilization in sigmoid and rectal resections-systematic review and meta-analysis. J Clin Med. 2018;7(11):E392.
49. Fukuoka A, Sasaki T, Tsukikawa S, Miyajima N, Ostubo T. Evaluating distribution of the left branch of the middle colic artery and the left colic artery by CT angiography and colonography to classify blood supply to the splenic flexure. Asian J Endosc Surg. 2017;10(2):148–53.
50. Boni L, Fingerhut A, Marzorati A, Rausei S, Dionigi G, Cassinotti E. Indocyanine green fluorescence angiography during laparoscopic low anterior resection: results of a case-matched study. Surg Endosc. 2017;31(4):1836–40.
51. Boni L, David G, Dionigi G, Rausei S, Cassinotti E, Fingerhut A. Indocyanine green-enhanced fluorescence to assess bowel perfusion during laparoscopic colorectal resection. Surg Endosc. 2016;30(7):2736–42.
52. Bornstein JE, Munger JA, Deliz JR, Mui A, Chen CS, Kim S, et al. Assessment of bowel end perfusion after mesenteric division: eye versus SPY. J Surg Res. 2018;232:179–85.
53. He H, Gruartmoner G, Ince Y, van Berge Henegouwen MI, Gisbertz SS, Geerts BF, et al. Effect of pneumoperitoneum and steep reverse-Trendelenburg position on mean systemic filling pressure, venous return, and microcirculation during esophagectomy. J Thorac Dis. 2018;10(6):3399–408.
54. Grasso M, Cimmino A, Sangiuliano N, Niglio A. How to save both transverse colon and continence after extensive left colon surgery: a case report of a new procedure. Int J Surg Case Rep. 2018;47:64–6.
55. Otani K, Nozawa H, Kiyomatsu T, Kawai K, Hata K, Tanaka T, et al. Laparoscopic Deloyers procedure to facilitate primary anastomosis after extended resection for synchronous cancers of transverse colon and rectum: easy to preform with good functional outcome. Tech Coloproctol. 2017;21(12):975–6.
56. Sciuto A, Grifasi C, Pirozzi F, Leon P, Pirozzi RE, Corcione F. Laparoscopic Deloyers procedure for tension-free anastomosis after extended left colectomy: technique and results. Tech Coloproctol. 2016;20(12):865–9.
57. Antona AD, Reggio S, Pirozzi F, Corcione F. Laparoscopic 3D high-definition Deloyers procedure: when, how, why? Updat Surg. 2016;68(1):111–3.
58. Deloyers L. Suspension of the right colon permits without exception preservation of the anal sphincter after extensive colectomy of the transverse and left colon (including rectum). Technic –indications- immediate and late results. Lyon Chir. 1964;60:404–13.
59. Dumont F, Da Re C, Goéré D, Honoré C, Elias D. Options and outcome for reconstruction after extended left hemicolectomy. Color Dis. 2013;15(6):747–54.
60. Manceau G, Karoui M, Breton S, Blanchet AS, Rousseau G, Savier E, et al. Right colon to rectal anastomosis (Deloyers procedure) as a salvage technique for low colorectal or coloanal anastomosis: postoperative and long-term outcomes. Dis Colon Rectum. 2012;55(3):363–8.
61. Ryan JA Jr, Oakley WC. Cecoproctostomy. Am J Surg. 1985;149(5):636–9.

62. Sarli L, Costi R, Sarli D, Roncoroni L. Pilot study of subtotal colectomy with antiperistaltic cecoproctostomy for the treatment of chronic slow-transit constipation. Dis Colon Rectum. 2001;44(10):1514–20.
63. Jones DW, Dimitrova M, Nandakumar G. Colonic salvage with antiperistaltic cecorectal anastomosis. Dis Colon Rectum. 2015;58(2):270–4.
64. Mishra A, Gosselink MP, Mortensen NJ, George BD, Cunningham C, Lindsey I, et al. Problem solving after marginal artery injury during splenic flexure mobilization – a video vignette. Color Dis. 2015;17(2):174–5.
65. Turnbull RB Jr, Cuthbertson A. Abdominorectal pull-through resection for cancer and for Hirschsprung's disease. Delayed posterior colorectal anastomosis. Cleve Clin Q. 1961;28:109–15.
66. Cutait DE, Figliolini FJ. A new method of colorectal anastomosis in abdominoperineal resection. Dis Colon Rectum. 1961;4:335–42.
67. Hallet J, Bouchard A, Drolet S, Milot H, Desrosiers E, Lebrun A, et al. Anastomotic salvage after rectal cancer resection using the Turnbull-Cutait delayed anastomosis. Can J Surg. 2014;57(6):405–11.
68. Hallet J, Milot H, Drolet S, Desrosiers E, Gregoire RC, Bouchard A. The clinical results of the Turnbull-Cutait delayed coloanal anastomosis: a systematic review. Tech Coloproctol. 2014;18(6):579–90.
69. Remzi FH, El Gazzaz G, Kiran RP, Kirat HT, Fazio VW. Outcomes following Turnbull-Cutait abdominoperineal pull-through compared with coloanal anastomosis. Br J Surg. 2009;96(4):424–9.
70. Davis BR. Overcoming technical challenges: prevention and managing complications. In: Ross H, Lee S, Mutch M, Rivadeneira D, Steele S, editors. Minimally invasive approaches to colon and rectal disease. New York: Springer International Publishing; 2015.
71. Ambrosetti P, Robert J, Mathey P, Rohner A. Left-sided colon and colorectal anastomoses: doppler ultrasound as an aid to assess bowel vascularization. A prospective evaluation of 200 consecutive elective cases. Int J Colorectal Dis. 1994;9:211–4.
72. Biondo S, Jaurrieta E, Jorba R, Moreno P, Farran L, Borobia F, et al. Intraoperative colonic lavage and primary anastomosis in peritonitis and obstruction. Br J Surg. 1997;84:222–5.
73. Bokey EL, Chapuis PH, Fung C, Hughes WJ, Koorey SG, Brewer D, et al. Postoperative morbidity and mortality following resection of the colon and rectum for cancer. Dis Colon Rectum. 1995;38:480–7.
74. Bouillot JL, Aouad K, Badawy A, Alamowitch B, Alexandre JH. Elective laparoscopic-assisted colectomy for diverticular disease. A prospective study in 50 patients. Surg Endosc. 1998;12:1393–6.
75. Burke P, Mealy K, Gillen P, Joyce W, Traynor O, Hyland J. Requirement for bowel preparation in colorectal surgery. Br J Surg. 1994;81:907–10.
76. Cornwell EE III, Velmahos GC, Berne TV, Murray JA, Chahwan S, Asensio J, et al. The fate of colonic suture lines in high-risk trauma patients: a prospective analysis. J Am Coll Surg. 1998;187:58–63.
77. De Wever I, Van de Moortel M, Stas M. Temporary colostomy in supralevator pelvic exenteration. A comparative study between stapled loop and loop colostomy. Eur J Surg Oncol. 1996;22:84–7.
78. Debus ES, Sailer M, Geiger D, Dietz UA, Fuchs KH, Thiede A. Long-term results after 75 anastomoses in the upper extraperitoneal rectum with the biofragmentable anastomosis ring. Dig Surg. 1999;16:55–9.
79. Deen KI, Smart PJ. Prospective evaluation of sutured, continuous, and interrupted single layer colonic anastomoses. Eur J Surg. 1995;161:751–3.
80. Dehni N, Schlegel RD, Cunningham C, Guiguet M, Tiret E, Parc R. Influence of a defunctioning stoma on leakage rates after low colorectal anastomosis and colonic J pouch-anal anastomosis. Br J Surg. 1998;85:1114–7.
81. Docherty JG, McGregor JR, Akyol AM, Murray GD, Galloway DJ. Comparison of manually constructed and stapled anastomoses in colorectal surgery. West of Scotland and Highland Anastomosis Study Group. Ann Surg. 1995;221:176–84.

82. Fingerhut A, Elhadad A, Hay JM, Lacaine F, Flamant Y. Infraperitoneal colorectal anastomosis: hand-sewn versus circular staples. A controlled clinical trial. French Associations for Surgical Research. Surgery. 1994;116:484–90.
83. Fingerhut A, Hay JM, Elhadad A, Lacaine F, Flamant Y. Supraperitoneal colorectal anastomosis: hand-sewn versus circular staples – a controlled clinical trial. French Associations for Surgical Research. Surgery. 1995;118:479–85.
84. Hallbook O, Pahlman L, Krog M, Wexner SD, Sjodahl R. Randomized comparison of straight and colonic J pouch anastomosis after low anterior resection. Ann Surg. 1996;224:58–65.
85. Hansen O, Schwenk W, Hucke HP, Stock W. Colorectalstapled anastomoses. Experiences and results. Dis Colon Rectum. 1996;39:30–6.
86. Hida J, Yasutomi M, Fujimoto K, Okuno K, Ieda S, Machidera N, et al. Functional outcome after low anterior resection with low anastomosis for rectal cancer using the colonic J-pouch. Prospective randomized study for determination of optimum pouch size. Dis Colon Rectum. 1996;39:986–91.
87. Iversen LH, Thomsen GH, Thorlacius-Ussing O. Systemic coagulation activation and anastomotic leakage after colorectal cancer surgery. Dis Colon Rectum. 1999;42:56–65.
88. Junger W, Junger WG, Miller K, Bahrami S, Redl H, Schlag G, et al. Early detection of anastomotic leaks after colorectal surgery by measuring endotoxin in the drainage Huid. Hepatogastroenterology. 1996;43:1523–9.
89. Karanjia ND, Corder AP, Bearn P, Heald RJ. Leakage from stapled low anastomosis after total mesorectal excision for carcinoma ofthe rectum. Br J Surg. 1994;81:1224–6.
90. Kessler H, Hermanek P Jr, Wiebelt J. Operative mortality in carcinoma of the rectum. Results of the German Multicentre Study. Int J Colorectal Dis. 1993;8:158–66.
91. Kockerling F, Rose J, Schneider C, Scheidbach H, Scheuerlein H, Reymond MA, et al. Laparoscopic colorectal anastomosis: risk of postoperative leakage: results of a multicenter study. Surg Endosc. 1999;13:639–44.
92. Kracht M, Hay JM, Fagniez PL, Fingerhut A. Ileocolonic anastomosis after right hemicolectomy for carcinoma: stapled or hand-sewn? A prospective, multicenter, randomized trial. Int J Colorectal Dis. 1993;8:29–33.
93. Mann B, Kleinschmidt S, Stremmel W. Prospective study of hand-sutured anastomosis after colorectal resection. Br J Surg. 1996;83:29–31.
94. Merad F, Hay JM, Fingerhut A, Yahchouchi E, Laborde Y, Pelissier E, et al. Is prophylactic pelvic drainage useful after elective rectal or anal anastomosis? A multicenter controlled randomized trial. French Associations for Surgical Research. Surgery. 1999;125:529–35.
95. Merad F, Hay JM, Fingerhut A, Flamant Y, Molkhou JM, Laborde Y. Omentoplasty in the prevention of anastomotic leakage after colonic or rectal resection: a prospective randomized study in 712 patients. French Associations for Surgical Research. Ann Surg. 1998;227:179 86.
96. Miller K, Arrer E, Leitner C. Early detection of anastomotic leaks after low anterior resection of the rectum. Dis Colon Rectum. 1996;39:1081–5.
97. Miller K, Moritz E. Circular stapling techniques for low anterior resection of rectal carcinoma. Hepatogastroenterology. 1996;43:823–31.
98. Moore JW, Chapuis PH, Bokey EL. Morbidity and mortality after single- and double-stapled colorectal anastomoses in patients with carcinoma of the rectum. Aust N Z J Surg. 1996;66:820–3.
99. Norris B, Solomon MJ, Evers AA, West RH, Glenn DC, Morgan BP. Abdominal surgery in the older Crohn's population. Aust N Z J Surg. 1999;69:199–204.
100. Pakkastie TE, Ovaska JT, Pekkala ES, Luukkonen PE, Jarvinen HJ. A randomized study of colostomies in low colorectal anastomoses. Eur J Surg. 1997;163:929–33.
101. Petersen S, Freitag M, Hellmich G, Ludwig K. Anastomotic leakage: impact on local recurrence and survival in surgery of colorectal cancer. Int J Colorectal Dis. 1998;13:160–3.
102. Redmond HP, Austin OM, Clery AP, Deasy JM. Safety of double-stapled anastomosis in low anterior resection. Br JSurg. 1993;80:924–7.
103. Sagar PM, Hartley MN, Macfie J, Mancey-Jones B, Sedman P, May J. Randomized trial of pelvic drainage after rectal resection. Dis Colon Rectum. 1995;38:254–8.

104. Santos JC Jr, Batista J, Sirimarco MT, Guimaraes AS, Levy CE. Prospective randomized trial of mechanical bowel preparation in patients undergoing elective colorectalsurgery. Br J Surg. 1994;81:1673–6.
105. Slim K, Pezet D, Riff Y, Clark E, Chipponi J. High morbidity after converted laparoscopic colorectal surgery. Br J Surg. 1995;82:1406–8.
106. Stewart BT, Woods RJ, Collopy BT, Fink RJ, Mackay JR, Keck JO. Early feeding after elective open colorectal resections: a prospective randomized trial. Aust N Z J Surg. 1998;68:125–8.
107. Tagart RE. Restorative rectal resection: an audit of 220 cases. Br J Surg. 1986;73:70–1.
108. Thompson GA, Cocks JR, Collopy BT, Cade RJ, Ewing HP, Rogerson JW, et al. Colorectal resection in Victoria: a comparison of hospital based and individual audit. Aust N Z J Surg. 1996;66:520–4.
109. Watson AJM, Krukowski ZH, Munro A. Salvage of large bowel anastomotic leaks. Br J Surg. 1999;86:499–500.
110. Wheeler JMD, Gilbert JM. Controlled intraoperative water testing of left-sided colorectal anastomoses: are ileostomies avoidable? Ann R Coll Surg Engl. 1999;81:105–8.
111. Vignali A, Giamotti L, Braga M, Radaelli G, Malvezzi L, Di Carlo V. Altered microperfusion at the rectal stump is predictive for rectal anastomotic leak. Dis Colon Rectum. 2000;43(1):76–82.
112. Schmidt O, Merkel S, Hohenberger W. Anastomotic leakage after low rectal stapler anastomosis: significance of intraoperative anastomotic testing. Eur J Surg Oncol. 2003;29:239–43.
113. Ishihara S, Watanabe T, Nagawa H. Intraoperative colonoscopy for stapled anastomosis in colorectal surgery. Surg Today. 2008;38(11):1063–5.
114. Lanthaler M, Biebl M, Mittermair R, Ofner D, Nehoda H. Intraoperative colonoscopy for anastomosis assessment in laparoscopically assisted left-sided colon resection: is it worthwhile? J Laparoendosc Adv Surg Tech A. 2008;18(1):27–31.
115. Shamiyeh A, Szabo K, Ulf Wayand W, Zehetner J. Intraoperative endoscopy for the assessment of circular-stapled anastomosis in laparoscopic colon surgery. Surg Laparosc Endosc Percutan Tech. 2012;22(1):65–7.
116. Ivanov D, Cvijanovic R, Gvozdenovic L. Intraoperative air testing of colorectal anastomoses. Srp Arh Celok Lek. 2011;139(5–6):333–8.
117. Lieto E, Orditura M, Castellano P, et al. Endoscopic intraoperative anastomotic testing may avoid early gastrointestinal anastomotic complications. A prospective study. J Gastrointest Surg. 2011;15(1):145–52.
118. Xiao L, Zhang WB, Jiang PC, et al. Can transanal tube placement after anterior resection for rectal carcinoma reduce anastomotic leakage rate? A single-institution prospective randomized study. World J Surg. 2011;35(6):1367–77.
119. Kamal T, Pai A, Velchuru VR, Zawadzki M, Park JJ, Marecik SJ, et al. Should anastomotic assessment with flexible sigmoidoscopy be routine following laparoscopic restorative left colorectal resection? Colorectal Dis. 2015;17(2):160–4.

31 Minimizing Conversion in Laparoscopic Colorectal Surgery: From Preoperative Risk Assessment to Intraoperative Strategies

John Byrn and Heather Yeo

Introduction and Rationale

More than 300,000 colorectal resections were performed in 2012 for benign and malignant conditions in the United States [1]. Since 1991, the use of laparoscopy for colorectal surgery has increased, reaching 22.7% in 2005 to 49.8% in 2014 [2]. This steady increase in adoption results from improvements in instrumentation, standardization of surgical techniques through training, as well as mounting evidence demonstrating the clinical benefits and oncologic safety of laparoscopy from randomized controlled trials (RCTs) [3]. Compared to open surgery, minimally invasive colorectal resections result in less pain, less blood loss, shorter hospital stay, and shorter recovery, with significant cost savings [4].

Over the last two decades, laparoscopic techniques and instrumentation have continued to improve. As laparoscopy continues to gain traction in colorectal surgery, it is important that surgeons become familiar with various techniques and tools available in their armamentarium in order to minimize the risk of conversion. Several factors, including unclear anatomy, bowel injury, and bleeding, can lead to conversion. Reactive conversion follows an intraoperative complication (i.e., a vascular, ureteral, or bowel injury), while preemptive conversion is performed to avoid complications (i.e., when there is difficulty with structural identification or a decision that performing a procedure will be too difficult laparoscopically) [5]. While no studies have evaluated the difference, it is our experience that reactive conversion leads to worse outcomes as it is in response to a complication, and preemptive

J. Byrn
Division of Colorectal Surgery, Department of Surgery, University of Michigan, Ann Arbor, MI, USA
e-mail: jcbyrn@med.umich.edu

H. Yeo (✉)
New York Presbyterian – Weill Cornell Medicine, Department of Surgery, New York, NY, USA
e-mail: Hey9002@med.cornell.edu

P. Sylla et al. (eds.), *The SAGES Manual of Colorectal Surgery*,
https://doi.org/10.1007/978-3-030-24812-3_31

conversion is done to avoid a complication. However, often a case that is difficult laparoscopically may also be difficult as an open procedure.

The overall impact of conversion has been well studied with demonstrated negative effects on costs, morbidity, and patient outcomes [6]. Several factors have been shown to impact rates of conversion; however, while conversion rates have decreased over time as experience with the minimally invasive technique has grown, the conversion rate is still 10–25% nationally, and, as a result, techniques to mitigate these consequences have important clinical benefit. In this chapter, we discuss preoperative considerations and intraoperative steps that may help to achieve the goal of decreasing conversion rates.

Indications and Contraindications

Laparoscopic and minimally invasive approaches to colon and rectal resections have become the preferred method over open surgery for nearly all colorectal surgical procedures. They can be used for benign and malignant disease and have lowered the morbidity and mortality of many procedures, especially colon resections, rectopexy, and procedures for fecal diversion. There are no absolute contraindications to laparoscopic colorectal procedures [7], but much of the decision depends on the surgeon's experience and comfort with laparoscopy. Extra caution should be taken in patients with a history of previous abdominal surgeries, a history of cardiopulmonary comorbidities, obese patients, pregnant patients, and patients with rectal cancer, where the use of laparoscopy is more controversial. Absolute contraindications are emergency patients with hemodynamic instability due to bleeding, sepsis, or trauma.

Principles and Benchmarks

While there are no benchmarks for conversion during laparoscopic surgery, most major RCTs have reported conversion rates ranging between 1% and 25% (Table 31.1). The conversion rates from these trials should be evaluated with the understanding that most of them included only experienced laparoscopists, so the numbers may be lower than many surgeons might see in their own practice.

The practicing surgeon can easily determine his or her own laparoscopic conversion to open colectomy or proctectomy rate using his or her own institutional data. This rough estimate may allow self-assessment and aids in determining if the surgeon is providing a certain measure of quality care. The COST trial conversion rate for colectomy (excluding transverse colectomy) was 21%, and in the Z6051 trial, the laparoscopic conversion to open proctectomy rate for rectal cancer was 11%. Both trials involved expert surgeons with significant laparoscopic experience (>20 lifetime laparoscopic colectomies) and more importantly had undergone a credentialing process for the study where a video was reviewed for evaluation of surgical technique.

An important consideration when evaluating conversion rates is the impact of conversion on patient outcomes. While reactive conversion, for example, due to iatrogenic colotomy with gross fecal contamination is necessary and associated with worse outcomes with respect to infectious complications, other conversions may not have as

Table 31.1 Major colorectal laparoscopy trials

Title	Design	Year	Study Comparison	# of institutions	Pnts # (Op/Lap)	Conversion rate (%)	Complications	LOS (Days)
Rectal procedure studies								
CLASICC trial [15, 19]	RCT	2007	Laparoscopic vs. open survival and recurrence	27	737 (253/484)	34%	13%	–
COREAN trial [20]	RCT	2014	Laparoscopic vs. open survival outcomes	3	340 (170/170)	1%	–	–
A randomized trial of laparoscopic versus open surgery for rectal cancer [7]	RCT	2015	Laparoscopic vs. open survival and recurrence	30	1044 (345/699)	16%	–	–
ACOSOG Z6051 [21]	RCT	2015	Laparoscopic vs. open pathological outcomes	35	462 (222/240)	11.3%	22%	7
ALaCaRT [22]	RCT	2015	Laparoscopic vs. open pathological outcomes	24	457 (237/238)	9%	–	–
Colon studies								
COST [16]	RCT	2004	Laparoscopic vs. open survival and recurrence	48	863 (428/435)	21%	21%	5
COLOR [23]	RCT	2005	Laparoscopic vs. open clinical outcomes	1	1082 (546/536)	19%	21%	8.2
CLASICC trial [15, 19]	RCT	2007	Laparoscopic vs. open survival and recurrence	27	737 (253/484)	25%	7%	–

(continued)

Table 31.1 (continued)

Title	Design	Year	Study Comparison	# of institutions	Pnts # (Op/Lap)	Conversion rate (%)	Complications	LOS (Days)
Laparoscopically assisted vs open colectomy for colon cancer [24]	Meta-analysis	2007	Laparoscopic vs. open survival outcomes		1536 (740/796)	19%		
Clinical outcomes and resource utilization associated with laparoscopic and open colectomy using a large national database [25]	Retrospective	2008	Laparoscopic vs. open clinical and economic outcomes	402	32,733 (21,689/11,044)	10.1%	26%	7
Elective open versus laparoscopic sigmoid colectomy for diverticular disease: A meta-analysis with the sigma trial [26]	Meta-analysis	2010	Laparoscopic vs. open clinical outcomes		10,898 (9360/1538)	8.4%	–	–
ALCCaS trial [27]	RCT	2018	Laparoscopic vs. open symptoms and QoL	Multicenter	425 (213/212)	15%	–	–

much of a deleterious effect. Hence, the decision to attempt a laparoscopic approach should balance the benefits of a laparoscopic approach, and the risks of complications including consequences of conversion to open surgery with the understanding that a preemptive conversion, before complications or injury arises, may mitigate the impact of conversion on outcomes. Although a laparoscopic approach may be highly desirable in complex cases based on the clinical benefits incurred from avoidance of a laparotomy, early and preemptive conversion should be considered in the face of failure to progress or impending complications. When conversion is performed early, it may mitigate the morbidity incurred from reactive conversion in the face of a complication. When interpreting the literature on the negative impact of conversion on oncologic and infectious outcomes, surgeons should not become discouraged from attempting laparoscopy for fear of conversion but be prepared for this possibility and realistic with respect to when to convert. This clinical judgment is part of the laparoscopic learning curve and can only be finessed through experience gained when attempting complex cases. As a general rule, surgeons should consider diagnostic laparoscopy, with a low threshold to convert when the risk of injury and/or prolonged operative time outweighs the benefits of persisting with a laparoscopic approach.

High conversion rates for any given surgeon should prompt careful review of case logs, with specific focus on patient selection and risk factors for conversion, case volume, and experience with specific cases. This will in turn identify areas for improvement and strategies to mitigate the risk of conversion.

Preoperative Planning, Patient Work-Up, and Optimization

Patients undergoing laparoscopic colorectal surgery need a detailed medical history, physical exam, and colorectal cancer staging if the pathology is a colorectal malignancy. Particular attention should be paid to the number and type of previous abdominal surgeries and any history of abdominal infections, radiation, or surgical complications. The operative reports from previous abdominal surgeries should be reviewed. Patients can then proceed with standard preoperative blood work-up, electrocardiogram, and chest X-ray as indicated. A focused physical abdominal exam will appreciate previous surgical scars, the approach to previous surgeries (Pfannenstiel vs. midline laparotomy), and the presence of incisional hernias. The most important findings on history and physical are related to cardiopulmonary debilitation. A patient with poor functional status and non-optimized cardiac and pulmonary comorbidity often needs further specialty care through cardiology and pulmonology before surgery. Increases in preoperative activity and smoking cessation, prehabilitation, are of proven benefit in surgical outcomes.

When considering segmental colectomy for malignant polyps or tumors, localization of the tumor is key and achieved through a combination of cross-sectional imaging and endoscopy. Colonoscopy reports are valuable, as endoscopic tattoo placement or clipping may be crucial to localizing the pathology and planning your resection during the procedure. Preoperative planning entails reviewing all images prior to surgery. A CT scan is not only useful to localize disease but is also helpful to assess the thickness of the abdominal wall, location of the top of the splenic flexure, and other important surgical landmarks, which can help in port planning.

Table 31.2 Risk factors for conversion

Patient related	Disease related	Surgeon related
Advanced age (>80) Male gender Obesity (BMI >30) ASA classification (class 4) Previous surgery Ascites Cardiopulmonary comorbidities	Anatomical site (rectum and transverse colon) Pathology (Crohn's disease) Presentation (emergency setting)	Experience (low volume)

Patient Risk Factors for Conversion (Table 31.2)

Studies on the patient-related risk factors for conversion have almost exclusively retrospective single institution case series but are still worth considering for anyone adopting laparoscopy into his or her practice. Patient-related factors that have been shown to increase risk of conversion include advanced age, obesity, gender, ASA classification, previous surgery, and cardiopulmonary comorbidity. For patients undergoing colectomy, those older than 80 have a 73% higher chance of conversion compared to patients younger than 50 [8]. Male gender is also associated with a higher risk of conversion in colectomy [9, 10]. Obese patients (BMI >30 kg/m^2) showed increasing the chance of conversion by 31% compared to patients with normal BMI [8]. While there is an increasing epidemic of obesity in the USA, the technical difficulty of performing laparoscopic colorectal resections increases with BMI, particularly in individuals with a BMI >40 or super obesity. In elective cases, we often council patients regarding weight loss strategies preoperatively, as this can significantly impact outcomes. Obesity contributes to difficulty with exposure as these patients often have a shortened mesentery and retraction of the small bowel can be difficult. Please refer to Chap. 32 on laparoscopic colorectal surgery in the obese and morbidly obese patient for more details on preoperative strategies and surgical techniques.

Patients with ascites have been found to be approximately three times more likely to require conversion as ascites may represent underlying primary liver disease or malignant ascites secondary to peritoneal carcinomatosis [8]. In addition, those with cardiopulmonary comorbidities are of increased risk of conversion, as the CO_2 pneumoperitoneum may lead to hemodynamic and pulmonary function alterations. Patients with Society of Anesthesiologists (ASA) class 4 have 68% increased odds of conversion when compared to patients with ASA class 1, hence the importance of patient selection and preoperative risk assessment.

Disease-Related Factors for Conversion

Conversion rates vary depending on the specific type of colectomy performed. In a review of National Inpatient Sample data from 2009 and 2010, it was found that proctectomy was associated with the highest rates of conversion (31.3%), followed by transverse colectomy (20.5%), with lower rates for left and right colectomy, sigmoid colectomy, and total colectomy [10]. Transverse colon and rectal lesions were originally excluded from laparoscopic trials, as they required advanced skills. These rates also vary depending on indications, with the highest rates of conversions in patients undergoing resection for Crohn's disease (20.2%) relative to other pathologies, including benign and malignant tumors, diverticulitis, and ulcerative colitis [10].

The nature of presentation of colorectal pathology also plays into the conversion rate. Patients admitted as an emergency are less likely to undergo emergency laparoscopic procedures. In one study, the percentage of surgeons using an open technique rose from 8% in an elective setting to 47% in an emergency setting [11].

Careful consideration should be given to patients presenting with Crohn's disease or diverticulitis with abscess/phlegmon, especially in reoperative cases. The risks of conversion are high, as well as that of inadvertent injury to the bowel or surrounding structures. In patients with visceral obesity and a short, bulky transverse colon mesentery, the surgeons should proceed cautiously during laparoscopic resection of transverse colon cancer as it may be difficult to obtain a high ligation on the middle colic vessels and an adequate lymphadenectomy in this patient habitus. Additionally, great care should be taken when performing laparoscopic procedure in the setting of large or small bowel obstruction, fulminant colitis, or toxic megacolon, with an increased risk of intraoperative perforation during laparoscopic manipulation of the bowel, which will increase the risk of serious post-operative infectious complications. Our recommendation is to conduct a careful diagnostic laparoscopy with a low threshold to convert.

Patients deemed to be at high risk for conversion should be counseled preoperatively with respect to the likelihood of requiring conversion and the risk of organ injury and other complications incurred from attempting laparoscopy in the face of one or more risk factors for conversion.

Surgeon-Related Factors

One of the factors that clearly plays a role in conversion during laparoscopic colorectal surgery is the surgeon's experience and comfort during complex laparoscopic colon or rectal resections. A recent study of laparoscopic colorectal procedures showed that regardless of the training, high-volume laparoscopic surgeons ($\geq$100 laparoscopic procedures) have lower rate of conversion compared to low-volume laparoscopic surgeons (<100 laparoscopic procedures) [5]. This trend was also seen in a nationwide study comparing high-volume surgeons (>15 procedures/year) with low-volume surgeons ($\leq$15 procedures/year), with high-volume surgeons not only having lower rates of conversion but also lower incidence of prolonged length of stay, bile duct injury, and mortality [12].

Bowel Preparation

While bowel preparation for colon and rectal surgery has waxed and waned in perceived efficacy to reduce surgical site infection, it remains widely adopted by many surgeons who find the colon easier to manage laparoscopically if the bowel has been prepped. Combined mechanical bowel preparation with oral antibiotics has recently been reinstituted into standard enhanced recovery protocols for colorectal procedures, as it has reduced surgical site infections and anastomotic leak rates compared to patients who did not receive either mechanical or antibiotic bowel prep [13]. A prepped bowel is easier to manipulate laparoscopically, and an additional benefit of operating on a prepped colon includes localization of the pathology, such as an unexpectedly inconspicuous tumor requiring direct palpation or intraoperative colonoscopy.

Ureteral Stents

Visualization and identification of the ureters before transection of the mesenteric vessels and the mesentery is crucial to prevent ureter injuries, and the inability to do so is a risk factor for conversion to open surgery. Intraoperative identification of the ureter can be challenging, especially in the setting of visceral obesity, inflammation, and during reoperative pelvic surgery. Some surgeons will opt for prophylactic ureteral stent placement to help with ureter identification and facilitate recognition of an inadvertent injury. However, their use is controversial because of the complications that accompany stenting, such as obstructive oliguria, ureteral injury, or urinary tract infection. In addition, there is no evidence that stents decrease the risk of ureteral injury, of conversion rates, but they may facilitate ureteral identification in difficult cases and help recognize ureteral injuries intraoperatively. Thus, for reoperative colorectal procedures, acute or complicated diverticular disease or Crohn's disease, bulky and locally advanced rectal or sigmoid cancers, we recommend prophylactic ureteral stent placement.

A ureter that is difficult to identify can slow progress significantly in laparoscopic colorectal surgery. Common scenarios are when dissecting inflamed mesentery off the left or right retroperitoneum. A medial to lateral approach to the mesentery is preferred where early identification of the correct anatomic planes, meticulous hemostasis, and careful dissection are your best ally. If oozing from the retroperitoneum is limiting progress, a lap pad or sponge introduced into the abdomen may allow for improved tamponade and visualization. If the patient is obese and there is difficulty with visualization medially, a lateral to medial approach can be used instead.

Key Point There should be a low threshold to call a urologist or colleague to assist in identification of the ureters if and when difficulty is encountered. Intraoperative ureteral stents can help with early laparoscopic identification of the ureters, and prophylactic stenting should be considered in complex colorectal cases.

Operative Setup and Operative Techniques

Patient Positioning

Patients must be placed securely in the supine or lithotomy position, depending on the planned procedure, and should be well padded. With patients positioned securely, the surgeon obtains the ability to place the patient into steep Trendelenburg or reverse Trendelenburg. Steep Trendelenburg position in particular makes it much easier to retract the small bowel out of the pelvis when approaching a rectal or sigmoid dissection. For almost all colon resections, the authors prefer the lithotomy position which allows for intraoperative colonoscopy for air leak testing and localization of the pathology when needed and for positioning of an operator between the patient's legs if needed. Regardless of positioning, patients' arms are usually tucked to the sides, allowing for safe frequent position changes that lead to successful laparoscopic surgery. Many other commercial products are available to help secure the patient; these may vary by institution and mimic a "bean bag" device that hold patients in place without sliding during extremes in left and right tilt as well as in Trendelenburg position.

One of the main obstacles in achieving and maintaining good exposure during laparoscopic colorectal procedures is adequate retraction of the small bowel. Patient positioning should use gravity to help expose the operative site; therefore, attention should be paid to padding and securing the patient to the table during steep position, especially for obese patients. Good exposure can be the difference between conversion and no conversion.

Key Point For obese patients, we prefer to use pink foam and tape to secure the patients to the operating table.

Pneumoperitoneum

Establishing pneumoperitoneum is a key first step in laparoscopic surgery, and it may result in vascular or visceral injury if not performed carefully. Adequate pneumoperitoneum can be established and maintained under an appropriate muscle relaxation. Usually, the intra-abdominal pressure should be between 10 and 12 mm Hg to provide sufficient laparoscopic visualization and working space.

Key Point We recommend starting with low-flow insufflation in any patient with cardiopulmonary disease to minimize the effect that it has on cardiac output.

Although there is no consensus regarding the best method to establish pneumoperitoneum, closed technique (Veress needle) method is the most frequently used. Although open Hasson technique is routinely used by some surgeons, it did not show any superior results regarding bowel injury [14]. However, it is primarily used in reoperative cases and when dense intra-abdominal adhesions are suspected. Another alternative to establish pneumoperitoneum is to use optical access trocar. The trocar used in this technique allows visualization of the dissected planes using the laparoscopic camera. It is best used in patients with a thick abdominal wall, where an "open" technique is difficult.

Key Point In reoperative cases where dense intra-abodminal adhesions are suspected, the Hasson technique is the preferred method for laparoscopic access.

Laparoscopic Exposure: Trocars

In most colorectal procedures, three to five trocars are typically used: one for the camera, two for the operating surgeon, and one or two for the assistant. Trocar placement is dependent on surgeon's preference, prior abdominal surgeries, body habitus, and type of procedure. Please see Figs. 31.1, 31.2, and 31.3 for our recommended port placement for (1) laparoscopic left colectomy (Fig. 31.1), (2) laparoscopic sigmoid colectomy (Fig. 31.2), and (3) laparoscopic rectal resection (Fig. 31.3). In most instances, the camera trocar is placed in the midline at the umbilicus, while the operating surgeon trocars are placed on the opposite side of the pathology under laparoscopic guidance. Additional consideration should be given to the distance between trocars, which should be at least 8 cm to ease the movement of the instruments. Additional care must be taken for lower abdominal trocars so that collision with the legs of the patient (this can occur in supine o lithotomy position) can be prevented.

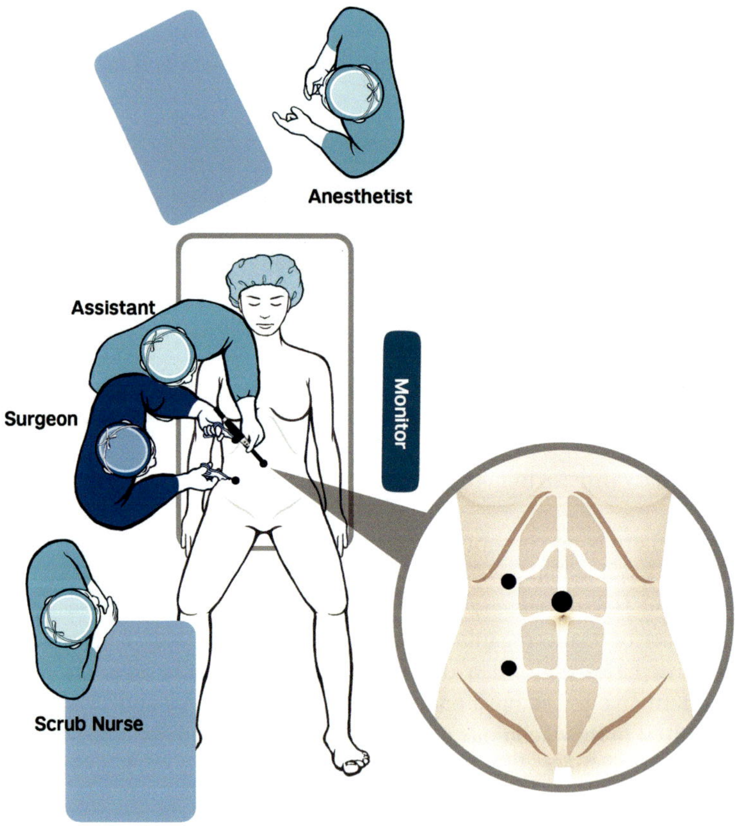

Fig. 31.1 Trocar placement for left colectomy. (Courtesy of Yuko Tonohira)

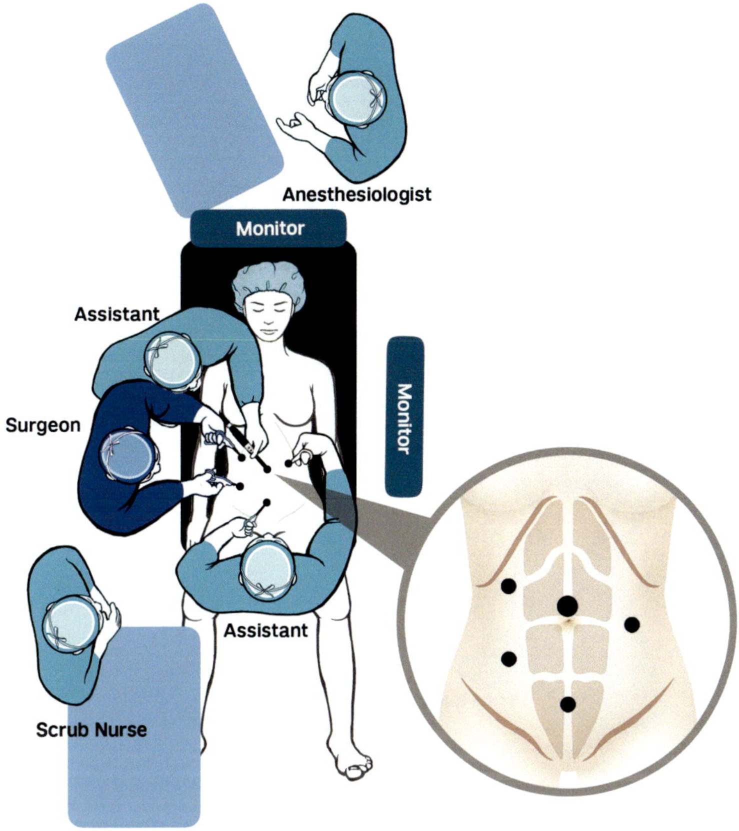

Fig. 31.2 Sigmoid colectomy port placement. Additional port for splenic flexure mobilization on the right. (Courtesy of Yuko Tonohira)

Key Point There is minimal morbidity with the addition of one or more 5 mm trocars. When struggling to achieve appropriate exposure laparoscopically, additional trocars should be placed.

Laparoscopic Adhesiolysis

For patients with complex adhesions, there are several tricks that our authors prefer using. Several instruments can be very beneficial, and one should be willing to add additional 5 mm ports where needed. For sharp adhesiolysis, we prefer the disposable microshears as these have a smaller cut length and are better for delicate dissection than traditional or reusable sheers (Fig. 31.4). In addition, the endo peanut is a good instrument to separate areas between the bowel and other areas where you do not want to perform sharp dissection (i.e., by the ureter). Adhesiolysis should be

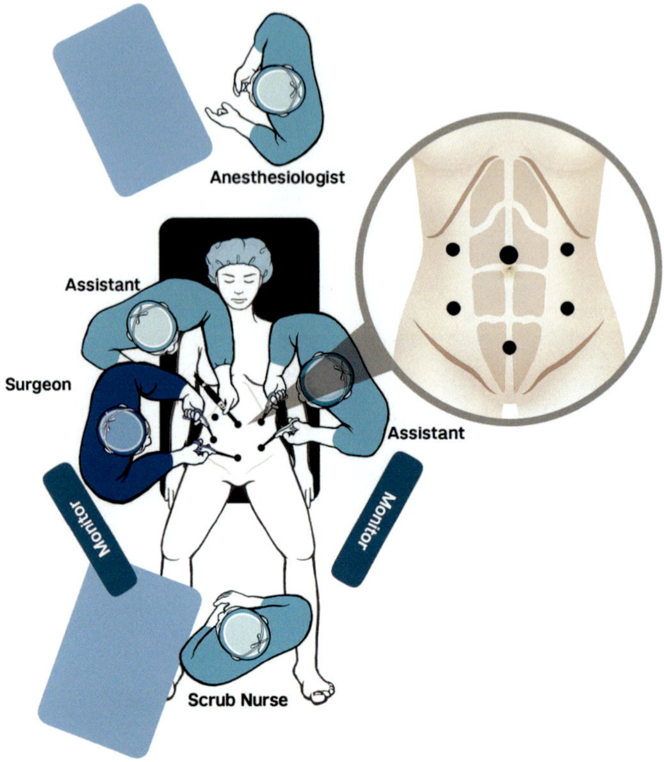

Fig. 31.3 Port placement for rectal resection. The suprapubic port is optional. (Courtesy of Yuko Tonohira)

Fig. 31.4 Laparoscopic lysis of adhesions facilitated by laparoscopic endo peanuts and cold endoshears. (Courtesy of Patricia Sylla, MD)

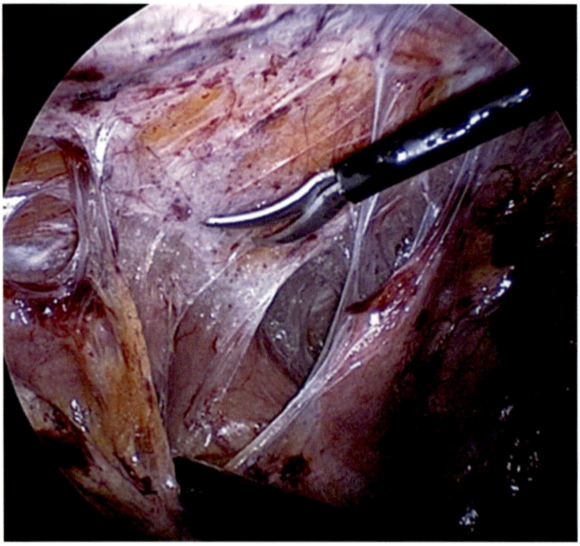

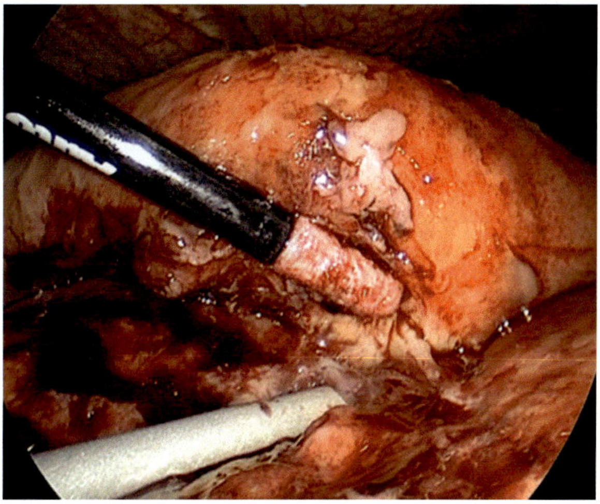

Fig. 31.5 Careful laparoscopic separation of inflamed bowel loops is facilitated by the use of endo peanuts. (Courtesy of Patricia Sylla, MD)

performed "cold" with no cautery to minimize the risk of burn injury and delayed enterotomy. The endo peanut used in a gentle twisting motion will often help separate even the most dense adhesions (Fig. 31.5). We also recommend achieving meticulous hemostasis and having the camera quite close to the dissection, as visibility of the correct planes is key to avoid injury (Fig. 31.6a, b).

Minimizing Incision Size

For more complex cases where surgeons are pushing the limits of their experience and learning curve, several options are available to minimize the extent of the open portion of the procedure when converting. The classic example of this scenario is in a low anterior resection, left or sigmoid colectomy to perform the major artery ligation and mobilization of the sigmoid and splenic flexure laparoscopically, while performing the rectal dissection open through a Pfannenstiel incision. In this scenario, the patient is saved a laparotomy through laparoscopic mobilization, but the surgeon is able to do high-risk portions of the procedure through the open exposure. Another opportunity for this would be with a difficult transverse colon during total colectomy where an upper midline hand port could be used to aid in laparoscopic mobilization and then open control of a short transverse colon mesentery. Lastly, an excellent option for very complex cases is to have a more experienced surgeon participate in the case. This could be an expert urologist who could help identify a left ureter matted in a diverticular phlegmon or a partner with a different training background or more diverse laparoscopic experience. Formal mentoring during a case or assistance is best addressed preoperatively and planned carefully, so neither party feels unsure of their role.

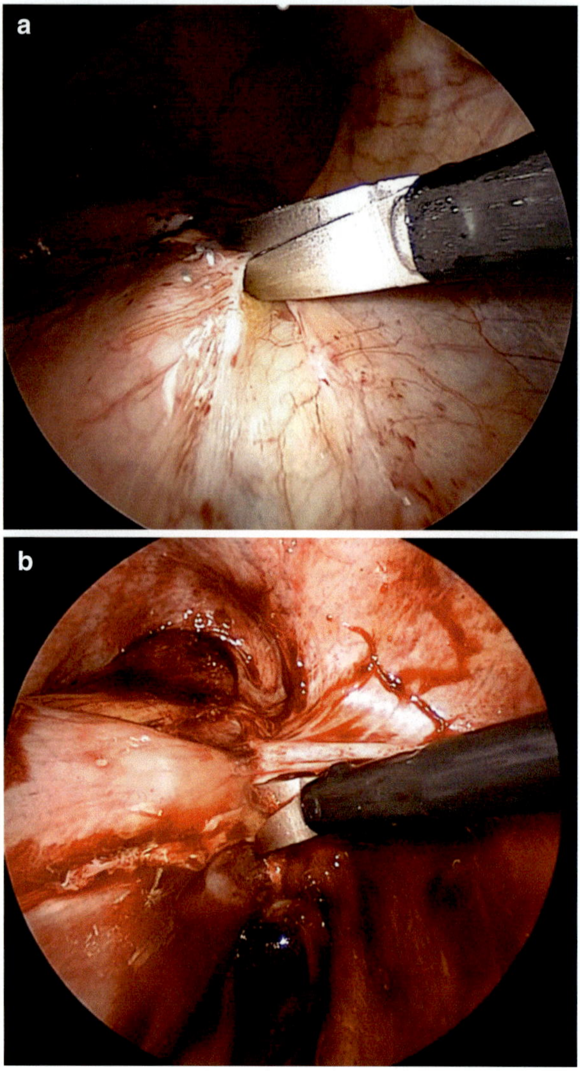

Fig. 31.6 (**a**, **b**) Pelvic side wall adhesions during ileoanal J pouch excision meticulously dissected sharply using endoshears. (Both: Courtesy of Patricia Sylla, MD)

Pitfalls and Troubleshooting

Common intraoperative pitfalls portending a conversion from laparoscopic to open colorectal resection include distortion of dissection planes due to inflammation or tumor, visceral obesity, and the challenge of laparoscopic handling of the transverse colon. We will discuss strategies below, but remedies include early conversion to open, hand-assist techniques, increased usage of assistants and assistant ports, and position changes.

Adhesions and Response to Injury

Obscuring of tissue planes during laparoscopic mobilization and handling of the colon mesentery can lead to bleeding, injury to surrounding structures, and conversion to open. Sometimes, very little can be done to combat this, and conversion to open is justified and preferred over prolonged operating times, excessive bleeding, and injury to other structures that would ultimately require conversion regardless.

Key Point In the event of acute bleeding during laparoscopic colorectal resection, an endo peanut or sponge can be used for tamponade, and/or a grasper can be used for clamping the vessel until hemostasis can be achieved.

Acute Inflammatory Process

When approaching a diverticular abscess or phlegmon or severely inflamed Crohn's ileitis, blunt and suction dissection can be useful and allow for the most progress with the less risk of injury. Inflammatory adhesions are, in our experience, one of the most common indications for open conversion. A defensive strategy is necessary when handling areas with intense inflammation (abscess or active disease). One approach is to first dissect away from the inflammation and identify important structures. These include the left ureter in sigmoid disease and the duodenum and adnexa in ileocolic disease. The surgeon may want to "circle the enemy" by working both medial and lateral, caudad and cephalad to the pathology, until maximal mobilization and dissection have been performed to identify anatomic landmark and the correct tissue planes. With this strategy, the most inflamed portion of the procedure is left for last. If dissection of the sigmoid off the left pelvic brim, for example, is not possible, assessment of the relationship between the inferior mesenteric artery (IMA) and left ureter for ligation and mobilization of the descending colon and splenic flexure may allow for completion of the procedure through an open technique, where the laparotomy length can be minimized, or a Pfannenstiel incision can be used.

A high ligation of the IMA, while not necessary for diverticular disease, does allow for handling of the mesentery outside of the inflammatory area and for establishing a clean plane to work off of when approaching the inflamed pelvic brim.

Key Point Avoid the area with abscess or inflammation until you have mobilized all surrounding structures and identified the correct tissue planes.

Traction Injuries

Excessive, unnecessary traction and counter traction may result in serosal tears or organ injuries, which may lead to conversion to open approach to fix these complications. In laparoscopic right hemicolectomy, injury to the middle colic vessels due to excessive traction or unclear anatomy can be a significant intraoperative complication and may lead the surgeon to convert.

Lateral Dissection

One of the most common errors to happen during right, left, or sigmoid surgery is dissection carried out too laterally onto the abdominal wall during lateral mobilization of the colon, which may result in retroperitoneal dissection and mobilization of the kidney and the ureter or pancreatic tail. During the dissection, our authors recommend staying close to the bowel mesentery or doing a medial to lateral approach.

Key Point You to not want to be in the retroperitoneal plane. Keep just anterior to that plane and dissect away from the bowel mesentery, not toward it, as this is more likely to pull the retroperitoneum up with you.

Bulky Tumors

If a bulky right colon tumor is approaching the duodenum, the most useful strategy is to employ a medial to lateral approach where this relationship is assessed early and conversion can be decided promptly. A bulky sigmoid lesion may require aggressive position changes and placement of additional trocars in order to provide the necessary retraction to achieve adequate exposure for IMA ligation and ureter identification.

Transverse Colectomy

Transverse colectomy, either in isolation for malignancy or as part of a total colectomy for a variety of indications, is a common pitfall of laparoscopic colorectal surgery. The transverse colon is redundant and can become unwieldy when encountered along with a bulky omentum. The transverse mesocolon can be treacherous as dissection of the middle colic vessels is carried out in close proximity to the superior mesenteric artery and vein. Additional trocar placement and retraction by additional assistants, position changes, use of hand-assist technique, and early conversions are the typical maneuvers that may be used to handle the difficult transverse colectomy.

Obesity

Visceral obesity often increases the technical difficulty of laparoscopic colorectal procedures but less consistently predicts conversion when compared to inflammation and mass. Stepwise approach to optimize exposure of the anatomy includes placement of additional trocars for additional levels of retraction, recruiting additional assistants to help with retraction, changes in patient positioning taking advantage of the effect of gravity on the bowel, and its mesentery.

Finally, in patients with difficult anatomy and where additional ports do not provide adequate exposure, conversion to a hand-assisted approach can help keep the case laparoscopic while avoiding conversion to a midline laparotomy. A hand-assist port can be placed as a midline (upper or lower) or as a Pfannenstiel. We prefer a Pfannenstiel as this has a lower rate of hernia and wound complications. Hand-assist techniques are necessary for the surgeon to have in his or her armamentarium and can apply to any situation (including inflammation and mass effect above) where the surgeon is struggling laparoscopically. Specifically, hand-assist techniques reduce conversions by improving retraction and augmenting the surgeon's ability to palpate the anatomy (Fig. 31.7a, b). The surgeon can assess fixity of a tumor to adjacent structures in order to confirm resectability, bluntly dissect inflammatory masses, control bleeding, and identify ureters. The hand also provides effective tissue retraction of redundant colon, bulky mesentery, or omentum to help expose the vascular pedicles in preparation for high ligation.

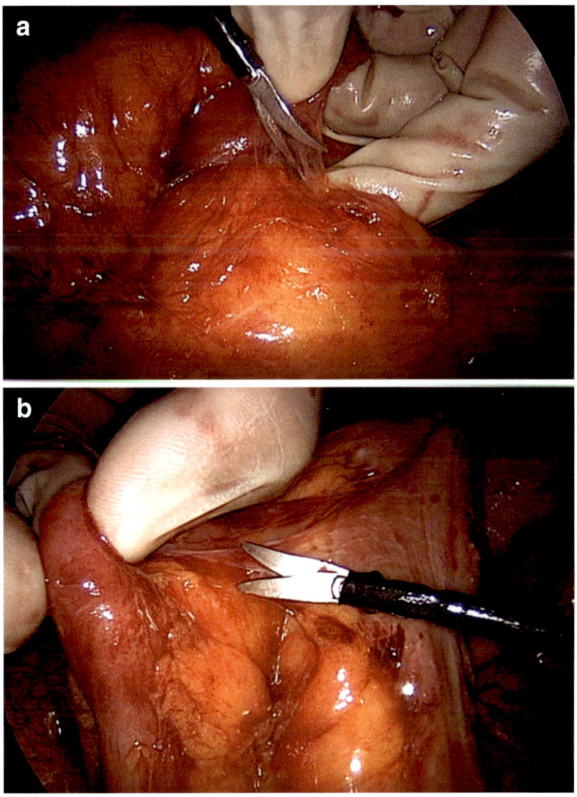

Fig. 31.7 (**a**, **b**) Hand-assisted laparoscopic lysis adhesions can be very helpful when extensive interloop adhesions are encountered. (Both: Courtesy of Patricia Sylla, MD)

Key Point Hand-assist techniques can facilitate laparoscopic completion of a complex colorectal resection that would otherwise require conversion to open laparotomy.

Outcomes

Available literature on outcomes of conversion of laparoscopic colon and rectal surgery to open surgery show worse outcomes with conversion relative to laparoscopic surgery or even open cases. Patients with colorectal cancer who underwent conversion during laparoscopic resection have been shown to have worse oncological outcomes, especially with respect to disease recurrence and overall mortality. As seen in the COST and MRC CLASICC trials [15, 16], there was a significant decrease in overall survival in converted patients with colorectal cancer. Although there are some caveats, as this was not a primary endpoint and the converted group had some worse preoperative parameters as well. Conversion is also associated with an increased need of blood transfusion and increased 30-day mortality [17].

Learning Curve

There is a clear learning curve in laparoscopic surgery. Studies have placed the learning curve in colorectal surgery in the range of 30–70 cases, with the learning curve for right colectomy being about 10 cases less than that for left or sigmoid colectomy [18]. For surgeons not trained laparoscopically, we recommend a training course as well as performing at least the first 30 with a more senior partner to gain experience.

Conclusions

Laparoscopic surgery has made significant strides over the last two decades. Improvements in technique have expanded indications. Conversion rates are due to both patient and physician factors. Careful preoperative preparation can help decrease conversion rates and give patients the best chance for an optimal recovery. Minimizing conversion whenever possible can help to improve patient outcomes. However, the surgeon should not delay conversion when laparoscopy is determined to be unsafe or if anatomy is unclear.

Acknowledgments The chapter authors would like to thank Yuko Tonohira for creating the three illustrations in this chapter.

References

1. Fingar KR, Stocks C, Weiss AJ, Steiner CA. Most frequent operating room procedures performed in U.S. hospitals, 2003–2012. Rockville: Agency for Healthcare Research and Quality; 2014. HCUP Statistical Brief #186.
2. Davis CH, Shirkey BA, Moore LW, Gaglani T, Du XL, Bailey HR, et al. Trends in laparoscopic colorectal surgery over time from 2005-2014 using the NSQIP database. J Surg Res. 2018;223:16–21.
3. Clinical Outcomes of Surgical Therapy Study Group, Nelson H, Sargent DJ, Wieand HS, Fleshman J, Anvari M, et al. A comparison of laparoscopically assisted and open colectomy for colon cancer. N Engl J Med. 2004;350(20):2050–9.
4. Crawshaw BP, Chien HL, Augestad KM, Delaney CP. Effect of laparoscopic surgery on health care utilization and costs in patients who undergo colectomy. JAMA Surg. 2015;150(5):410–5.
5. Massarotti H, Rodrigues F, O'Rourke C, Chadi SA, Wexner S. Impact of surgeon laparoscopic training and case volume of laparoscopic surgery on conversion during elective laparoscopic colorectal surgery. Color Dis. 2017;19(1):76–85.
6. Moghadamyeghaneh Z, Masoomi H, Mills SD, Carmichael JC, Pigazzi A, Nguyen NT, et al. Outcomes of conversion of laparoscopic colorectal surgery to open surgery. JSLS. 2014;18(4):e2014.
7. Bonjer HJ, Deijen CL, Abis GA, Cuesta MA, van der Pas MHGM, de Lange-de Klerk ESM, et al. A randomized trial of laparoscopic versus open surgery for rectal cancer. N Engl J Med. 2015;372:1324–32.
8. Bhama AR, Charlton ME, Schmitt MB, Cromwell JW, Byrn JC. Factors associated with conversion from laparoscopic to open colectomy using the National Surgical Quality Improvement Program (NSQIP) database. Color Dis. 2015;17(3):257–64.
9. Thorpe H, Jayne DG, Guillou PJ, Quirke P, Copeland J, Brown JM, et al. Patient factors influencing conversion from laparoscopically assisted to open surgery for colorectal cancer. Br J Surg. 2018;95(2):199–205.
10. Masoomi H, Moghadamyeghaneh Z, Mills S, Carmichael JC, Pigazzi A, Stamos MJ. Risk factors for conversion of laparoscopic colorectal surgery to open surgery: does conversion worsen outcome? World J Surg. 2015;39(5):1240–7.
11. Cameron IC. Management of acute cholecystitis in UK hospitals: time for a change. Postgrad Med J. 2004;80(943):292–4.
12. Csikesz NG, Singla A, Murphy MM, Tseng JF, Shah SA. Surgeon volume metrics in laparoscopic cholecystectomy. Dig Dis Sci. 2010;55(8):2398–405.
13. Midura EF, Jung AD, Hanseman DJ, Dhar V, Shah SA, Rafferty JF, et al. Combination oral and mechanical bowel preparations decreases complications in both right and left colectomy. Surgery. 2018;163(3):528–34.
14. Hashizume M, Sugimachi K. Needle and trocar injury during laparoscopic surgery in Japan. Surg Endosc. 1997;11(12):1198–201.
15. Green BL, Marshall HC, Collinson F, Quirke P, Guillou P, Jayne DG, et al. Long-term follow-up of the Medical Research Council CLASICC trial of conventional versus laparoscopically assisted resection in colorectal cancer. Br J Surg. 2013;100(1):75–82.
16. Fleshman J, Sargent DJ, Green E, Anvari M, Stryker SJ, Beart RW, et al. Laparoscopic colectomy for cancer is not inferior to open surgery based on 5-year data from the COST study group trial. Ann Surg. 2007;246(4):655–62.
17. Clancy C, O'Leary DP, Burke JP, Redmond HP, Coffey JC, Kerin MJ, et al. A meta-analysis to determine the oncological implications of conversion in laparoscopic colorectal cancer surgery. Color Dis. 2015;17(6):482–90.

18. Tekkis PP, Senagore AJ, Delaney CP, Fazio VW. Evaluation of the learning curve in laparoscopic colorectal surgery: comparison of right-sided and left-sided resections. Ann Surg. 2005;242(1):83–91.
19. Jayne DG, Thorpe HC, Copeland J, Quirke P, Brown JM, Guillou PJ. Five-year follow-up of the Medical Research Council CLASICC trial of laparoscopically assisted versus open surgery for colorectal cancer. Br J Surg. 2010;97(11):1638–45.
20. Jeong SY, Park JW, Nam BH, Kim S, Kang SB, Lim SB, et al. Open versus laparoscopic surgery for mid-rectal or low-rectal cancer after neoadjuvant chemoradiotherapy (COREAN trial): survival outcomes of an open-label, non-inferiority, randomized controlled trial. Lancet Oncol. 2014;15(7):767–74.
21. Fleshman J, Branda M, Sargent DJ, Boller AM, George V, Abbas M, et al. Effect of laparoscopic-assisted resection vs open resection of stage II or III rectal cancer on pathologic outcomes: the ACOSOG Z6051 randomized clinical trial. JAMA. 2015;314(13):1346–55.
22. Stevenson AR, Solomon MJ, Lumley JW, Hewett P, Clouston AD, Gebski VJ, et al. Effect of laparoscopic-assisted resection vs open resection on pathological outcomes in rectal cancer: the ALaCaRT randomized clinical trial. JAMA. 2015;314(13):1356–63.
23. Veldkamp R, Kuhry E, Hop WC, Jeekel J, Kazemier G, Bonjer HJ, et al. Laparoscopic surgery versus open surgery for colon cancer: short-term outcomes of a randomized trial. Lancet Oncol. 2005;6(7):477–84.
24. Bonjer HJ, Hop WC, Nelson H, Sargent DJ, Lacy AM, Castells A, et al. Laparoscopically assisted vs open colectomy for colon cancer: a meta-analysis. Arch Surg. 2007;142(3):298–303.
25. Delaney CP, Chang E, Senagore AJ, Broder M. Clinical outcomes and resource utilization associated with laparoscopic and open colectomy using a large national database. Ann Surg. 2008;247(5):819–24.
26. Siddiqui MR, Sajid MS, Khatri K, Cheek E, Baiq MK. Elective open versus laparoscopic sigmoid colectomy for diverticular disease: a meta-analysis with the Sigma trial. World J Surg. 2010;34(12):2883–901.
27. McCombie AM, Frizelle F, Bagshaw PF, Framptom CM, Hewett PJ, McMurrick PJ, et al. The ALCCaS trial: a randomized controlled trial comparing quality of life following laparoscopic versus open colectomy for colon cancer. Dis Colon Rectum. 2018;61(10):1156–62.

32 Laparoscopic Colorectal Surgery in the Obese and Morbidly Obese Patient: Preoperative Strategies and Surgical Techniques

Matthew T. Brady and Joseph C. Carmichael

Introduction and Rationale

Obesity is described by the Center for Disease Control and Prevention (CDC) as being common, serious, and costly. With a prevalence of 39.8% between 2015 and 2016 in the United States (US) and an estimated 93.3 million affected adults, obesity is a diagnosis all health-care professionals will encounter frequently [1]. Furthermore, obesity is a risk factor for the development of colorectal adenomas and carcinomas [2–4], Clinicians performing colon and rectal surgery must have a plan in place for surgery in obese patients. The surgical care of obese patients presents challenges to the individual surgeon. Surgery on patients affected by obesity can be more technically challenging resulting in longer operative times and increased complication rates [5–7]. With these challenges, along with an overall increased requirement for medical care associated with obesity-related comorbidities, it is not surprising that per capita medical spending is on average $1429 higher per year for obese patients [8].

Obesity is defined by the CDC as having a body mass index (BMI) greater than or equal to 30. Further classifications are described for stratifying patients with BMIs greater than or equal to 30: class I obese (BMI ≥ 30 and <35), class II obese (BMI ≥ 35 and <40), and class III Obese (BMI ≥ 40) [9]. Though BMI is often the most common term utilized when classifying patient outcomes with regard to

M. T. Brady (✉) · J. C. Carmichael
Division of Colon and Rectal Surgery, Department of Surgery, University of California at Irvine, Orange, CA, USA
e-mail: mtbrady@uci.edu; jcarmich@uci.edu

P. Sylla et al. (eds.), *The SAGES Manual of Colorectal Surgery*,
https://doi.org/10.1007/978-3-030-24812-3_32

weight, some have argued that other factors, specifically visceral fat, may be even more predictive [10]. Whichever classification is used, it is important to identify obesity preoperatively, consider its effect on the planned surgery, adjust the operative plan as needed, and counsel the patient accordingly as to potential increased risks.

While minimally invasive surgery may provide advantages for obese patients considering colorectal surgery, obesity remains a risk factor for many postoperative complications and creates technical challenges for the surgeon [11, 12]. Overall obese patients have longer operative times, higher rates of postoperative morbidity, and higher rates of anastomotic leak when compared with nonobese cohorts [13]. Patient outcomes in complex operations, such as ileal pouch-anal anastomosis, are also significantly worse in obese patients when compared with nonobese, with obesity being described as an independent risk factor for pouch-related complications [14]. Considering the increased rates of postoperative complications in obese patients, as well as increased costs of caring for those complications, a plan for preoperative weight loss may be advantageous in obese patients, though it is important to keep in mind that many disorders in the field of colon and rectal surgery cannot be delayed to allow for significant preoperative weight loss. Colon and rectal cancer, for example, require timely definitive treatment in order to best care for the patient. Additionally, complications arising from inflammatory bowel disease, both Crohn's and ulcerative colitis, often require prompt surgical intervention. Consideration for preoperative weight loss can occur in others though, for example, those with polyposis syndromes and patients with medically managed IBD considering future resections for long-term management of their disease. Currently, there is no literature investigating the use of weight loss surgery prior to planned colorectal resections.

In this chapter, we will review minimally invasive surgery techniques for colon and rectal surgery and prior literature that highlights the use of minimally invasive surgery in the treatment of colorectal disease and specifically highlight the technical challenges presented by obesity and strategies aimed to minimize complications.

Indications and Contraindications of Minimally Invasive Surgery in Obese Patients and Principles and Quality Benchmarks

Indications for surgery in colon and rectal surgery are similar regardless of the approach used, whether laparoscopic, robotic, or open. Each technique has its advantages and disadvantages. The choice of technique rests largely with the skill set of the surgeon along with the capabilities of the operating room. Additionally, disease pathology and anatomic considerations can weigh heavily into the choice of technique. Principles of laparoscopic colorectal surgery are not unique and mirror the principles of open surgery. For example, when approaching colon cancer cases, performing an R0 resection with an appropriate lymphadenectomy is essential. When considering rectal cancer, adhering to the principles of total mesorectal excision (TME) is critical regardless of the approach used. In all cases, careful attention is paid to meticulous dissection, maintaining an adequate blood supply to the preserved intestine, and proper anastomotic construction. Minimally invasive techniques in colorectal surgery have been shown to be as efficacious in treatment of colon and rectal cancer when compared to open techniques. No differences in oncologic outcomes have been seen in colon cancer when comparing laparoscopic and open techniques [15, 16]. Similarly, in rectal cancer, multiple trials have shown no significant differences between the two techniques with regard to local recurrence or survival [17, 18]. If there is concern during surgery that a quality resection cannot be achieved minimally invasively, this should prompt conversion to an open surgery.

Two recent trials were not able to designate laparoscopic approach non-inferior compared with open surgery with respect to immediate pathologic outcome; however, similar to prior studies, long-term follow-up did not demonstrate differences with regard to disease-free survival or recurrence [19–21]. Laparoscopic techniques have also been associated with improved outcomes for patients with Crohn's and ulcerative colitis [22]. Given the challenges of operating in the pelvis, conversion to open has been higher when comparing laparoscopic proctectomy with colectomy. In select patients, specifically obese and male patients, use of a robotic surgery platform has been associated with decreased rates of conversion [23]. Its use produces similar outcomes when compared with laparoscopic proctectomy when performed by surgeons proficient in either technique. Again, the indications for surgery, and principles adhered to, do not differ between laparoscopic, robotic, and open surgery. Not surprisingly, open surgery has not been shown to be superior to minimally invasive approaches in colon and rectal surgery. Given the many patient-derived benefits using a minimally invasive approach, it should be considered when appropriate.

Preoperative Planning, Patient Work-Up, and Optimization

Preoperative assessment of patients undergoing colon and rectal surgery focuses on the disease being treated and the patient as a whole. Obesity remains a risk factor for many other systemic diseases including hypertension, diabetes, ventricular hypertrophy, cardiac failure, obstructive sleep apnea, and overall decreases in respiratory function [24]. Careful attention to their preoperative functional capacity and medical history should help guide preoperative evaluation and optimization. Proper communication with the anesthesia team preoperatively can also help in their preoperative planning and intraoperative strategy.

Enhanced recovery after surgery (ERAS) protocols are not contraindicated in obese patients. Attention should be paid to their individual comorbidities. Of particular interest to ERAS, obese patients have been shown to have the same gastric emptying characteristics as nonobese patients [25]. Obese patients can have high rates of insulin resistance or diabetes. Postoperative insulin resistance is improved with administration of preoperative oral carbohydrates [26]. For patients with insulin resistance, it is important to continue their diabetic medications when preoperative carbohydrate loading is employed to avoid preoperative hyperglycemia.

Patients should be appropriately screened for medical comorbidities preoperatively. Screening for cardiac disease can be difficult in the obese. Symptoms such as dyspnea on exertion can be related to weight as opposed to poor cardiac or pulmonary function. Physical exam findings such as jugular venous distension and lower extremity edema can also be masked. Obese patients may have decreased physical exercise tolerance as a result of their increased weight. All patients should be screened for their risk of perioperative cardiovascular morbidity. Assessment tools such as the Revised Cardiac Risk Index (RCRI) and the Duke Activity Status Index (DASI) can help identify patients who would benefit from preoperative cardiac testing if it will impact management [27]. Obese patients with no risk factors may not require further testing.

Obese patients can have respiratory dysfunction. Obesity results in an increased work of breathing as a result of increased airway resistance and reduced respiratory compliance [28]. Screening for obstructive sleep apnea is important in the patient cohort as it has been shown to decrease intensive care unit admissions postoperatively in obese patients [29]. The snoring, tiredness, observed apnea, high blood pressure, BMI, age, neck circumference, and male gender (STOP-BANG) questionnaire is once effective screening tool to identify patients at risk for sleep apnea who would benefit from preoperative testing as they may require continuous positive airway pressure (CPAP) postoperatively.

Trendelenburg positioning is common in colorectal resections and has the potential to exacerbate poor respiratory compliance by increased load on the diaphragms intraoperatively. Inability to tolerate Trendelenburg positioning may be a reason to convert to an open surgery or delay surgery in non-urgent cases. While increased conversion rates have been described in obese patients undergoing laparoscopic colorectal surgery, the majority of these conversions are described to be due to operative factors such as adhesions, visualization, and tumor invasiveness as opposed to ability to tolerate Trendelenburg positioning [30]. Gradual positioning changes can help ensure the patient does not slide on the bed due to their increased weight and maintains adequate ventilation. Communication with the anesthesia team during positioning is critical in these cases in order to optimize outcomes.

With regard to disease-focused preoperative planning, it is critical to ensure patients are adequately prepared for the operating room. Malignant diseases, colon and rectal cancer, require the appropriate staging work-ups consisting of chest, abdomen, and pelvis computed tomography (CT) scans, serum CEA assessment, and locoregional staging of the pelvis for rectal cancer. Magnetic resonance imaging (MRI) is the preferred modality for assessment of locoregional disease in rectal cancer and best assesses the need for neoadjuvant therapy [31]. Obtaining an MRI can potentially be challenging in some obese patients due to table weight limitations and aperture diameter [32]. Open MRI may be able to accommodate patients, though image resolution can be poorer compared with closed MRI [32]. In patients who cannot undergo a staging MRI, endorectal ultrasound, while less accurate, should be performed [33].

In certain cases, a conversation regarding preoperative weight loss should be held when considering elective cases where patients can delay their colon surgery. As is well described in the bariatric surgery literature, weight loss by diet alone or by pharmaceutical means is relatively ineffective when compared with bariatric surgery [34]. Additionally, beyond weight loss, bariatric surgery has the benefit of providing resolution of many associated comorbidities. While there is an emerging body of literature in support of "prehabilitation" prior to colorectal surgery [35], prehabilitation research focuses on increasing a patient's functional capacity in the few weeks prior to surgery and not intentional preoperative weight loss. The effect of intentional preoperative weight loss prior to colon and rectal surgery to improve outcomes has not been studied, though benefits have been seen in the transplant literature where there is some limited evidence for using bariatric surgery as a bridge to cardiac transplantation in patients with advanced heart failure and morbid obesity [36]. While having patients undergo bariatric surgery prior to colon resection is not well described in the literature, given how much obesity can impact postoperative patient outcomes, both in the short and long term, referral to a weight loss surgery specialist seems reasonable in non-urgent cases. Additionally, referral patterns for bariatric surgery can vary widely; despite the known benefits, some studies have demonstrated very low rates of bariatric surgery referrals by primary care physicians [37]. Having a discussion with patients preoperatively regarding weight loss surgery may be the first opportunity they have had to consider the opportunity to undergo bariatric surgery.

An increased risk of venous thromboembolism (VTE) has been associated with obesity in some series, though this finding is not consistent in literature focusing on postoperative complications in obese and nonobese patients [38]. *The American Society of Colon and Rectal Surgeons Clinical Practice Guidelines for the Prevention of Venous Thromboembolic Disease in Colorectal Surgery* offers multiple strategies aimed at decreased VTE risk [39]. Obesity is noted as a risk factor for VTE in those guidelines. Early mobility and the use of pharmacological thromboprophylaxis are also strongly recommended for patients who are moderate to high risk for VTE and not high risk for bleeding complications. Also, consideration of high-risk patients for an extended VTE prophylaxis regimen following discharge is also strongly recommended.

Operative Technique: Surgical Steps

Numerous strategies and approaches for laparoscopic colectomy exist; the authors present their preferred strategies which highlight a totally laparoscopic approach. This approach avoids the use of a hand port, involves performing an intracorporeal anastomosis, and allows the surgeon to preferentially use a Pfannenstiel incision in order to minimize the risk of postoperative incisional hernia.

Laparoscopic Right Colectomy

The patient is positioned in either supine or lithotomy depending on the indications for surgery and the surgeon's preference. Some surgeons advocate for lithotomy position because they are able to stand between the legs during mesenteric mobilization; however, in a morbidly obese patient, this may not be possible. If the indication for surgery is an ileocolectomy for Crohn's disease, lithotomy may be the preferred position so that an unanticipated ileo-sigmoid fistula could be more easily addressed by allowing transanal anastomotic stapling if needed. Given that obesity and lithotomy position appear to be risk factors for peripheral motor nerve injury in colorectal surgery [40], we place obese patients in the supine position whenever possible. If lithotomy is required, it is imperative to ensure all pressure points are adequately padded (Fig. 32.1). Generally, both arms are tucked at the patient's sides; however, in the morbidly obese patient, sometimes it is only possible to tuck the patient's left arm, and it needs to be left outstretched; alternatively, an arm sled can be used. Pressure points are padded, and we prefer to have the patient on a soft foam or egg crate that is fixed to the table. This helps to create a "friction hold" between the patient's back and the table when using steep Trendelenburg position and should minimize pressure points that could lead to

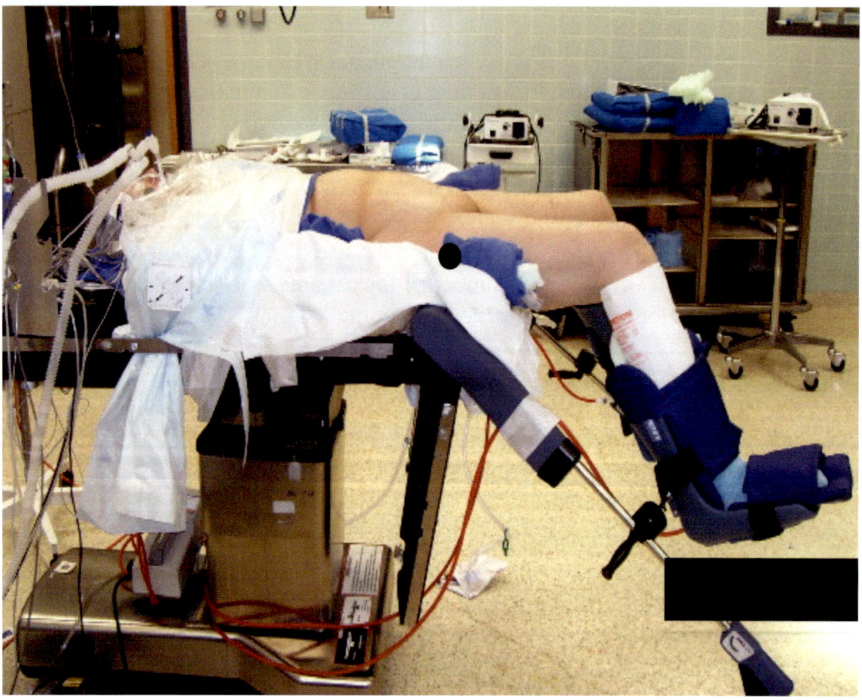

Fig. 32.1 Lithotomy position

nerve injury. We also employ padded straps around the patient's thighs (in supine position) and chest to minimize sliding during extreme table tilt. Additional padding behind the shoulders can further prevent sliding of the patient in Trendelenburg position (Fig. 32.2).

For laparoscopic right colectomy, a Veress needle insertion is used at Palmer's point in the left upper quadrant to gain insufflation. We utilize a four-port laparoscopic technique, but even within our practice, some variation in port placement does occur. In general, the laparoscopic ports should be separated by 10–12 cm. Figure 32.3 depicts a typical port placement scenario. Initially, a trocar is placed in the center of the abdomen equidistant from the pubic symphysis and the xiphoid process. Trocar size at this location will depend on the surgeon's preference regarding camera size (5 vs. 10 mm). The lower midline port is placed 10–12 cm below the central camera port, and sometimes there is the opportunity to place this through the intended Pfannenstiel extraction site. The left lower quadrant port is placed between the camera port and the anterior superior iliac spine. Finally, the left upper quadrant 5 mm port is placed (Fig. 32.3). In this port arrangement, the left lower quadrant 12 mm port site can also be enlarged for specimen extraction depending on the preference of the surgeon.

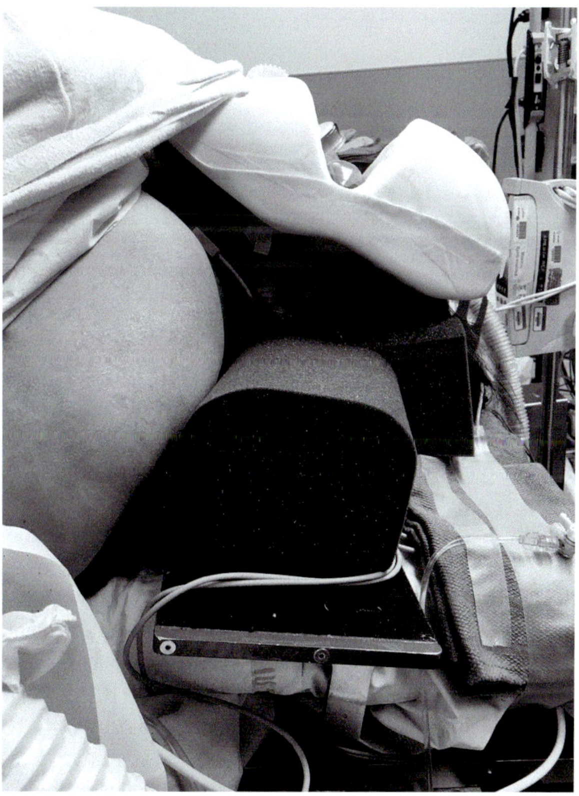

Fig. 32.2 Shoulder support during laparoscopic surgery

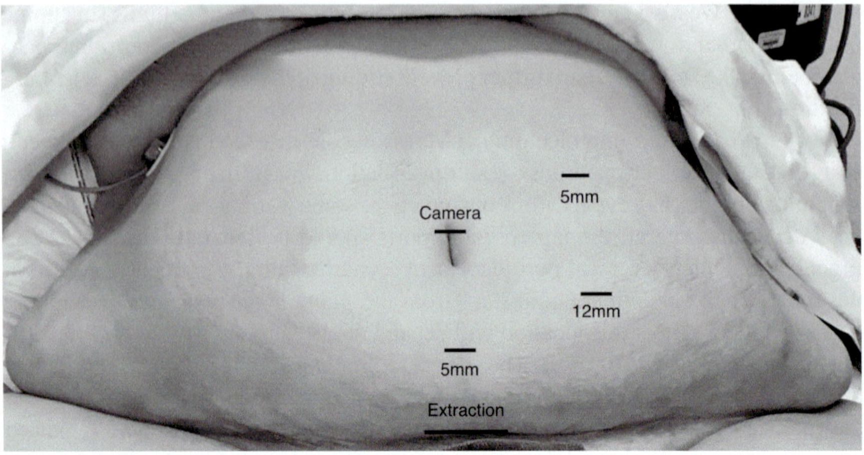

Fig. 32.3 Right colectomy port placement

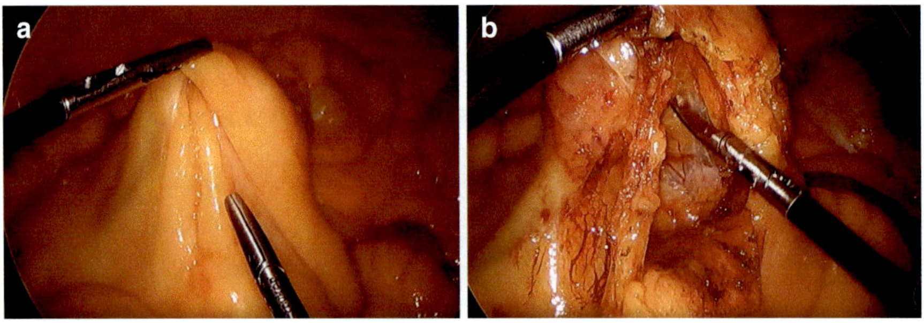

Fig. 32.4 (**a**, **b**). Medial to lateral approach: the mesentery is scored below the ileocolic pedicle (**a**), and the retromesenteric plane is dissected bluntly (**b**) (Both: Courtesy of Daniel Popowich, MD)

The patient is placed in Trendelenburg position with the left side down. The small bowel is swept to the patients left to expose the ileocolic pedicle which is further defined by having the assistant elevate the cecum anteriorly and inferiorly. For a medial to lateral approach, the mesentery is scored below the ileocolic pedicle, and the plane is developed bluntly to separate the mesocolon from the retroperitoneum (Fig. 32.4a, b). The duodenum is identified and protected, and the ileocolic pedicle is divided (Fig. 32.5a, b). The omentum is then freed from the transverse colon, and the hepatic flexure is taken down from a medial to lateral fashion. Finally, the white line of Toldt is released, and the ileal mesentery is freed from its posterior attachments. The mesentery of the transverse colon and ileum are divided with the energy device and the bowel divided with laparoscopic staplers.

We prefer an intracorporeal anastomosis (ICA) in all patients, and evidence suggests that ICA in obese patients is associated with a reduced risk of postoperative incisional hernia presumably because the specimen is not being removed via a midline incision [41]. For the intracorporeal anastomosis, multiple techniques can be

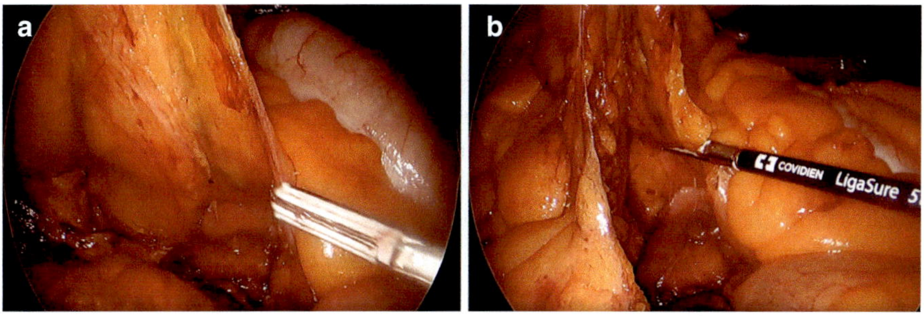

Fig. 32.5 (**a**, **b**) Medial to lateral approach: the second portion of the duodenum is visualized and serves as an anatomic landmark (**a**). The ileocolic pedicle is subsequently divided (**b**) (Both: Courtesy of Daniel Popowich, MD)

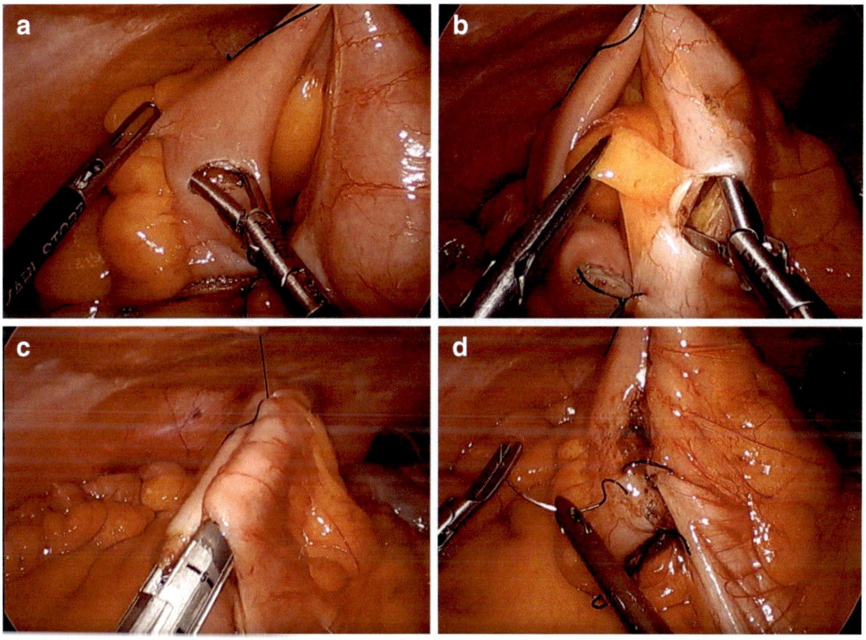

Fig. 32.6 (**a–d**) Laparoscopic stapled intracorporeal anastomosis following right hemicolectomy (All: Courtesy of Daniel Popowich, MD)

applied. The anastomosis can be set up antiperistaltic or isoperistaltic. In both techniques, the ends of the colon and ileum are aligned side by side. Enterotomies are created in the ileum and colon using a hook electrocautery. The laparoscopic stapler is used to create a common channel. For closure of the common enterotomy, an additional staple fire can be used; this technique is reproducible, is reliable, and mirrors the open technique of a totally stapled side-to-side anastomosis. Alternatively, the common enterotomy can be closed with sutures (Fig. 32.6a–d). An intracorporeal handsewn closure of the common enterotomy is also effective and has the benefit of cost savings compared with stapled closure.

Once the anastomosis is complete, a small Pfannenstiel incision is made, and the specimen is extracted through a wound protector. Alternatively, the left lower quadrant port site may be enlarged via a muscle splitting incision and the specimen removed via that site. Please refer to Chap. 14 on options for ileocolonic reconstruction for more details on various anastomotic techniques.

Laparoscopic Left Colectomy

For left colectomy, the room is set up to facilitate all personnel and provide access to the rectum. Abdominal insufflation is again gained through a Veress needle technique. The camera port placement is identical to what is described above. The 12 mm port is placed now 10–12 cm from the camera port on a diagonal line from the camera to the right anterior superior iliac spine. Five millimeter ports are next placed 10–12 cm from the camera port in the right upper quadrant midclavicular line and superior midline below the xiphoid process (Fig. 32.7).

Next, the dissection can begin either above or below the level of the inferior mesenteric artery (IMA). The authors prefer to begin above the level of the IMA at the inferior mesenteric vein (IMV). The dissection is begun by incising the peritoneum just below the IMV, which is found adjacent to the ligament of Treitz (Fig. 32.8). Again, blunt dissection is used to separate the mesocolon from the retroperitoneum. As the dissection progresses, the IMV is clipped and divided which will allow for complete mobilization of the splenic flexure. The attachments of the splenic flexure are released in a medial to lateral fashion as well. This is performed by dissecting over the anterior surface of the pancreas and entering the lesser sac.

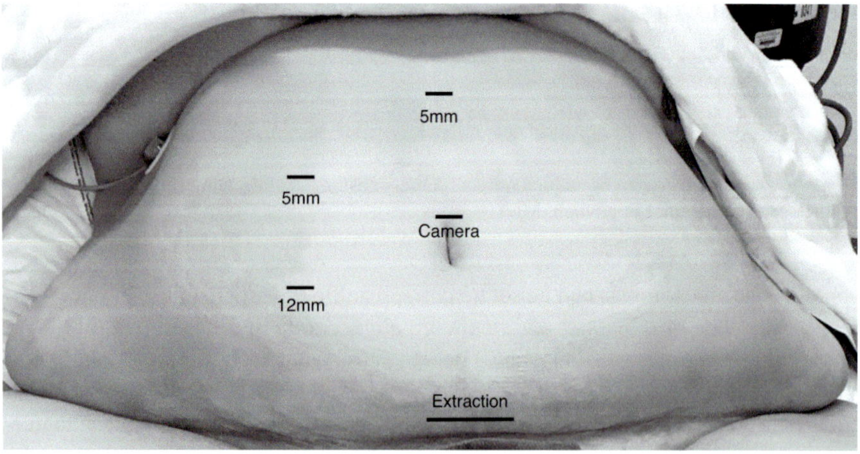

Fig. 32.7 Left colectomy port placement

Anecdotally, we have found that this seems to be an easier approach to splenic flexure mobilization in obese patients; however, care must be taken not to open a plane posterior to the pancreas and risk splenic vein injury. All attachments of the distal transverse colon and splenic flexure can be safely divided with this technique.

The dissection is next moved to below the level of the IMA. The sigmoid colon is elevated to the abdominal wall and the IMA put on stretch to aid in identification. The mesentery below the IMA is scored from the IMA to the sacral promontory and blunt dissection again utilized to free the mesocolon from the retroperitoneum (Fig. 32.9a, b). Here, the ureter and gonadal vessels must be identified prior to IMA division. Following division of the IMA, the white line of Toldt is incised to release the colon from the abdominal wall, and the omentum is elevated off the transverse colon as needed. The mesorectum and rectum are divided intracorporeally as this

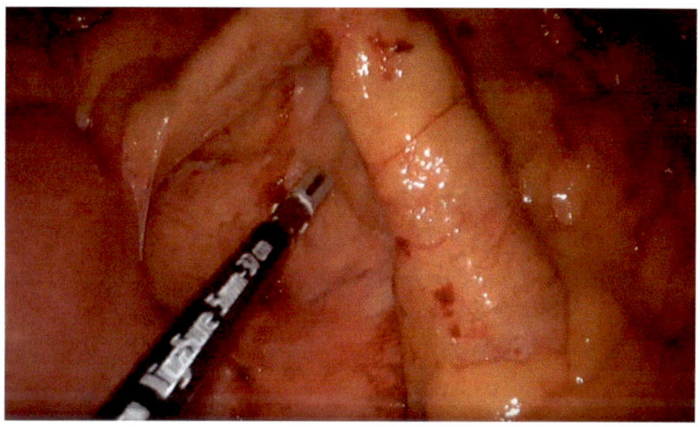

Fig. 32.8 Dissection under the inferior mesenteric vein in an obese patient (Courtesy of Daniel Popowich, MD)

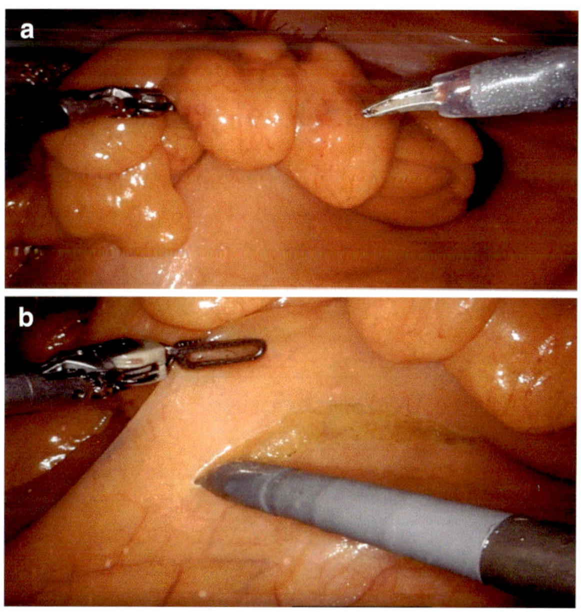

Fig. 32.9 (**a**, **b**) Medial to lateral approach: the rectosigmoid mesentery is retracted superiorly (**a**), and the mesentery below the IMA is scored starting just above the sacral promontory (**b**) (Both: Courtesy of Daniel Popowich, MD)

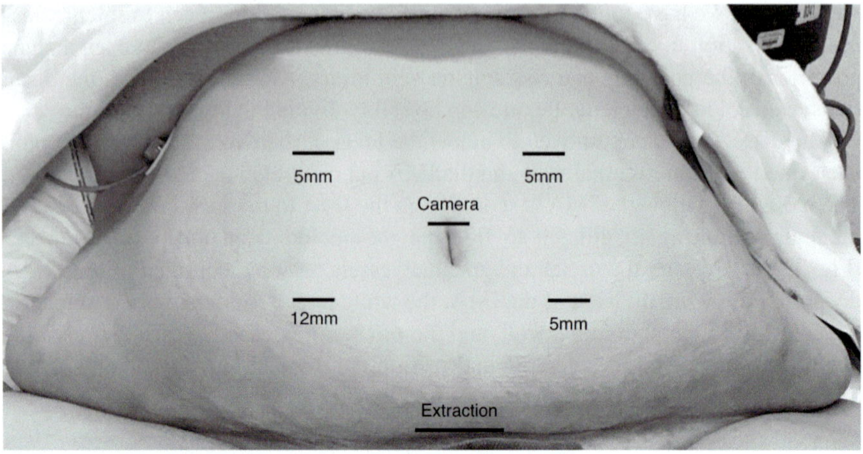

Fig. 32.10 Total colectomy port placement

approach is straightforward, and this can be very challenging to perform extracorporeally via the Pfannenstiel incision in obese patients. Similarly, the proximal mesocolon is divided intracorporeally as this would also be very challenging to divide extracorporeally via the Pfannenstiel incision in an obese patient.

A Pfannenstiel extraction site is created, a wound protector placed, and the distal end of the specimen is brought out. Field isolation is employed, and the colon is divided at the proximal margin extracorporeally. An anvil is secured in the proximal colon, and it is returned to the abdomen. Next, a transanal circular stapler is used to anastomose the colon and rectum. Flexible endoscopy is used to test the anastomosis for bleeding and air leak testing.

Laparoscopic Total Colectomy

For laparoscopic total colectomy, our ports are typically placed in a box configuration as depicted in Fig. 32.10. This configuration allows for access to all four abdominal quadrants, allows for both the surgeon and assistant to work simultaneously, and is similar to port placements for both the right and left laparoscopic colectomies.

Pitfalls and Troubleshooting

Port Placement

Laparoscopic colectomy often involves working in multiple quadrants within the abdomen (Fig. 32.11). Improper port placement can severely limit your ability to access each quadrant of the abdomen without undue stress put on the

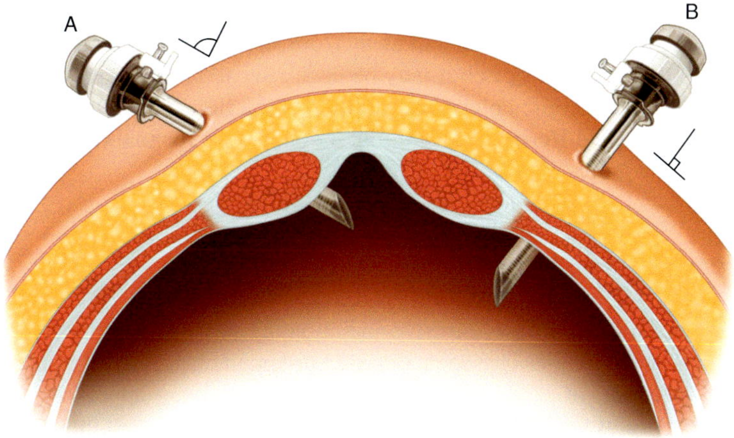

Fig. 32.11 Proper port placement

patient's abdominal wall as well as the surgeon. It is critical to consider the trajectory of the laparoscopic port during placement. The patient's abdomen exists as a dome once insufflated; the surgeon's goal should be to have their port placement be exactly perpendicular to the skin and abdominal wall at the point of insertion. This insertion results in the least amount of trauma to surrounding tissue and the most ergonomic positioning for working in multiple quadrants within the abdomen. One technique that can help achieve this positioning is to push trocars directly forward until the tip of the trocar engages the fascia. After that, it is appropriate to begin twisting motion required of spreading trocars for insertion. Twisting prior to engaging the fascia can often result in skiving tangentially in the subcutaneous fat prior to engaging the fascia. It is easier to skive the trocar in obese patients given the greater distance between the skin and abdominal wall.

Identification of Anatomic Landmarks

Proper identification of vascular landmarks and critical structures such as the ureters is essential for successfully completing a laparoscopic or open colectomy. However, obesity can challenge identification of these landmarks secondary to a thickened and shortened mesentery. Indeed, some studies have shown that it is the presence of excessive visceral fat, rather than BMI, that is highly predictive of postoperative complications in colon resection [42, 43]. Furthermore, men tend to carry the obesity in the mesentery rather than the subcutaneous tissue [44]. This can generally make for a more challenging colon resection. In the event it is difficult to expose a given vascular pedicle, i.e., the ileocolic pedicle, inferior mesenteric vein, or inferior mesenteric artery, the surgeon should always review factors that can assist exposure. Proper bed positioning can often be critical for exposing vascular anatomy. Proper positioning will allow the small bowel to fall away from structures of interests. Adequate assistance is also critical, often it may be necessary to use an extra 5 mm assistant port for laparoscopic colectomy to aid in retraction. Those two factors can often make a large difference in avoiding a conversion for inability to progress during a laparoscopic colectomy.

Failure to Progress

If in the course of a minimally invasive operation the surgeon determines that there has been failure to progress based on disease burden, unclear anatomy, unfavorable anatomy, bleeding, or other factors, conversion to an open approach is recommended. Advocates for hand-assisted laparoscopy (HALS) suggest this may reduce the risk of conversion to an open surgery. With regard to HALS in obese patients, a retrospective single-center study did demonstrate a decreased conversion to open procedure in patients, BMI > 30, undergoing hand-assisted laparoscopy when compared with conventional laparoscopic resection [45]. Subgroup analysis in that study demonstrated this benefit was only statistically significant in patients undergoing right colectomy. Interestingly, differences in conversion rate did not reach statistical significance in the left colectomy, sigmoid colectomy, total colectomy, proctocolectomy, low-anterior resection, or abdominoperineal resection subgroups.

Minimally Invasive Proctectomy: A Word of Caution

Minimally invasive total mesorectal excision in an obese male patient is generally regarded as one of the most challenging surgeries that a colorectal surgeon will face. The choice of which minimally invasive approach a surgeon should take (laparoscopic, robotic, transanal TME) depends on what the surgeon is comfortable performing and what the surgeon has the most experience in performing. In the UK Medical Research Council (MRC), trial of conventional vs. laparoscopic-assisted surgery in colorectal cancer (CLASICC), surgeons were required to have performed at least 20 laparoscopic resections to enter the study [46]. Over the study period, the rate of conversion to open surgery fell from 38% to 16% suggesting that an experience of 20 cases was not enough. Given a general surgeon in the United States performs an average of 11 colon resections annually [47], and that not all cases are candidates for laparoscopic surgery, it could take a surgeon years to gain adequate experience to perform these cases.

In addition, it has been demonstrated that the hospital experience with minimally invasive proctectomy also matters. In the Colon Cancer Laparoscopic or Open Resection (COLOR) trial, "high-volume" hospitals that performed more than 10 laparoscopic proctectomy procedures per year had a lower conversion rate compared with "low-volume" hospitals that performed fewer than five cases per year (9% conversion vs. 24% conversion) [48]. High-volume hospitals also had more lymph nodes recovered, fewer complications, shorter hospital stay, and shorter operative time independent of surgeon experience. What this means for the surgeon is that experience matters for both the individual and the institution.

As noted previously, there appears to be some evidence that robotics offers benefit over laparoscopy in obese male proctectomy patients in terms of decreased risk of conversion to open surgery [23]. At least two articles have suggested the robotic learning curve for proctectomy has three phases and could be achieved within 25 cases [49, 50]. A direct comparison of the laparoscopic proctectomy learning curve vs. the robotic proctectomy learning curve is difficult to find. However, one study from South Korea noted that while tasks like splenic flexure mobilization and IMA dissection had similar learning curves between laparoscopic and robotic surgery, TME had a shorter learning curve when performed robotically [51]. In this study, TME showed consistently shorter operative times for robotics after 22 cases. For the surgeon who is new to minimally invasive proctectomy, robotic surgery may prove to be easier to learn than a laparoscopic approach. The literature regarding transanal TME is developing, but currently it would seem prudent for this to only be performed by high-volume experts in proctectomy.

Tips and Tricks to Successful Minimally Invasive Colorectal Surgery in Obese Patients

Regarding minimally invasive proctectomy and colectomy in the obese patient, we have several recommendations for the surgeon:

1. Be clear with patients regarding your experience level. It is important to manage patients' expectations regarding the duration of surgery and risk of conversion to open surgery. As you gain experience, the duration of surgery and risk of conversion will improve.
2. Understand that obesity significantly increases the challenge of minimally invasive surgery, and these are not good learning cases, particularly in male patients who tend to have central obesity rather than subcutaneous obesity. However, extensive minimally invasive surgical experience, even if not specific to colectomy or proctectomy, is very helpful.
3. Be well prepared for a challenging case. These are not cases to perform post-call or at the end of a long operative day. Mental preparation and understanding elective conversion to open surgery in a case that is not progressing is not a failure. Reasons to convert to open include failure to identify the ureter in a left

colectomy, inability to safely retract the small bowel out of the field, and generally failure of the case to progress.

4. It may be simpler to staple the vascular pedicle rather than divide it with an energy device in a patient with obesity. For example, when performing a left colectomy for colon cancer and a high ligation of the IMA, the small bowel may be falling into the surgical field periodically. If this happens when your energy device is halfway across the IMA, it can cause significant problems. With stapling, the stapling device can be safely placed across the IMA and closed without committing to vascular ligation. Once it appears safe to staple, the surgeon can proceed. Regarding the vascular division, it is important to always reidentify the left ureter prior to vascular division.
5. When dividing the rectum intracorporeally, it is important to remember that an obese patient may require a thicker stapler load than what you are typically used to using. If the stapler is hard to close, it would be wise to select a stapler load capable of handling thicker tissue.

Outcomes

Minimally invasive approaches to colon and rectal surgery are sound strategies when considering surgery in the obese patient population. Laparoscopy has many benefits when compared with open colectomy in obese patients. These benefits include decreased hospital length of stay, decreased long-term complications, and improvement in patient postoperative quality of life [30, 52]. Obesity poses a significant risk for incisional hernia development following colorectal resection. However, laparoscopic colectomy can have decreased incisional hernia rates compared with open surgery, especially when Pfannenstiel incisions are utilized [53]. While conversion rates can be higher in obese patients compared with nonobese patients, conversion to open surgery is not associated with worse outcomes relative to patients who undergo laparotomy as a planned procedure [30].

Results from a small number of studies focusing on postoperative outcomes following laparoscopic and open colectomy are summarized in Table 32.1. They suggest that there does not appear to be any increase in anastomotic leak rate between these two techniques. Overall, minimally invasive approaches to colorectal surgery in obese patients are safe and can provide many advantages.

It is important to recognize the obvious limitations of these reports: a BMI up to 35 has become the new "baseline," and there is consensus that in the hands of experienced surgeons, the operative management and outcomes in this patient population are similar to that of normal BMI patients. The unanswered question remains whether superobesity (BMI > 40) allows for the same quality surgery as would be expected in normal BMI patients.

Table 32.1 Studies comparing outcomes between laparoscopic and open colectomy specifically in obese patients

Authors	Year	Number of patients (laparoscopic vs. open)	Definition of obesity	Operations	OR time mean (min) (laparoscopic vs. open)	Conversion rate in laparoscopic arm (%)	Overall morbidity % (laparoscopic vs. open)	Surgical site infection (laparoscopic vs. open)	Anastomotic leak (laparoscopic vs. open)	Incisional hernia %	Length of stay (mean days)
Vignali et al. [54]	2013	98 vs 98	BMI > 30 kg/m^2	Laparoscopic vs. open right and left colectomy	193 vs. 164*	13.3	27.6 vs. 33.7	8.2 vs 15.4	7.1 vs. 5.1	17.3 vs 31.6*	8 vs. 10.4*
Cai et al. [55]	2013	64 vs. 102	BMI > 28 kg/m^2	Right colectomy, left colectomy, low-anterior resection	*183* vs. *167**	4.7	NR	17 vs. 31*	5 vs 6	NR	12 vs. 15
Hardiman et al. [56]	2013	4925 vs. 6412	BMI > 30 kg/m^2	Ileocolectomy, partial colectomy with anastomosis	NR	NR	OR 0.61; 95% CI 0.55–0.67	Superficial OR 0.44 (95% CI 0.31–0.61); Deep OR 0.61 (95% CI 0.49–0.78)	NR	NR	NR
Delaney et al. [30]	2005	94 vs. 94	BMI > 30 kg/m^2	Colorectal resections	123 vs. 112	29.7	21.2 vs. 24.4	NR	2 vs. 1	NR	3.8 vs 5.8*

*$p < 0.05$; *NR* not reported, *OR* odd's ratio, *CI* confidence interval

Conclusions

Obesity rates are on the rise, and obesity is a significant risk factor for the development of colorectal adenomas and carcinomas. Therefore, the busy colon and rectal surgeon must have a strategy in place for the surgical approach to these patients. While obese patients have increased risks of complications in colon and rectal surgery, minimally invasive surgical techniques have proven benefit in obese patients in terms of wound complications, length of stay, hernia rates, and quality of life.

References

1. Hales CM, Carroll MD, Fryar CD, Ogden CL. Prevalence of obesity among adults and youth: United States, 2015–2016. NCHS Data Brief. 2017;(288):1–8.
2. Shapero TF, Chen GI, Devlin T, Gibbs A, Murray IC, Tran S, et al. Obesity increases prevalence of colonic adenomas at screening colonoscopy: a Canadian community-based study. Can J Gastroenterol Hepatol. 2017;2017:8750967.
3. Seo IK, Kim BJ, Kim B, Choi CH, Kim JW, Kim JG, et al. Abdominal fat distribution measured using computed tomography is associated with an increased risk of colorectal adenoma in men. Medicine. 2017;96(37):e8051.
4. Dong Y, Zhou J, Zhu Y, Luo L, He T, Hu H, et al. Abdominal obesity and colorectal cancer risk: systematic review and meta-analysis of prospective studies. Biosci Rep. 2017;37(6).
5. Alizadeh RF, Moghadamyeghaneh Z, Whealon MD, Hanna MH, Mills SD, Pigazzi A, et al. Body mass index significantly impacts outcomes of colorectal surgery. Am Surg. 2016;82(10):930–5.
6. He Y, Wang J, Bian H, Deng X, Wang Z. BMI as a predictor for perioperative outcome of laparoscopic colorectal surgery: a pooled analysis of comparative studies. Dis Colon Rectum. 2017;60(4):433–45.
7. Poelemeijer YQM, Lijftogt N, Detering R, Fiocco M, Tollenaar R, Wouters M. Obesity as a determinant of perioperative and postoperative outcome in patients following colorectal cancer surgery: a population-based study (2009–2016). Eur J Surg Oncol. 2018;44(12):1849–57.
8. Finkelstein EA, Trogdon JG, Cohen JW, Dietz W. Annual medical spending attributable to obesity: payer-and service-specific estimates. Health Aff (Millwood). 2009;28(5):w822–31.
9. Available from: https://www.cdc.gov/obesity/adult/defining.html.
10. Tsujinaka S, Konishi F, Kawamura YJ, Saito M, Tajima N, Tanaka O, et al. Visceral obesity predicts surgical outcomes after laparoscopic colectomy for sigmoid colon cancer. Dis Colon Rectum. 2008;51(12):1757–65; discussion 65–7.
11. Amri R, Bordeianou LG, Sylla P, Berger DL. Obesity, outcomes and quality of care: body mass index increases the risk of wound-related complications in colon cancer surgery. Am J Surg. 2014;207(1):17–23.
12. Wahl TS, Patel FC, Goss LE, Chu DI, Grams J, Morris MS. The obese colorectal surgery patient: surgical site infection and outcomes. Dis Colon Rectum. 2018;61(8):938–45.
13. Senagore AJ, Delaney CP, Madboulay K, Brady KM, Fazio VW. Laparoscopic colectomy in obese and nonobese patients. J Gastrointest Surg. 2003;7(4):558–61.
14. Klos CL, Safar B, Jamal N, Hunt SR, Wise PE, Birnbaum EH, et al. Obesity increases risk for pouch-related complications following restorative proctocolectomy with ileal pouch-anal anastomosis (IPAA). J Gastrointest Surg. 2014;18(3):573–9.
15. Clinical Outcomes of Surgical Therapy Study Group, Nelson H, Sargent DJ, Wieand HS, Fleshman J, Anvari M, et al. A comparison of laparoscopically assisted and open colectomy for colon cancer. N Engl J Med. 2004;350(20):2050–9.

16. Jayne DG, Thorpe HC, Copeland J, Quirke P, Brown JM, Guillou PJ. Five-year follow-up of the Medical Research Council CLASICC trial of laparoscopically assisted versus open surgery for colorectal cancer. Br J Surg. 2010;97(11):1638–45.
17. Jeong SY, Park JW, Nam BH, Kim S, Kang SB, Lim SB, et al. Open versus laparoscopic surgery for mid-rectal or low-rectal cancer after neoadjuvant chemoradiotherapy (COREAN trial): survival outcomes of an open-label, non-inferiority, randomised controlled trial. Lancet Oncol. 2014;15(7):767–74.
18. Bonjer HJ, Deijen CL, Abis GA, Cuesta MA, van der Pas MH, de Lange-de Klerk ES, et al. A randomized trial of laparoscopic versus open surgery for rectal cancer. N Engl J Med. 2015;372(14):1324–32.
19. Fleshman J, Branda M, Sargent DJ, Boller AM, George V, Abbas M, et al. Effect of laparoscopic-assisted resection vs open resection of stage II or III rectal cancer on pathologic outcomes: the ACOSOG Z6051 randomized clinical trial. JAMA. 2015;314(13):1346–55.
20. Stevenson AR, Solomon MJ, Lumley JW, Hewett P, Clouston AD, Gebski VJ, et al. Effect of laparoscopic-assisted resection vs open resection on pathological outcomes in rectal cancer: the ALaCaRT randomized clinical trial. JAMA. 2015;314(13):1356–63.
21. Fleshman J, Branda ME, Sargent DJ, Boller AM, George VV, Abbas MA, et al. Disease-free survival and local recurrence for laparoscopic resection compared with open resection of stage II to III rectal cancer: follow-up results of the ACOSOG Z6051 randomized controlled trial. Ann Surg. 2019;269(4):589–95.
22. Tan JJ, Tjandra JJ. Laparoscopic surgery for Crohn's disease: a meta-analysis. Dis Colon Rectum. 2007;50(5):576–85.
23. Jayne D, Pigazzi A, Marshall H, Croft J, Corrigan N, Copeland J, et al. Effect of robotic-assisted vs conventional laparoscopic surgery on risk of conversion to open laparotomy among patients undergoing resection for rectal cancer: the ROLARR randomized clinical trial. JAMA. 2017;318(16):1569–80.
24. Cullen A, Ferguson A. Perioperative management of the severely obese patient: a selective pathophysiological review. Can J Anaesth. 2012;59(10):974–96.
25. Gustafsson UO, Scott MJ, Schwenk W, Demartines N, Roulin D, Francis N, et al. Guidelines for perioperative care in elective colonic surgery: enhanced recovery after surgery (ERAS((R))) society recommendations. World J Surg. 2013;37(2):259–84.
26. Wang ZG, Wang Q, Wang WJ, Qin HL. Randomized clinical trial to compare the effects of preoperative oral carbohydrate versus placebo on insulin resistance after colorectal surgery. Br J Surg. 2010;97(3):317–27.
27. Wijeysundera DN, Pearse RM, Shulman MA, Abbott TEF, Torres E, Ambosta A, et al. Assessment of functional capacity before major non-cardiac surgery: an international, prospective cohort study. Lancet. 2018;391(10140):2631–40.
28. Hodgson LE, Murphy PB, Hart N. Respiratory management of the obese patient undergoing surgery. J Thorac Dis. 2015;7(5):943–52.
29. Hallowell PT, Stellato TA, Petrozzi MC, Schuster M, Graf K, Robinson A, et al. Eliminating respiratory intensive care unit stay after gastric bypass surgery. Surgery. 2007;142(4):608–12; discussion 12 e1.
30. Delaney CP, Pokala N, Senagore AJ, Casillas S, Kiran RP, Brady KM, et al. Is laparoscopic colectomy applicable to patients with body mass index >30? A case-matched comparative study with open colectomy. Dis Colon Rectum. 2005;48(5):975–81.
31. Group MS. Diagnostic accuracy of preoperative magnetic resonance imaging in predicting curative resection of rectal cancer: prospective observational study. BMJ. 2006;333(7572):779.
32. Tao W, Lagergren J. Clinical management of obese patients with cancer. Nat Rev Clin Oncol. 2013;10:519.
33. Garcia-Aguilar J, Pollack J, Lee SH, Hernandez de Anda E, Mellgren A, Wong WD, et al. Accuracy of endorectal ultrasonography in preoperative staging of rectal tumors. Dis Colon Rectum. 2002;45(1):10–5.
34. Buchwald H, Avidor Y, Braunwald E, Jensen MD, Pories W, Fahrbach K, et al. Bariatric surgery: a systematic review and meta-analysis. JAMA. 2004;292(14):1724–37.

35. Mayo NE, Feldman L, Scott S, Zavorsky G, Kim DJ, Charlebois P, et al. Impact of preoperative change in physical function on postoperative recovery: argument supporting prehabilitation for colorectal surgery. Surgery. 2011;150(3):505–14.
36. Lim C-P, Fisher OM, Falkenback D, Boyd D, Hayward CS, Keogh A, et al. Bariatric surgery provides a "bridge to transplant" for morbidly obese patients with advanced heart failure and may obviate the need for transplantation. Obes Surg. 2016;26(3):486–93.
37. Avidor Y, Still CD, Brunner M, Buchwald JN, Buchwald H. Primary care and subspecialty management of morbid obesity: referral patterns for bariatric surgery. Surg Obes Relat Dis. 2007;3(3):392–407.
38. Geiger TM, Muldoon R. Complications following colon rectal surgery in the obese patient. Clin Colon Rectal Surg. 2011;24(4):274–82.
39. Fleming F, Gaertner W, Ternent CA, Finlayson E, Herzig D, Paquette IM, et al. The American Society of Colon and Rectal Surgeons clinical practice guideline for the prevention of venous thromboembolic disease in colorectal surgery. Dis Colon Rectum. 2018;61(1):14–20.
40. Al-Temimi MH, Chandrasekaran B, Phelan MJ, Pigazzi A, Mills SD, Stamos MJ, et al. Incidence, risk factors, and trends of motor peripheral nerve injury after colorectal surgery: analysis of the National Surgical Quality Improvement Program Database. Dis Colon Rectum. 2017;60(3):318–25.
41. Vignali A, Elmore U, Lemma M, Guarnieri G, Radaelli G, Rosati R. Intracorporeal versus extracorporeal anastomoses following laparoscopic right colectomy in obese patients: a case-matched study. Dig Surg. 2018;35(3):236–42.
42. Kuritzkes BA, Pappou EP, Kiran RP, Baser O, Fan L, Guo X, et al. Visceral fat area, not body mass index, predicts postoperative 30-day morbidity in patients undergoing colon resection for cancer. Int J Color Dis. 2018;33(8):1019–28.
43. Cecchini S, Cavazzini E, Marchesi F, Sarli L, Roncoroni L. Computed tomography volumetric fat parameters versus body mass index for predicting short-term outcomes of colon surgery. World J Surg. 2011;35(2):415–23.
44. Maurovich-Horvat P, Massaro J, Fox CS, Moselewski F, O'Donnell CJ, Hoffmann U. Comparison of anthropometric, area- and volume-based assessment of abdominal subcutaneous and visceral adipose tissue volumes using multi-detector computed tomography. Int J Obes. 2007;31(3):500–6.
45. Heneghan HM, Martin ST, Kiran RP, Khoury W, Stocchi L, Remzi FH, et al. Laparoscopic colorectal surgery for obese patients: decreased conversions with the hand-assisted technique. J Gastrointest Surg. 2013;17(3):548–54.
46. Guillou PJ, Quirke P, Thorpe H, Walker J, Jayne DG, Smith AMH, et al. Short-term endpoints of conventional versus laparoscopic-assisted surgery in patients with colorectal cancer (MRC CLASICC trial): multicentre, randomised controlled trial. Lancet. 2005;365(9472):1718–26.
47. Hyman N. How much colorectal surgery do general surgeons do? J Am Coll Surg. 2002;194(1):37–9.
48. Group CS. Impact of hospital case volume on short-term outcome after laparoscopic operation for colonic cancer. Surg Endosc. 2005;19(5):687–92.
49. Bokhari MB, Patel CB, Ramos-Valadez DI, Ragupathi M, Haas EM. Learning curve for robotic-assisted laparoscopic colorectal surgery. Surg Endosc. 2011;25(3):855–60.
50. Foo CC, Law WL. The learning curve of robotic-assisted low rectal resection of a novice rectal surgeon. World J Surg. 2016;40(2):456–62.
51. Melich G, Hong YK, Kim J, Hur H, Baik SH, Kim NK, et al. Simultaneous development of laparoscopy and robotics provides acceptable perioperative outcomes and shows robotics to have a faster learning curve and to be overall faster in rectal cancer surgery: analysis of novice MIS surgeon learning curves. Surg Endosc. 2015;29(3):558–68.
52. Braga M, Frasson M, Vignali A, Zuliani W, Civelli V, Di Carlo V. Laparoscopic vs. open colectomy in cancer patients: long-term complications, quality of life, and survival. Dis Colon Rectum. 2005;48(12):2217–23.

53. Singh R, Omiccioli A, Hegge S, McKinley CJSE. Does the extraction-site location in laparoscopic colorectal surgery have an impact on incisional hernia rates? Surg Endosc. 2008;22(12):2596–600.
54. Vignali A, De Nardi P, Ghirardelli L, Di Palo S, Staudacher C. Short and long-term outcomes of laparoscopic colectomy in obese patients. World J Gastroenterol. 2013;19(42):7405–11.
55. Cai Y, Zhou Y, Li Z, Xiang J, Chen Z. Surgical outcome of laparoscopic colectomy for colorectal cancer in obese patients: a comparative study with open colectomy. Oncol Lett. 2013;6(4):1057–62.
56. Hardiman K, Chang ET, Diggs BS, Lu KC. Laparoscopic colectomy reduces morbidity and mortality in obese patients. Surg Endosc. 2013;27(8):2907–10.

Part VI

Other Colorectal Resections and Advanced Techniques

33 The Challenge of the Transverse Colon Tumor: Laparoscopic Techniques and Strategies

Izi Obokhare and Kelly A. Garrett

Introduction and Rationale

Laparoscopic techniques for colon cancer resections have significant benefits over open techniques as evidenced by earlier return of bowel function, shorter length of stay, and reduced postoperative pain. In recent years, enhanced recovery after surgery (ERAS) protocols have dramatically changed the perioperative care of surgical patients by reducing morbidity and mortality while at the same time reducing healthcare cost and patient length of stay. The incidence of transverse colon and splenic flexure tumors is lower than that of right- and left-sided colon cancer. At the same time, the prognosis of transverse colon tumors is also significantly poorer compared to left-sided and right-sided colon cancers. The reason for this difference is not completely known; however, it is postulated that due to the late presentation of symptoms and proximity to other organs such as the stomach, liver, gallbladder, and pancreas, the symptoms are misdiagnosed. Until recently, the laparoscopic approach to transverse colon cancer had not been well studied. Previous research comparing open to laparoscopic colectomy for cancer had excluded transverse colon tumors due to the increased difficulty of laparoscopic lymph node dissection around the middle colic artery and vein, as well as the proximity of the transverse mesocolon to structures such as the duodenum, pancreas, spleen, and the superior mesenteric artery (SMA).

I. Obokhare (✉)
Texas Tech University Health Sciences Center, Department of Surgery, Amarillo, TX, USA
e-mail: Izi.obokhare@ttushsc.edu

K. A. Garrett
Weill Cornell Medicine/New York Presbyterian Hospital, Department of Surgery, Division of Colon and Rectal Surgery, New York, NY, USA
e-mail: Keg9034@med.cornell.edu

P. Sylla et al. (eds.), *The SAGES Manual of Colorectal Surgery*,
https://doi.org/10.1007/978-3-030-24812-3_33

There appears to be a renewed interest in analyzing minimally invasive surgery for transverse colon tumors as evidenced by recent publications comparing oncologic outcomes of the open and laparoscopic approach. This may be due to the increased use of laparoscopy and robotic technology for colon resections. A recent 2017 meta-analysis by Athanasiou showed laparoscopic transverse colectomy had a longer operative time, conversion rates of 1.9% to 16.7%, faster oral intake, and reduced length of stay while at the same time providing equivalent mortality and morbidity as well as overall disease-free survival (DFS) when compared to the open approach [1]. With regard to short- and long-term outcomes, Kim and colleagues studied 102 consecutive patients who underwent laparoscopic-assisted colectomy for stage II and III transverse colon cancer [2, 3]. In this study, laparoscopic surgery had better short-term outcomes compared to open surgery; however, both had similar long-term outcomes. The oncological outcomes were also similar for both groups with similar lymph node harvest which is a well-known important benchmark for completeness of resection.

Indications and Contradictions

Minimally invasive transverse colon resection is indicated for patients who are candidates for general laparoscopic surgery. Patients with severe pulmonary and cardiovascular comorbidities are not ideal candidates for laparoscopic transverse colectomy and are to be excluded due to the hemodynamic effects of prolonged carbon dioxide abdominal insufflation. Multiple previous extensive abdominal surgery as well as large or multiple ventral hernias requiring repair may preclude a laparoscopic approach.

Laparoscopic transverse colectomy may be indicated for patients with early-stage colon cancer, impending obstruction, and massive or recurrent colorectal bleeding. Matching the medically optimized surgical candidate to the laparoscopic surgeon with appropriate skill and training is the key to achieving the ideal patient outcome.

Principles and Quality Benchmarks

The quality benchmarks of laparoscopic transverse colectomy include (a) negative proximal and distal margin of resection, (b) ligation of the middle colic vessels at the base to achieve adequate lymph node sampling, (c) similar or reduced wound and anastomotic complications as compared to open transverse colectomy, and finally (d) similar morbidity and mortality as compared to open resection.

An important point to consider in the management of a transverse colon tumor is that tumors located at the proximal transverse colon or close to the hepatic flexure can be managed by a right colectomy taking the right branch of the middle colic vessels. Tumors in the mid-transverse colon may also be managed by performing an extended right colectomy or a transverse colectomy. In both instances, a high ligation of the middle colic vessels must be performed in order to achieve a complete oncologic resection. However, several different approaches have been advocated for transverse tumors close to the splenic flexure. One may consider a segmental transverse colectomy involving the splenic flexure or a more aggressive subtotal colectomy with an anastomosis between the terminal ileum and the descending colon. Another option is an extended left colectomy with ligation of the left branch of the middle colic, the marginal artery of Roland, and left colic artery at their origins to remove nodes that may be involved [3, 4].

The individualized choice of the best oncologic resection procedure matching the skill level of the surgeon is crucial to ensure an excellent outcome. Patients with increased body mass index (BMI), cardiac and pulmonary comorbid conditions, and multiple previous abdominal surgical procedures will be considered rather complex and should only be managed by surgeons with extensive colorectal minimal invasive surgery experience to prevent undue mortality and morbidity.

Preoperative Planning, Patient Workup, and Optimization

Preoperative evaluation with colonoscopy and tattooing of the lesion and staging CT scans of the chest abdomen and pelvis to assess for resectability and for metastatic disease are crucial for preoperative staging.

In case of advanced disease, i.e., stage IV transverse colon cancer, neoadjuvant 5-FU-based chemotherapy should be considered. For patients with local invasion of nearby structures such as the stomach, pancreas, and spleen, surgical intervention for cure should not be performed if en bloc resection is not feasible.

Preparing patients for laparoscopic transverse colectomy calls for risk optimization. The concept of prehabilitation is especially vital for patients with extensive comorbid conditions. All patients are encouraged to increase physical activity, vitamin/nutritional supplementation, and smoking cessation prior to surgical intervention. In some cases, cardiac and pulmonary risk optimization is necessary, and the patient is sent for consultation with a cardiologist and/or pulmonologist before surgical intervention. Oral antibiotics and mechanical bowel preparation have been shown in randomized studies to reduce infectious complications and also aid in reducing the fecal load within the colon hence making laparoscopic manipulation easier.

Operative Setup

As part of ERAS protocols, patients are given a promotility agent (mu-opioid receptor antagonist) and preoperative pain management prior to surgical intervention. A dose of intravenous antibiotics should be given within 1 hour of incision. Deep vein thrombosis prevention including sequential compression devices placed on the lower extremities and subcutaneous heparin is beneficial prior to induction of general anesthesia. The patient should be positioned on a nonslip mat to prevent movement during extremes of positioning. Both arms should be tucked and all pressure points padded. A Foley catheter can be placed for bladder decompression.

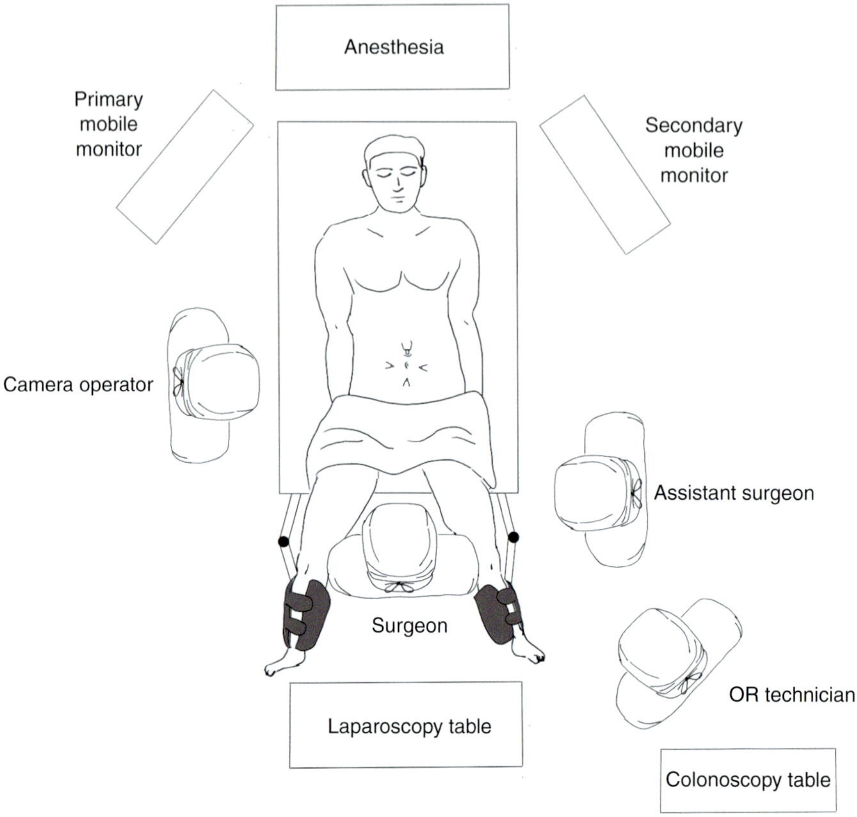

Fig. 33.1 Patient positioning and operating room setup. (Used with permission of Jeremy Moon)

The patient can be positioned on the operating table in a supine fashion; however, the lithotomy or split-leg position provides better ergonomics for the operating surgeon (Fig. 33.1). Having the ability to stand between the legs during mobilization of the splenic flexure reduces back and neck strain of the surgeon and enhances to reach of the laparoscopic instruments. This positioning can be helpful to prevent musculoskeletal strain on the part of the surgeon during prolonged laparoscopic surgery. The viewing screen should be positioned at the head of the bed at an adequate comfort level for the surgeon and the surgical assistants.

Operative Technique

After the abdomen is prepped and draped, trocars are placed. The choice of sentinel trocar placement technique is dictated by the preference of the surgeon. Several techniques exist such as the Veress needle, the Visiport/Optiview trocar technique, the Hasson and the open cutdown technique, or a hybrid of several techniques. Utilizing the laparoscopic principle of triangulation, most surgeons favor the use of multiple 5 mm trocars placed just lateral to the epigastric vessels bilaterally (Figs. 33.2 and 33.3). This reduces the risk of bleeding from the rectus abdominis and the epigastric vessels while at the same time alleviating the risk of abdominal

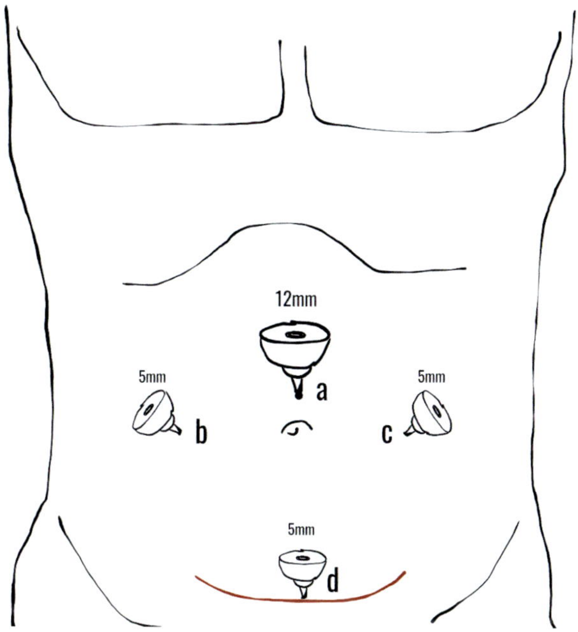

Fig. 33.2 Laparoscopic trocar placement with Pfannestiel extraction. (Used with permission of Jeremy Moon)

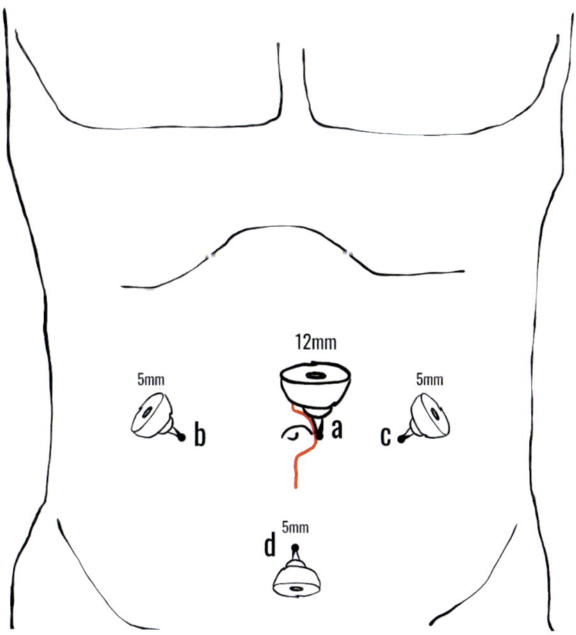

Fig. 33.3 Laparoscopic trocar placement with midline extraction. (Used with permission of Jeremy Moon)

wall hernias and providing adequate reach to the target area. In addition, a 12 mm trocar is required when using the laparoscopic stapler. The ideal location to place the laparoscopic 12 mm stapler trocar is in the umbilical area as this area can be used for extracorporeal anastomosis creation and specimen extraction. However, in the setting of an intracorporeal anastomosis, the 12 mm trocar can be placed anywhere on the abdomen depending on surgeon preference. The use of the articulating endoscopic stapler is useful as it allows the stapler to be fired from almost any angle. The major advantage of an intracorporeal anastomosis is the extraction site can be placed at the Pfannestiel site.

To ensure adequate exposure of the transverse colon, the operating table is placed in a slight reverse Trendelenburg position at about 10 degrees, and the procedure is begun with a diagnostic exploration of the abdominal cavity to determine the extent of the disease. The liver, peritoneal surface, and primary transverse colon tumor location are carefully inspected. Biopsies of the liver or peritoneal surface are obtained with request for frozen sections made when appropriate. If the patient is found to have stage IV disease with peritoneal implants and hepatic metastatic disease, the surgical plan is modified to reduce mortality and morbidity in the perioperative period. For patient with stage IV disease, a palliative resection with a colostomy or a diverting ostomy without resection may be a better option. However, in the absence of metastatic disease, the oncologic procedure can proceed as planned. The anatomic position of the transverse colon mesentery is verified and the proposed resection margins clearly noted (Fig. 33.4a, b).

Adequate exposure is provided by reflecting the omentum in a cephalad position over the liver (Fig. 33.5). The small bowel is retracted gently into the pelvis. A

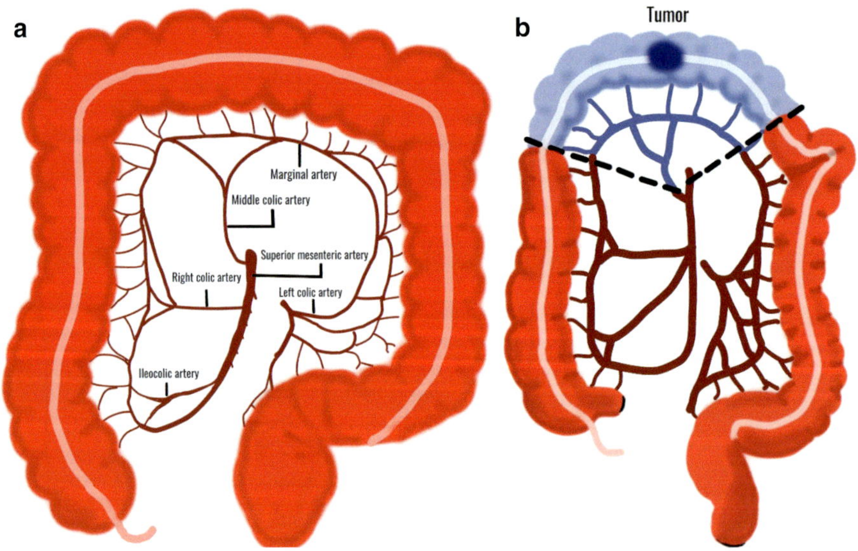

Fig. 33.4 (**a**, **b**) Anatomic considerations of the transverse colon. (**a**, **b**: Used with permission of Jeremy Moon)

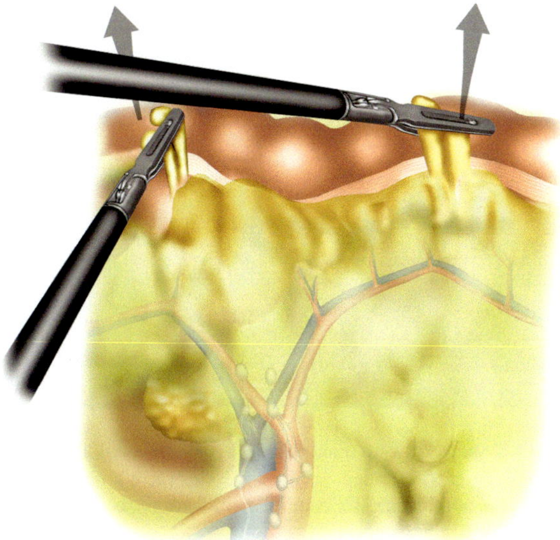

Fig. 33.5 Transverse colon mesentery exposure. (Used with permission of Yuko Tonohira, Medical Illustrator, Dept of Surgery, Weill Cornell Medical Center)

gauze can be placed in the abdominal cavity to provide exposure with gentle traction on the small bowel caudally, as well as to help with hemostatic control during the operative procedure. The small bowel, stomach, and colon should be grasped with an atraumatic bowel grasper to reduce the risk of undue tension and iatrogenic bowel injury during the procedure. Using an energy device of the surgeon's preference, the gastrocolic ligament is incised separating the colon from the stomach and entering the lesser sac (Fig. 33.6a, b). The splenic flexure is mobilized by taking down the lateral attachments of the colon along the white line of Toldt. The hepatic flexure is also mobilized with care taken to preserve the gallbladder, duodenum, and kidney from harm. The mesocolic dissection is performed by providing gentle traction on the transverse colon. The middle colic vessel exposure is provided by gentle upward retraction using a long atraumatic grasper providing adequate tension of the vascular base (Figs. 33.5 and 33.7a, b).

It is not necessary to ligate the inferior mesenteric vein (IMV) during the splenic flexure mobilization. This will prevent devascularization and congestion of the left colon. High ligation of the middle colic vessel can be performed between clips, a vascular stapler load or vessel sealing device. After ligation of the middle colic vessels, the specimen can be extracted through a small midline incision at the level of the umbilicus. A suprapubic incision may also be used for extraction which has the added benefit of reduction of abdominal wall hernias and less postoperative pain. This requires adequate mobilization, however, to ensure reach. A wound protector should be used to prevent abdominal wall tumor seeding and to reduce the risk of wound infections. An extracorporeal side-to-side anastomosis can be created using a linear stapler and can be ideally performed via the upper midline incision. The common enterotomy can be closed using a linear stapler or suturing. Reinforcing the anastomosis with another layer of suture can

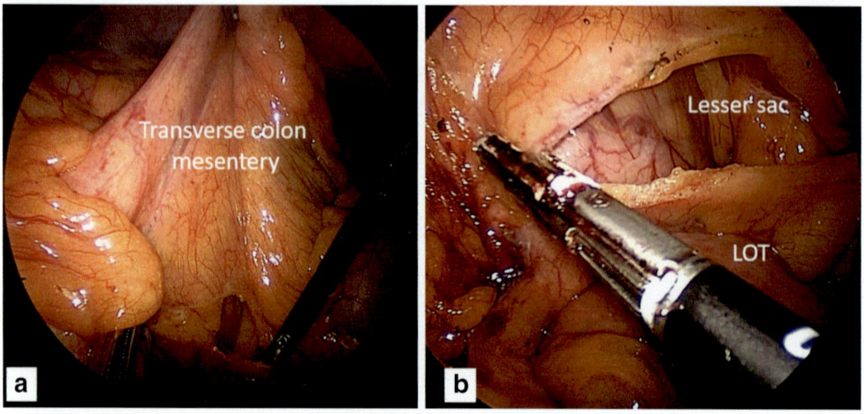

Fig. 33.6 (**a**, **b**) Upward traction on the transverse colon mesentery exposes the base of the middle colic vessels and the lesser sac (**a**). The lesser sac is entered and the gastrocolic ligament is divided. *LOT* ligament of Treitz, *MCA* middle colic artery (**b**). (Courtesy of Patricia Sylla, MD)

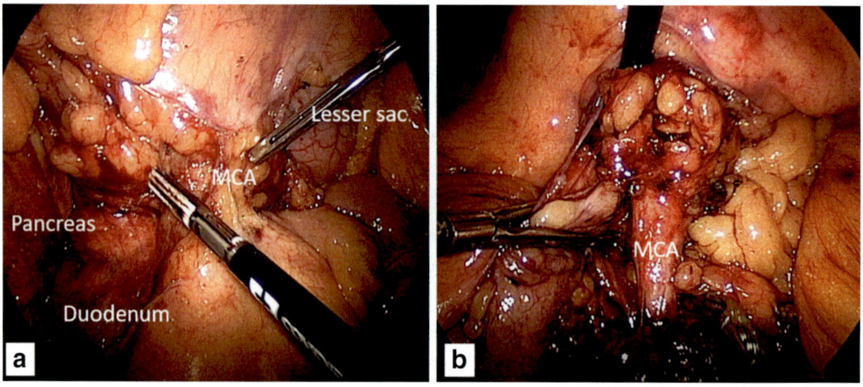

Fig. 33.7 (**a**, **b**) The middle colic artery is carefully dissected and subsequently divided. (Courtesy of Patricia Sylla, MD)

be done based on the preference of the surgeon. Prior to performing the anastomosis, the surgeon may elect to use indocyanine green (ICG) angiography to evaluate the vascularity of the proposed sites for the anastomosis. Obtaining surgical margins of at least 5 cm macroscopically is also crucial to prevent local recurrence at the anastomotic site. Depending on the experience and preference of the surgeon, laparoscopic intracorporeal isoperistaltic colo-colonic anastomosis (Fig. 33.8) can be performed using the appropriate laparoscopic endostapler based on tissue thickness. An important advantage of the intracorporeal anastomosis is that it avoids undue tension on the two bowel limbs and the extraction of the specimen can be performed at the Pfannestiel site.

The robotic approach tends to provide enhanced dexterity for intracorporeal anastomosis.

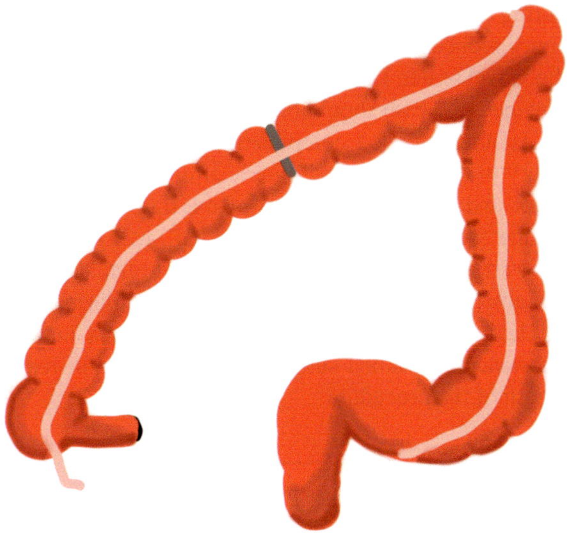

Fig. 33.8 Post resection and expected anastomotic configuration. (Used with permission of Jeremy Moon)

Pitfalls and Troubleshooting

One common pitfall of laparoscopic transverse colectomy includes not adequately mobilizing the hepatic and splenic flexure of the colon. This creates difficulty with extracting the specimen for extracorporeal colo-colonic anastomosis especially in obese patients with a short and bulky mesentery. This may also produce undue tension at the anastomosis or creates bleeding of the colonic mesentery. Another pitfall is performing an anastomosis between poorly vascularized segments of the colon. The splenic flexure is a watershed zone, therefore ensuring adequate vascularity between the two proposed sites of anastomosis is crucial to prevent anastomotic leaks. The vascularity of the colon can be ascertained by a variety of techniques. Direct visual inspection of the colon can identify the transition point between ischemic (blue) and well vascularized bowel (pink) prior to transection. The presence of arterial bleeding at the stapled colonic margins and ICG angiography are also very helpful to assess adequate perfusion. Finally, another pitfall is not having an adequately prepped bowel. Failure to perform a mechanical prep results in a bulky transverse colon, and a partially prepped bowel without oral antibiotics may result in spillage of colonic contents during the anastomosis.

One major complication of the surgical procedure is bleeding either from the spleen or from the middle colic pedicle [4–6]. Pulsatile arterial bleeding can obscure the surgical field. The use of suction and surgical gauze can help to tamponade the bleeding while adequate exposure and subsequent hemostasis is achieved. Using a hemoclip or endoloop can further secure the vascular pedicle without the application of thermal energy which can cause delayed injury to underlying structures such as the duodenum, pancreas, and superior mesenteric artery. Providing upward traction during exposure of the middle colic vessels and gently reducing the traction during the sealing phase with the vessel sealer can extend the compression time and hence reduce the risk of premature breakage or inadequate sealing of the vessels by the vessel sealer. Ultimately, if adequate control of the bleeding cannot be promptly obtained, the case should be converted to open surgery.

Another dreaded complication of this procedure is pancreatitis and possible injury to the superior mesenteric artery. These two vital structures are located posterior and medial to the base of the transverse colon mesentery. Placing a gauze behind the transverse colon, working layer by layer when transecting the middle colic artery, and working from known surgical dissection planes to unknown planes can ameliorate the risk of such iatrogenic injuries.

Having adequate experience with complex laparoscopic procedures as well as assistance by trained surgical staff will help to reduce complications and overall length of the procedure.

Outcomes

Due to the heterogeneity of various studies comparing the outcomes of laparoscopic versus open transverse colectomy, head-to-head compression of the data is somewhat difficult to achieve. However, across all the studies evaluated, the 5-year overall survival (OS) and disease-free survival (DFS) between laparoscopic and open transverse colectomy showed no statistically significant difference. Recent meta-analysis by Athanasiou and colleagues showed a mortality rate of 0.4% across several studies examined. As expected, laparoscopic resections took a longer time to complete reflecting the difficulty of laparoscopic dissection and the variability of the mesenteric vasculature. Yamaguchi showed a significantly higher rate of wound infection 9.7% vs. 6.4% when comparing open surgery to laparoscopic surgery; however, meta-analysis of multiple studies did not support this [1, 7].

A conversion rate of 4.5%–6.3% was also reported by Yamaguchi and Kim and colleagues mostly due to severe adhesions, advanced cancer, and bleeding. Postoperative ileus was reported at 2.6% for laparoscopic and 4.1% for open surgery. As expected, there was no statistically significant difference in the reoperation rate between the laparoscopic and open colectomy groups. With respect to the length of stay, the laparoscopic group had a significantly shorter length of stay and time to oral intake without any statistically significant difference with respect to local recurrence

Table 33.1 Outcomes. Short-term outcomes of laparoscopic (LAC) vs. open (OC) resection for transverse colon cancer

	LAC ($n = 79$)	OC ($n = 23$)	P value
Mean operating time (mins)	332.5	241.3	0.000
Time to flatus	3.5	3.3	0.119
LOS (mean)	12	15.9	0.000
Bleeding	2	0	
Conversion	6.3%		

Data from: Kim et al. [2]

disease-free survival and distant metastatic disease [1–3, 7]. *A brief description of patient outcomes is presented in* Table 33.1 *from a study by Kim and colleagues* [2].

Conclusion

Overall, the evidence suggests that laparoscopic colectomy for transverse colon cancer is feasible and safe when performed by an experienced surgeon. Similar to other laparoscopic colon resection techniques, it provides earlier return to baseline function and reduces pain, postoperative length of stay, and postoperative complications such as pneumonia and postoperative ileus. Transverse colectomy can be performed safely with the appropriate skill level and proper preparation of the patient. Complications such as anastomotic leak, splenic injury, mesenteric bleeding, pancreatitis, and gastric and bowel injury can be reduced significantly with adequate exposure during the surgical procedure [7, 8].

References

1. Athanasiou CD, Robinson J, Yiasemidou M, Lockwood S, Markides GA. Laparoscopic vs open approach for trasnsverse colon cancer. A systematic review and meta-analysis of short and long term outcomes. Int J Surg. 2017;41:78–85.
2. Kim MK, Won DY, Lee JK, Kang WK, Kye BH, Cho HM. Laparoscopic surgery for transverse Colon Cancer: short- and long-term outcomes in comparison with conventional open surgery. J Lapendosc Adv Surg Tech A. 2015;25(12):982–9.
3. Okuda J, Yamamoto M, Tanaka K, Masubuchi S, Uchivama K. Laparoscopic resection of transverse colon cancer at splenic flexture: technical aspects and results. Updates Surg. 2016;68(1):71–5.
4. Wu Q, Ye Z, Bi L, Zheng E, Hu T, Gu C, et al. Laparoscopic colectomy versus open colectomy for treatment of transverse Colon cancer: a systematic review and meta-analysis. J Laproendosc Adv Surg Tech A. 2017;27(10):1038–50.
5. Carlini M, Spoletini D, Castaldi F, Giovannini C, Passaro U. Laparoscopic resection of splenic flexure tumors. Updat Surg. 2016;68(1):77–83.
6. Reddavid R, Esposito L, Evangelista A, Sofia S, Degiuli M. Non-anatomical colonic resections: splenic flexure and transverse colectomy. Central vascular ligation is crucial for survival. Minerva Chir. 2019;74(2):176–86.
7. Yamaguchi S, Yamaguchi S, Tashiro J, Araki R, Okuda J, Hanai T, et al. Laparoscopic versus open resection for transverse and descending colon cancer: short-term and long term outcomes of a multicenter retrospective study of 1830 patients. Asian J Endosc Surg. 2017;10(3):268.
8. Mistrangelo M, Allaix M, Cassoni P, Giraudo G, Arolfo S, Morino M. Laparoscopic vs open resection for transverse colon cancer. Surg Endosc. 2015;29(8):2196–202.

34 Laparoscopic Total Abdominal Colectomy for Emergent and Elective Indications: Perioperative Considerations and Techniques

Meagan Costedio and Luca Stocchi

Introduction and Rationale

In hemodynamically stable patients, the laparoscopic approach is associated with decreased length of stay, blood loss, and morbidity [1, 2]. Laparoscopic total abdominal colectomy (TAC) is currently performed for a number of indications including malignant and benign disease. The short-term benefits of decreased length of stay, blood loss, and pain are well established laparoscopically versus the open approach. Malignant indications include patients with synchronous carcinomas and/or polyps and/or with a background of familial adenomatous polyposis (FAP) or hereditary nonpolyposis colorectal cancer (HNPCC). Benign indications include inflammatory bowel disease (IBD), *Clostridium difficile* (*C. diff.*) colitis, and colonic inertia. Typically, TAC when performed in the setting of medically refractory ulcerative colitis (UC) results in the creation of an end-ileostomy and preservation of the rectum or rectosigmoid stump. This is the most common reason for emergent or urgent TAC. Initially these cases were performed open, but recent data support short-term recovery benefits of laparoscopy in skilled hands despite the emergent nature of the surgery. When TAC is performed for Crohn's disease (CD) or slow transit constipation, a restorative procedure can be performed with creation of an ileorectal anastomosis.

M. Costedio (✉)
Department of Colorectal Surgery, Ahuja Medical Center of University Hospitals, Beachwood, OH, USA

L. Stocchi
The Story-Garschina Chair in Colorectal Surgery, Cleveland Clinic Department of Colorectal Surgery, Digestive Disease and Surgery Institute, Cleveland, OH, USA
e-mail: stocchl@ccf.org

P. Sylla et al. (eds.), *The SAGES Manual of Colorectal Surgery*,
https://doi.org/10.1007/978-3-030-24812-3_34

Indications and Contraindications

An increasing number of patients undergoing surgery for UC require a TAC without anastomosis, which has become the most common initial operation for UC [3, 4]. This procedure is most often performed laparoscopically [5]. In a substantial proportion of cases, the procedures are performed urgently after patients have been admitted with either severe or fulminant UC (Table 34.1). When patients are acutely ill and on high-dose steroids, immediate total proctocolectomy with ileal pouch-anal anastomosis has an increased incidence of leak and pelvic sepsis [6, 7]. The operation of choice is an initial TAC with creation of an end-ileostomy and preservation of the rectum or rectosigmoid stump to reduce postoperative morbidity while preserving the anatomy and dissection planes in the pelvis. Most of these patients are suitable for a delayed, elective completion proctectomy and ileal pouch-anal anastomosis after a 3–6 month recovery period. Other candidates for an initial TAC are those patients who have become progressively anemic or malnourished as a result of a combination of severe disease and prolonged treatment with high doses of steroids or other immunosuppressive medications.

The indication for initial total abdominal colectomy in patients with medically refractory UC who have received biologic medications within the last 3 months preceding surgery is more controversial [8]. There are data, however, indicating that the increased morbidity associated with an immediate total proctocolectomy and ileal pouch-anal anastomosis [9, 10] can be mitigated by an initial TAC [11].

Another relative indication for initial TAC is in morbidly obese patients with central adiposity who can be offered the opportunity to reduce their weight to maximize the reach of the pouch increasing the chance of successful surgery.

Crohn's disease (CD) can also manifest as severe acute colitis requiring total abdominal colectomy due to unresponsiveness to medical management, although this is less common than in UC. In some cases, an initial TAC may be preferable regardless of the severity of inflammatory bowel disease (IBD) to clarify the diagnosis of CD versus UC or indeterminate colitis and therefore guide subsequent management and counseling. Patients with Crohn's colitis and rectal sparing who

Table 34.1 Preoperative risk factors for urgent or emergent surgery for ulcerative colitis and Crohn's disease and the risk of immediate stage 2 (TPC-IPAA) versus stage 3 (TAC) pouch surgery

Preoperative risk factors	TAC	TPC-IPAA
Steroids >20 mg	Preferred	Avoid
Malnutrition >10% weight loss	Preferred	With caution
Anemia	Safe	Safe
Morbid obesity	Safe	Risk of reach issues
Pregnancy	With caution	Avoid
Unclear diagnosis	Safe	Avoid in CD
Biologics	Safe	With caution
Multiple risk factors	Preferred	Avoid

TAC total abdominal colectomy, *TPC-IPAA* total proctocolectomy with ileal pouch-anal anastomosis, *CD* Crohn's disease become unresponsive to medical management or develop complications of disease such as colonic strictures precluding colonoscopic cancer surveillance or fistulae are also candidates for laparoscopic TAC with IRA.

Laparoscopic TAC with IRA is a viable option for patients with colonic inertia after workup and aggressive trial of prokinetic medications. Initially, patients should have a colonoscopy confirming no intraluminal pathology and blood work ruling out endocrine or metabolic abnormalities. Patients should have manometry looking for the rectoanal inhibitory reflex. Barium or MR defecography can help determine if the patient has pelvic floor outlet dysfunction. If pelvic floor dysfunction is diagnosed then pelvic floor physical therapy is recommended. If the sitz marker test shows greater than 20% retention of markers at 5 days off laxatives, the test is consistent with slow transit. If the patient fails aggressive medical therapies, then laparoscopic TAC with IRA is warranted (Fig. 34.1).

Laparoscopic TAC is warranted in FAP when there is relative rectal sparing (less than 20) or when rectal polyps are amenable to endoscopic excision. Prophylactic surgery is recommended in patients with a known mutation or phenotype of disease in their early 20s or at a younger age in the case of symptoms or high-grade dysplasia. Patients with significant rectal polyp burden or rectal cancer should proceed with total proctocolectomy with reconstruction [12]. Patients with a significant family history of colon or rectal cancer or patients known to have HNPCC are watched closely, but if they do develop a colon cancer, TAC is the operation of choice.

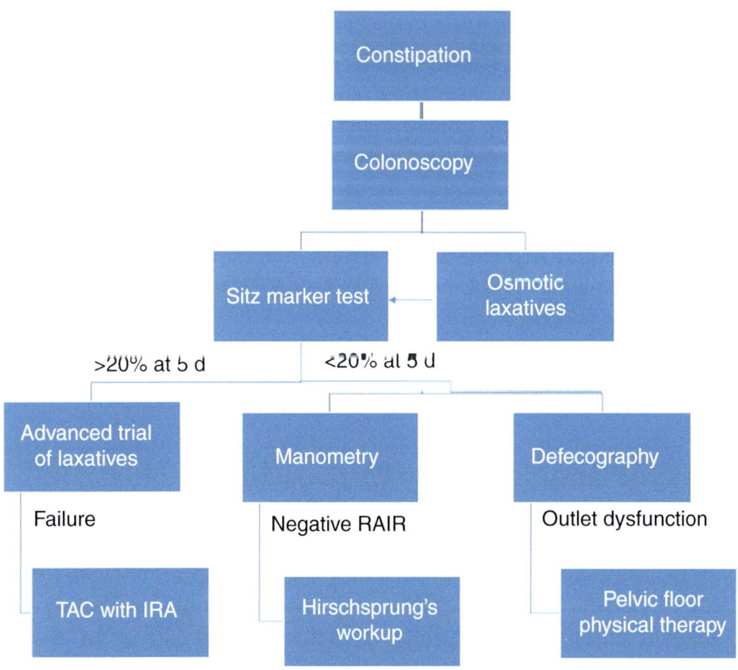

Fig. 34.1 Algorithm for decision-making for the treatment of constipation. TAC total abdominal colectomy, RAIR rectoanal inhibitory reflex, IRA ileorectal anastomosis

Laparoscopy is the approach of choice when the patient is stable and the surgeon feels comfortable with the approach. Relative contraindications to laparoscopy include massive bleeding, colonic perforation with fecal peritonitis, and toxic megacolon. A TAC is an accepted option for obstructing left-sided colon cancer, but again the degree of colonic dilatation can become a significant obstacle in the conduct of a laparoscopic operation, particularly where high ligation of the vessels is essential. There are also insufficient data to support laparoscopy in the pregnant patients developing severe acute UC requiring surgery [13]. In addition, there may be circumstances in which the surgeon can make an individual judgment that poor quality and friability of the tissues excessively increase the risk of intra-abdominal colonic injury during laparoscopy, thus making an open approach preferable. The role of TAC in the management of *C. difficile* colitis is covered in Chap. 35.

Principles and Quality Benchmarks

Laparoscopic TAC can be performed with technical variations based on the specific indication. If the indication is management of a biopsy-proven carcinoma, polyp, or dysplasia it is necessary to perform high vascular ligation with oncologic mesenteric dissection throughout the colon. Ligation at the origin of the lymphovascular pedicles is not necessary for benign disease, which can facilitate and expedite the conduct of the operation. The ileorectal anastomosis should be typically performed at the level of the upper rectum, recognized by the confluence of the teniae, which frequently occurs at the level of the sacral promontory. Some surgeons prefer to leave a shorter segment of rectum if the indication is colonic inertia to facilitate bowel function, which remains controversial. In CD the specific length of residual rectosigmoid is based on the principle that the large intestine left in place should have minimal or absent gross disease. In the case of nonrestorative procedures, the inflamed upper rectum can be transected laparoscopically to create a longer defunctionalized rectosigmoid segment which can be implanted in the subcutaneous tissues or left just underneath the abdominal fascia. Overall morbidity and pelvic sepsis rates are comparable regardless of whether the rectal stump is left under the fascia or secured above the fascia; therefore the decision is at the individual surgeon's discretion [14].

Preoperative Planning, Patient Workup, and Optimization

Preoperative planning and workup largely depend on the individual diagnosis and urgency of the indications for TAC. The following paragraph is relevant for patients undergoing elective resection. A complete colonoscopy should be ideally performed in all patients requiring TAC. It is imperative that patients with a history of colitis for more than 8 years undergo surveillance if medically feasible, to ensure that there is no dysplasia prior to proceeding with planned colectomy without high ligation of the vessels. Nutrition assessment is essential in operative planning to make sure that patients are optimized prior to surgery when there is time to postpone surgery. Also, an anemia workup should be performed and iron and B12 replaced prior to surgery to optimize blood levels. Patients should be seen by a specialist to mark the appropriate site for a stoma, optimally in the right lower or upper quadrant. For patients on biologics who are doing poorly, if possible, it is optimal to wait close to the timing of the next dose of medication to have the lowest serologic levels of drug while the patient retains some benefits from the medication. When performing a TAC for UC, the authors choose to leave patients on the dose of steroids where the patient can best function, as forcing a decrease in steroids can lead to fulminant colitis. Severe acute IBD is a relative contraindication to complete colonoscopy due to increased risk of perforation, in which case a sigmoidoscopy can be sufficient to confirm the severity of disease as well as perform biopsies to rule out CMV infection. Infectious causes of diarrhea should be excluded. Stool studies for *Clostridium difficile*, ova and parasites, and bacterial pathogens should be performed. Computed tomography (CT) or magnetic resonance (MR) enterography can be performed to rule out small bowel CD when the diagnosis of colitis is in question. For patients hospitalized with fulminant colitis, giving intravenous iron can help build up stores for postoperative recovery. There is no demonstrated benefit in delaying colectomy to give preoperative parenteral nutrition [15].

Patients with colonic malignancy should be adequately staged with CT of the chest abdomen and pelvis and a CEA level. In patients who are younger than 50 or with a strong family history of colorectal, ovarian, endometrial, or renal cancer, genetic counseling is recommended preoperatively, as the patient may want to consider concomitant preventative surgery such as hysterectomy and oophorectomy. Concurrent conditions within hereditary syndromes should be assessed and addressed as well. A type and screen is encouraged in all of these patients as it is common for patients to be anemic as well as have antibodies to blood with IBD. A mechanical bowel preparation with oral antibiotics is recommended in all hemodynamically stable patients to help decrease the risk of surgical site infection.

Operative Setup

The patient is positioned on the operating room table in the supine split-leg or lithotomy position. This positioning is helpful for two reasons: the operating surgeons can stand between the legs, and the surgeon has access to the rectum for the anastomosis or to help define the anatomy by inserting a rectal probe. The OR mattress should be taped to the bed base and nonslip padding, or bean bags can be used to prevent movement of the patient during surgery. If an ileorectal anastomosis is planned, the perineum needs to be positioned over the end of the bed to allow for any cephalad sliding which might occur with steep Trendelenburg tilt. Both arms are tucked, and the patient is secured to the table to minimize sliding. Ensuring that the patient has adequate IV access and two blood pressure cuffs on can help to prevent untucking the arms later in the case. Two laparoscopic monitors that are mobile are helpful as the operation progresses in all four quadrants of the abdomen. Prophylactic antibiotics that cover aerobes and anaerobes such as a third-generation cephalosporin or ciprofloxacin and metronidazole are administered within 1 hour of incision. A prophylactic subcutaneous heparin dose is administered even if the patient is anemic preoperatively. This is an important step as the majority of the patients needing a TAC will have IBD or cancer and are at increased risk for venous thromboembolism (VTE). The benefit of stress dose intravenous steroids should be discussed with the anesthesia team prior to surgery if the patient has been taking steroids within the preceding 6 months.

Operative Technique: Surgical Steps

Port placement varies based on the surgeon's preference and indication for surgery. An umbilical trocar is placed that will house the laparoscopic camera (5 or 10 mm based on surgeon preference). Classically ports in the midclavicular line in the right and left lower and upper quadrants are used (Fig. 34.2). In many cases the patient will need an end or diverting loop ileostomy, so it is preferable to place a 12 mm port in the right lower quadrant position at the previously marked stoma site if a laparoscopic stapler will be used, so that the fascial defect will not need to be closed. If the patient does not need a stoma, then the extraction site, which is at the discretion of the surgeon, can be used for the 12 mm port site as well. Alternatively, it is possible to start with the stoma or extraction site and place a wound protector with a 12 mm port held in place with a Penrose drain and penetrating towel clamps, or a specialized port with a wound protector, as it is easier to enter the peritoneal cavity through a larger incision. If the surgeon feels comfortable with single incision laparoscopic surgery (SILS), then the stoma site or extraction site can be used (Fig. 34.3). Another option for port placement keeping the extraction site off the midline would be to place the extraction incision in the suprapubic site and

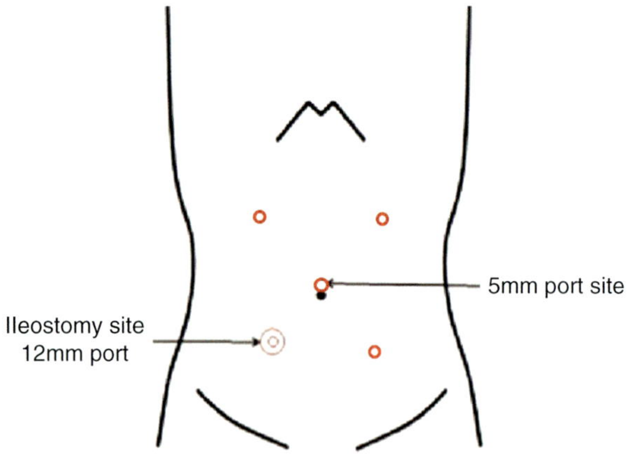

Fig. 34.2 Laparoscopic port placement for TAC

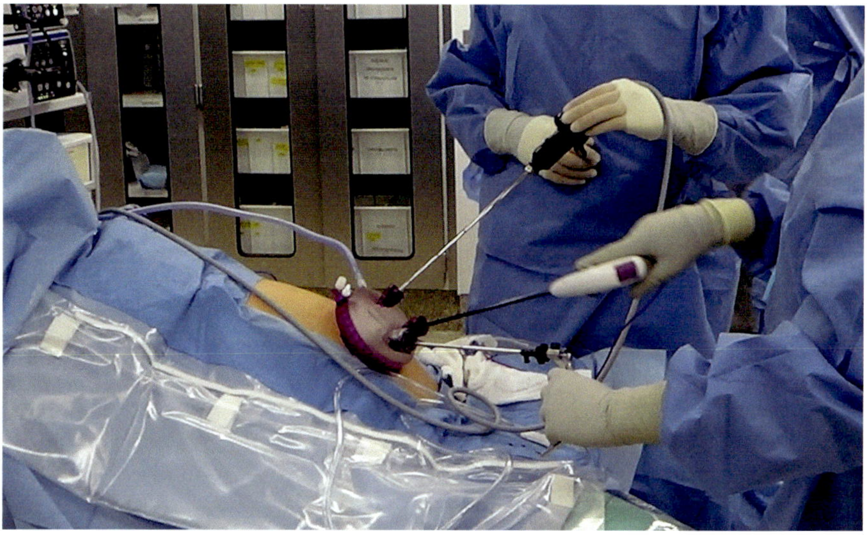

Fig. 34.3 Single incision laparoscopic port placement in the right lower quadrant ileostomy site

use that as a either a SILS port or a hand-assist port for patients with a bulky mesentery. Additional 5 mm ports can be added as necessary to complete the surgery safely.

Total Abdominal Colectomy for Benign Disease

After safe port placement, in cases of colitis, the small bowel is briefly inspected to ensure that there is no gross evidence of CD. The camera is placed in the umbilical port, and the operating surgeon stands on the left side of the patient and operates through the left-sided ports or the right lower quadrant and left lower quadrant ports. With the patient placed in Trendelenburg and left side down position, the mesentery is grasped just under the ligament of Treves and retracted laterally and anteriorly. The terminal ileum is positioned in the pelvis, and the remainder of the small bowel falls into the left abdomen. This will tent up the ileocolic artery and vein. The groove under the ileocolic vessels is then scored, and blunt dissection is used to dissect the posterior aspect of the mesentery from the retroperitoneum and anterior duodenum (Fig. 34.4a, b). Finding the plane just anterior to the duodenum ensures the correct avascular dissection up to the hepatic flexure. When the ileocolic vessels are divided, a high ligation is not necessary in benign disease but can facilitate reach for an ileoanal anastomosis if that is planned for a later date. In UC cases, the authors prefer high ligation of the ileocolic vessels so that the J-pouch operation is always the same whether it is performed for malignancy or benign disease as far as reach maneuvers and blood supply, although this remains at the discretion of the individual surgeon.

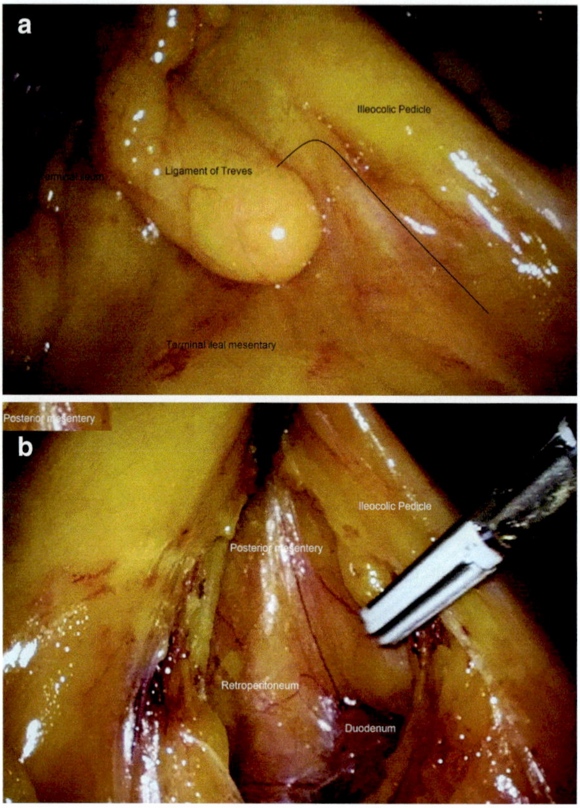

Fig. 34.4 (**a**) Ileocolic pedicle when the ligament of Treves is retracted anterolaterally. The black line depicts the plane between the retroperitoneum and the posterior mesentery. (**b**) Once the peritoneum is scored, this photo demonstrates how to identify the anterior duodenum, which will lead the surgeon to the correct avascular plane between the posterior right mesocolon/mesentery and retroperitoneum

The mesentery is dissected free from the retroperitoneum up to the hepatic flexure and laterally to the abdominal wall. The terminal ileum is then retracted cephalad and anteriorly. There is an avascular plane between the small bowel mesentery and the retroperitoneum containing the ureter and gonadal vessels. That avascular plane is scored and the prior dissection is joined (Fig. 34.5a, b). Often the surgeon can see a dark/red area behind the mesentery which corresponds to the previously dissected space. Once the dissections are joined, the lateral attachments of the right colon are divided with monopolar cautery or a vessel sealer up to the hepatic flexure. The operating surgeon then changes the table position to the reverse Trendelenburg and left side down position and moves to operate between the legs from the RLQ and LLQ ports. The hepatocolic attachments are taken with care to avoid the duodenum and stomach. If the surgeon chooses to spare the omentum, the omentum is retracted over the colon and dissected free from the transverse colon eventually entering the lesser sac closer to the splenic flexure. The previously dissected mesentery of the right colon is retracted anteriorly and caudally to demonstrate the transverse colon mesentery (Fig. 34.6). In cases where it is difficult to dissect the lesser omentum from the transverse mesocolon, the lesser omentum can be taken with the transverse colon mesentery close to the colon wall across the

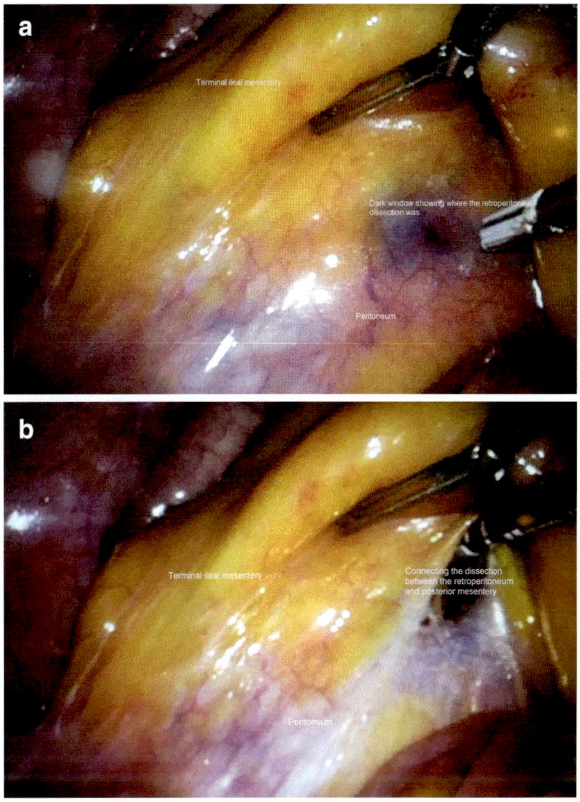

Fig. 34.5 (**a**) The terminal ileal mesentery is retracted anteriorly and cephalad showing a dark area which is the previously dissected space between the mesentery and retroperitoneum. (**b**) The peritoneum is scored, and the prior dissection plane is entered ensuring identification of the correct plane, after which the right lateral attachments can be expeditiously taken down

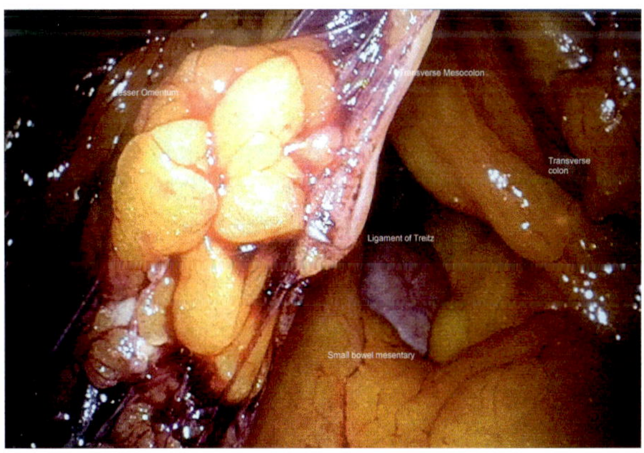

Fig. 34.6 With the patient in reverse Trendelenburg position and the middle colic vessels and lesser omentum tented over a grasper, the transverse mesocolon is above the ligament of Treitz and can be taken close to the colon wall in benign disease

transverse colon and the omentum removed with the colon. The patient is then transitioned into the reverse Trendelenburg and right side down position. Once the transverse mesocolon starts to curve to become the descending colon mesentery, the lesser sac is entered, and the lesser omentum is taken off the splenic flexure (Fig. 34.7). The splenic flexure is then retracted caudally, and the splenocolic

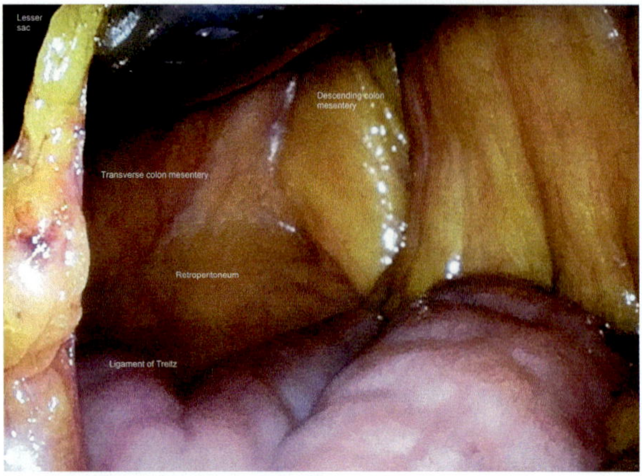

Fig. 34.7 The transverse mesocolon comes to an end as it sweeps around to become the descending mesocolon. The lesser sac must be entered and dissected off the splenic flexure to the abdominal wall so that the descending colon can then be medialized and the mesocolon dissected off Gerota's fascia and taken close to the colon wall

attachments are taken. The left colon attachments are taken as well, and the descending colon is medialized off Gerota's fascia. The left colon is dissected free from the retroperitoneum, and the mesentery can be taken close to the wall of the left colon. The sigmoid is dissected from the retroperitoneum, ensuring the left ureter and gonadal vessels are kept retroperitoneally. The authors prefer to keep the dissection of the mesocolon anterior to the superior hemorrhoidal vessels to ensure adequate blood flow to the proximal rectum. Patients with IBD or *C. diff.* on high-dose steroids and biologics, severely malnourished, and/or having severe rectal inflammation, are at increased risk of staple line breakdown. In this case, the mesorectum is then taken to the rectal wall at the rectosigmoid junction in an area that will reach up to the suprapubic abdominal wall to prevent intra-abdominal rectal stump leak. A small horizontal extraction site is created in the suprapubic area splitting the rectus muscles. The terminal ileum is transected and grasped, and the colon is removed through this site through a wound protector. The rectosigmoid is stapled either intracorporeally or extracorporeally, and the rectal stump mesentery can be sutured to the surrounding fascia, and the skin can be closed or left open. If the patient is on less than 20 mg of prednisone/day or 100 mg of hydrocortisone, with normal nutrition and tissue integrity, then the mesentery is taken up to the rectal wall close to the peritoneal reflection, and the rectum is transected with a laparoscopic stapler. This will minimize the amount of inflamed rectum left in place. A common practice is to leave a rectal tube to decrease the pressure on the staple line until the patient is able to mobilize and try to evacuate air and mucous on their own. A potential side effect of pelvic surgery is decreased fecundity; it is important to minimize dissection near the ovaries and irrigate and remove any blood products to prevent scarring near the fallopian tubes in female patients. Once assured that the mesentery is appropriately oriented without twists, the specimen and the terminal ileum are delivered through the wound protector at the stoma site and matured.

In the case of a subtotal colectomy for slow transit constipation, the laparoscopic colectomy portion of the operation is the same, but the mesentery is taken to the top of the proximal rectum, approximately 7–9 cm from the anterior peritoneal reflection. The rectosigmoid is transected using a laparoscopic stapler, and a circular stapler, anvil, is secured into the terminal ileum using a purse-string suture through the extraction site. The correct mesenteric orientation is again ensured, and an end-to-end anastomosis is created intracorporeally and checked with air leak testing. For patients with Crohn's colitis, a point of normal colon or rectum is chosen for the anastomosis. If the patient is young and has a normal colon, an ileosigmoid anastomosis can be performed. It can be difficult to get the EEA stapler to the end of the transected sigmoid colon, so in these cases, a handsewn end-to-end anastomosis is preferred for ease of small bowel endoscopic surveillance. A diverting loop ileostomy is always an option for patients on >20 mg of prednisone daily or who have lost greater than 10% of their body weight.

Total Abdominal Colectomy for Malignancy/Dysplasia

The laparoscopic setup is the same as described for benign disease. The operation proceeds as in the benign setting, but a complete mesocolic excision is required for the entire colon (Fig. 34.8). When the ileocolic vessels are identified, they are dissected back above the duodenum and taken at the bifurcation at the last branch of the superior mesenteric artery (SMA). The hepatic flexure is taken down as described in the benign section. The patient is placed in the reverse Trendelenburg position, and the omentum is retracted over the colon, and the lesser sac is then entered in the mid-transverse colon, and the omentum is dissected free from the colon to the splenic flexure. The posterior aspect of the stomach is dissected from the transverse mesocolon toward the right to facilitate high ligation of the middle colic vessels. The middle colic vessels can then be taken in a high ligation with care to avoid the fourth portion of the duodenum as it courses through the transverse mesocolon. The transverse mesocolon is then taken just above the ligament of Treitz ensuring a high

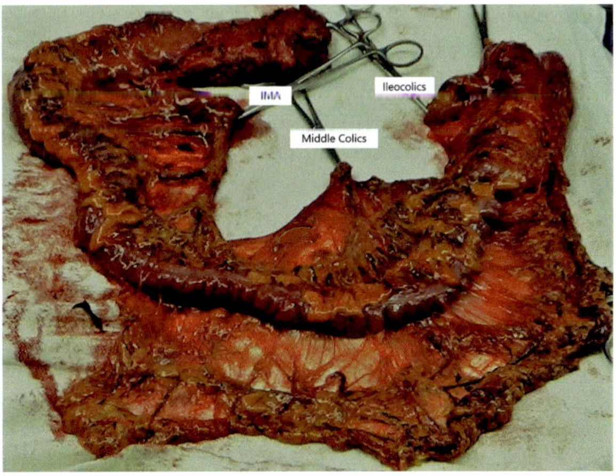

Fig. 34.8 Complete mesocolic excision is required for the entire colon for TAC for malignancy/dysplasia

ligation. The splenic flexure can be released at this point, but the authors prefer to transition to the left colon in a medial to lateral approach for a high ligation of the inferior mesenteric artery (IMA) and vein (IMV). The patient is placed back into the Trendelenburg and right side down position. The superior hemorrhoidal vessels are identified and tented up, and the plane between the posterior mesorectum and presacral fascia is identified, sweeping the inferior hypogastric nerves, ureters, and gonadal vessels posteriorly. The superior hemorrhoidal artery is traced back to the base of the IMA, and the IMA is taken close to the aorta to ensure a high ligation. The posterior aspect of the left colon mesentery is dissected free from the retroperitoneum. The IMV is then taken in a high ligation, and the previous dissection from the transverse mesocolon and splenic flexure should be met. The lateral attachments of the left colon are taken down to the pelvis.

Following division of the IMA, the blood supply to the rectum relies on middle rectal artery backflow. It is essential for adequate blood supply as well as for oncologic reasons that the true rectum be transected rather than the distal sigmoid. The authors select a transection point along the rectum, approximately 7–9 cm proximal to the peritoneal reflection for a planned end-to-end anastomosis. Drains are not routinely used for total abdominal colectomy. If the rectal stump is implanted suprapubically, the authors routinely close the skin as only 15% will blow out and become a mucous fistula [14]. Rarely the rectum will be so inflamed it will not hold sutures or staples, in which case it should be matured as a mucous fistula.

Pitfalls and Troubleshooting

Common Errors: Injury to the Fragile Colon/Mesentery

A dreaded and common complication of this surgery is perforation of the colon and intraperitoneal stool contamination. It is essential that the colon is grasped as little as possible for retraction. Utilization of steep table positioning as well as tenting of the mesentery for retraction can obtain adequate visualization without grasping the colon wall. The authors use an open bowel grasper under the mesentery to adequately expose planes posterior to the colon with minimal tension on the weakened colon wall.

In cases of IBD, the mesentery is often thickened and fragile and bleeds easily. The authors chose to stay in the avascular planes posterior to the thickened mesentery and use a vessel sealing device with multiple firings to control this fragile and thickened mesentery. While most procedures can be completed with minimal blood loss, surgeons should be prepared for the possibility of severe bleeding from the fragile Crohn's mesentery.

Intraoperative Difficulties: Megacolon and Microperforation

Megacolon was initially considered a contraindication to laparoscopy. Since laparoscopic equipment and experience have increased, that is no longer the case, and laparoscopy can provide short-term recovery benefits even under emergent circumstances. If the patient has significant small bowel or colonic dilation, then open surgery may still be required, as there may not be sufficient domain to maneuver laparoscopically. As long as the megacolon is caused by benign pathology, there are tricks to performing this surgery safely, and in experienced hands, the risk of colonic perforation during laparoscopic TAC in this setting is equivalent to that during open surgery.

A medial to lateral approach is often not possible due to bowel dilation. In this case steep table positioning can be helpful to move the dilated and often heavy colon, and great care is taken to grasp or tent the mesentery rather than the dilated colon to help avoiding perforation. Gauze can be used to retract and manipulate the bowel. The patient is placed in the steep Trendelenburg and left side down position. The terminal ileal mesentery is retracted cephalad and toward the abdominal wall and the avascular plane between the posterior aspect of the mesentery, and the retroperitoneum is developed to the hepatic flexure. The terminal ileum can be transected laparoscopically and the mesentery divided with a vessel sealing device at the level at the colon wall and the lateral attachments taken all while tenting the colon and mesentery upward. The patient is then positioned in reverse Trendelenburg, left side down, and once the colon has fallen into the pelvis, then the procedure can be performed as described as for benign disease, for the remainder of the colon as the lateral to medial dissection is safer in this case. For benign disease, particularly if the right side of the colon is the most dilated, if pneumoperitoneum is inadequate, the surgeon can transect the transverse colon using a laparoscopic stapler and remove the proximal, dilated bowel through a wound protector to reduce a portion of dilated colon and improve exposure and maneuverability.

Management of Intraoperative Complications: Tips and Tricks, Salvage, and When to Convert

Perforation

As alluded to above, acutely ill patients with UC are at a very high risk for intraoperative perforation both open and laparoscopically. Just grasping the colon or sometimes even putting pressure on the colonic wall can cause perforation. The authors attempt to tent under the colon and mesentery to avoid putting pressure on the fragile colon wall. If a perforation is encountered with stool spillage, a suction irrigator is needed to control fecal soilage, and either sutures or a laparoscopic stapler can be used to control further fecal contamination. If the surgeon is unable to contain fecal spillage, they should convert to open.

Bleeding

The authors use a vessel sealing device to control the major colonic vessels. If bleeding is encountered, the vessel is occluded with a bowel grasper or Maryland grasper, and the blood vessel can be controlled with a repeat application of the vessel sealing device, assuming the surrounding structures are safely out of harm, clips, or intracorporeal suturing. If the surgeon cannot gain control of the vessel, then conversion to open is appropriate.

Injury to Other Organs

Small bowel injury most often occurs during adhesiolysis. As long as the small bowel is mobilized and freed from other adhesions, often the entire small bowel can be run through a stoma or extraction site. The surgeon can pull up the concerning area and place a stitch on the area extracorporeally and then run the entire bowel and repair any areas of concern without having to formally covert to open. Injury to the ureters should prompt a urology consult and may require conversion to open based on the experience of the consulting urologic surgeon. Injury of the duodenum can be repaired laparoscopically or open based on the comfort of the individual surgeon. Splenic injury is a rare laparoscopic complication but can happen, and its management can range from use of hemostatic agents to splenectomy, based again on the comfort of the surgeon. A very rare but concerning complication of a total colectomy would be injury to the superior mesenteric artery or superior mesenteric vein (SMA, SMV) which could compromise small bowel viability. In this scenario, the authors recommend conversion to open with repair and intraoperative consultation with a vascular surgeon.

Level of Difficulty of Particular Approach, Prerequisite Skills, Learning Curve

Total colectomy is a difficult procedure which requires knowledge of the anatomy over the entire abdominal cavity as the surgeon is working in all four quadrants. There is a significant learning curve for efficient retraction in this case as well. If the surgeon is well versed in right, extended right, and left colectomy, then TAC for benign disease is reasonable. For cases of dysplasia or malignancy, the surgeon needs specific training for complete mesocolic excision with high ligation of the ileocolic, middle colic, and inferior mesenteric vessels. If the surgeon does not feel comfortable with these techniques, then additional training or proctoring should be sought.

Outcomes

The largest available evidence on the outcomes of laparoscopic TAC comes from the evaluation of large administrative databases. There is evidence that the laparoscopic technique is more commonly performed for constipation and IBD compared with neoplasm in the assessment of 744 patients included in the American College of Surgeons National Surgical Quality Improvement Program (NSQIP) undergoing

TAC, including any indication for surgery, both laparoscopic and open techniques and both restorative and nonrestorative procedures. Median operative times were longer for laparoscopic surgery (230 vs. 178 min, $p < 0.001$), and the difference remained similar regardless of the diagnosis. The laparoscopic approach resulted in a significant decrease in the median length of hospital stay among patients with neoplasm or IBD (6 vs. 8 days, $p < 0.001$, and 7 vs. 9 days, $p < 0.001$, respectively), but not in patients operated on for colonic inertia [16]. In another series limited to restorative procedures, 326 patients undergoing laparoscopic TAC and ileorectal anastomosis for any indications were compared with an equivalent number of patients who underwent an open procedure. The laparoscopic technique was again associated with a significantly longer mean operative time (242 minutes versus 202 minutes, $p < 0.001$) but a significantly shorter length of hospital stay (9.4 versus 13.3 days, $p < 0.001$) and decreased rates of ileus (24% versus 31%, $p = 0.04$). The morbidity and mortality rates were comparable, in particular anastomotic leak rates (5.2% in each group) and sepsis rates (5.2% after laparoscopic surgery vs. 8.9% after open surgery, $p = 0.07$) [17]. There is evidence from a single institution indicating that TAC with ileorectal anastomosis is associated with increased morbidity when carried out for colonic inertia compared with neoplasm. However, when assessing the specific subgroup of patients undergoing laparoscopic surgery, the rates of anastomotic leakage and postoperative abscess were statistically similar, and the difference in readmission and overall morbidity favoring patients operated on for neoplasm was statistically borderline ($p = 0.05$) [18]. The comparison of morbidity rates after TAC according to specific diagnosis in the abovementioned NSQIP study did not indicate significant differences, in particular for septic complications, except for increased urinary tract infection rates and neurologic and renal complication in constipation patients when compared to IBD [16]. Contemporary results of laparoscopic TAC for IBD from individual institutions are reported in Table 34.2. The laparoscopic approach has been generally associated with recovery

Table 34.2 Selected series of laparoscopic total abdominal colectomy and end-ileostomy for severe acute inflammatory bowel disease

Author	Year	Patients (*n*)	Laparoscopic technique used	Overall morbidity (%)	LOS (days)
Ouaïssi [23]	2008	23	Standard	35	9.3
Chung [24]	2009	37	HALS and standard	51	5
Watanabe [25]	2009	30	HALS	37	23
Telem [26]	2010	29	Standard	28	4.5/10.3[a]
Bartels [27]	2012	36	HALS and standard	17	N/A
Parnaby [28]	2013	32	Standard	72	7
Frid [29]	2013	42	Standard	43	6
Gu [30]	2014	197	HALS and standard	40	6
Messenger [31]	2014	131	Standard	31	7 (median)
Buchs [32]	2017	117	Standard	32	10.5

LOS length of hospital stay. LOS reported as means, *HALS* hand-assisted laparoscopic surgery
[a]Reported separately for patients with unremarkable postoperative course and experiencing postoperative complications

benefits when compared with open TAC while maintaining similar postoperative morbidity, as also confirmed by a systematic review and meta-analysis [19]. Within the subgroup of TAC for colonic inertia, a number of single institutional series have also demonstrated earlier return of bowel function, reduced postoperative pain, and shorter length of hospital stay after laparoscopic surgery [20]. With respect to anorectal function, it is generally accepted that laparoscopic TAC is associated with similar function to their open counterparts, although a recent small series indicated improved function after laparoscopic surgery [21] for still unclear reasons. There is also evidence based on the Nationwide Inpatient Sample (NIS) database that laparoscopic TAC is associated with decreased hospital charges. In an analysis of 26,721 patients who underwent elective TAC between 2009 and 2012, almost 63% had an open operation, while slightly more than 37% had a minimally invasive approach including a less than 1% rate of robotic surgery. The most common indication for surgery was UC. While the conversion rate for laparoscopic surgery was significantly higher than that of robotic TAC (13.3 versus 1.5%, $p < 0.01$), patients undergoing laparoscopic surgery have significantly lower total hospital charges compared to patients who underwent open surgery. Total hospital charges for the robotic approach were also significantly higher than for the laparoscopic approach [22]. While this retrospective analysis remains associated with possible selection bias when comparing different surgical approaches and assessed charges rather than direct hospital costs, its results corroborate the widespread use of laparoscopic surgery for TAC.

Conclusions

Laparoscopic TAC is associated with recovery advantages when compared to open surgery and can be successfully performed for a number of indications. Besides recovery benefits, laparoscopic TAC is also associated with substantial cost savings when compared to open surgery. Laparoscopic surgery is the established technique of choice for TAC for both benign and malignant disease. With technical advancement and increased experience, laparoscopic TAC can be considered as the initial approach even in emergent situations, depending of the individual surgeon comfort.

References

1. Keller DS, Pedraza R, Flores-Gonzalez JR, LeFave JP, Mahmood A, Haas EM. The current status of emergent laparoscopic colectomy: a population-based study of clinical and financial outcomes. Surg Endosc. 2016;30(8):3321–6.
2. Sujatha-Bhaskar S, Alizadeh RF, Koh C, Inaba C, Jafari MD, Carmichael JC, et al. The growing utilization of laparoscopy in emergent colonic disease. Am Surg. 2017;83(10):1068–73.
3. Geltzeiler CB, Lu KC, Diggs BS, Deveney KE, Keyashian K, Herzig DO, et al. Initial surgical management of ulcerative colitis in the biologic era. Dis Colon Rectum. 2014;57(12):1358–63.

4. Bikhchandani J, Polites SF, Wagie AE, Habermann EB, Cima RR. National trends of 3- versus 2-stage restorative proctocolectomy for chronic ulcerative colitis. Dis Colon Rectum. 2015;58(2):199–204.
5. Causey MW, Stoddard D, Johnson EK, Maykel JA, Martin MJ, Rivadeneira D, et al. Laparoscopy impacts outcomes favorably following colectomy for ulcerative colitis: a critical analysis of the ACS-NSQIP database. Surg Endosc. 2013;27(2):603–9.
6. Ritter KA, Burke JP, Stocchi L, Aiello A, Holubar S, Ashburn JH, et al. Postoperative steroid taper is associated with pelvic sepsis after ileal pouch-anal anastomosis. Inflamm Bowel Dis. 2019; 25(8):1383–9.
7. Zittan E, Wong-Chong N, Ma GW, McLeod RS, Silverberg MS, Cohen Z. Modified two-stage ileal pouch-anal anastomosis results in lower rate of anastomotic leak compared with traditional two-stage surgery for ulcerative colitis. J Crohns Colitis. 2016;10(7):766–72.
8. Kulaylat AS, Kulaylat AN, Schaefer EW, Tinsley A, Williams E, Koltun W, et al. Association of preoperative anti-tumor necrosis factor therapy with adverse postoperative outcomes in patients undergoing abdominal surgery for ulcerative colitis. JAMA Surg. 2017;152(8):e171538.
9. Selvasekar CR, Cima RR, Larson DW, Dozois EJ, Harrington JR, Harmsen WS, et al. Effect of infliximab on short-term complications in patients undergoing operation for chronic ulcerative colitis. J Am Coll Surg. 2007;204(5):956–62; discussion 62–3.
10. Mor IJ, Vogel JD, da Luz Moreira A, Shen B, Hammel J, Remzi FH. Infliximab in ulcerative colitis is associated with an increased risk of postoperative complications after restorative proctocolectomy. Dis Colon Rectum. 2008;51(8):1202–7; discussion 7–10.
11. Gu J, Remzi FH, Shen B, Vogel JD, Kiran RP. Operative strategy modifies risk of pouch-related outcomes in patients with ulcerative colitis on preoperative anti-tumor necrosis factor-alpha therapy. Dis Colon Rectum. 2013;56(11):1243–52.
12. Wu JS, Paul P, McGannon EA, Church JM. APC genotype, polyp number, and surgical options in familial adenomatous polyposis. Ann Surg. 1998;227(1):57–62.
13. Ooi BS, Remzi FH, Fazio VW. Turnbull-Blowhole colostomy for toxic ulcerative colitis in pregnancy: report of two cases. Dis Colon Rectum. 2003;46(1):111–5.
14. Gu J, Stocchi L, Remzi F, Kiran RP. Intraperitoneal or subcutaneous: does location of the (colo)rectal stump influence outcomes after laparoscopic total abdominal colectomy for ulcerative colitis? Dis Colon Rectum. 2013;56(5):615–21.
15. Salinas H, Dursun A, Konstantinidis I, Nguyen D, Shellito P, Hodin R, et al. Does preoperative total parenteral nutrition in patients with ulcerative colitis produce better outcomes? Int J Colorectal Dis. 2012;27(11):1479–83.
16. Alves-Ferreira PC, de Campos-Lobato LF, Zutshi M, Hull T, Gurland B. Total abdominal colectomy has a similar short-term outcome profile regardless of indication: data from the National Surgical Quality Improvement Program. Am Surg. 2011;77(12):1613–8.
17. Onder A, Benlice C, Church J, Kessler H, Gorgun E. Short-term outcomes of laparoscopic versus open total colectomy with ileorectal anastomosis: a case-matched analysis from a nationwide database. Tech Coloproctol. 2016;20(11):767–73.
18. Reshef A, Gurland B, Zutshi M, Kiran RP, Hull T. Colectomy with ileorectal anastomosis has a worse 30-day outcome when performed for colonic inertia than for a neoplastic indication. Colorectal Dis. 2013;15(4):481–6.
19. Bartels SA, Gardenbroek TJ, Ubbink DT, Buskens CJ, Tanis PJ, Bemelman WA. Systematic review and meta-analysis of laparoscopic versus open colectomy with end ileostomy for non-toxic colitis. Br J Surg. 2013;100(6):726–33.
20. Tillou J, Poylin V. Functional disorders: slow-transit constipation. Clin Colon Rectal Surg. 2017;30(1):76–86.
21. Khan M, Jayne D, Saunders R. Comparison of defecatory function after laparoscopic total colectomy and ileorectal anastomosis versus a traditional open approach. Ann R Coll Surg Engl. 2018;100(3):235–9.
22. Moghadamyeghaneh Z, Hanna MH, Carmichael JC, Pigazzi A, Stamos MJ, Mills S. Comparison of open, laparoscopic, and robotic approaches for total abdominal colectomy. Surg Endosc. 2016;30(7):2792–8.

23. Ouaissi M, Lefevre JH, Bretagnol F, Alves A, Valleur P, Panis Y. Laparoscopic 3-step restorative proctocolectomy: comparative study with open approach in 45 patients. Surg Laparosc Endosc Percutan Tech. 2008;18(4):357–62.
24. Chung TP, Fleshman JW, Birnbaum EH, Hunt SR, Dietz DW, Read TE, et al. Laparoscopic vs. open total abdominal colectomy for severe colitis: impact on recovery and subsequent completion restorative proctectomy. Dis Colon Rectum. 2009;52(1):4–10.
25. Watanabe K, Funayama Y, Fukushima K, Shibata C, Takahashi K, Sasaki I. Hand-assisted laparoscopic vs. open subtotal colectomy for severe ulcerative colitis. Dis Colon Rectum. 2009;52(4):640–5.
26. Telem DA, Vine AJ, Swain G, Divino CM, Salky B, Greenstein AJ, et al. Laparoscopic subtotal colectomy for medically refractory ulcerative colitis: the time has come. Surg Endosc. 2010;24(7):1616–20.
27. Bartels SA, Vlug MS, Henneman D, Ponsioen CY, Tanis PJ, Bemelman WA. Less adhesiolysis and hernia repair during completion proctocolectomy after laparoscopic emergency colectomy for ulcerative colitis. Surg Endosc. 2012;26(2):368–73.
28. Parnaby CN, Ramsay G, Macleod CS, Hope NR, Jansen JO, McAdam TK. Complications after laparoscopic and open subtotal colectomy for inflammatory colitis: a case-matched comparison. Colorectal Dis. 2013;15(11):1399–405.
29. Frid NL, Bulut O, Pachler J. Acceptable short-term outcome of laparoscopic subtotal colectomy for inflammatory bowel disease. Dan Med J. 2013;60(6):A4645.
30. Gu J, Stocchi L, Remzi FH, Kiran RP. Total abdominal colectomy for severe ulcerative colitis: does the laparoscopic approach really have benefit? Surg Endosc. 2014;28(2):617–25.
31. Messenger DE, Mihailovic D, MacRae HM, O'Connor BI, Victor JC, McLeod RS. Subtotal colectomy in severe ulcerative and Crohn's colitis: what benefit does the laparoscopic approach confer? Dis Colon Rectum. 2014;57(12):1349–57.
32. Buchs NC, Bloemendaal ALA, Wood CPJ, Travis S, Mortensen NJ, Guy RJ, et al. Subtotal colectomy for ulcerative colitis: lessons learned from a tertiary centre. Colorectal Dis. 2017;19(5):O153–o61.

35 Organ-Preserving Strategies in the Management of Fulminant *Clostridium difficile* Colitis

Ari Grinspan and Marylise Boutros

Introduction and Rationale

Clostridium difficile infection (CDI) is a major cause of morbidity and mortality for hospitalized patients and is a leading cause of nosocomial infections and antibiotic-associated diarrhea [1]. In the United States, there are an estimated 500,000 cases of CDI each year with 29,000 deaths within 30 days of initial diagnosis [1]. The incidence of CDI has been rising since 1996 and has been estimated to cost up to 4.8 billion dollars per year in the United States [1–4]. Of the patients who get CDI, 3–10% develop severe or fulminant CDI which carries a 35–57% mortality rate [5–7].

CDI is diagnosed by the presence of symptoms and an objective marker of toxigenic *Clostridium difficile*. CDI should be suspected in patients with unexplained acute diarrhea (≥3 unformed bowel movements per day) with risk factors such as recent antibiotic exposure and/or health-care exposure [8]. Stool tests should then be submitted to confirm diagnosis in suspected cases. There are three readily available stool tests for CDI with varying degrees of sensitivity and specificity: glutamate dehydrogenase (GDH) immunoassays, enzyme immunoassays (EIA) detecting toxin, and nucleic acid amplification test (NAAT) detecting the toxin gene. GDH and NAAT have high negative predictive value, but a positive result does not distinguish

A. Grinspan
Mount Sinai Hospital, The Dr. Henry D. Janowitz Division of Gastroenterology, New York, NY, USA

Icahn School of Medicine at Mount Sinai, The Dr. Henry D. Janowitz Division of Gastroenterology, New York, NY, USA
e-mail: Ari.grinspan@mountsinai.org

M. Boutros (✉)
Jewish General Hospital, Division of Colorectal Surgery, Montreal, QC, Canada

McGill University, Department of Surgery, Montreal, QC, Canada

P. Sylla et al. (eds.), *The SAGES Manual of Colorectal Surgery*,
https://doi.org/10.1007/978-3-030-24812-3_35

Table 35.1 *Clostridium difficile* infection severity classification

Classification	Definition
Non-severe	WBC <15 and Cr <1.5
Severe	WBC ≥15 and/or Cr ≥1.5
Fulminant	Hypotension, shock, ileus, megacolon

Data from: McDonald et al. [8]

active infection from colonization. Toxin EIA has the highest positive predictive value, but its sensitivity is less than GDH and NAAT. The most accurate way to diagnose CDI is to use a multistep algorithm, such as GDH plus toxin EIA followed by a confirmatory test with NAAT [8].

Recent guidelines from the Infectious Diseases Society of America have redefined the severity classification of CDI: non-severe, severe, and fulminant [8] (Table 35.1). Fulminant *Clostridium difficile* colitis (FCDC) is characterized by hypotension, shock, ileus, or megacolon [8]. Toxic megacolon is a clinical and radiographic diagnosis defined as total or segmental nonobstructive colonic dilation greater than 6 cm accompanied by systemic toxicity. General management strategies include continued enteral nutrition, fluid resuscitation, discontinuation of other antibiotics if possible, and initiation of appropriate anti-CDI antibiotics [8, 9]. Treatment for fulminant CDI includes vancomycin 500 mg orally 4 times daily and metronidazole 500 mg intravenously every 8 hours. In cases of ileus, vancomycin retention enemas can be administered every 6 hours, though data to support this therapy are sparse [10]. Adjunct treatments including intravenous immunoglobulin and other antibiotic regimens have not been shown to improve outcomes in fulminant CDI [11–13]. For some patients, the appropriate course of action is surgery, but identifying these patients is challenging. Multiple studies have looked at risk factors of failing medical therapy including shock, pressor requirement, end organ failure, and laboratory abnormalities including leukocyte count and lactate [5, 6, 14, 15]. The mortality rate reported with colectomy in patients with fulminant CDI range from 30% to 50% [14]. Several studies have identified predictors for poor outcome with surgical treatment including respiratory insufficiency, renal insufficiency, age > 60, peripheral vascular disease, congestive heart failure, and coagulopathy [3, 5, 14–16]. Long-term outcomes after standard of care total abdominal colectomy (TAC) for CDI are poor with mean survival of 18.1 months and median survival of 3.2 months [17]. Mounting evidence suggests early intervention is key, which may reduce mortality in these patients [6, 7, 18–21].

Given the poor outcomes with current medical and surgical approaches to fulminant CDI, alternate treatment approaches have been explored. In this chapter, we will explore organ-preserving strategies in the management of fulminant CDI.

Currently, the standard of care for FCDC is timely TAC with end ileostomy. However, despite this early intervention, mortality rates remain high ranging from 35% to 57% [16, 18, 22, 23]; thus TAC for FCDC is usually reserved as a measure of last resort for many patients. This is in part due to the absence of absolute indications for surgery such as the rare events of colonic ischemia and perforation and the lack of clear guidelines on the optimal timing of surgical intervention for FCDC. Furthermore, patients who survive a TAC for FCDC often face a difficult and prolonged recovery, with significant morbidity [17]. Moreover, the majority of patients are left with a permanent ileostomy, as is demonstrated by the low gastrointestinal restoration rates following TAC for FCDC in the literature [17, 24].

However, in spite of the high mortality and morbidity associated with TAC, many studies have reported improved mortality for patients with FCDC who underwent early operative intervention [16, 19, 25]. Even though these studies were limited by retrospective designs, a recent systematic review confirmed that this procedure still provides a survival advantage compared to medical management alone [7].

Furthermore, a recent study by Stokes and coauthors reported a significantly decreased mortality in patients with CDI admitted under the care of gastrointestinal surgeons compared to patients admitted under general medical services [26]. Sailhamer and coauthors similarly reported a decreased mortality rate in patients admitted under the care of the surgical department compared to medical departments, with a shorter time from admission to operation and a trend toward a higher rate of operation [18]. These data show that timely surgical intervention improves survival as it prevents the development of multi-organ system failure.

Operative Interventions

Loop Ileostomy and Colonic Lavage

Indications and Contraindications

Loop ileostomy and colonic lavage for FCDC involve the creation of a loop ileostomy, an intraoperative colonic lavage with warmed polyethylene glycol (PEG) via the ileostomy, and postoperative antegrade instillation of vancomycin flushes into the diseased colon via the ileostomy (Fig. 35.1a, b) [27]. First described by Neal and coauthors in 2011, this single institution, single surgeon series compared 42 patients who underwent loop ileostomy and colonic lavage for FCDC with 42 historical patients who had undergone a TAC. Indications for operative management included a diagnosis of CDI either by endoscopy, toxin assay, or evidence of colitis on imaging with any sign of clinical worsening. These included signs of peritonitis, worsening abdominal distention, sepsis, new onset ventilator requirement, new or increasing vasopressor requirement, altered mental status, unexplained change in clinical status, non-improving leukocytosis, or bandemia, despite appropriate antibiotic therapy.

Absolute contraindications for loop ileostomy and colonic lavage include the rare situations of FCDC presenting with colonic perforation or ischemia. In addition, patients with toxic megacolon may not tolerate the lavage required for this procedure.

Principles and Quality Benchmarks of the Approach

The primary endpoint was resolution of clinical signs associated with CDI and normalization of peripheral leukocyte count. Both the historical TAC and experimental groups were comparably critically ill as evidenced by similarities in their

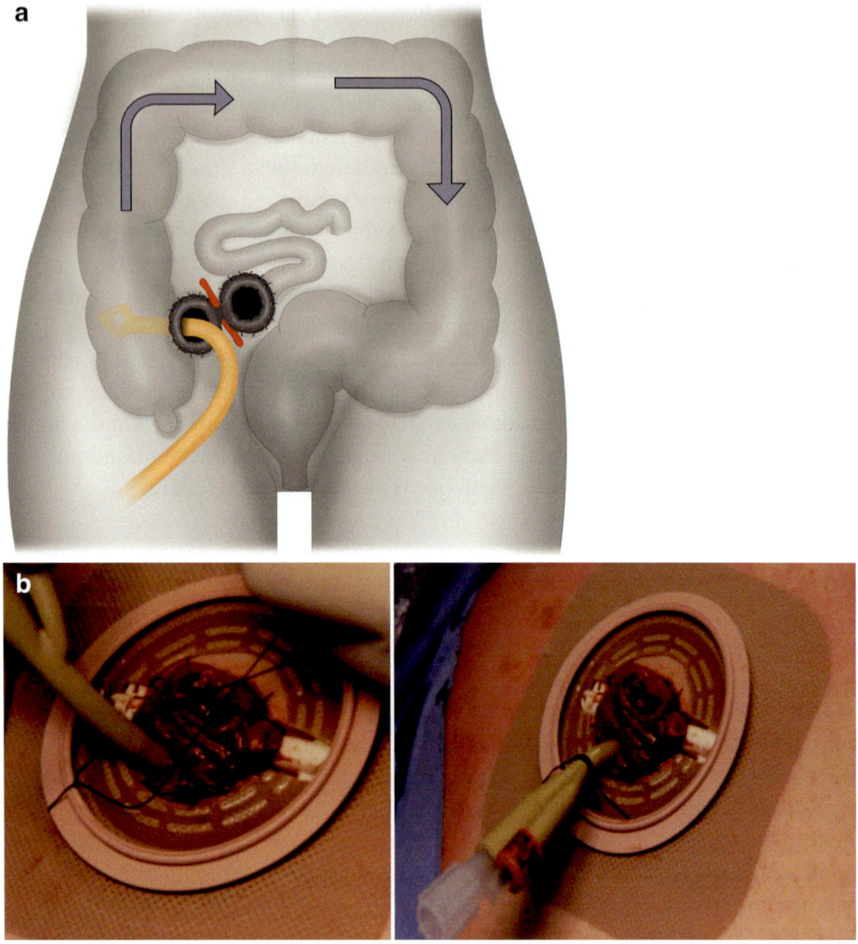

Fig. 35.1 (**a**) Schematic illustration of loop ileostomy with lavage technique (**a**: Used with permission of Wolters Kluwer Health, Inc., from Neal et al. [27]). (**b**) Securing the Foley catheter. The Foley can be secured to the ileostomy appliance as shown here. Alternatively, it can be secured to the rod, or a tie around the catheter can be left long and held in place by the stoma bag

APACHE-II scores, white blood cell counts, intensive care unit admission, preoperative intubation, need for vasopressors, and pharmacologic immunosuppression. The authors found that all patients achieved resolution of disease, with a significant reduction in the 30-day mortality in the loop ileostomy group compared to the historical control group who underwent a TAC (19% vs 50%, respectively; $p = 0.006$). In addition to the survival benefit, there was an increase in ileostomy reversal rates (reported at 79% at 6 months), which is considerably higher than the reported 20% rate of gastrointestinal restoration rates following TAC [24]. The authors were also able to perform the lavage laparoscopically in the majority of patients (83%). In their series, one patient required immediate conversion to TAC due to persistent abdominal compartment syndrome (ACS) that was not improved with the lavage, and one patient developed ACS 12 hours after the lavage and required conversion to TAC. In their series of 42 patients, only one patient had recurrent vasopressor requirement 12 days after surgery and required conversion to a TAC. Thus, in a minority of patients who undergo a lavage, a second surgery may be necessary. The authors' hypotheses for the success of the lavage were that a diverting loop ileostomy poses minimal surgical stress for the critically ill patient and that since the fecal stream is diverted and the colonic lumen deprived of nutrition, mechanical lavage and local vancomycin delivery would result in successful removal of the bacteria and toxin.

Operative Technique

Exploratory laparotomy or diagnostic laparoscopy is carried out first to confirm the diagnosis and ensure that there is no colonic necrosis or perforation. A laparoscopic approach is preferable if the patient is a good candidate and if the surgeon is comfortable with the procedure; otherwise it can be undertaken using an open approach.

The second step involves the creation of a loop ileostomy. The loop ileostomy is ideally created 20 cm from the ileocecal valve so that an 18Fr Foley catheter, inserted into the distal limb of the ileostomy, can be positioned in the cecum. The Foley should be secured to the ileostomy at the end of the procedure using a 0-silk suture (Fig. 35.1b). Lavage of the colon is then performed with 8 liters of polyethylene glycol (PEG) solution warmed to 37 °C. The colonic lavage is performed with the use of the Foley catheter connected to a bag with the PEG solution using urological connection tubing, similar to the one used in cystoscopy. A rectal tube or management device should be inserted into the rectum and attached to a large drainage bag until the lavage is complete. The PEG solution is administered in increments, liter by liter, ensuring that effluent drainage is collected in the rectal tube. If the procedure is performed laparoscopically, pneumoperitoneum can be maintained at 7–10 mmHg during lavage. Laparoscopic bowel graspers may be used to aid in pushing the fluid along the colon. If performed by a laparotomy, the abdomen is kept open, and the surgeon can manually aid the movement of the fluid through the colon. If trouble is encountered getting fluid through the colon, the patient may be moved into the Trendelenburg/reverse Trendelenburg positions as well as left side up/down and right side up/down to move the fluid along the colon. Alternatively, though rarely required, the hepatic and/or splenic flexures may be mobilized. Due to fluid sequestration in the diseased and atonic colon, an ACS may occur during or after the operation. Although the authors do not recommend routinely monitoring for ACS, the surgeon should be aware of this possibility. The surgeon may choose to leave a drain in the paracolic gutters to drain excessive ascites and potentially reduce the risk of an ACS. Postoperatively, vancomycin flushes (500 mg in 500 mL of Lactated Ringers) are delivered to the diseased colon through the Foley catheter that was left in the efferent limb of the ileostomy. The first vancomycin flush is given after completion of the PEG flushes, and administration should be continued every 8 hours for 10 days or until the patient is clinically well.

Table 35.2 Summary table comparing total abdominal colectomy vs. loop ileostomy and colonic lavage for fulminant *Clostridium difficile* colitis

Procedure	Pros	Cons
Loop ileostomy and colonic lavage	Minimally invasive option Apparent survival benefit Higher gastrointestinal restoration rates	Limited available data to support use, especially regarding recurrence rates May fail and some patients would require reoperation
Total abdominal colectomy	Definitive management, rare recurrence	High morbidity and mortality Low gastrointestinal restoration rates

Outcomes

Since earlier time to operation in patients with FCDC has been associated with faster recovery and better outcomes, the success of this procedure could be attributed to earlier time in surgical intervention. As such, this might encourage surgeons to intervene at the first signs of severe or complicated disease, using this minimally invasive procedure, rather than delaying to the point where a TAC is the last resort (Table 35.2) [28].

Since the first description of this novel procedure, Ferrada and coauthors conducted the first multicenter study comparing TAC with loop ileostomy in the treatment of CDI [20]. This study retrospectively compared 77 patients who underwent TAC to 21 patients who underwent loop ileostomy and lavage for FCDC. The authors demonstrated that management of FCDC with loop ileostomy carried a significantly lower mortality rate than TAC (17.2% vs 39.7%). Further research is currently being undertaken in the form of a prospective national Canadian registry [29]. This registry will also collect information on strain of *C. difficile* to establish whether patients infected with some strains will be more likely to fail this minimally invasive operative management or suffer higher recurrence rates. Moreover, the registry will also allow for evaluation of the patient's quality of life and documentation of long-term outcomes, including recurrence of CDI.

Turnbull-Blowhole Procedure

The Turnbull-Blowhole procedure was described as a less invasive option, compared to TAC, for critically ill patients with inflammatory bowel diseases. The procedure involves colonic decompression by a skin level colostomy and a loop ileostomy for toxic megacolon [30]. The goal of this operation is to divert the fecal stream and thereby deprive the colonic mucosa of nutrition without the stress of a radical operation.

In their publication in 1971, Turnbull and colleagues described a diverting loop ileostomy and a transverse colostomy (Fig. 35.1a, b). The authors recommended a sigmoid colostomy be created if the sigmoid remained significantly dilated. Although this procedure has been used by surgeons for cases of FCDC, evidence to support its use is lacking. The authors believe this procedure could be an alternative in severely ill patients in whom intestinal lavage may lead to colonic perforation.

Non-operative Interventions

Nasojejunal Lavage

Drawing from the success of the colonic lavage proposed by Neal and colleagues, some surgeons described the use of nasojejunal PEG irrigation as an alternative to surgical intervention. The authors consider this procedure an option for the management of early severe disease, albeit without entirely replacing loop ileostomy and colonic lavage or TAC. To date, the specific indication(s) for this intervention are not clear, and the outcomes of this method have not yet been determined. However, it is a possible alternative for patients who are not surgical candidates or who refuse surgery. A randomized trial of nasojejunal intestinal lavage for the treatment of *C. difficile* is underway and will provide evidence on this procedure as a potential early alternative to surgical intervention [31].

Fecal Microbiota Therapy (FMT)

Another non-operative approach for FCDC, fecal microbiota transplant (FMT), aims to recolonize the colon with normal intestinal flora. FMT was first introduced in the English language [technically first introduced in fourth century China] with a four person case series in 1958 [32]. Subsequently there have been numerous reports and randomized trials that show FMT is a successful and safe treatment for recurrent CDI [33–36].

Indications and Contraindications

Current guidelines from both gastrointestinal and infectious disease societies recommend using FMT after three recurrences of CDI [8, 37]. While there are no guidelines on the use of FMT in FCDC, several groups have recently reported successful treatment of severe and fulminant CDI with FMT with 1 month survival of 70–100% [38–42]. The exact timing of FMT in this disease process remains unknown, but Hocquart and colleagues showed that a single FMT performed 48 hours after severe CDI diagnosis was associated with significant mortality benefit at 3 months compared to standard-of-care (17% vs 69%, $p < 0.0001$) [42]. Based on the available data, FMT for FCDC should be considered in patients not responding to standard of care antibiotics for 48 hours. A multidisciplinary approach is paramount with these patients to coordinate plan of care. Patients with bowel perforation or evidence of colonic ischemia should not undergo FMT. Relative contraindications to performing FMT include patients with severe immunocompromised status, though recent case reports have shown FMT to be successful in these patients [43–45]. It is recommended not to pursue FMT in patients who are on concomitant non-CDI antibiotics for other conditions.

Principles and Quality Benchmarks of the Approach

Our current understanding of the disease pathogenesis is that a disruption in the host intestinal flora and metabolic pathways allows *Clostridium difficile* to proliferate and produce a diarrhea-causing toxin [46–48]. FMT is the process of transferring healthy stool containing colonic microbes and metabolic products from a healthy individual into a patient with disease. FMT has been shown to restore microbial diversity and richness as well as bile acid metabolism in patients with CDI, leading to clinical cure [49, 50].

Preoperative Planning, Patient Work-Up, and Optimization

A multidisciplinary approach should be used in these patients with input from infectious disease, surgery and gastroenterology services. Prior to FMT, potential donors undergo screening including laboratory testing as outlined by FMT Working Group [51]. In the cases of fulminant CDI, there is not enough time to screen donors. In these cases, stool should be easily available and accessible to be administered within 48 hours of patient presentation. The majority of practitioners now use frozen stool either from a local donor or from a stool bank, such as OpenBiome (Somerville, MA, USA). Standard-of-care antibiotics can be held for 6–12 hours before the procedure, though there is no consensus on this practice. Colonic bowel preparation with 4 L of PEG solution is recommended if there is no ileus or bowel obstruction, though there is no consensus on this practice.

Operative Setup and Technique

While FMT can be administered via upper or lower gastrointestinal (GI) tract, it is recommended to perform via lower GI tract with either flexible sigmoidoscopy or colonoscopy in these patients. FMT can be performed at bedside, operating room, or endoscopy suite.

Upper GI route includes delivery via nasogastric tube, nasoduodenal tube, push enteroscopy, percutaneous gastrostomy tube, and percutaneous jejunotomy tube. Lower GI delivery includes colonoscopy, flexible sigmoidoscopy, or enema. In patients with ileus, it is advisable to administer FMT via lower GI delivery. FMT via upper GI route should be administered at the most distal site and with a maximum of 100 cc of product. FMT via lower GI route should be administered at the most proximal extent of exam [terminal ileum or colon] with approximately 250 cc of product. While any of the above delivery mechanisms can be utilized with similar rates of efficacy [75–90%], for patients with fulminant CDI, it is recommended to perform via flexible sigmoidoscopy or colonoscopy in order to assess for pseudomembranous colitis. If pseudomembranes are visualized, vancomycin should be restarted within 24 hours (Fig. 35.2). Serial FMTs, using the above approach, are performed every 3–5 days until pseudomembranes are resolved (Fig. 35.3).

Pitfalls and Troubleshooting

If severe pseudomembranous colitis is encountered during colonoscopy, we recommended using minimal air insufflation to avoid air trapping and perforation, and

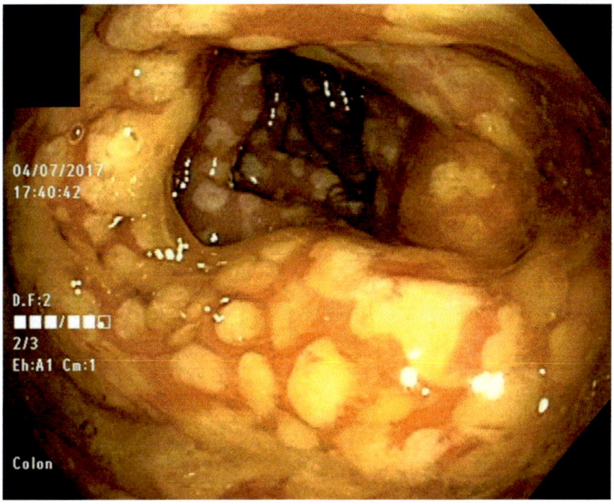

Fig. 35.2 Pseudomembranes visualized endoscopically

Fig. 35.3 The approach to the administration of serial FMT

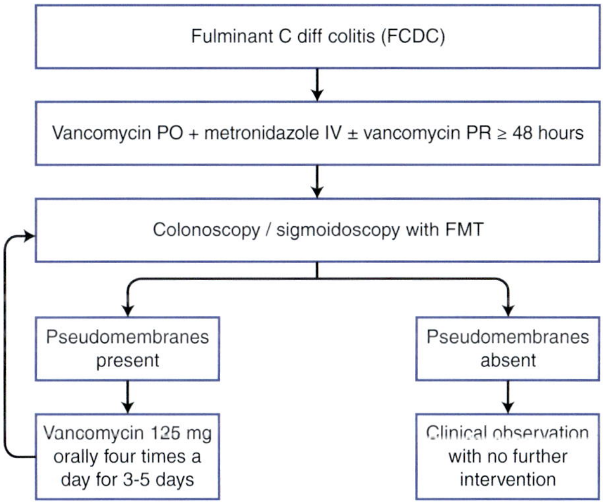

only advancing the scope to the splenic flexure or where the endoscopist feels most comfortable advancing. Ideally carbon dioxide should be used to minimize the risk of bowel perforation. Patients with WBC > 20, albumin <2.5, pseudomembranous colitis on index colonoscopy, and use of non-CDI antibiotics during admission are more likely to require multiple FMTs. Serial FMTs performed every 3–5 days, until resolution of pseudomembranous colitis, have been shown to be effective in these patients [38, 39]. Administering FMT via upper GI tract in patients with fulminant CDI may be ineffective given the high prevalence of ileus in these patients and subsequent risk of fecal aspiration [52].

Table 35.3 Use of FMT in severe and fulminant CDI

Study	Patients	Severity of CDI	Intervention	Administration	Outcomes
Fischer et al. [38, 53]	57	Severe and fulminant	Serial FMT	Colonoscopy	Cure rate = 91% Survival at 1 month = 94.7%
Aroniadis et al. [40]	17	Severe and fulminant	1 or 2 FMT	Colonoscopy	Cure rate = 88% Survival at 1 month = 100%
Ianiro et al. [39]	56	Severe and fulminant	Single FMT vs. multiple FMT	Colonoscopy	Survival at 1 month = 100%
Zainah et al. [41]	14	Severe	Single FMT	NGT	Cure rate = 79% Survival at 1 month = 71%
Hocquart et al. [42]	34	Severe	Single FMT	NGT	Survival at 3 months = 87%

NGT nasogastric tube

Outcomes

The existing literature shows FMT to be a very promising treatment strategy for patients with FCDC (Table 35.3). Using an endoscopic response-guided FMT strategy achieved clinical cure in 90% of patients with 1 month survival >90% and no significant adverse event profile [38, 53]. Given the positive results, favorable risk profile, and ease of administration with frozen stool, FMT is a practical organ-preserving strategy in the management of fulminant *Clostridium difficile* colitis.

Conclusion

Overall, colon-preserving options for FCDC have been shown to improve survival and gastrointestinal restoration/preservation rates while minimizing complications and facilitating earlier intervention for FCDC. However, despite these minimally invasive surgical alternatives such as loop ileostomy with colonic lavage, or non-operative interventions such as nasojejunal lavage or FMT, some patients will still require a TAC. Furthermore, the patient and disease selection criteria for each of these approaches have yet to be definitively determined. While evidence for these new techniques is still emerging, the anticipated results from ongoing prospective trials will outline their specific roles in the management of FCDC (Fig. 35.4).

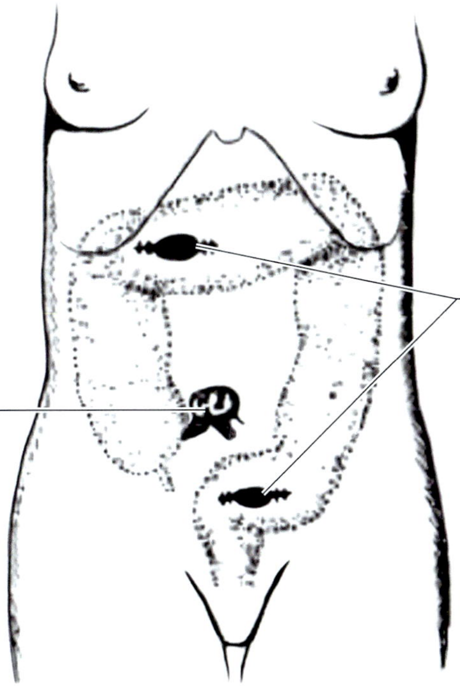

Fig. 35.4 Diverting loop ileostomy and decompression colostomies. (Used with permission of Elsevier from Turnbull et al. [30])

References

1. Lessa FC, Mu Y, Bamberg WM, Beldavs ZG, Dumyati GK, Dunn JR, et al. Burden of Clostridium difficile infection in the United States. N Engl J Med. 2015;372(9):825–34.
2. Kelly CP, LaMont JT. Clostridium difficile—more difficult than ever. N Engl J Med. 2008;359(18):1932–40.
3. Halabi WJ, Nguyen VQ, Carmichael JC, Pigazzi A, Stamos MJ, Mills S. Clostridium difficile colitis in the United States: a decade of trends, outcomes, risk factors for colectomy, and mortality after colectomy. J Am Coll Surg. 2013;217(5):802–12.
4. Hall AJ, Curns AT, McDonald LC, Parashar UD, Lopman BA. The roles of Clostridium difficile and norovirus among gastroenteritis-associated deaths in the United States, 1999–2007. Clin Infect Dis. 2012;55(2):216–23.
5. Bhangu A, Nepogodiev D, Gupta A, Torrance A, Singh P, Collaborative WMR. Systematic review and meta-analysis of outcomes following emergency surgery for Clostridium difficile colitis. Br J Surg. 2012;99(11):1501–13.
6. Butala P, Divino CM. Surgical aspects of fulminant Clostridium difficile colitis. Am J Surg. 2010;200(1):131–5.
7. Stewart D, Hollenbeak C, Wilson M. Is colectomy for fulminant Clostridium difficile colitis life saving? A systematic review. Colorectal Dis. 2013;15(7):798–804.
8. McDonald LC, Gerding DN, Johnson S, Bakken JS, Carroll KC, Coffin SE, et al. Clinical practice guidelines for Clostridium difficile infection in adults and children: 2017 update by

the Infectious Diseases Society of America (IDSA) and Society for Healthcare Epidemiology of America (SHEA). Clin Infect Dis. 2018;66(7):e1–e48.
9. Kautza B, Zuckerbraun BS. The surgical management of complicated Clostridium Difficile infection: alternatives to colectomy. Surg Infect (Larchmt). 2016;17(3):337–42.
10. Malamood M, Nellis E, Ehrlich AC, Friedenberg FK. Vancomycin enemas as adjunctive therapy for Clostridium difficile infection. J Clin Med Res. 2015;7(6):422.
11. McPherson S, Rees CJ, Ellis R, Soo S, Panter SJ. Intravenous immunoglobulin for the treatment of severe, refractory, and recurrent Clostridium difficile diarrhea. Dis Colon Rectum. 2006;49(5):640–5.
12. Salcedo J, Keates S, Pothoulakis C, Warny M, Castagliuolo I, LaMont J, et al. Intravenous immunoglobulin therapy for severe Clostridium difficile colitis. Gut. 1997;41(3):366–70.
13. Herpers BL, Vlaminckx B, Burkhardt O, Blom H, Biemond-Moeniralam HS, Hornef M, et al. Intravenous tigecycline as adjunctive or alternative therapy for severe refractory Clostridium difficile infection. Clin Infect Dis. 2009;48(12):1732–5.
14. Dudukgian H, Sie E, Gonzalez-Ruiz C, Etzioni DA, Kaiser AM. C. difficile colitis—predictors of fatal outcome. J Gastrointest Surg. 2010;14(2):315–22.
15. Byrn JC, Maun DC, Gingold DS, Baril DT, Ozao JJ, Divino CM. Predictors of mortality after colectomy for fulminant Clostridium difficile colitis. Arch Surg. 2008;143(2):150–4; discussion 5.
16. Pepin J, Vo TT, Boutros M, Marcotte E, Dial S, Dube S, et al. Risk factors for mortality following emergency colectomy for fulminant Clostridium difficile infection. Dis Colon Rectum. 2009;52(3):400–5.
17. Dallas KB, Condren A, Divino CM. Life after colectomy for fulminant Clostridium difficile colitis: a 7-year follow up study. Am J Surg. 2014;207(4):533–9.
18. Sailhamer EA, Carson K, Chang Y, Zacharias N, Spaniolas K, Tabbara M, et al. Fulminant Clostridium difficile colitis: patterns of care and predictors of mortality. Arch Surg. 2009;144(5):433–9; discussion 9–40.
19. Ali SO, Welch JP, Dring RJ. Early surgical intervention for fulminant pseudomembranous colitis. Am Surg. 2008;74(1):20–6.
20. Ferrada P, Callcut R, Zielinski MD, Bruns B, Yeh DD, Zakrison TL, et al. Loop ileostomy versus total colectomy as surgical treatment for Clostridium difficile–associated disease: an Eastern Association for the Surgery of Trauma multicenter trial. J Trauma Acute Care Surg. 2017;83(1):36–40.
21. Seder CW, Villalba MR, Robbins J, Ivascu FA, Carpenter CF, Dietrich M. Early colectomy may be associated with improved survival in fulminant Clostridium difficile colitis: an 8-year experience. Am J Surg. 2009;197(3):302–7.
22. Lamontagne F, Labbe AC, Haeck O, Lesur O, Lalancette M, Patino C, et al. Impact of emergency colectomy on survival of patients with fulminant Clostridium difficile colitis during an epidemic caused by a hypervirulent strain. Ann Surg. 2007;245(2):267–72.
23. Dallal RM, Harbrecht BG, Boujoukas AJ, Sirio CA, Farkas LM, Lee KK, et al. Fulminant Clostridium difficile: an underappreciated and increasing cause of death and complications. Ann Surg. 2002;235(3):363–72.
24. Miller AT, Tabrizian P, Greenstein AJ, Dikman A, Byrn J, Divino C. Long-term follow-up of patients with fulminant Clostridium difficile colitis. J Gastrointest Surg. 2009;13(5):956–9.
25. Markelov A, Livert D, Kohli H. Predictors of fatal outcome after colectomy for fulminant Clostridium difficile colitis: a 10-year experience. dr.markelov@gmail.com. Am Surg. 2011;77(8):977–80.
26. Stokes AL, Bible A, Hollenbeak CS, Stewart DB Sr. Clostridium difficile infection is associated with lower inpatient mortality when managed by GI surgeons. Dis Colon Rectum. 2016;59(9):855–61.
27. Neal MD, Alverdy JC, Hall DE, Simmons RL, Zuckerbraun BS. Diverting loop ileostomy and colonic lavage: an alternative to total abdominal colectomy for the treatment of severe, complicated Clostridium difficile associated disease. Ann Surg. 2011;254(3):423–7; discussion 7–9.

28. Hall JF, Berger D. Outcome of colectomy for Clostridium difficile colitis: a plea for early surgical management. Am J Surg. 2008;196(3):384–8.
29. ClinicalTrials.gov. Loop ileostomy with colonic lavage for fulminant Clostridium difficile colitis. 2017. Available from: https://clinicaltrials.gov/show/NCT02347280.
30. Turnbull RB Jr, Hawk WA, Weakley FL. Surgical treatment of toxic megacolon. Ileostomy and colostomy to prepare patients for colectomy. Am J Surg. 1971;122(3):325–31.
31. ClinicalTrials.gov. Intestinal lavage for the treatment of severe C. difficile infections. 2015. Available from: https://clinicaltrials.gov/ct2/show/NCT02466698.
32. Eiseman Á, Silen W, Bascom G, Kauvar A. Fecal enema as an adjunct in the treatment of pseudomembranous enterocolitis. Surgery. 1958;44(5):854–9.
33. Van Nood E, Vrieze A, Nieuwdorp M, Fuentes S, Zoetendal EG, de Vos WM, et al. Duodenal infusion of donor feces for recurrent Clostridium difficile. N Engl J Med. 2013;368(5):407–15.
34. Kassam Z, Lee CH, Yuan Y, Hunt RH. Fecal microbiota transplantation for Clostridium difficile infection: systematic review and meta-analysis. Am J Gastroenterol. 2013;108(4):500.
35. Cammarota G, Masucci L, Ianiro G, Bibbò S, Dinoi G, Costamagna G, et al. Randomised clinical trial: faecal microbiota transplantation by colonoscopy vs. vancomycin for the treatment of recurrent Clostridium difficile infection. Aliment Pharmacol Ther. 2015;41(9):835–43.
36. Kelly CR, Khoruts A, Staley C, Sadowsky MJ, Abd M, Alani M, et al. Effect of fecal microbiota transplantation on recurrence in multiply recurrent Clostridium difficile infection: a randomized trial. Ann Intern Med. 2016;165(9):609–16.
37. Surawicz CM, Brandt LJ, Binion DG, Ananthakrishnan AN, Curry SR, Gilligan PH, et al. Guidelines for diagnosis, treatment, and prevention of Clostridium difficile infections. Am J Gastroenterol. 2013;108(4):478–98; quiz 99.
38. Fischer M, Sipe B, Rogers N, Cook G, Robb B, Vuppalanchi R, et al. Faecal microbiota transplantation plus selected use of vancomycin for severe-complicated Clostridium difficile infection: description of a protocol with high success rate. Aliment Pharmacol Ther. 2015;42(4):470–6.
39. Ianiro G, Masucci L, Quaranta G, Simonelli C, Lopetuso L, Sanguinetti M, et al. Randomised clinical trial: faecal microbiota transplantation by colonoscopy plus vancomycin for the treatment of severe refractory Clostridium difficile infection—single versus multiple infusions. Aliment Pharmacol Ther. 2018;48(2):152–9.
40. Aroniadis OC, Brandt LJ, Greenberg A, Borody T, Kelly CR, Mellow M, et al. Long-term follow-up study of fecal microbiota transplantation for severe and/or complicated Clostridium difficile infection. J Clin Gastroenterol. 2016;50(5):398–402.
41. Zainah H, Hassan M, Shiekh-Sroujieh L, Hassan S, Alangaden G, Ramesh M. Intestinal microbiota transplantation, a simple and effective treatment for severe and refractory Clostridium difficile infection. Dig Dis Sci. 2015;60(1):181–5.
42. Hocquart M, Lagier JC, Cassir N, Saidani N, Eldin C, Kerbaj J, et al. Early fecal microbiota transplantation improves survival in severe Clostridium difficile infections. Clin Infect Dis. 2018;66(5):645–50.
43. Shogbesan O, Poudel DR, Victor S, Jehangir A, Fadahunsi O, Shogbesan G, et al. A systematic review of the efficacy and safety of fecal microbiota transplant for Clostridium difficile infection in immunocompromised patients. Can J Gastroenterol Hepatol. 2018;2018:1394379.
44. Kelly CR, Ihunnah C, Fischer M, Khoruts A, Surawicz C, Afzali A, et al. Fecal microbiota transplant for treatment of Clostridium difficile infection in immunocompromised patients. Am J Gastroenterol. 2014;109(7):1065.
45. Lin SC, Alonso CD, Moss AC. Fecal microbiota transplantation for recurrent Clostridium difficile infection in patients with solid organ transplants: an institutional experience and review of the literature. Transpl Infect Dis. 2018;20:e12967.
46. Leffler DA, Lamont JT. Clostridium difficile infection. N Engl J Med. 2015;372(16):1539–48.
47. Brandt LJ. American Journal of Gastroenterology Lecture: intestinal microbiota and the role of fecal microbiota transplant (FMT) in treatment of C. difficile infection. Am J Gastroenterol. 2013;108(2):177.

48. Allegretti JR, Kearney S, Li N, Bogart E, Bullock K, Gerber GK, et al. Recurrent Clostridium difficile infection associates with distinct bile acid and microbiome profiles. Aliment Pharmacol Ther. 2016;43(11):1142–53.
49. Khoruts A, Sadowsky MJ. Understanding the mechanisms of faecal microbiota transplantation. Nat Rev Gastroenterol Hepatol. 2016;13(9):508.
50. Weingarden AR, Dosa PI, DeWinter E, Steer CJ, Shaughnessy MK, Johnson JR, et al. Changes in colonic bile acid composition following fecal microbiota transplantation are sufficient to control Clostridium difficile germination and growth. PLoS One. 2016;11(1):e0147210.
51. Bakken JS, Borody T, Brandt LJ, Brill JV, Demarco DC, Franzos MA, et al. Treating Clostridium difficile infection with fecal microbiota transplantation. Clin Gastroenterol Hepatol. 2011;9(12):1044–9.
52. Wang S, Xu M, Wang W, Cao X, Piao M, Khan S, et al. Systematic review: adverse events of fecal microbiota transplantation. PLoS One. 2016;11(8):e0161174.
53. Fischer M, Sipe B, Cheng Y-W, Phelps E, Rogers N, Sagi S, et al. Fecal microbiota transplant in severe and severe-complicated Clostridium difficile: a promising treatment approach. Gut Microbes. 2017;8(3):289–302.

Optimizing Stoma Function and Quality of Life: Best Practices in Planned and Unplanned Stoma Creation

36

Lisa M. Cannon and Dana M. Hayden

Introduction

Intestinal diversion refers to a surgical operation in which a bowel segment is diverted to an artificial opening through the abdominal wall. Permanent or temporary intestinal diversion is necessary in the management of a number of colon and rectal disorders, such as trauma, fecal incontinence, malignancy, inflammatory bowel disease (IBD), diverticular disease, postsurgical complications, and functional bowel disorders. The overall incidence and prevalence of ostomies are difficult to approximate since the procedure is often bundled within other operations, and there is no national registry of ostomates in the United States. However, a Danish study in 2016 created a database that extrapolated an incidence of 4000 stomas created per year and a prevalence of 10–12,000 people living with stomas in that country at one time [1]. It is estimated that more than 120,000 intestinal stomas are created annually in the United States [2].

The type of stoma and its reversibility are extremely variable. Over 80% of rectal cancer patients undergoing proctectomy undergo fecal diversion at their initial operation, with approximately 20% undergoing abdominoperineal resection (APR) with permanent colostomy [3]. Up to 25% of patients undergoing sphincter-preserving surgery for rectal cancer never undergo ileostomy reversal. In the trauma population, 10% of patients with hollow viscus injury require a stoma, and of these, 25% will not have been reversed at 5 years [4]. Approximately half of patients undergoing emergency surgery for diverticulitis will receive a colostomy or ileostomy, compared to only 15% of those undergoing elective resection [5]. Only one half of patients

L. M. Cannon (✉)
University of Chicago, Chicago, IL, USA

D. M. Hayden
Division of Colon and Rectal Surgery, Rush University Medical Center, Department of General Surgery, Chicago, IL, USA

P. Sylla et al. (eds.), *The SAGES Manual of Colorectal Surgery*,
https://doi.org/10.1007/978-3-030-24812-3_36

undergoing Hartmann's procedure (HP) for diverticulitis will be reversed, whereas over 90% of diverting loop ileostomies performed at primary resection with anastomosis will be reversed [6, 7]. Fecal diversion is occasionally used in the management of Crohn's colitis and severe perianal disease; while this is often planned as temporary strategy, long-term bowel restoration is successful in only 17% of these patients [6].

While stomas may decrease postoperative complications, improve quality of life, and may even be lifesaving, they are undeniably life-altering. Proper site selection and marking, adherence to proper technique when maturing a colostomy or ileotomy, enhanced stoma education, and knowledge of postoperative support in stoma care are essential to any general surgeon who performs colon or rectal surgery.

Indications and Contraindications

The indications for fecal diversion are broad and are summarized in Box 36.1. There are no firm contraindications for ostomy formation, only relative contraindications in regard to the type of diversion selected. Emergency indications for stoma formation include traumatic or iatrogenic intestinal injury, reoperation for anastomotic leak, perforated diverticulitis, large bowel obstruction (LBO), and toxic megacolon such as with *Clostridium difficile* colitis, ulcerative colitis or Crohn's colitis, and colonic volvulus when anastomosis is not indicated. Unplanned stoma creation is most often seen during intraoperative consultation for iatrogenic injury or for anastomotic protection when unanticipated operative findings or events such as bleeding or bowel ischemia have made an anastomosis unexpectedly tenuous. Elective stoma creation can be used as definitive management after resection for rectal cancer and planned anastomotic protection for high-risk anastomoses, as a last resort for fecal incontinence or constipation and in the management of congenital intestinal anomalies.

Box 36.1 Indications for Fecal Diversion

Trauma
Diverticulitis
Rectal cancer
Fecal incontinence
Ulcerative colitis
Crohn's disease
Constipation
Volvulus
Toxic megacolon
Mesenteric ischemia
Anastomotic protection
Obstruction
Congenital anomalies
Radiation proctitis

It is important to stress that stoma formation is not always indicated in each of the above circumstances, and patient- and disease-specific factors should guide the decision-making process. Both ileostomy and colostomy formation, temporary or permanent, are associated with an array of complications including peristomal skin complications, dehydration, infectious complications, obstruction, hernia, reduced quality of life, prolapse, stenosis, and retraction, all resulting in increased health-care costs and decreased quality of life.

Principles and Quality Benchmarks

There are multiple options of diversion depending on the disease process, so thoughtful decisions in regard to current and future surgeries are integral. When large bowel obstruction requires diversion, sigmoid loop colostomy is preferred if the obstruction is distal, within the rectosigmoid. This allows the loop colostomy site to be easily resected with the primary pathology at the time of planned resection, without a separate anastomosis. If the obstruction is more proximal, a transverse loop colostomy should be considered. In the setting of LBO, ileostomy should be created cautiously if the ileocecal valve is competent as this can lead to a closed loop obstruction. These operative approaches possess different complication profiles. Wound infection, sepsis, and stoma prolapse are more common with transverse loop colostomy, while loop ileostomy patients have higher rates of dehydration, readmission, and obstructive complications after closure [7]. Resection with a primary anastomosis with or without loop ileostomy is emerging as a favorable alternative to Hartmann's procedure for Hinchey III and IV diverticulitis [8, 9]. Subspecialty referral may lead to a higher likelihood of primary anastomosis during a left-sided resection in the emergent setting without increased morbidity or mortality [10]. All diverting ostomies are associated with significant morbidity, so this decision should be carefully scrutinized for individual patients, weighing patient- and disease-specific factors.

Types of Stomas

There are four main types of intestinal stomas, which may be created with either the small or large intestine. These are end stoma, loop stoma, end-loop (also called Prasad type, defunctioned loop or divided loop) stoma, and pseudo-loop (also called loop-end) stoma. These are illustrated in Fig. 36.1a–d. An end-loop stoma is utilized as a means to reduce the morbidity of subsequent re-establishment of intestinal continuity by bringing both the proximal and distal bowel loops through the same abdominal wall aperture. It can be created with remote intestinal segments following bowel resection. The end-loop technique is preferred to the formation of an end stoma and mucus fistula through two separate abdominal wall apertures or leaving a long Hartmann's pouch in situ, which can lead to catastrophic Hartmann's pouch blowout. When this technique is used, stoma closure can often

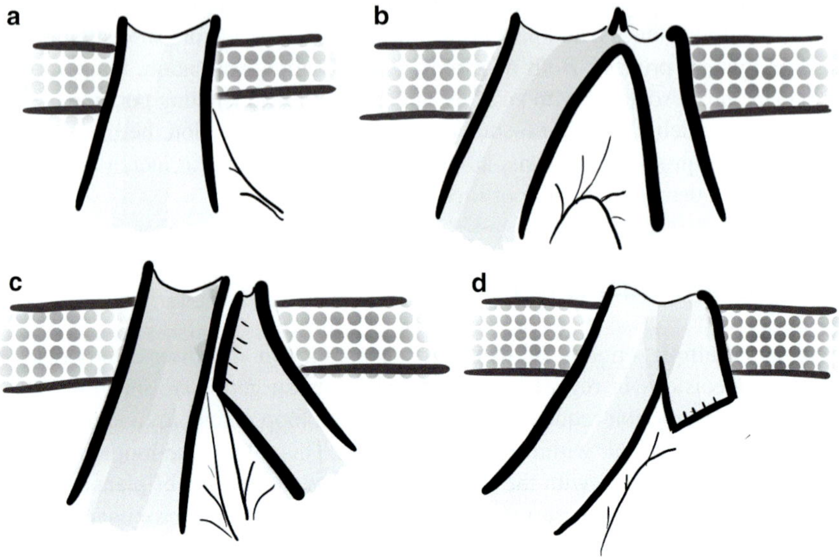

Fig. 36.1 Types of intestinal stomas. (**a**) End stoma, (**b**) loop stoma, (**c**) end-loop (Prasad, defunctioned loop, divided loop) stoma, (**d**) pseudo-loop (loop-end) stoma

be performed without the need for laparotomy [11]. A pseudo-loop stoma is used when it is difficult to create a well-perfused, tension-free end stoma. The distal end of the bowel is stapled off, and the antimesenteric border of the bowel 2–5 cm upstream is brought up through the stoma aperture and matured. This can gain a few additional centimeters of bowel reach and be less traumatizing on the mesentery. Pseudo-loop stoma creation is most often required after sigmoid colectomy; however, it is occasionally necessary when maturing an end ileostomy or colostomy in a morbidly obese patient.

Preoperative Planning, Patient Workup, and Optimization

Stoma Site Selection and Marking

All patients scheduled for colon or rectal surgery with planned or potential stoma creation should undergo a dedicated outpatient visit with an experienced wound, ostomy, and continence nurse (WOCN) and be marked preoperatively. The American Society of Colon and Rectal Surgeons (ASCRS) and the WOCN Society have published a joint position statement on proper site marking for fecal diversion [12]. While site selection is a priority during the visit, the WOCN can assist in setting expectations, addressing misconceptions and anxieties about stomas, and directing patients toward adequate support and resources available after surgery [13].

In addition to the preoperative marking and education by the WOCN, the surgeon's role is important to optimize stoma function at the time of creation. The ostomy should be meticulously constructed to allow for easy pouching and reduction in the risk of stoma complications and peristomal skin irritation [7]. Anatomical considerations and the disease process requiring surgery guide proper site selection for stoma formation. Firstly, the bowel segment selected for stoma creation will influence its location (ileum, transverse, or sigmoid colon). Secondly, it is desirable to lead the bowel through the rectus muscle. Thirdly, the patient's body habitus and pannus size, folds, divots, and their clothing preferences should be taken into consideration.

The "ostomy triangle" is used to guide both preoperative marking and unplanned stoma creation at the time of surgery. It is the zone defined by the umbilicus, the anterior superior iliac spine, and the pubic tubercle. If the stoma is too close to a bony prominence such as the iliac spine or the costal margin, this may push off the faceplate during normal wear. The stoma will sit ideally on the apex of an abdominal fold and be at least 5 cm away from skin creases and folds the umbilicus and prior surgical scars. Having the patient lean over while sitting will accentuate abdominal creases. The site should be assessed with the patient in sitting, standing, and supine positions. If possible, the stoma is placed below the beltline to allow for more concealed wear. However, lower quadrant placement may not be possible or advisable in some circumstances. Obese patients with their large lower abdominal panniculi can be particularly challenging. The weight of the panniculus can substantially shift the location of the stoma site and move it over the patient's visual horizon on their abdominal wall (Fig. 36.2). If the surgery is elective, the patient should be instructed to sit up in order to select a stoma location that they can see and access. A more cephalad location should be chosen to allow for visualization and reach. The upper abdomen is also beneficial since the abdominal wall is comparably thinner and positional shift is less impactful. Unfortunately, appropriate marking does not completely eliminate other stoma risks in obese patients, who are more prone to stoma necrosis, retraction, and pouching difficulty [14].

Nonobese patients are also at risk of stoma complications, including parastomal hernia. Traditional teaching recommends that the stoma should be sited within the borders of the rectus muscle to reduce the incidence of parastomal hernia formation. However, a recent Cochrane review of 9 retrospective cohort studies with a total of 761 patients failed to show a reduced hernia formation with the transrectus approach compared to lateral pararectus stoma placement [15].

Unplanned Stoma Creation

An unplanned stoma creation may be necessary under emergency conditions (e.g., colon perforation, large bowel obstruction, ischemia, etc.) or in case of a complication from a previously undiverted distal surgery (e.g., anastomotic leak, recto-vaginal/recto-urinary fistula). Creation of a stoma under such difficult circumstances has been associated with an increased rate of stoma complications and pouching difficulty. A prospective audit of 3970 stomas created across multiple sites in the

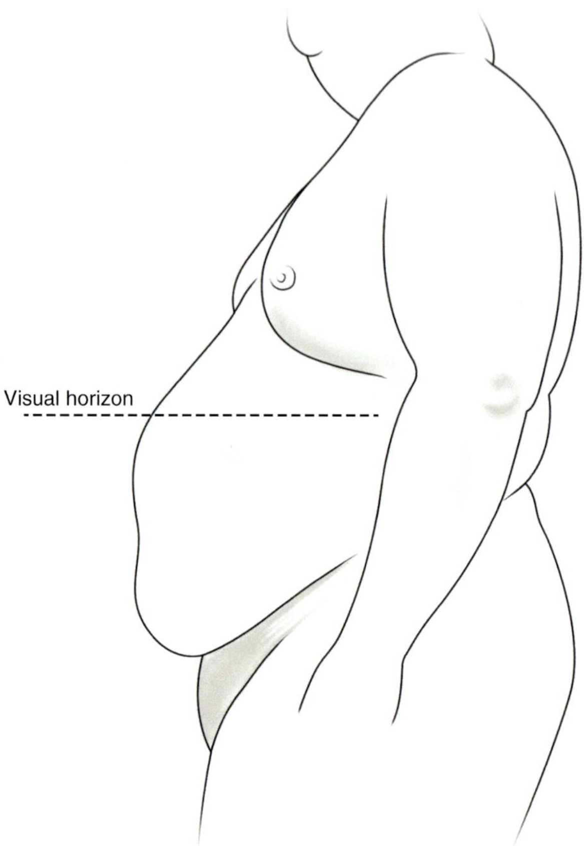

Fig. 36.2 Site selection in the upper abdomen in an obese patient

United Kingdom revealed that insufficient stoma height <10 mm, loop ileostomies, and those created in an emergency setting were more likely to be problematic, requiring increased stoma care and pouching system changes. Problems included retraction, mucocutaneous separation, poor sitting causing pouching difficulty, necrosis, and prolapse [16]. A similar study in 2011 identified colostomy, short stoma, BMI >30, emergency surgery, and lack of marking as risk factors for a problematic stoma (Fig. 36.3) [17]. If emergency surgery is unavoidable, consideration should be given as to whether there is a safe alternative to stoma creation.

While preoperative stoma site marking is a must for all elective cases, the patient undergoing emergency surgery may not be in a condition to allow for marking, or the patient's abdominal contour immediately prior to emergency surgery (e.g., LBO, fluid retention, or anasarca) may not reflect the true body habitus and may obscure even deep abdominal creases and folds.

In the obese patient undergoing emergency surgery, intertriginous skin pathology from chronic moisture may highlight skin creases that should be avoided.

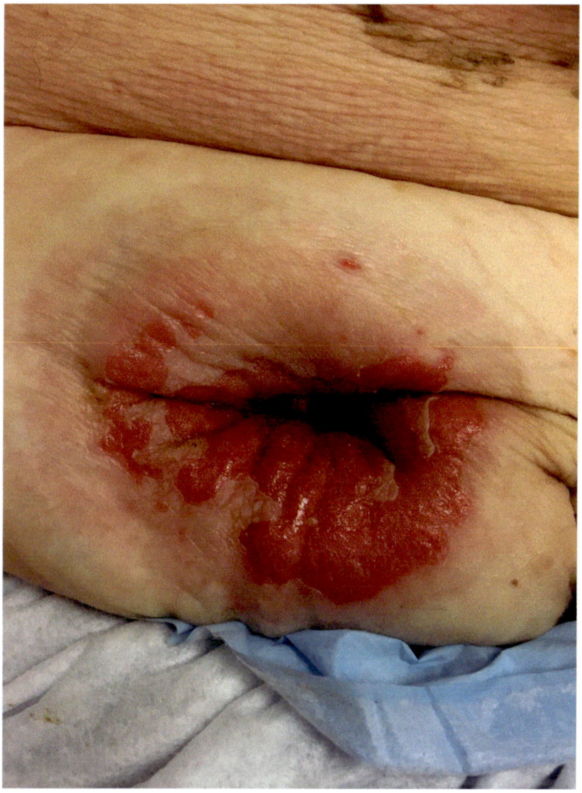

Fig. 36.3 A poorly sited stoma in an obese patient. This stoma is both retracted and in a skin crease, causing pouching difficulty and chemical burn. (Courtesy of M. Kaplon-Jones, APRN)

Stoma placement should be planned much higher than in a thinner patient, typically in a supraumbilical location. An oversized fascial and skin aperture will help prevent congestion and ischemia; although it is likely to lead to peristomal hernia and stoma prolapse in the long-term, these are less morbid outcomes (Fig. 36.4). For emergency colostomy, adequate mobilization from retroperitoneal attachments is important to prevent retraction or ischemia. Another option would be a pseudo-loop (also called loop-end) colostomy since the antimesenteric border has slightly more reach and may require a smaller aperture. The small bowel or colon is pulled up as a loop just proximal to the staple line, and stapled end is left within the abdomen (Fig. 36.1d). This procedure facilitates leaving most of the fatty mesentery within the abdomen and decreases the risk of tearing the mesentery off the bowel wall as it is being pulled through the stoma site. Also, a small wound protector can be placed through the stoma site which puts stretch on the aperture and compresses the wall. With the addition of sterile lubrication, the colon can be more easily pulled through a thick abdominal wall [18].

In a patient with LBO, the distended and fragile colon may be difficult to handle and get to the abdominal wall. Venous compression at the fascial aperture adds to the challenge as it can lead to ischemia in this tenuous bowel. The

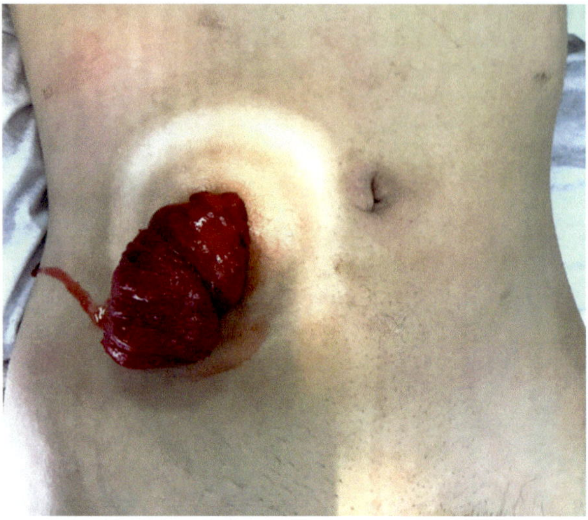

Fig. 36.4 Acute prolapse of an end ileostomy requiring operative reduction and pexy. (Courtesy of Patricia Sylla, MD)

surgeon should assess the cecum and right colon in a left-sided obstruction in case there is vascular compromise or wall compromise due to shear stress. Colonic decompression should be considered early as it greatly facilitates the manipulation of the colon and reduces the risk of rupture and stool spillage. A purse-string suture can be placed at the anticipated site of the colostomy to decompress the colon in a controlled manner. This should facilitate a smaller colostomy aperture and ease pulling the colon through the abdominal wall. Rarely, it may be the case that only the antimesenteric side of the colon can be matured, leading to a stoma that does not fully divert the fecal stream and may require revision later [18].

Operative Setup and Surgical Techniques

Intestinal diversion, if it is not the primary procedure, is typically performed as the concluding stage of an operative procedure. Both colostomy and ileostomy maturation can be accomplished with the patient in any supine or semi-supine position. Patients in high lithotomy will need to be repositioned into low lithotomy or modified low lithotomy. Patients in prone or left lateral decubitus position will require repositioning and redraping. For laparoscopic stoma creation, the patient is placed in lithotomy with arms tucked at the sides.

Routine mechanical or antibiotic bowel preparation prior to ileostomy formation is not required but should be performed prior to colostomy formation. Preoperative antibiotic prophylaxis covering gastrointestinal flora is administered prior to the procedure. Sequential compression stockings are utilized throughout the case. An oral gastric tube and Foley catheterization are not required. If stoma formation is part of a longer operative case, the above considerations should be dictated by the primary procedure being performed.

Aperture Creation When the Primary Operation Has Been Performed Through a Midline Incision

1. A Kocher clamp is placed on the fascial edge to keep the abdominal wall in alignment. A folded dry laparotomy pad is then placed intra-abdominally.
2. A circular disk of skin is excised at the site previously marked. The skin aperture for ileostomy should be 2 cm in diameter and slightly larger for colostomy. There are two techniques to excise the skin aperture; the first is to grasp the central portion of this skin with a second Kocher clamp and pull and excise the tented skin and dermis. The second technique is to use cutting cautery or scalpel to develop a cruciate incision into the subcutaneous tissue and then excise the "dog ears" to create a circular incision.
3. The subcutaneous tissue is divided down to and through Scarpa's fascia until the anterior rectus sheath is exposed. Army-navy, curved S, or appendiceal retractors will assist in exposing the fascia.
4. A vertical incision is then made in the anterior rectus sheath. This aperture should be slightly larger than the skin aperture, or about 3 cm. A small 1 cm cruciate incision is made laterally. The operating surgeon will now place their supinated nondominant hand under the laparotomy pad and apply some upward pressure for improved exposure.
5. The rectus muscle is split in the direction of its muscle fibers, and the retractors are advanced into the incision to now expose the posterior rectus sheath. The posterior sheath is now incised with cutting cautery to expose the intra-abdominal laparotomy pad, thus avoiding bowel injury. The defect should be approximately 2 fingerbreadths in diameter for ileostomies and 3 fingerbreadths for colostomies.
6. The previously divided bowel is then delivered through the aperture that has been created in the abdominal wall. A Babcock clamp can facilitate delivery of the ileum or colon but is important to push the bowel out, rather than pull it, as the bowel and mesentery are easily injured.
7. The bowel is then carefully oriented to ensure the mesentery is straight. The mesentery should be oriented in the cephalad direction.
8. The midline incision is then closed using the preferred technique and then either dressed or covered with an operative towel before the stoma is Brooked [19].

Primary Aperture Creation Without a Secondary Incision

Note: This technique is identical to the above technique with the following modifications:

1. The technique begins with excision of the circular disk of skin at the previously marked site.
2. Once the retractors are advanced into the incision to expose the posterior rectus sheath, the posterior sheath is grasped with two tonsil clamps and elevated, and Metzenbaum scissors are utilized to open the posterior sheath and peritoneum.

Stoma Maturation for End Ileostomy or Colostomy

1. Care must be taken to ensure that the planned stoma does not change its orientation while attention may be turned to closing other incisions or port sites first. If the end of the bowel has been stapled to control enteric spillage, this staple line is removed. Care is taken not to allow the stoma to drop back into the abdominal cavity or for enteric contents to seep into the aperture.
2. Four to five absorbable sutures (3-0 or 4-0, either chromic catgut or braided suture, on a small tapered needle such as an SH or CV-23) are then used to evert or "Brooke" the stoma. The first suture is passed from mucosa-to-serosa on the antimesenteric side of the bowel, and then a seromuscular bite is taken 3–4 cm proximal to the cut edge of the bowel, then through a subcuticular layer of skin. Passage of the suture through the epidermis can result in peristomal skin complications, such as persistent mucosal islands or scarring. Of note, The ASCRS practice guidelines recommend that whenever possible, both ileostomies and colostomies should be fashioned to protrude above the skin surface [7].
3. This process is repeated as Brooke sutures are placed at each cardinal location on the bowel. The small end of an army-navy retractor or the back of an Adson tissue forceps is then used to evert the bowel wall as these sutures are sequentially tied down.
4. Additional intervening sutures are then placed to approximate the mucocutaneous junction. These need not be numerous, and should not include the seromuscular bite.
5. If desired, the stoma can be digitized to confirm an adequately patent fascial aperture and a finger placed alongside the stoma to ensure the aperture is not too tight. A pouching system is placed.

Stoma Maturation for Loop Ileostomy or Colostomy

1. The appropriate length of colon or ileum is identified. If the stoma is meant to be a terminal loop ileostomy, the site of stoma maturation is approximately 20 cm proximal to the ileocecal valve.
2. It is recommended to mark this length of bowel and to indicate which direction is distal. This can be achieved through dyed and undyed suture or long- and short-tailed marking sutures, with cautery or with a tip of a sterile marking pen used intra-corporeally.
3. To deliver the bowel through the abdominal wall, a Penrose, umbilical tape or 14F red rubber catheter can be passed just under the mesenteric side of the bowel.
4. The bowel is now carefully oriented to ensure the afferent and efferent limbs are identified by the previously placed suture or mark, and with direct visualization.
5. If desired, the red rubber catheter can be secured to the deep dermis using 3-0 nylon suture.

6. Approximately 80% circumference of the antimesenteric portion of the bowel is opened with a horizontal incision using cutting cautery. This should not be at the apex of the exposed loop but on the distal end.
7. The proximal end of the stoma (efferent into the stoma appliance) is matured similarly as above using cardinal everting Brooke sutures.
8. The distal edges are secured to dermal edge with simple sutures, again excluding the epidermis, to complete the maturation, and a pouching system is applied.

Operative Technique for Laparoscopic Stoma Creation

1. Enter the abdomen using the Optiview port under direct visualization at Palmer's point in the left upper quadrant. Alternatively the abdomen can be entered at the planned site of stoma creation using an open cutdown technique.
2. Once intra-peritoneal and the abdomen is insufflated, perform diagnostic exploration of the abdomen to assess for adhesions or carcinomatosis. Plans for either ileostomy or colostomy will dictate port placement. For ileostomy creation, a 5 mm port will be placed infra-umbilically, and a second 5 mm port will be placed in the left lower quadrant for triangulation. Often, however, a two-port technique is feasible when simply pulling up a loop ileostomy.
3. The cecum and terminal ileum are identified, and the small intestine is lifted and run proximally for about 10–20 cm from the ileocecal valve. Look for excess mobility of the ileal mesentery to reach the abdominal wall where the patient was previously marked. If the mesentery is stuck, some lysis of adhesions or mobilization of the cecum can be performed. This can be done sharply, so advanced energy devices are not necessary. The surgeon should avoid creating the ileostomy too close to the ileocecal valve, to allow for easy mobilization and a tension-free, well-vascularized small bowel anastomosis at the time of ileostomy reversal. However, creating the stoma too proximal may increase the risk of high ileostomy output.
4. Once the site is chosen, use an intracorporeal suture to mark the proximal and distal direction of the small bowel. Clamp the small bowel with a padded grasper.
5. The stoma aperture is created at the previously marked site. See "Primary aperture creation without a secondary incision."
6. Pneumoperitoneum is maintained with a finger placed through the stoma site intraperitoneally until it is widened enough to fit two fingers. As pneumoperitoneum is maintained with two fingers in place, a Babcock is inserted between the fingers, and, under laparoscopic visualization, the small intestine is lifted to the Babcock and then grasped. It is carefully pulled through the abdominal wall without twisting the mesentery. De-sufflate and confirm that there is no excessive tension on the bowel and its mesentery.
7. Once pulled through, a hemostat is pushed through the mesentery just underneath the bowel wall and then replaced with a 14-18F red rubber or stoma bar. If there is minimal to no tension on the stoma, consideration can be given to avoiding the use of a supporting bar or rod.

8. The abdomen is re-insufflated and explored again to make sure the mesentery is straight and under no tension. One last check is that a finger will fit along the side of the stoma within the aperture and the ports are removed under direct visualization and pneumoperitoneum is released.
9. The skin incisions are irrigated and closed with subcuticular sutures, and the abdomen is covered except for the stoma.
10. The stoma is matured identically to the open approach for loop ileostomy.
11. Note: For laparoscopic colostomy creation, the steps are very similar. The part of the colon used for the stoma is the most variable aspect of the operation. This decision depends on the reason for stoma creation, abdominal adhesions, mobility, presence of carcinomatosis, diameter of the colon, fatty mesentery or epiploica, and preoperative marking. Generally, we try to bring up the sigmoid colon or the most distal aspect of the colon that is mobile. Without a redundant sigmoid, the left colon may need to be mobilized by taking down the white line of Toldt. If a more proximal colostomy is created, such as at the distal transverse, the omentum should be taken down and mobilization performed both proximal and distal to the site of the planned colostomy. More mobilization performed laparoscopically will allow for more length, easier reach, and less tissue to be pulled through the abdominal wall. We routinely Brooke our colostomies, so the same steps listed above for ileostomy are carried out during colostomy creation.

The minimally invasive approach to colon and rectal surgery in general and stoma creation is widely supported. Particularly in conjunction with an enhanced recovery program, there has been decreased morbidity, decreased length of stay, and increased patient satisfaction [7]. Laparoscopic approach to ileostomy or colostomy creation is safe and can be a fast and minimally morbid operation.

During laparoscopic stoma creation, it is particularly important to maintain proper bowel orientation. A retrospective review of 161 patients undergoing laparoscopic loop ileostomy formation demonstrated a 5% rate of obstructive complications, owing to improper orientation, adhesive kinking of the ileostomy, or tight fascia [20]. Re-insufflation and peritoneal exploration after exteriorization of the bowel should be employed to reduce twisting, and the stoma should be digitized to judge appropriate size of the fascial aperture. If proper orientation during loop colostomy creation is in question, endoscopy should be performed.

Single-incision "scarless" technique in the setting of stoma creation for temporary fecal diversion has also been described [21–24]. The technique begins by developing the cylindrical trephine stoma incision at the site previously chosen and marked by an enterostomal therapist. For this reason, the single-incision approach is not appropriate when multiple sites of stoma maturation have been marked and are being considered. A commercially available single-incision port device is then introduced, or a "glove port" can be fashioned by securing a sterile glove around a small wound protector. Laparoscopy is then used to grasp the appropriate length of terminal ileum or colon, and great care is taken to keep this oriented while delivering it through the stoma aperture.

Use of a Stoma Bridge

A stoma bridge is a temporary tool meant to prevent stoma retraction and is more commonly used for the creation of a loop colostomy than an ileostomy. Common techniques to establish the stoma bridge include commercially available stoma rods, use of a red rubber catheter as a ring-rod, and placement of a subcutaneously placed bridge device, among others [25–28]. Bridges tend to interfere with the application of the flange which can lead to leakage and pouching difficulty. Furthermore, plastic stoma rods can cause pressure necrosis of the underlying skin. Use of a “ring-rod” instead of a conventional bar eliminates the risk of peristomal pressure ulceration (Fig. 36.5) [29]. In some studies, a bridge was associated with an increased rate of stomal necrosis, congestion, edema, and readmission; but often times these complications are more likely the result of a challenging body habitus and bowel condition [30].

In summary, a stoma bridge is not universally beneficial and should be used on a selective basis and may not be necessary for loop ileostomies. If a bridge is felt to be necessary, ring-rod construction is preferred. Removal of the bridge is typically done after 2–3 weeks when sufficient bonding of the bowel with the abdominal wall has occurred but can be removed as early as 3–5 days after stoma construction if the bowel appears to be intact well above the abdominal wall.

Peristomal Adhesion Barrier Membranes for Temporary Ostomies

A temporary ileostomy or colostomy may be constructed as a means to defunctionalize a lower rectal anastomosis in oncologic resections, ileal pouch-anal anastomoses in ulcerative colitis or for damage control and avoidance of intra-abdominal anastomoses in the setting of trauma, feculent peritonitis, hemodynamic instability,

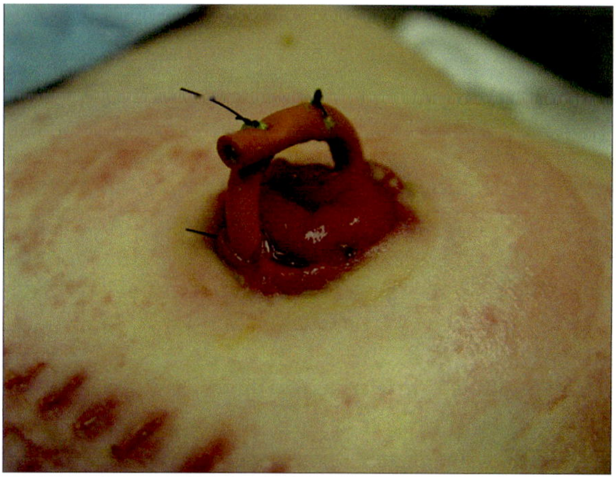

Fig. 36.5 A ring-rod type stoma bridge fashioned from a 14F red rubber catheter. The rod is secured to the dermis with 3-0 nylon. (Courtesy of J. Colwell, RN)

and severe protein-calorie malnutrition. These ostomies are typically closed 6 weeks to 3 months after the initial operation.

A number of studies have sought to determine whether placement of a peristomal anti-adhesion barrier facilitates these stoma closure operations. These bioresorbable barrier membranes are placed on the stoma-bearing bowel segment as it is pulled through the abdominal wall. They are made of sodium hyaluronate and carboxymethylcellulose, which may reduce peristomal adhesions in the subcutaneous space and immediate pre-aperture peritoneum and fascial edge. Aside from a rare allergy, these barrier membranes are considered to be safe [31–34]. The closure of the temporary stoma may come easier, faster, and safer when less adhesiolysis is required.

Postoperative Pouching Considerations

Goals of selecting a proper pouching system (Fig. 36.6) include good adherence with consistent wear time, release of flatus with no odor, comfort, and ease of application [35]. The choice of product depends on stoma-specific factors, peristomal skin health, and self-care abilities [36]. In addition, periodic reassessment of the pouching system in the immediate perioperative period as well as after major weight changes is appropriate.

A large number of pouching manufacturers and products to collect stoma effluent are available. They all utilize a solid skin barrier, also called the faceplate. This is a one- or two-piece adhesive hydrocolloid wafer that provides a wide seal between the skin and pouch. As the hydrocolloid adhesive erodes with moisture, the recommended pouch wear time is generally limited to a maximum of 4 days. The solid skin barrier may be cut-to-fit or precut to a prescribed aperture. If necessary, a convex barrier is utilized to flatten peristomal creases (Fig. 36.7a, b).

The solid barrier seal is augmented with any number of additional skin barriers. A moldable hydrocolloid washer may enhance the appliance seal. These can be stretched to fit and provide a slight convexity when a flat faceplate is utilized. In a limited resource setting, stockage of a universal cut-to-fit solid barrier seal accommodating 22–64 mm diameter stomas as well as a skin barrier ring will allow for successful pouching in the large majority of patients with stomas [13]. Skin barrier paste can be best thought of as "stoma caulk" and is used to fill uneven areas near the stoma, for example, in the case of mucocutaneous separation. Application of barrier paste requires a fair amount of manual dexterity and is not a good choice for patients with limited ability to self-care. Barrier powder helps secure a seal when the peristomal skin irritated, ulcerated, or weeping. It is sprinkled onto the moist, denuded peristomal skin and then gently brushed away. Liquid skin barriers (acrylate copolymer or cyanoacrylate clear film) can be placed over skin barrier powder to protect the skin from stoma effluent or adhesive stripping. Liquid barriers must be allowed to dry before application of the solid barrier. Elastic skin barrier strips add extra security in sealing the outer rim of the pouching system. Finally, a number of accessory products including belts,

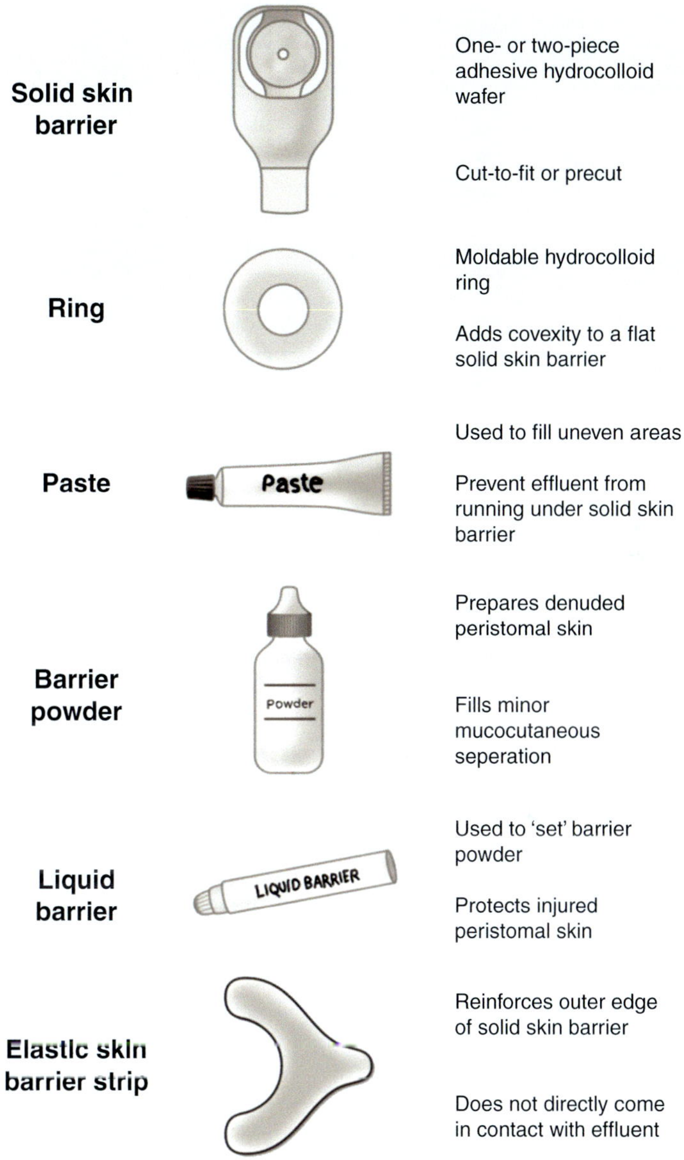

Fig. 36.6 Elements of a proper pouching system

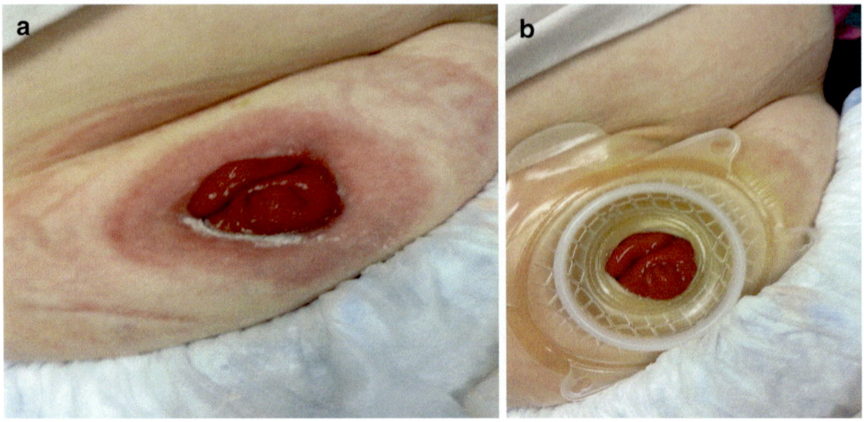

Fig. 36.7 (**a**) A peristomal skin crease interfering with successful pouching. (**b**) Application of a convex appliance flattens this crease. (Both: Courtesy of J. Colwell, RN.)

pouch covers, deodorants, and absorbent products provide additional comfort and discretion for ostomates.

After supplies are gathered, the soiled pouch is gently removed with the help of an adhesive remover wipe or spray. The peristomal skin is gently cleansed and dried. If indicated, peristomal hair is clipped; shaving can contribute to mechanical trauma and folliculitis and should be avoided. The solid barrier is cut-to-fit if necessary using a prior stoma template. If needed, skin barrier paste or the barrier ring is applied to the peristomal skin or to the solid barrier. The solid barrier is then pressed into place, using the hands to create a bit of warmth to "set" the barrier and improve seal [37].

Prolonged wearing of a pouch without change when the output is not solid allows for the hydrocolloid barrier to break down, which may lead to chronic moisture and ultimately a condition called pseudoverrucous epitheliomatous hyperplasia (PEH). This can cause increasing pouching difficulty (Fig. 36.8) as it interferes with maintaining a seal. Occasionally, surgical excision may be required [13]. Patients with colostomies, which have more solid stool, can consider extending frequency of changes to every 4–7 days.

Pitfalls and Troubleshooting

Short-Term and Long-Term Complications

Short- and long-term complications of stomas are numerous and vary in terms of their severity and morbidity to the patient. Their incidence and management are covered in Tables 36.1 and 36.2.

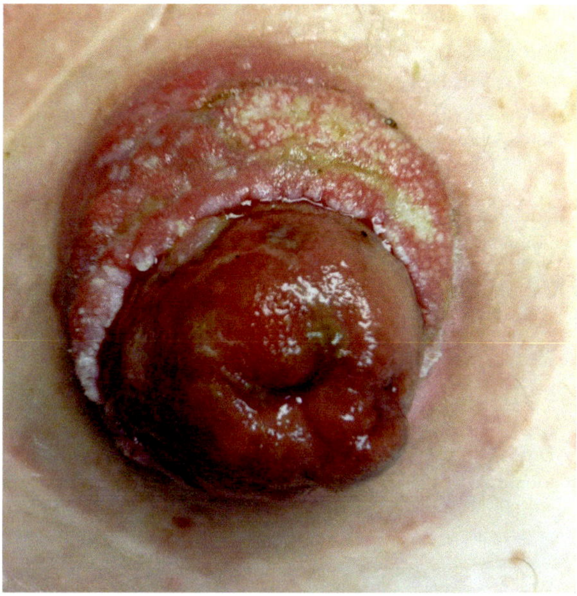

Fig. 36.8 Raised pseudoverrucous epitheliomatous hyperplasia due to improperly sized solid skin barrier aperture. (Used with permission of Georg Thieme Verlag KG from Steinhagen et al. [39])

Table 36.1 Short-term complications of stomas: incidence and management

Short-term complications	Incidence	Management
Dehydration [60]	17% readmission rate with ileostomy	Preventative education on signs of dehydration. Dietary modification including thickening foods and seperating solid from liquid intake. Initiation of loperamide. Oral rehydration solution. IV hydration and high-output stoma management for refractory cases
Stomal ischemia [38, 61]	13%, most commonly with colostomy	Preventative measures including adequate mesenteric length and fascial aperture. Distinguish mucosal from full-thickness ischemia. Distinguish subfascial from suprafascial ischemia. Manage mucosal and suprafascial ischemia expectantly, anticipating retraction, and/or stenosis. Full-thickness, subfascial necrosis requires operative revision
Stoma retraction [61]	Up to 30%, most commonly with colostomy and emergency stoma	Preventative measures including adequate mobilization of the mesentery. Distinguish subfascial from suprafascial retraction. Manage suprafascial retraction expectantly, anticipating stenosis. Subfascial retraction requires operative revision
Obstruction [62]	~3% readmission rate	Most often due to inadequate fascial aperture or improper dietary choices. If fascia-level obstruction, trial gentle irrigation. Remove stoma rod if present. Low threshold for operative re-exploration to rule out volvulus around stoma as fixed point through abdominal wall, which can lead to devastating small bowel loss

(continued)

Table 36.1 (continued)

Short-term complications	Incidence	Management
Mucocutaneous separation [39]	Extremely common	Local wound care, irrigation of fibrinous slough, and application of skin barrier powder. Even circumferential mucocutaneous separation typically will heal with expectant management
Suture sinus and granuloma	Varies	Avoid suturing through the epidermis which can create mucosal islands. Remove any visible suture. Treat granulomas with topical silver nitrate. Recalcitrant suture sinus may require operative exploration
Leakage/chemical irritation [39, 63]	Up to 34% of ileostomy patients	Prevention with proper site selection and stoma maturation with good protrusion. Evaluation with enterostomal therapy to ensure proper pouching practices. Topical hydrocolloid powder. Once leak is corrected, skin tends to heal rapidly
Allergic contact dermatitis	Varies	Transition to nonallergenic alternative pouching system may require topical aerosolized corticosteroids and rarely systemic steroids
Peristomal folliculitis	Varies	Instruct patient to clip, not shave, hair under appliance. Cleanse with antibacterial soap

Table 36.2 Long-term complications of stomas: incidence and management

Long-term complications	Incidence	Management
Parastomal hernia [64]	Up to 30% for ileostomy, up to 50% for colostomy	75% rate of recurrence after local repair. Various open and laparoscopic repair options with mesh are available. Prophylactic mesh reinforcement for permanent stoma formation should be offered
Stoma prolapse [38]	3% for ileostomy, 2% for colostomy	Prevention with appropriate fascial aperture. Reduce at bedside with aid of sugar and ice. If incarcerated will require operative resection and rematuration. If it is a loop stoma, convert a loop stoma to a divided "end-loop" stoma. If stoma is temporary, consider reversal surgery
Parastomal varices [38]	Rare, associated with portal hypertension	Avoid long-term stoma creation in portal hypertensive patients. Manage systemic portal hypertension with transjugular intrahepatic portosystemic shunt. Percutaneous embolization of mesenteric veins. Circumferential incision 1 cm from mucocutaneous junction with division of varices and closure of skin incision can provide short-term control
Stoma stenosis [38]	Up to 9%	Sequelae of ischemia and/or retraction. Preventative measures including adequate mesenteric length and fascial aperture. If stoma is temporary, serial dilation to bridge to reversal surgery. If stoma is permanent, local revision with rematuration is possible once the stoma is well-established
Pyoderma gangrenosum [65]	0.6% associated with inflammatory bowel disease (IBD)	Minimize skin trauma. Topical steroids. Escalate to topical tacrolimus. Ensure underlying IBD is under control. Reestablish intestinal continuity if possible
Pressure ulcer [39]	Varies, associated with parastomal hernia	Change to flexible pouching system. Treat full-thickness wounds with alginate or hydrocolloid dressing. Correct parastomal hernia

Salvaging a Borderline Stoma in the Postoperative Period

Intestinal ischemia, stoma retraction, and mucocutaneous separation are fairly common and likely underreported in the literature [16, 38]. Mucocutaneous separation may arise from excessive tension, impaired wound healing, or infection. Ischemia, diabetes, immunosuppression, and chemotherapy are risk factors. Mucocutaneous separation is a common cause of pouching difficulties in the early postoperative period. Fortunately, most cases can be treated successfully with fastidious wound care. The areas of separation are cleansed and then filled with barrier powder prior to application of the pouching system to protect the wound from stoma effluent. Even circumferential separation can usually be salvaged, though it may take substantial time and contribute to stoma retraction and subsequent stenosis (Fig. 36.9) [39].

Mucosal ischemia is common, especially during resuscitation after emergency surgery. Vascular congestion can impede venous drainage, causing the stoma to swell and turn blue or purple, and possibly slough. Mucosal ischemia alone rarely causes long-term sequela such as stenosis. Stoma necrosis, on the other hand, involves full-thickness ischemia and is a result of devascularization of the bowel conduit. This may have occurred through overzealous removal of the peristomal

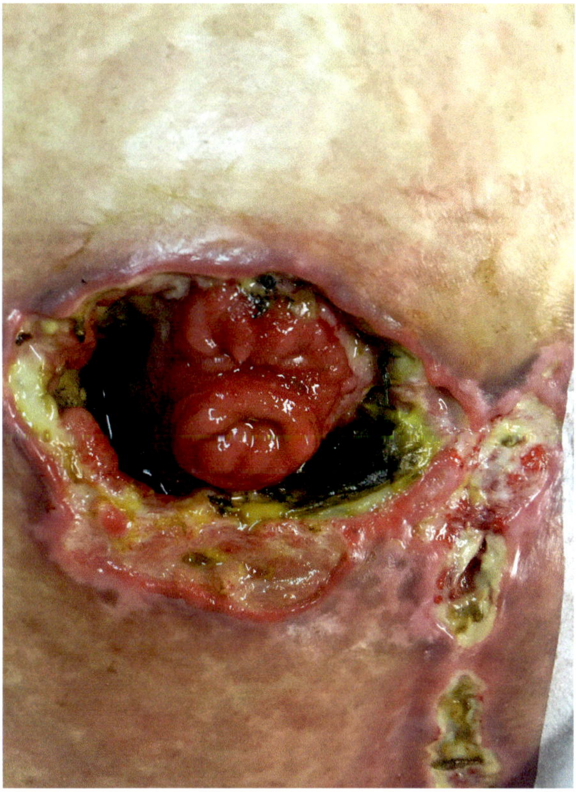

Fig. 36.9 Deep, circumferential mucocutaneous separation. (Courtesy of M. Kaplon-Jones, APRN)

mesentery during maturation, improper ligation of an important collateral vessel during mobilization, avulsion of the mesentery when the bowel is pulled through the fascia, or strangulation at the fascia level. If the ischemia is limited to a suprafascial level, the situation is not life-threatening, and the stoma can often be managed conservatively during the acute perioperative period (Fig. 36.10a). This usually results in retraction and stricture, which may be acceptable for the limited time of a temporary stoma. However, if the stoma is meant to be permanent, a revision is necessary when the intra-abdominal condition has improved, and the mesentery has relaxed somewhat. Serial dilations may be required as a bridge through the postoperative

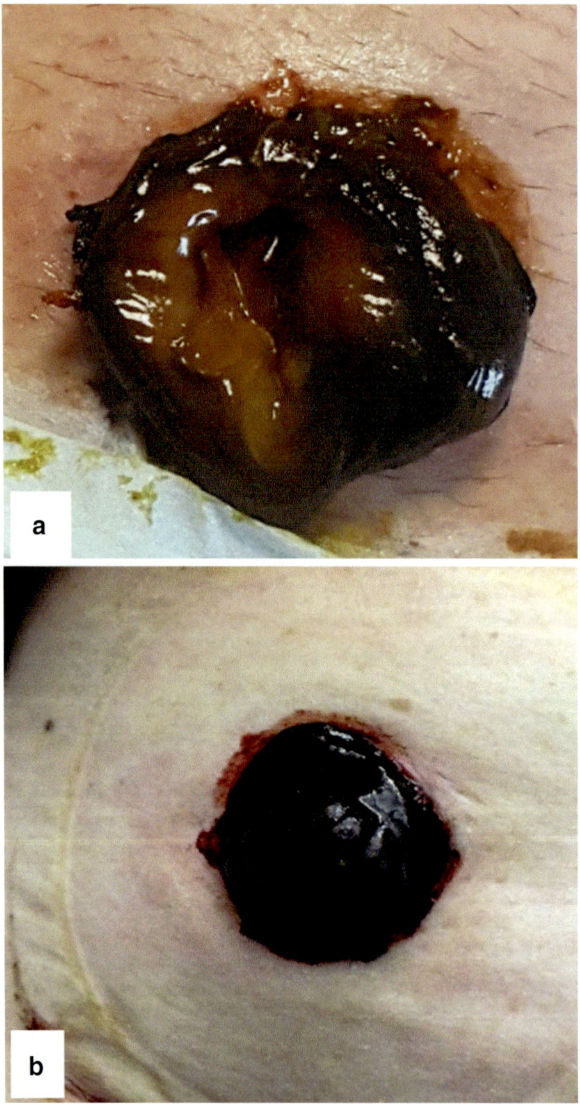

Fig. 36.10 (**a**) Mucosal ischemia and necrosis that, on test-tube exam, did not extend below the fascia and was successfully managed nonoperatively but resulted in stenosis that will later require revision. (Courtesy of Y. Vignaswaran, MD); (**b**) Stoma necrosis extending to below the fascia, and required revision. (Courtesy of Patricia Sylla, MD)

period to either revision or reversal. In contrast, extension of the full-thickness ischemia to a subfascial level represents an urgent situation requiring immediate re-exploration and stoma revision as the necrosis may lead to perforation and feculent peritonitis (Fig. 36.10b). A pinprick test using an 18-guage needle can help distinguish between mucosal and muscular ischemia: if blood emanates from this area of trauma, the ischemia is likely only mucosal. The classic "test-tube" or better a flexible endoscopy evaluation is more common and more reliable in determining the extent of ischemia [18, 38].

The same principles outlined above apply to stoma retraction. Stoma retraction is most commonly due to inadequate mobilization and mucocutaneous tension. If the stoma retracts below the fascia, immediate re-exploration and revision are indicated. If the retraction remains suprafascial, efforts may center on salvaging the stoma with local wound care. Circumferentially retracted stomas will likely require a revision or takedown whereby the timing is a matter of the individual circumstances (Fig. 36.11) [38].

During the operation, the surgeon should always mobilize more colon than may be necessary. It can be frustrating and inefficient if there is not enough reach to the abdominal wall, and pneumoperitoneum has to be reestablished to perform more

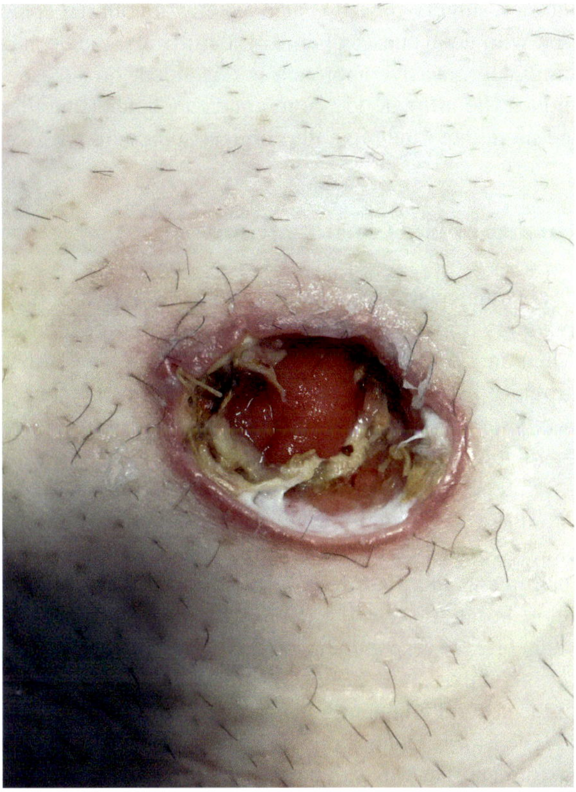

Fig. 36.11 Circumferential mucocutaneous separation with retraction. (Courtesy of M. Kaplon-Jones, APRN)

mobilization. If the colon looks ischemic or there seems to be tension, believe it and perform more mobilization, and avoid "hoping the stoma will look good" after the operation is complete. The most mobile part of the colon should be utilized, keeping in mind any future surgeries and potential reversal. Parastomal hernia or prolapse is less morbid than stoma ischemia, necrosis, or retraction; thus, the results of enlargement of the aperture may outweigh the risks of tension or vascular comprise.

Outcomes

Laparoscopic and Single-Incision Stoma Creation

Outcomes are generally good with a low rate of conversion to standard multiport or open technique, most often owing to adhesions [40]. Because delivering the bowel through the incision is performed with a pull rather than push technique, care must be taken to create an adequate fascial aperture to reduce trauma to the bowel or mesentery to decrease the potential for ischemia. The rate of bowel ischemia with this technique can be as high as 25% which should be taken into consideration when counseling the patient and planning the intervention [24].

There have also been reports of using the stoma site as a means to conduct single-incision surgery for IBD, such as total abdominal colectomy or ileal-pouch formation with good success [41, 42]. Ultimately, the decision to create a stoma using a minimally invasive approach is dependent on surgeon proficiency with this technique. The ultimate location, appearance, and functionality of the resulting stoma are more important than the surgical approach.

Quality of Life Considerations

Evaluating quality of life in an ostomate is a complex and contextual process. Findings from multiple studies suggest that health-related QoL is often impaired when an ostomy has been created [43]. However, there are also a non-negligible group of patients who chose to have a stoma created to overcome functional incapacitation (incontinence, colonic dysmotility) and see a dramatic improvement in their QoL after ostomy formation.

A generic (QoL) instrument is not entirely sufficient to appropriately evaluate ostomates as they do not include aspects that are important to stoma patients, for example, odor or concern about appliance leak. However, utilization of generic instruments is important in order to compare QoL to the general population. The Short Form 36 version 2 (SF36v2) is one such generic health-related QoL tool. A study of 2329 respondents, 40% with a colostomy and 44% with an ileostomy, demonstrated that physical health limited ostomates to an extent greater than that seen in the general population [44].

The Stoma Quality of Life Scale (SQoLS) is a 21-item condition-specific QoL instrument that was validated in 2003 and features a work/social function scale, a sexuality/body image scale, a stoma functional scale, and a measure of the financial impact on ostomates as well as skin irritation [45]. The City of Hope Quality of Life Ostomy (COHQoL-O) tool is a 90-item condition-specific tool with a very broad scope. Validation of this tool has demonstrated that married ostomates, those who identify with a support system, and those who are active in the workforce have higher QoL compared to other ostomates without these identifiers [46]. There are other stoma-related instruments that are disease-specific to either cancer or inflammatory bowel disease [47, 48]. Utilization of such instruments can be used to administer targeted patient education, manage expectations, and compare surgical options that may or may not include permanent stoma formation.

Several factors impact health-related QoL in ostomates. Quality of life is most severely impaired in the immediate postoperative period, but dramatically improves by 3 months, and subsequently stabilizes [49]. Persons who have difficulty paying for ostomy supplies experience a lower quality of life [50]. Quality of life considerations also extend to the spouses of ostomates, with these individuals reporting significantly increased time spent at home and decline or complete dissolution of sexual activity [51].

Though not well studied, patients with a temporary stoma have some unique QoL considerations. Knowing the stoma is temporary may interfere with adaptation to the ostomy. It has been reported that patients with temporary stomas feel a decreased sense of control, put social and work life on hold, and restrict disclosure of the presence of the stoma, even to spouses [52]. Further, stoma closure becomes a strong anchoring event for these patients, and any uncertainty related to the timing of closure becomes a source of great angst [53].

New ostomates find themselves burdened by the rigors of stoma self-care, coping issues, real and perceived physical activity limitations, new challenges in personal hygiene, frustration, helplessness, and other negative feelings [54]. Structured preoperative and inpatient education have a positive effect on health-related QoL [55]. The addition of targeted post-discharge educational sessions and stoma support groups focusing on topics such as everyday life with a stoma, sexuality and intimacy, and return to work may lead to more rapid improvement in QoL after stoma formation [56].

Finally, proper stoma site marking and maturation are crucial to preserved health-related QoL. Patients who were not marked preoperatively, or those who otherwise have an inappropriately sited stoma, report significantly lower QoL scores in several studies [57–59].

Conclusions

Most ostomates, regardless of whether the diversion is temporary or permanent, will experience a profound effect on their quality of life. It may be negative, especially in the first few months after creation. However, preoperative marking and education by a WOCN specialist, careful construction by the surgeon, and rigorous postoperative support and education will dampen any negative impact on a patient's quality of life. A properly sited, adequately protruding stoma will ease the burden of daily pouching and maintenance. In circumstances where emergency unplanned stoma formation is required, one must anticipate and manage postoperative complications including ischemia, retraction, stenosis, and subsequent pouching difficulty.

Acknowledgments Special thanks to Jan Colwell, RN, MS, CWOCN, FAAN, Michele Kaplon–Jones, MSN, RN, ANP-BC, CWOCN, and Dr. Yalani Vignaswaran, MD, for their photo contributions.

References

1. Danielsen AK, Christensen BM, Mortensen J, Voergaard LL, Herlufsen P, Balleby L. Establishment of a regional Danish database for patients with a stoma. Color Dis. 2014;17:27–33.
2. Turnbull G. The ostomy files: ostomy statistics: the $64,000 question. Ostomy Wound Manage. 2003;49:22–3.
3. Warschkow R, Ebinger SM, Brunner W, Schmied BM, Marti L. Survival after abdominoperineal and sphincter-preserving resection in nonmetastatic rectal cancer: a population based time trend and propensity score-matched SEER analysis. Gastroenterol Res Pract. 2017;6058907 https://doi.org/10.1155/2017/6058907; epub ahead of print.
4. Godat L, Kobayashi L, Chang DC, Coimbra R. Do trauma stomas ever get reversed? J Am Coll Surg. 2014;219:70–8.
5. Salem L, Anaya DA, Flum DR. Temporal changes in the management of diverticulitis. J Surg Research. 2005;124:318–23.
6. Singh S, Ding NS, Mathis KL, Dulai PS, Farrell AM, Pemberton JH, et al. Systematic review with meta-analysis: faecal diversion for management of perianal Crohn's disease. Aliment Pharmacol Ther. 2015;42(7):783–92.
7. Hendren S, Hammond K, Glasgow SC, Perry WB, Buie WD, Steele SR, et al. Clinical practice guidelines for ostomy surgery. Dis Colon Rectum. 2015;58(4):375–87.
8. Gachabayov M, Oberkofler CE, Tuech JJ, Hahnloser D, Bergamaschi R. Resection with primary anastomosis vs nonrestorative resection for perforated diverticulitis with peritonitis: a systematic review and meta-analysis. Color Dis. 2018 Sep;20(9):753–70.
9. Schmidt S, Ismail T, Puhan MA, Soll C, Breitenstein S. Meta-analysis of surgical strategies in perforated left colonic diverticulitis with generalized peritonitis. Langenbeck's Arch Surg. 2018;403(4):425–33.
10. Gibbons G, Tan CJ, Bartolo DCC, Filgate R, Makin G, Barwood N, et al. Emergency left colonic resection on an acute surgical unit: does subspecialization improve outcomes? ANZ J Surg. 2015;85:739–43.
11. Cataldo PA. Technical tips for stoma creation in the challenging patient. Clin Colon and Rectal Surg. 2008;21(1):17–22.
12. Berry K, Carmel J, Gutman N, Link M, Markt B, Metzger B, et al. ASCRS and WOCN joint position statement on the value of preoperative stoma marking for patients undergoing fecal ostomy surgery. J Wound Ostomy Continence Nurs. 2007;34(6):627–8.
13. Thorson AG. Preoperative considerations. In: Cataldo PA, Mackeigan JM, editors. Intestinal stomas: principles, techniques and management. 2nd ed. New York: Marcel Dekker, Inc; 2004. p. 57–64.
14. Colwell JC. The role of obesity in the patient undergoing colorectal surgery and fecal diversion: a review of the literature. Ostomy Wound Manage. 2014;60(1):24–8.
15. Hardt J, Meerpohl JJ, Metzendorf MI, Kienle P, Post S, Herrle F. Lateral pararectal versus transrectal stoma placement for prevention of parastomal herniation. Cochrane Database Syst Rev. 2013;(11):CD009487.
16. Cottam J, Richards K, Hasted A, Blackman A. Results of a nationwide prospective audit of stoma complications within 3 weeks of surgery. Color Dis. 2007;9:834–8.

17. Parmar KL, Zammit M, Smith A, Kenyon D, Lees NP. A prospective audit of early stoma complications in colorectal cancer treatment throughout the Greater Manchester and Cheshire colorectal cancer network. Color Dis. 2011;13:935–8.
18. Cataldo P. Technical tips for the difficult stoma. In: Cataldo PA, Mackeigan JM, editors. Intestinal stomas: principles, techniques and management. 2nd ed. New York: Marcel Dekker, Inc; 2004. p. 411–25.
19. Hyman NH. End ileostomy. In: Cataldo PA, Mackeigan JM, editors. Intestinal Stomas: Principles, techniques and management. 2nd ed. New York: Marcel Dekker, Inc; 2004. p. 159–64.
20. Ng KH, Ng DC, Cheung HY, Wong JC, Yau KK, Chung CC, et al. Obstructive complications of laparoscopically created defunctioning ileostomy. Dis Colon Rectum. 2008;51:1664–8.
21. Hasegawa J, Hirota M, Min Kim H, Mikata S, Shimizu J, Soma Y, et al. Single-incision laparoscopic stoma creation: experience with 31 consecutive cases. Asian J Endosc Surg. 2013;6:181–5.
22. Shah A, Moftah M, Hadi Nahar Al-Furaji H, Cahill RA. Standardized technique for single port laparoscopic ileostomy and colostomy. Color Dis. 2014;16:0248–O252.
23. Subhas G, Kim E, Gupta A, Mittal VK, Mckendrick A. Laparoscopic loop ileostomy with a single-port stab incision technique. Tech Coloproctol. 2011;15:337–9.
24. Zaghiyan KN, Murrell Z, Fleshner PR. Scarless single-incision laparoscopic loop ileostomy: a novel technique. Dis Colon Rectum. 2011;54(12):1542–6.
25. Baloyiannis I, Christodoulidis G, Symeonidis D, Hatzinikolaou I, Spyridakis M, Tepetes K. Loop stomas with a subcutaneously placed bridge device. Tech Coloproctol. 2010;14(S1):S75–6.
26. Branco AM, Saraiva AC. Loop colostomy with a suprafascial bridge device. Dig Surg. 2009;26:282–4.
27. Harish K. The loop stoma bridge: a new technique. J Gastrointest Surg. 2008;12:958–61.
28. Milner CS, Sutton C, Hemingway D. The skin bridge loop colostomy. Tech Coloproctol. 2006;10:137–8.
29. Scarpa M, Sadocchi L, Ruffolo C, Iacobone M, Filosa T, Prando D, et al. Rod in loop ileostomy: just an insignificant detail for ileostomy related complications? Langenbeck's Arch Surg. 2007;392:149–54.
30. Franklyn J, Varghese G, Mittal R, Rebekah G, Jesudason MR, Perakath B. A prospective randomized controlled trial comparing early postoperative complications in patients undergoing loop colostomy with and without a stoma rod. Color Dis. 2017;19:675–80.
31. Tang CL, Seow-Choen F, Fook-Chong S, Eu K-W. Bioresorbable adhesion barrier facilitate early closure of the defunctioning ileostomy after rectal excision: a prospective, randomized trial. Dis Colon Rectum. 2003;46(9):1200–7.
32. Kawamura YJ, Kakizawa N, Tan KY, Mizokami K, Sasaki J, Tsujinaka S, et al. Sushi-roll wrap of Seprafilm for ileostomy limb facilitates ileostomy closure. Tech Coloproctol. 2009;13:211–4.
33. Bertoni DM, Hammond KL, Beck DE, Hicks TC, Whitlow CB, Vargas HD, et al. Use of sodium hyaluronate/carboxymethylcellulose bioresorbably membrane in loop ileostomy construction facilitates stoma closure. Ochsner Journal. 2017;17:146–9.
34. Salum M, Wexner SD, Nogueras JJ, Weiss E, Koruda M, Behrens K, et al. Does sodium hyaluronate- and carboxymethylcellulose-based bioresorbably membrane (seprafilm) decrease operative time for loop ileostomy closure? Tech Coloproctol. 2006;10:187–91.
35. Slater R. Quality of life for ostomates. BJN. 2013;22(9):504.
36. Colwell JC. Selection of a pouching system. In: Carmel JE, Colwell JC, Goldberg MT, editors. WOCN society core curriculum: ostomy management. Philadelphia: Wolters Kluwer; 2016. p. 120–30.
37. Lavery IC, Erwin-Toth P. Stoma therapy. In: Cataldo PA, Mackeigan JM, editors. Intestinal stomas: principles, techniques and management. 2nd ed. New York: Marcel Dekker, Inc; 2004. p. 259–66.
38. Krishnamurty DM, Blatnik J, Mutch M. Stoma Complications. Clin Colon Rectal Surg. 2017;30:193–200.

39. Steinhagen E, Colwell J, Cannon LM. Intestinal stomas: postoperative stoma care and peristomal skin complications. Clin Colon Rectal Surg. 2017;30(3):184–92.
40. Luchtefeld M. Minimally invasive stomas. In: Cataldo PA, Mackeigan JM, editors. Intestinal stomas: principles, techniques and management. 2nd ed. New York: Marcel Dekker, Inc; 2004. p. 259–66.
41. Fichera A, Zoccali M, Gullo R. Single incision ("Scarless") laparoscopic total abdominal colectomy with end ileostomy for ulcerative colitis. J Gastrointest Surg. 2011;15:1247–51.
42. Olson CH, Bedros N, Hakiman H, Araghizaheh FY. Single-site laparoscopic surgery for inflammatory bowel disease. JSLS. 2014;18(2):258–64.
43. Pittman J, Kozell K, Gray M. Should WOC nurses measure health-related quality of life in patients undergoing intestinal ostomy surgery? J Wound Ostomy Continence Nurs. 2009;36(3):254–65.
44. Nichols TR. Quality of life in US residents with ostomies as assessed using the SF36v2. J Wound Ostomy Continence. 2015;42(1):71–8.
45. Baxter NN, Novotny PJ, Jacobson T, Maidl JL, Sloan J, Young-Fadok TM. A stoma quality of life scale. Dis Colon Rectum. 2006;49:205–12.
46. Grant M, Ferrell B, Dean G, Uman G, Chu D, Krouse R. Revision and psychometric testing of the city of hope quality of life ostomy questionnaire. Qual Life Res. 2004;13:1445–7.
47. Kluka S, Kristjanson LJ. Development and testing of the ostomy concerns scale: Measuring ostomy-related concerns of cancer patients and their partner. J Wound Ostomy Continence Nurs. 1996;23:166–70.
48. Olbrisch ME, Ziegler SW. Psychological adjustment and patient information in inflammatory bowel disease: development of two assessment instruments. J Chronic Dis. 1982;35:649–58.
49. Marquis P, Marrel A, Jambon B. Quality of life in patients with stomas: the Montreux study. Ostomy Wound Manage. 2003;49(2):48–55.
50. Coons SJ, Chongpison Y, Wendel CS, Grant M, Krouse RS. Overall quality of life and difficulty paying for ostomy supplies in the veterans affairs ostomy health-related quality of life study: an exploratory analysis. Med Care. 2007;45(9):891–5.
51. Cakmak A, Aylaz G, Kuzu A. Permanent stoma not only affects patients' quality of life but also that of their spouses. World J Surg. 2010;34:2872–6.
52. Smith DM, Loewenstein G, Jankovich A, Ubel PA. Happily hopeless: adaptation to a permanent, but not to a temporary, disability. Health Psychol. 2009;28(6):787–91.
53. Danielsen AK, Soerensen EE, Burchart K, Rosenberg J. Impact of a temporary stoma on patients' everyday lives: feelings of uncertainty while waiting for closure of the stoma. J Clin Nursing. 2013;22:1343–52.
54. Lim SH, Chan SWC, He HG. Patients' experiences of performing self-care of stomas in the initial postoperative period. Cancer Nurs. 2015;38(3):185–93.
55. Danielsen AK, Bucharth J, Rosenberg J. Patient education has a positive effect in patients with a stoma: a systematic review. Color Dis. 2013;15:e276–83.
56. Danielsen AK, Rosenberg J. Health related quality of life may increase when patients with a stoma attend patient education: a case-control study. PLoS One. 2014;9(3):e90354.
57. Mahjoubi B, Kiani Goodarzi K, Mohammad-Sadeghi H. Quality of life in stoma patients: appropriate and inappropriate stoma sites. World J Surg. 2010;34:147–52.
58. McKenna LS, Taggart E, Stoelting J, Kirkbride G, Forbes GB. The impact of preoperative stoma marking on health-related quality of life: a comparison cohort study. J Wound Ostomy Continence Nurs. 2016;43(1):57–61.
59. Person B, Ifargan R, Lachter J, Duek SD, Kluger Y, Assalia A. The impact of preoperative stoma site marking on the incidence of complications, quality of life, and the patient's independence. Dis Colon Rectum. 2012;55:783–7.
60. Messaris E, Sehgal R, Deiling S, Koltun WA, Stewart D, McKenna K, et al. Dehydration is the most common indication for readmission after diverting ileostomy creation. Dis Colon Rectum. 2012;55:175–80.
61. Harris DA, Egbeare D, Jones S, Benjamin H, Woodward A, Foster ME. Complications and mortality following stoma formation. Ann R Coll Surg Engl. 2005;87(6):427–31.

62. LI W, Stocchi L, Cherla D, Liu G, Agostinelli A, Delaney CP, et al. Factors associated with hospital readmission following diverting ileostomy creation. Tech Coloproctol. 2017;21:641–8.
63. Leong APK, Londono-Schimmer EE, Philips RKS. Life table analysis of stomal complications following ileostomy. Br J Surg. 1994;81:727–9.
64. Hotouras A, Murphy J, Thaha M, Chan CL. The persistent challenge of parastomal herniation: a review of the literature and future developments. Color Dis. 2013;15(5):e202–e-214.
65. Lyon CC, Smith AJ, Griffiths CE, Beck MH. The spectrum of skin disorders in abdominal stoma patients. Br J Dermatol. 2000;143:1248–60.

37 Prophylactic Approaches for Parastomal Hernia Formation During Laparoscopic Creation of Permanent End Stomas: Rationale, Techniques, and Outcomes

Sami A. Chadi and Steven D. Wexner

Introduction and Rationale

A parastomal hernia (PSH) is defined as an incisional hernia at the site of an ostomy, usually created for urine or fecal diversion. The recent Association of Coloproctology of Great Britain and Ireland (ACPGBI) Delphi exercise identified PSH to be one the second most important non-cancer concern to be addressed [1]. The incidence of PSH varies from 1% to as high as 50% of patients [2, 3] depending on the method and criteria used for diagnosis. Although categorizations of PSH subtypes have been proposed, none have been validated or used consistently in clinical trials [4–6]. Both size of the PSH defect and the presence of a concomitant incisional hernia can affect the type of repair used. As such, the European Hernia Society proposed an additional classification system that takes both of these factors into account [7]. Most PSH will develop in the first few years after stoma creation; however, there are reports of PSH developing over 20 years later [8, 9]. Although the majority of patients are asymptomatic [10] diagnosed radiologically or clinically [11], close to 30% of patients develop significant symptoms including pain or discomfort,

S. A. Chadi (✉)
Division of Surgical Oncology, Department of Surgery, University Health Network and Princess Margaret Hospital, Toronto, ON, Canada

University of Toronto, Department of Surgery, Toronto, ON, Canada
e-mail: Sami.chadi@uhn.ca

S. D. Wexner
Cleveland Clinic Florida, Department of Colorectal Surgery, Weston, FL, USA

Cleveland Clinic Lerner College of Medicine of Case Western Reserve University, Cleveland, FL, USA

Charles E. Schmidt College of Medicine, Florida Atlantic University, Boca Raton, FL, USA

Herbert Wertheim College of Medicine, Florida International University, Miami, FL, USA
e-mail: wexners@ccf.org

P. Sylla et al. (eds.), *The SAGES Manual of Colorectal Surgery*,
https://doi.org/10.1007/978-3-030-24812-3_37

parastomal bulging, nausea and vomiting, bowel obstruction, or rarely fistulization [2]. Furthermore, there are established effects on the quality of life of patients with significant impact on peristomal discomfort, physical function, general health, and overall shame associated with the associated bulge [12].

The etiology of PSH has been investigated in various institutional datasets. In general, there are patient and technical factors to be considered, similar to incisional hernias. Patient factors include obesity, malnutrition, sources of increased intra-abdominal pressure (ascites, chronic coughing, constipation, benign prostatic hyperplasia, and urinary retention), increased age, malignancy, and immunosuppressant use [2, 10, 13]. Various technical factors have been proposed from the preoperative setting (stoma therapist consultation, stoma site selection) to intraoperative aspect of the procedure (size of the trephine in the abdominal wall, fixation of the stoma to the abdominal wall, intraperitoneal vs. extraperitoneal course), as well as the elective or emergent nature of the procedure [2].

Stoma Position

Stoma placement was traditionally left to the preference of the surgeon, with some stomas being brought through the midline incisions and other through the umbilicus, less common nowadays given the increased frequency of midline incisions versus the previously performed paramedian incisions [14]. As surgeons realized the decreased rates of parastomal herniation by using the bulk of the rectus muscle to both surround and secure the stoma, this principle became further established in surgical technique [15, 16]. Interestingly, equipoise continued to exist with lateral pararectus abdominis and intrarectus abdominis approaches to stoma creation, whereby the stoma is brought through the abdominal wall lateral to the rectus abdominis muscle or through the body of muscle, respectively [17]. Hardt and colleagues performed a single-centered randomized controlled trial of both stoma positions, the PATRASTOM trial, where 30 patients were randomized to each approach, and no significant difference was identified in PSH rates or EORTC quality of life outcomes [18]. Given the low number of patients recruited, the authors acknowledge that a small difference in PSH rates between the two groups cannot be ruled out, and, as such, the available literature does not support that pararectal location further increases PSH rates.

Stoma Aperture Size

Varying sizes of abdominal wall apertures have been recommended for different stoma types usually based on the fingerbreadths of the trephine window created. Turnbull recommended 1 fingerbreadth for end ileostomies and 2 fingerbreadths for loop ileostomies [15], where Babcock discussed 2 fingerbreadths for end ileostomies [19]. These varying diameters of fingerbreadths led to recommendations based on size. Nguyen recommended a 1.5 cm aperture for colostomies and a 2 cm aperture for loop ileostomies [20]. This proposal was supported by a regression model assessing predictors of PSH in a sample of 108 patients, in which trephine size was found to be significant, although the size cutoff was not defined [21].

The prevalence of PSH has led surgeons to seek preventative approaches at the time of stoma creation. Manook and colleagues described the use of a fascial securing "Hepworth hitch" to prevent further fascial separation [22]. Furthermore, an extraperitoneal course to the stoma was proposed as early as 1958 so as to avoid a linear tract through the abdominal wall, thereby decreasing the likelihood of a PSH [23]. The use of a prophylactic mesh is being increasingly investigated in the literature but is not novel as reports of prophylactic mesh use were reported over 30 years ago [24], reported to allow for a strengthening of the adjacent fascia. Varying approaches have been proposed including the Sugarbaker technique [25], the keyhole approach [26], and the SMART (Stapled Mesh Stoma Reinforcement Technique) approach [27].

Indications and Contraindications

Extraperitoneal Stomas

Although no established indications exist for the use of added measures to prevent PSH in patients, recommendations vary in the literature regarding the approach. The evidence supporting an extraperitoneal course of permanent stomas remains largely retrospective in nature with only two small randomized controlled trials [28, 29]. Meta-analyses of these data suggest a significantly lower rate of PSH with extraperitoneal approaches (risk ratio 0.36; 95% CI 0.21–0.62; $p < 0.001$) [30]. The indications for this technique would be center-specific in that certain programs routinely employ such preventative tactics [31, 32]. Furthermore, in centers wishing to start using a prophylactic technique for PSH formation, the extraperitoneal approach lends itself well when cost implications of mesh as well as concerns regarding mesh complications are factored in. The authors do not routinely employ extraperitoneal stoma creation as the data continue to mature in the literature (Table 37.1), but the technique has been performed for quite some time and has more recently been adapted to laparoscopic procedures. Explicit contraindications have not been published; however, performing these procedures in emergent cases where exposure and patient stability are of concern is likely not optimal. Furthermore, the mesocolon or mesentery in these emergent cases or in patients with inflammation due to Crohn's disease can be robust, edematous, and foreshortened. Crohn's patients are also more likely to require reoperative surgery or to develop fistulizing disease. This can make it difficult to bring the intestinal conduit of the stoma through the extraperitoneal space. Additionally, patients with prior abdominal wall reconstructive procedures or multiple previous laparotomies (disruption of the parietal peritoneum) may not be amenable to an extraperitoneal stoma creation.

Table 37.1 Review of studies of extraperitoneal versus transperitoneal stoma creation in minimally invasive surgery

Author (year)	Type of study	Sample size TPS/EPS		Primary surgery	Median follow-up (months)	Outcomes (TPS vs. EPS)
Hamada et al. (2012) [32]	Retrospective	37		APR	24	33.3 vs. 4.5%
		15	22			($p = 0.031$)
Leroy et al. (2012) [31]	Retrospective	22		APR	N/A	33.3 vs. 0%
		12	10			($p = 0.02$)
Funahashi et al. (2014) [55]	Retrospective	80		APR/TPE	31	34.8 vs. 17.6%
		46	34			($p < 0.01$)
Heiying et al. (2014) [29]	Randomized trial	36		APR	17	11.1 vs. 0%
		18	18			($p = 0.15$)
Hino et al. (2017) [56]	Retrospective	59		APR/	21	41 vs. 13%
		29	30	Hartmann's		($p = 0.02$)

EPS extraperitoneal stoma, *TPC* transperitoneal stoma, *APR* abdominoperineal resection, *TPE* total pelvic exenteration

Prophylactic Mesh Use

Select reports have supported the routine use of prophylactic mesh based on the available published literature [33]. Ultimately, prophylactic mesh placement has been shown to have a low complication profile in long-term follow-up studies [34], suggesting the procedure to be safe in these clean-contaminated procedures. The use of prophylactic mesh should thus be left to the surgeon's judgment; however, patients with elevated BMI, diabetes, or undergoing surgery for malignancy may be at an increased risk, further supporting the use of prophylactic mesh [35].

Contraindications would mainly include those patients with diffuse fecal or purulent contamination for concern of mesh infection. These include situations where significant contamination has occurred during an emergent procedure or due to visceral injury, as well as patients with peritoneal carcinomatosis or short-life expectancy.

Preoperative Planning, Patient Workup, and Optimization

In the setting of elective procedures, it is important to ensure that modifiable patient factors have been optimized in preparation for surgery. Preoperative planning is the same whether the surgeon is planning an extraperitoneal approach or the use of prophylactic mesh. Most patients who will require a permanent stoma will require surgery on a semi-urgent or urgent basis for indications such as inflammatory bowel disease or malignancy. As such, there is often an insufficient amount of time to optimize many modifiable factors including smoking status, obesity, and nutritional status among others. Various pre-habilitative programs have been proposed to prepare patients for abdominal surgical procedures but none in particular to optimize the outcomes related to the creation of a permanent end stoma. Abdominal imaging with computed tomography (CT) will often have been performed for disease-specific purposes. This imaging can be used to visualize abdominal wall anatomy and the intactness of the various muscular and fascial layers, which can be particularly important in patients with previous abdominal surgical procedures.

Although preoperative bowel preparations and intravenous antibiotics have been shown to decrease the likelihood of a surgical site infection, there has not been any correlation with a decreased risk of infectious peristomal complications. Bowel preparation can help mitigate intra-abdominal contamination during laparoscopy although some surgeons believe that the liquidity of intracolonic contents can make spillage more likely with an intraoperative colonic injury.

Preoperative assessment of the patient's abdominal wall is crucial to identify the optimal site for stoma creation. This is usually performed by a trained enterostomal therapy (ET) nurse. Various factors are taken into account including naturally occurring skin creases in the seated and supine positions, surgical scars, the patient's belt line, the width of the rectus muscles, the type of stoma being created, the patient's abdominal wall adiposity, as well as factors such as manual dexterity, location of a seatbelt, and others. It is important to protect the skin marking, often by marking the skin and placing a watertight adhesive on top to prevent the marking from being washed off. Furthermore, informing your ET nurse of the potential location of incisions for the laparoscopic procedure may allow for proposed stoma sites to be incorporated into incisions. Additionally, in complex cases, selection of bilateral or four-quadrant stoma locations can also provide the surgeon with more options at the time of stoma creation, especially with obese abdominal walls and difficulty bring through the intestinal segment. For additional details on optimizing stoma function, please refer to Chap. 36 on best practices in planned and unplanned stoma creation.

Operative Setup

Procedures can be performed using a laparoscopic approach. Ensuring the drapes are sufficiently laterally positioned is important to allow for exposure of the skin for the lateral fixation sutures. Placing the lateral drapes just medial to the anterior axillary line will allow for sufficient lateral access.

Extraperitoneal Stoma Creation

Principles and Quality Benchmarks

A number of techniques are available to allow for the creation of an extraperitoneal tract. When performed laparoscopically, the maneuver tends to be technically challenging. The challenge lies in the ability to create the intraperitoneal opening as well as the supraperitoneal tunnel under visualization while maintaining pneumoperitoneum. In the view of the authors, this approach has little role during the creation of temporary stomas. The decision that needs to be made is the position of the stoma

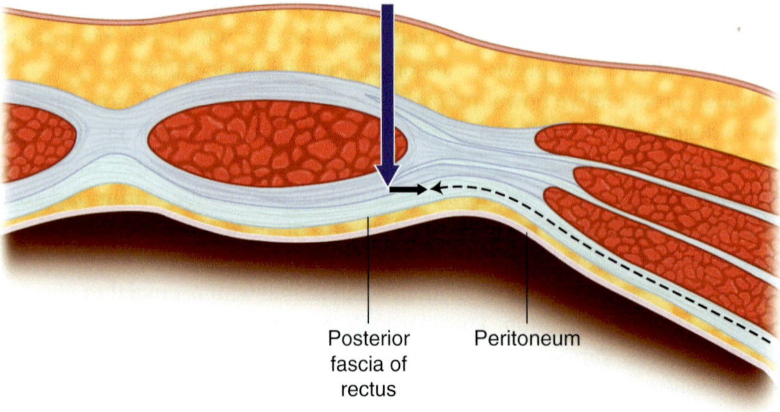

Fig. 37.1 Cross-sectional image of the abdominal wall delineating a retrorectus extraperitoneal tract for a permanent stoma to prevent parastomal hernias

relative to the various abdominal wall layers. One of the more common approaches is to bring the colostomy anterior to the parietal peritoneum, below all the abdominal wall structures [31, 32, 36] (Fig. 37.1) or, less commonly, below the transversalis muscle but anterior to the transversalis fascia and parietal peritoneum [37]. Furthermore, a dissector is needed to create the extraperitoneal tunnel from the peritoneum at the level of the skin aperture to the window created intraperitoneally. Some surgeons have used the curve of a Kelly clamp to gently separate the appropriate layers. Leroy and colleagues discuss the EndoH® retractor (Karl Storz® (Tuttlingen, Germany) [31], whereas others have used the Covidien® Endo Retract™ Maxi 10 mm device (Mansfield, MA, USA) [36].

Operative Technique

Individual techniques vary, but consistently, the resectional aspect of the procedure is completed first, and the proximal transection margin is stapled off. In abdominoperineal resections (APR), if the perineal dissection is being performed supine, the specimen is often removed through the perineum and the perineal wound closed prior to reinsufflation. If the perineal is approach prone, the colostomy is fashioned first.

During this approach, it is important to mobilize the descending colon slightly more proximally to allow for sufficient mobility of the colonic conduit that is to be brought through the extraperitoneal space. If an assistant port has been placed at the proposed stoma site, the port is removed, and a disc of skin is excised corresponding to the proposed stoma site. This aperture can vary between 20 and 25 mm depending on the width of the lumen and type of stoma being created. It is up to the surgeon to decide if the underlying subcutaneous fat is to be resected or separated. The anterior rectus sheath is identified and can be incised either in a cephalocaudal axis or in a cruciate fashion, after which the rectus muscle fibers are separated. It is important to ensure a perpendicular approach through the abdominal wall is being followed. The posterior rectus sheath, if present, is then identified and carefully incised to expose the intact peritoneum. The dissection of the extraperitoneal tract is often and more easily performed in an external to internal fashion. The width of the tract should be approximately 2 fingerbreadths or 5 cm and taken laterally to the paracolic gutter or smaller with end ileostomies. This is also performed with laparoscopic observation and guidance. The tunnel may often have to be angled in a slight cephalad fashion to accommodate the path along which the colon and mesocolon/mesentery must be brought along. Laparoscopically, the peritoneum is then incised laterally at the proposed entry site of the intestinal conduit of the end stoma. It is important to ensure that the size of the path being created accounts for the bulk of the mesentery/mesocolon. Leroy and colleagues report placing an absorbable suture loop around the distal end of the stoma that is then grasped by the laparoscopic grasper placed through the trephine opening [31]. The intestinal segment is gently pulled through, at times requiring digital assistance. The lateral parietal peritoneal opening may sometimes be narrowed down using intracorporeally placed absorbable sutures (3-0) to minimize the likelihood of a potential for herniation of intestinal content.

Tulina and colleagues rejuvenated the Goligher approach by creating the extraperitoneal tract along the retrorectus plane, anterior to the transversalis fascia and peritoneum [37]. They describe using the assistant trocar at the site of the stoma by gradually pulling it back from the intraperitoneal space to the appropriate abdominal wall level and then connecting the laparoscopic insufflation to assist with the separation of the planes using pneumodissection. The plane can be created during delivery of the bowel through the stoma aperture.

Pitfalls and Troubleshooting

In slim patients, the parietal peritoneum may be violated. In such situations, if the defect is too large, a different tract can be created, which when formally complete can then allow for the disrupted segment of peritoneum to be closed with laparoscopically placed sutures. Alternatively, the retrorectus plane described by Tulina and colleagues can be followed instead [37].

It is important to ensure the tract is sufficiently wide to allow for the intestinal segment and its mesentery to be passed through without tension or excessive narrowing. Lowering intra-abdominal pressures can decrease tension on the abdominal wall. The cut-edge of the mesentery or mesocolon should be kept in consideration as tension on this as the segment is being pulled through the tract may result in tears and bleeding. Bleeding can often be addressed with laparoscopic techniques but care must be taken not to affect the vascular inflow of the conduit. Conduits appearing ischemic at the time of stoma creation should be observed briefly in a non-insufflated state to ensure it is not a tension-related phenomenon; if there is no improvement in the appearance, adjuncts such as indocyanine green angiography can be used to objectively assess perfusion. Frankly ischemic stomas should be revised. Conversion to an open procedure should be based on the comfort of the surgeon to revise and manage these issues laparoscopically.

Caution should be taken in considering this for patients with Crohn's disease. The mesenteric bulk and fistulizing nature of the disease as well as the frequent need for reoperations may result in intraperitoneal complications and abdominal wall inflammatory in case of recurrence.

Outcomes

A number of retrospective reports and two prospective randomized controlled trials have been reported, which are well summarized in a recently published meta-analysis comparing transperitoneal and extraperitoneal approaches for stoma creation [30]. In this review, the authors report lower rates of PSH (risk ratio 0.36; 95% CI 0.21–0.62; $p < 0.001$) and stoma prolapse (risk ratio 0.21; 95% CI 0.06–0.73; $p < 0.01$) with no difference in the rate of stoma necrosis. Well-designed randomized trials are pending at this time. No cost-effectiveness data are available. The published data on the comparative outcomes of extraperitoneal techniques in minimally invasive surgery are summarized in Table 37.1.

Prophylactic Mesh Placement

Principles and Quality Benchmarks for Prophylactic Mesh Placement for Permanent End Colostomies and Ileostomies

There are a number of approaches to the application of prophylactic mesh to decrease the likelihood of PSH and stoma prolapse with an end stoma. The main questions that should be asked are the following: (1) What type of mesh will be used? (2) Which technique and location of mesh placement will be employed?

As will be described in the outcomes section, the use of biologic mesh is not currently supported by the published data [38, 39]. Most of the published evidence describes outcomes following the placement of a retromuscular segment of nonabsorbable synthetic mesh in an open fashion. The focus of our discussion is on the laparoscopic placement, and as such, the main procedures would be a modified-Sugarbaker or a keyhole approach, both of which are the intraperitoneal techniques. Comparative trials of the keyhole and Sugarbaker techniques have focused on the therapeutic management of PSH. A number of trials have been published assessing these two approaches in the therapeutic treatment of PSH with no data available on their comparative efficacies in the prophylactic setting. These trials have noted improved results with the Sugarbaker approach, compared to keyhole approach, which has led surgeon to preferentially opt for the former approach [40, 41]. The senior author (SDW) performs the keyhole technique as it is his preferred method of therapeutic rather than prophylactic mesh placement, whereas the corresponding author prefers a Sugarbaker technique for the above reasons.

Most of trials included the use of lightweight macroporous polypropylene mesh, often with a single or dual composite component when used intraperitoneally. As reflected in the outcomes section (Table 37.2), most assessments of the efficacy of biologic mesh have failed to demonstrate any role in prophylaxis against PSH development. The jury is still out on the efficacy of heavy versus lightweight meshes although both authors prefer dual-layer composite lightweight macroporous mesh. The mesh is prepared externally and should be cut with the objective of a 10 cm overlap both medially and laterally.

The first step is both mesh orientation and fixation. When used intraperitoneally with either the Sugarbaker or the keyhole technique, the mesh should be fixed with either absorbable or nonabsorbable sutures or absorbable or nonabsorbable tacks to allow for preplacement and optimal final securing of the mesh (Fig. 37.2). One of the authors (SDW) favors the use of a barbed suture to hold mesh but occasionally uses tacks, whereas alternatively proposed (SAC) approaches include the use of permanent polypropylene sutures (2–0), followed by a double-crown placement of tacks. These sutures are preplaced on the mesh prior to the introduction into the abdomen. Small 2 mm skin incisions are made at the proposed sites of fixation (usually 4 points), and the sutures are brought through with a suture passer, such as a Carter-Thompson® device (Cooper Surgical, Trumbull, CT, USA). A number of technical pearls have been identified to improve the efficacy of these procedures.

For both techniques, a number of procedural pearls can be focused on to decrease the likelihood of recurrence. Although the overview and conclusions presented by Muysoms, Winkel, and Ramaswamy were aimed to describe parastomal hernia repair, these same principles are applicable to the prophylactic placement of mesh [42]. The following are some of the main recommendations:

- Clear the abdominal wall lateral to the fascial aperture to allow for the appropriate lateralization of the bowel segment. The authors also recommend tacking sutures of the segment of bowel leading to the fascial aperture to the abdominal wall to ensure it is appropriately linearized. Mesh placement can often retract medially due to abdominal wall forces resulting in lateral sites of recurrence. The above maneuver helps address this. This lateral segment extends down to the paracolic gutter, but usually, only a portion of this will be covered by the mesh. One of the authors (SAC) clears the peritoneum for 10 cm lateral to the aperture.
- Ensuring the stoma aperture is not too wide to provide the greatest surface area adjacent to the intestinal segment on the peritoneum and the fascia for mesh ingrowth.
- Although this point is not widely taught, the authors recommend stripping the peri-aperture abdominal wall of its peritoneum and fascia to allow the mesh to securely attach to the fascia or muscle fibers, thereby further encouraging ingrowth of the mesh.
- Maximize the overlap of the mesh by ensuring at least 5 cm of contact overlap between the mesh and the surrounding fascia. Some authors, as do the chapter authors, recommend 10 cm of overlap, especially lateral to the aperture as this is the most frequent site of hernia recurrence.

Table 37.2 Review of large (>50 patients) randomized controlled studies of mesh prevention strategies for parastomal hernias

Author (year)	*n*	Mesh type	Mesh position	Technique	Outcome assessment	Follow-up	Outcome (no mesh vs. mesh)
Serra-Aracil et al. (2009) [57]	55	Synthetic, nonabsorbable	Sublay	Open	Clinical/CT	29 (median)	40.7 vs. 14.8 ($p = 0.03$)
Cui et al. (2009) [58]	60	Synthetic, nonabsorbable	Intraperitoneal	Open	Clinical/CT/ultrasound	36 (mean)	26.7 vs. 0% ($p < 0.01$)
Fleshman et al. (2014) [39]	113	Biologic	Intraperitoneal	Open	Clinical; CT if suspicion of PSH	24 (mean)	13.2 vs. 12.2% (p – NS)
Vierimaa et al. (2015) [59]	70	Synthetic, nonabsorbable	Intraperitoneal	Laparoscopic	Clinical/CT	12 (mean)	32.3 vs. 14.3% ($p = 0.049$)
Lambrecht et al. (2016) [60]	58	Synthetic, nonabsorbable	Sublay	Open	Clinical/CT	40 (median)	46 vs. 5% ($p < 0.001$)
Lopez-Cano et al. (2016) [61]	52	Synthetic, nonabsorbable	Intraperitoneal	Laparoscopic	Clinical/CT	26 (median)	64.3 vs. 25% ($p = 0.005$)
Brandsma et al. (2017) [43]	133	Synthetic, nonabsorbable	Sublay	Open	Clinical/CT	12 (median)	24.2 vs. 4.5% ($p = 0.0011$)
Odensten et al. (2019) [50]	211	Synthetic, nonabsorbable	Sublay	Open	Clinical/CT	12 (median)	30 vs. 29% ($p = 0.866$)

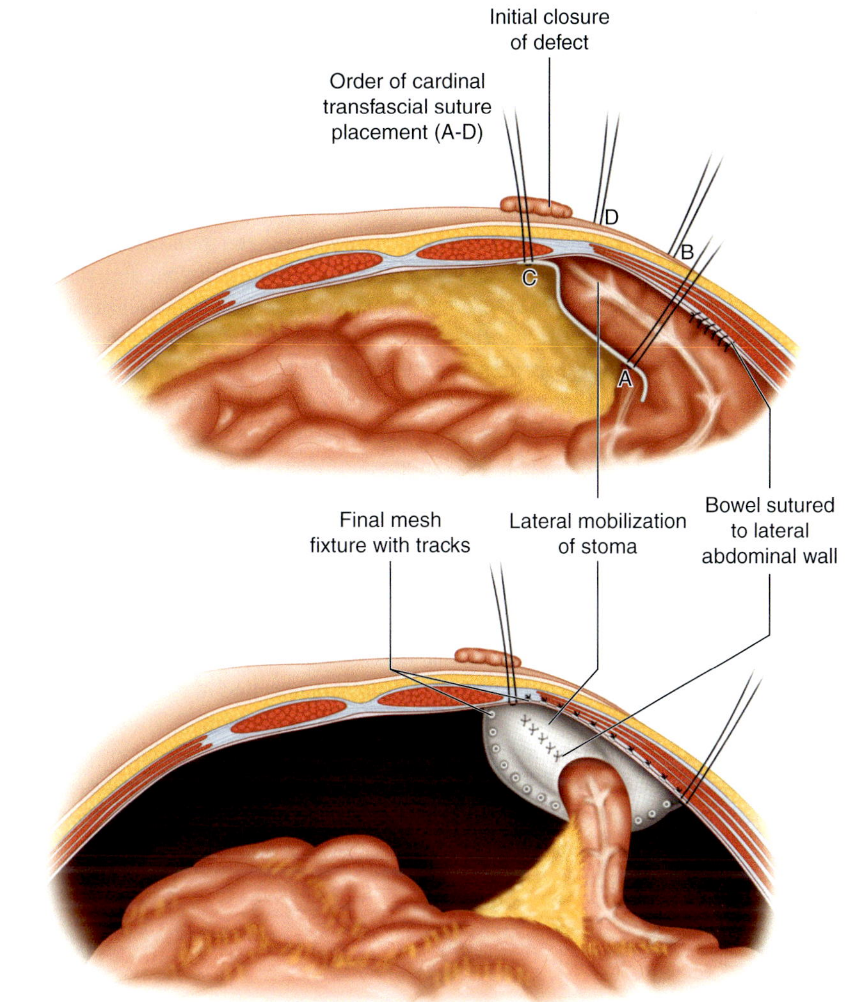

Fig. 37.2 Placement of the nonabsorbable segment of mesh using a modified-Sugarbaker technique, with lateral suturing the bowel segment to the abdominal wall. The tacks should be applied after the transfascial sutures have been tied down. These are down in a double crown configuration

- In addition to double-crown placement of tacks, transabdominal fixation sutures should be tied down in a lateral to medial sequence as described above.

Operative Technique for the Laparoscopic Sugarbaker Approach

Please refer to the "Operative Technique" section in regarding the resectional aspects of the procedure. A disc of skin measuring 20–25 mm in diameter is excised at the proposed stoma site. The underlying fat can be resected or transected at the surgeon's preference. The anterior rectus sheath is exposed which is incised in a cephalocaudal axis or as a cruciate. The muscle fibers are separate along their course medially and laterally exposing the underlying posterior sheath and peritoneum. This is incised exposing the intra-abdominal space and is dilated to ~20 mm diameter. The intestinal segment is brought through the abdominal wall and secured to the skin, protruding by 10–20 mm.

After ensuring that the bowel has been sufficiently mobilized to the lateral abdominal wall, some authors will recommend placing individual interrupted absorbable or nonabsorbable tacking sutures with seromuscular bites of the intestinal segment to the parietal peritoneum, thus linearizing the segment and allowing the surgeon to clearly visualize its course. The mesh is prepared by selecting the appropriate size initially. Usually mesh of 20 cm in diameter will allow for a 5 cm minimum overlap with the surround fascia when the size and width of the intestinal segment is also taken into account. Furthermore, with single-sided composite mesh, it is important to mark the non-composite side with a nonsymmetrical mark or letter to allow its identification intracorporeally; additionally, drawing a line along the long axis of the mesh can help clarify orientation. Cardinal sutures are placed on the medial and lateral aspects of the mesh prior to its insertion into the abdominal cavity. Prior to insertion of the segment of mesh, it often helps to roll it with the composite side on the inside of the roll. This allows for the mesh to be unrolled onto the abdominal wall with the composite side exposed to the abdomen. The long axis of the mesh is unrolled in a medial to lateral fashion to allow for maximal coverage of the intestinal segment. A suture passer is used through small 2–3 mm abdominal incisions to pull through the tacking sutures which can then be tied down (Fig. 37.3). A snap or toothed forced can be used to retract on the skin in this area to prevent the edge from being pulled down to the fascia

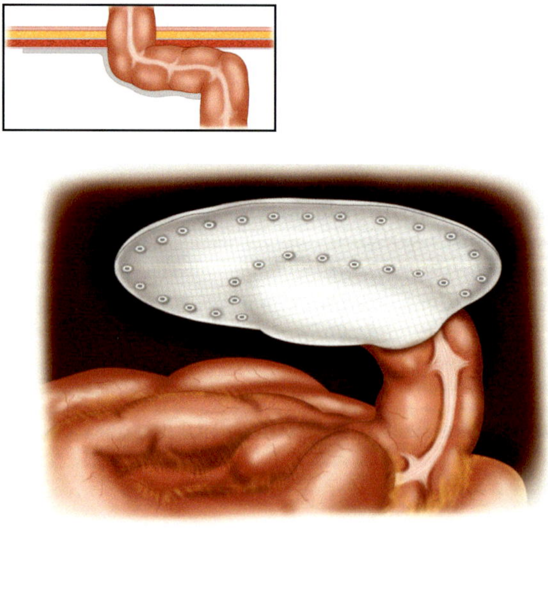

Fig. 37.3 Ultimate appearance of a modified-Sugarbaker mesh application for prophylaxis against parastomal hernia formation

with the suture. Subsequently, double-crown placement of tacks is applied to the mesh around the stoma to ensure that there are no gaps through which a segment of intestine can enter. Counterpressure externally with manual pressure on the abdominal wall can help ensure the tacks are well placed. It is important to ensure that the sutures and tacks are placed in a less insufflated state. We prefer to decrease intra-abdominal pressures to 6 mmHg, allowing for adequate visualization but not overstretching the mesh; this allows for its placement in a more physiologically natural state (Fig. 37.4). When this is complete, the abdomen is desufflated and the skin at the port sites closed (including the fascia of any larger port sites), after which the stoma is matured. This is performed in a Brooke fashion with absorbable sutures, 3-0 in size, ensuring approximately a 10 mm protrusion of the colonic mucosa.

Operative Technique for the Laparoscopic Keyhole Approach

The above pearls and recommendations with regard to preparation of the stoma aperture, the intestinal segment, and the introduction of the mesh apply for this approach as well. With this technique, it is important to ensure that the "non-slit" side of the

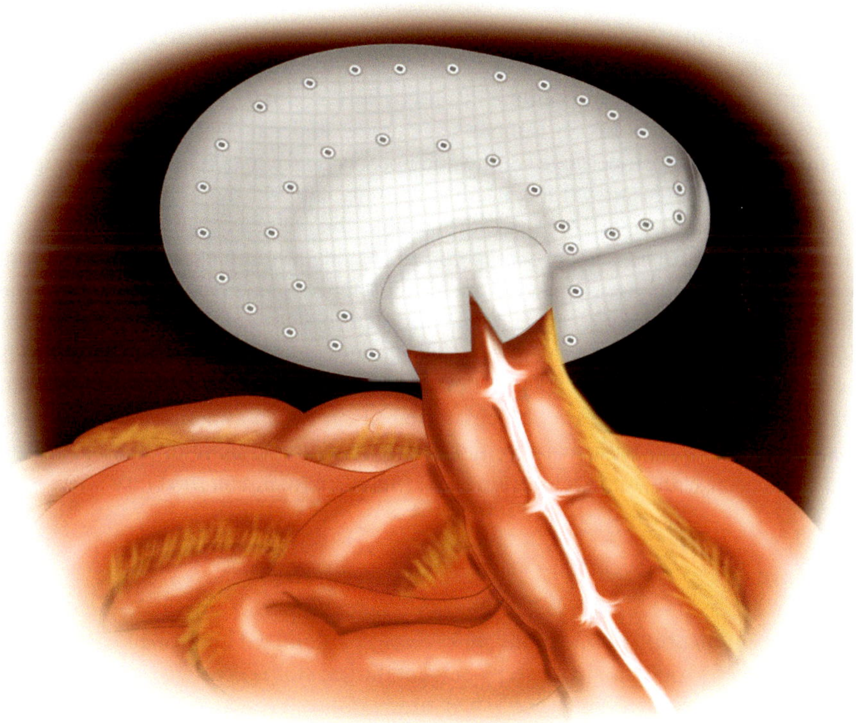

Fig. 37.4 Placement of a keyhole segment of mesh using a double-crown technique to secure the mesh in place

mesh be positioned laterally to ensure the area at highest risk for recurrence, i.e., the lateral side, is covered. Overlapping the two limbs should be done in a way to ensure the aperture of the mesh at the level of the intestinal conduit is not too tight to avoid stenosis but not more than 1 cm to avoid herniation of any other intra-abdominal structures between the mesh and intestine. Overlap of these limbs can be performed by pre-placing a stay suture on one limb while bringing a suture passer transabdominally, through both limbs, grasping the suture and then securing it. A second line of fixation of both the limbs and the mesh itself can then be performed with a tracking device. It is the authors' preference to use permanent tacks in these circumstances.

Pitfalls and Troubleshooting

A complete double crown of absorbable or permanent tacks will ensure there are no gaps for loops of the small intestine to enter through. Although rare, it is possible for the abdominal tacks to be placed through the intestinal segment. If this were to occur, the risks of fecal contamination of the segment of mesh would be too high. As such, taking down the mesh, repairing the injury to the intestinal segment, and proceeding without placement of the prophylactic mesh would be most appropriate. Furthermore, the tack may cause a bleeding-related injury to the abdominal wall or the mesentery/mesocolon. In such a situation, a segment of gauze can be inserted laparoscopically, and pressure can be applied to the area for 5–10 minutes. It is generally best to apply this pressure in a less insufflated state to ensure that the resolution of bleeding occurs in a more physiologic and natural anatomic state that would mimic the postoperative setting and not secondary to tamponade from higher intra-abdominal pressures. If the bleeding does not subside, the surgeon will need to take down part of the mesh to expose the area bleeding to allow for it to be addressed. This can be performed with an energy device or using a suture passer to suture ligate the vessel. It is also important to ensure the mesh is not placed too tightly around the stomal conduit that may result in bowel obstruction. Mesh erosion, fistulization, or infection generally requires excision of mesh with stoma relocation. The bowel is often quite adherent to this area, at times necessitating a resection of the involved intestinal segment. There are rare circumstances in which a mesh infection can be successfully treated with incision and drainage and/or antibiotics, but in general mesh excision with stoma relocation is the preferred treatment modality.

Outcomes

Since the publication of one of the most recent randomized controlled trial assessing the use of prophylactic mesh placement during stoma creation [43], a number of meta-analyses have been published summarizing the data, all of which have commented on a decrease in the rate of PSH when using prophylactically placed mesh at the time of the original procedure [11, 44–49]. These publications are summarized in Table 37.2. These meta-analyses have not accounted for the results of a more recent well-designed randomized trial that did not identify any differences in outcomes between the mesh and non-mesh groups [50]. Most studies commented on the fact that there remains heterogeneity between studies with respect to detection methods for PSH, whether clinically, radiologically, or both, as well as with regard to the type of mesh (biologic vs. synthetic) and the technique in which it was applied (retromuscular, intraperitoneal onlay – modified Sugarbaker or keyhole). The Cochrane review by Jones and colleagues reports a decrease in the likelihood of a PSH with mesh placement by more than 50% (relative risk of 0.53, 95% Confidence Interval 0.43–0.56) although the I^2 value indicative of inter-study heterogeneity was 69%, which is high [48]. One such source of inter-study heterogeneity is the method by which the PSH is diagnosed. In an attempt to control for this heterogeneity, the meta-analysis by Patel and colleagues found a pooled odds ratio of 0.21 (95% confidence interval 0.11–0.38) for a PSH when prophylactic mesh was used, with an I^2 value of 0% [11], indicating the outcome of PSH is almost 80% less likely with mesh prophylaxis. Furthermore, consistent with the findings of the individual studies, the odds ratio (OR) was found to be 0.16 (95% confidence interval 0.09–0.27) when studies including synthetic mesh were selected for in a subgroup analysis (greater than 95% less likely chance of PSH with synthetic mesh versus no mesh), with no significant effect in the studies using biologic mesh [38, 39]. Reassuringly, there were no differences in overall adverse event rates or stoma-related complications (such as fistulization, stenosis, or bleeding) between the mesh and non-mesh groups. Additionally, in assessing the cost-effectiveness of the data, Findlay and colleagues identified that the use of prophylactic synthetic mesh was cost-effective in preventing PSH, whereas the use of composite mesh was cost-neutral. Furthermore, given the more expensive nature of biologic mesh and the negative results of studies, biologic meshes were found to be more costly [51].

The publications summarized in Table 37.2 are largely associated with a demonstrable prophylactic effect of mesh use on the outcome of PSH. The recent 2019 publication by Odensten and colleagues presents data to the contrary [50]. At this juncture, the authors do not routinely use mesh to prevent PSH. But based on the demonstrated preventative effect of mesh use against the occurrence of PSH, the low rate of stoma-related and general adverse outcomes and the cost-effective nature of this approach have led societies such as the European Hernia Society to strongly recommend placement of prophylactic mesh at the time of surgery with a permanent colostomy [52].

With respect to the learning curve associated with the use of prophylactic mesh to prevent PSH, there are no published data that have investigated this. At this point, the authors would strongly recommend that the first few procedures performed by any surgeon be appropriately proctored by a local expert to ensure outcomes are optimal for the patient. Safe and proctored implementation of this technique is likely to ensure patients experience optimal outcomes of PSH prophylaxis.

Upcoming Procedures: SMART Procedure

Recently, the Stapled Mesh Stoma Reinforcement Technique (SMART) was developed by Williams and colleagues [27]. Although prophylactic mesh placement seems advisable based upon the ever-increasing body of literature, certain cost constraints as well as technical challenges may be the factors which have limited the application of this recommendation. During this procedure, the anterior rectus sheath is exposed and incised. The rectus muscle fibers are separated and the posterior sheath and peritoneum are entered. The anvil of the 28 mm stapler is placed intra-abdominally and is connected through the posterior sheath, peritoneum, and anterior sheath defects to the spike of the body of the stapler. Usually a 28 mm circular end-to-end stapler was used with the stapler placed through the stoma itself and the anvil of the stapler within the distal most end of bowel to be matured into a stoma. The fully extended spike of the body of the circular stapler is connected to the anvil. The spike will have had the circular segment of the biologic mesh pre-loaded (10 cm diameter circular configuration). The stapler is deployed resulting in a stapled incorporation of the mesh into the anterior rectus sheath, standardizing the trephine size. The outer edges of the mesh are sewn to the anterior rectus sheath after which the conduit is brought through (Fig. 37.5). The technique was developed to further enhance the strength of the adjacent fascial defect. Other authors have commented on the fact that the use of biologic mesh is not well-supported in the literature, in addition to the fact that these staples do have the ability to further separate, allowing for the mesh to release and the aperture to distend further. Long-term follow-up and well-designed prospective trials are necessary to better evaluate the efficacy of this technique.

The outcomes from this technique remain preliminary at this time. In a cohort study of 22 SMART patients and 11 controls, the rate of PSH was 19% (4 patients) in the SMART group and 73% in the control [53] with similar age and BMI distributions between both groups. This report was provided by the center that first reported the technique. A second report from a different center of 29 patients undergoing SMART and 38 undergoing a transperitoneal non-mesh approach was reported with no difference in patient demographics and a median follow-up of 27 months. The rate of PSH in the SMART group was 13.8% with a rate of 29.5% in the control group ($p = 0.029$) [54]. Both of these studies are preliminary with other reports published in abstract format. The authors have not employed nor recommend this technique at the time of writing but identify it as a potential future option for PSH prophylaxis.

Conclusions

A number of techniques, varying in invasiveness, are available to minimize the likelihood of PSH formation with the creation of end stomas. Laparoscopic and other minimally invasive approaches do not preclude the use of various approaches,

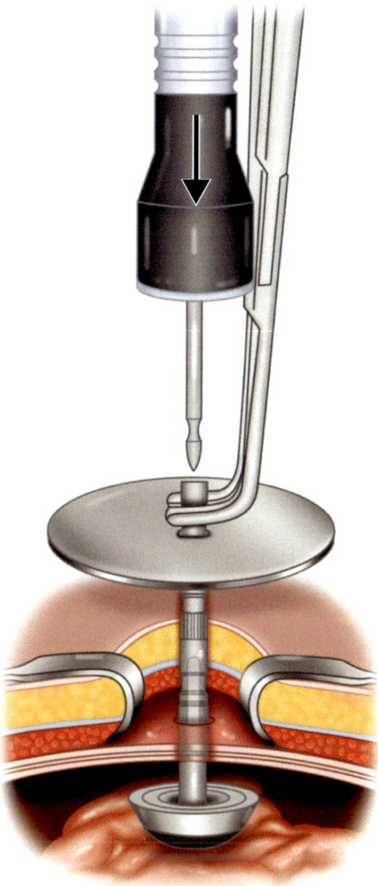

Fig. 37.5 The Stapled Mesh Stoma Reinforcement Technique (SMART) utilizing a circular stapler to fixate a segment of biologic mesh to the anterior rectus sheath

including the creation of extraperitoneal routes and the application of prophylactic mesh techniques. The use of these techniques does have significant support from published evidence, with some heterogeneity in the literature remaining. Given the implications of complications with these procedures, authors should be comfortable with their minimally invasive skillsets prior to performing these additional techniques and should optimally ensure they have been through the appropriate training pathways and proctorship networks.

References

1. Tiernan J, Cook A, Geh I, George B, Magill L, Northover J, et al. Use of a modified Delphi approach to develop research priorities for the association of coloproctology of Great Britain and Ireland. Color Dis. 2014;16(12):965–70.
2. Carne PWG, Robertson GM, Frizelle FA. Parastomal hernia. Br J Surg. 2003;90(7):784–93.

3. Andersen RM, Klausen TW, Danielsen AK, Vinther A, Gögenur I, Thomsen T. Incidence and risk factors for parastomal bulging in patients with ileostomy or colostomy: a register-based study using data from the Danish stoma database capital region. Color Dis. 2018;20(4):331–40.
4. Moreno-Matias J, Serra-Aracil X, Darnell-Martin A, Bombardo-Junca J, Mora-Lopez L, Alcantara-Moral M, et al. The prevalence of parastomal hernia after formation of an end colostomy. A new clinico-radiological classification. Color Dis. 2009;11(2):173–7.
5. Seo SH, Kim HJ, Oh SY, Lee JH, Suh KW. Computed tomography classification for parastomal hernia. J Korean Surg Soc. 2011;81(2):111–4.
6. Gil G, Szczepkowski M. A new classification of parastomal hernias--from the experience at Bielański Hospital in Warsaw. Pol Przegl Chir. 2011;83(8):430–7.
7. Smietanski M, Szczepkowski M, Alexandre JA, Berger D, Bury K, Conze J, et al. European Hernia Society classification of parastomal hernias. Hernia. 2014;18(1):1–6.
8. Leong AP, Londono-Schimmer EE, Phillips RK. Life-table analysis of stomal complications following ileostomy. Br J Surg. 1994;81(5):727–9.
9. Londono-Schimmer EE, Leong AP, Phillips RK. Life table analysis of stomal complications following colostomy. Dis Colon Rectum. 1994;37(9):916–20.
10. Pearl RK. Parastomal hernias. World J Surg. 1989;13(5):569–72.
11. Patel SV, Zhang L, Chadi SA, Wexner SD. Prophylactic mesh to prevent parastomal hernia: a meta-analysis of randomized controlled studies. Tech Coloproctol. 2016;21(1):5–13.
12. van Dijk SM, Timmermans L, Deerenberg EB, Lamme B, Kleinrensink G-J, Jeekel J, et al. Parastomal Hernia: impact on quality of life? World J Surg. 2015;39(10):2595–601.
13. Leslie D. The parastomal hernia. Surg Clin North Am. 1984;64(2):407–15.
14. Thorlakson RH. Technique of repair of herniations associated with colonic stomas. Surg Gynecol Obstet. 1965;120:347–50.
15. Turnbull RB. Intestinal stomas. Surg Clin North Am. 1958;38(5):1361–72.
16. Sjödahl R, Anderberg B, Bolin T. Parastomal hernia in relation to site of the abdominal stoma. Br J Surg. 1988;75(4):339–41.
17. Hardt J, Meerpohl JJ, Metzendorf M-I, Kienle P, Post S, Herrle F. Lateral pararectal versus transrectal stoma placement for prevention of parastomal herniation. Cochrane Database Syst Rev. 2013;49(10):1559–1.
18. Hardt J, Seyfried S, Weiß C, Post S, Kienle P, Herrle F. A pilot single-centre randomized trial assessing the safety and efficacy of lateral pararectus abdominis compared with transrectus abdominis muscle stoma placement in patients with temporary loop ileostomies: the PATRASTOM trial. Color Dis. 2016;18(2):O81–90.
19. Babcock G, Bivins BA, Sachatello CR. Technical complications of ileostomy. South Med J. 1980;73(3):329–31.
20. Nguyen MH, Pittas F. How large should a skin trephine be for an end stoma? Aust N Z J Surg. 1999;69(9):675–6.
21. Hong SY, Oh SY, Lee JH, Kim DY, Suh KW. Risk factors for parastomal hernia: based on radiological definition. J Korean Surg Soc. 2013;84(1):43–7.
22. Manook M. "Hepworth hitch": parastomal hernia prevention by simple modifications of operative techniques. Tech Coloproctol. 2018;22(6):461–3.
23. Goligher JC. Extraperitoneal colostomy or ileostomy. Br J Surg. 1958;46(196):97–103.
24. Bayer I, Kyzer S, Chaimoff C. A new approach to primary strengthening of colostomy with Marlex mesh to prevent paracolostomy hernia. Surg Gynecol Obstet. 1986;163(6):579–80.
25. Hansson BME, Morales-Conde S, Mussack T, Valdes J, Muysoms FE, Bleichrodt RP. The laparoscopic modified Sugarbaker technique is safe and has a low recurrence rate: a multicenter cohort study. Surg Endosc. 2013;27(2):494–500.
26. Mizrahi H, Bhattacharya P, Parker MC. Laparoscopic slit mesh repair of parastomal hernia using a designated mesh: long-term results. Surg Endosc. 2012;26(1):267–70.
27. Williams NS, Nair R, Bhan C. Stapled mesh stoma reinforcement technique (SMART) – a procedure to prevent parastomal herniation. Ann R Coll Surg Engl. 2011;93(2):169.

28. Dong L-R, Zhu Y-M, Xu Q, Cao C-X, Zhang B-Z. Clinical evaluation of extraperitoneal colostomy without damaging the muscle layer of the abdominal wall. J Int Med Res. 2012;40(4):1410–6.
29. Heiying J, Yonghong D, Xiaofeng W, Hang Y, Kunlan W, Bei Z, et al. A study of laparoscopic extraperitoneal sigmoid colostomy after abdomino-perineal resection for rectal cancer. Gastroenterol Rep (Oxf). 2014;2(1):58–62.
30. Kroese LF, de Smet GHJ, Jeekel J, Kleinrensink G-J, Lange JF. Systematic review and meta-analysis of xtraperitoneal versus Transperitoneal colostomy for preventing parastomal hernia. Dis Colon Rectum. 2016;59(7):688–95.
31. Leroy J, Diana M, Callari C, Barry B, D'Agostino J, Wu HS, et al. Laparoscopic extraperitoneal colostomy in elective abdominoperineal resection for cancer: a single surgeon experience. Color Dis. 2012;14(9):e618–22.
32. Hamada M, Ozaki K, Muraoka G, Kawakita N, Nishioka Y. Permanent end-sigmoid colostomy through the extraperitoneal route prevents parastomal hernia after laparoscopic abdominoperineal resection. Dis Colon Rectum. 2012;55(9):963–9.
33. Muysoms FE, Dietz UA. Prophylactic meshes in the abdominal wall. Chirurg. 2017;88(Suppl 1):34–41.
34. Jänes A, Cengiz Y, Israelsson LA. Preventing parastomal hernia with a prosthetic mesh: a 5-year follow-up of a randomized study. World J Surg. 2009;33(1):118–21; discussion 122–3.
35. Lambrichts DPV, de Smet GHJ, van der Bogt RD, Kroese LF, Menon AG, Jeekel J, et al. Incidence, risk factors and prevention of stoma site incisional hernias: a systematic review and meta-analysis. Color Dis. 2018;20(10):O288–303.
36. Akamoto S, Noge S, Uemura J, Maeda N, Ohshima M, Kashiwagi H, et al. Extraperitoneal colostomy in laparoscopic abdominoperineal resection using a laparoscopic retractor. Surg Today. 2013;43(5):580–2.
37. Tulina IA, Kitsenko YE, Ubushiev MN, Efetov SK, Wexner SD, Tsarkov PV. Laparoscopic technique of modified extraperitoneal (retrotransversalis) end colostomy for abdominoperineal excision. Color Dis. 2018;20(8):O235–8.
38. Hammond TM, Huang A, Prosser K, Frye JN, Williams NS. Parastomal hernia prevention using a novel collagen implant: a randomised controlled phase 1 study. Hernia. 2008;12(5):475–81.
39. Fleshman JW, Beck DE, Hyman N, Wexner SD, Bauer J, George V, et al. A prospective, multicenter, randomized, controlled study of non-cross-linked porcine acellular dermal matrix fascial sublay for parastomal reinforcement in patients undergoing surgery for permanent abdominal wall ostomies. Dis Colon Rectum. 2014;57(5):623–31.
40. Asif A, Ruiz M, Yetasook A, Denham W, Linn J, Carbray J, et al. Laparoscopic modified Sugarbaker technique results in superior recurrence rate. Surg Endosc. 2012;26(12):3430–4.
41. Hansson BME, Slater NJ, van der Velden AS, Groenewoud HMM, Buyne OR, de Hingh IHJT, et al. Surgical techniques for parastomal hernia repair: a systematic review of the literature. Ann Surg. 2012;255(4):685–95.
42. Muysoms F, Winkel N, Ramaswamy A. The Achilles' heel of Sugarbaker. Hernia. 2016;21(3):477–9.
43. Brandsma H T, Hansson BME, Aufenacker TJ, van Geldere D, Lammeren FMV, Mahabier C, et al. Prophylactic mesh placement during formation of an end-colostomy reduces the rate of parastomal hernia. Ann Surg. 2017;265(4):663–9.
44. Wang S, Wang W, Zhu B, Song G, Jiang C. Efficacy of prophylactic mesh in end-colostomy construction: a systematic review and meta-analysis of randomized controlled trials. World J Surg. 2016;40(10):2528–36.
45. Cross AJ, Buchwald PL, Frizelle FA, Eglinton TW. Meta-analysis of prophylactic mesh to prevent parastomal hernia. Br J Surg. 2017;104(3):179–86.
46. Chapman SJ, Wood B, Drake TM, Young N, Jayne DG. Systematic review and meta-analysis of prophylactic mesh during primary stoma formation to prevent parastomal hernia. Dis Colon Rectum. 2017;60(1):107–15.

47. Pianka F, Probst P, Keller A-V, Saure D, Grummich K, Büchler MW, et al. Prophylactic mesh placement for the PREvention of paraSTOmal hernias: the PRESTO systematic review and meta-analysis. PLoS One. 2017;12(2):e0171548–15.
48. Jones HG, Rees M, Aboumarzouk OM, Brown J, Cragg J, Billings P, et al. Prosthetic mesh placement for the prevention of parastomal herniation. Cochrane Database Syst Rev. 2018;265(4):663–70.
49. Wijeyekoon SP, Gurusamy K, El-Gendy K, Chan CL. Prevention of parastomal herniation with biologic/composite prosthetic mesh: a systematic review and meta-analysis of randomized controlled trials. J Am Coll Surg. 2010;211(5):637–45.
50. Odensten C, Strigård K, Rutegård J, Dahlberg M, Ståhle U, Gunnarsson U, et al. Use of prophylactic mesh when creating a colostomy does not prevent parastomal hernia. Ann Surg. 2019;269(3):427–31.
51. Findlay JM, Wood CPJ, Cunningham C. Prophylactic mesh reinforcement of stomas: a cost-effectiveness meta-analysis of randomised controlled trials. Tech Coloproctol. 2018;22(4):265–70.
52. Antoniou SA, Agresta F, Alamino JMG, Berger D, Berrevoet F, Brandsma HT, et al. European Hernia Society guidelines on prevention and treatment of parastomal hernias. Hernia. 2017;22(1):183–98.
53. Williams NS, Hotouras A, Bhan C, Murphy J, Chan CL. A case-controlled pilot study assessing the safety and efficacy of the Stapled Mesh stomA Reinforcement Technique (SMART) in reducing the incidence of parastomal herniation. Hernia. 2015;19(6):949–54.
54. Canda AE, Terzi C, Agalar C, Egeli T, Arslan C, Altay C, et al. Preventing parastomal hernia with modified stapled mesh stoma reinforcement technique (SMART) in patients who underwent surgery for rectal cancer: a case–control study. Hernia. 2018;22(2):379–84.
55. Funahashi K, Suzuki T, Nagashima Y, Matsuda S, Koike J, Shiokawa H, et al. Risk factors for parastomal hernia in Japanese patients with permanent colostomy. Surg Today. 2013;44(8):1465–9.
56. Hino H, Yamaguchi T, Kinugasa Y, Shiomi A, Kagawa H, Yamakawa Y, et al. Relationship between stoma creation route for end colostomy and parastomal hernia development after laparoscopic surgery. Surg Endosc. 2016;31(4):1966–73.
57. Serra-Aracil X, Bombardo-Junca J, Moreno-Matias J, Darnell A, Mora-Lopez L, Alcantara-Moral M, et al. Randomized, controlled, prospective trial of the use of a mesh to prevent parastomal hernia. Ann Surg. 2009;249(4):583–7.
58. Cui J, Xiang J, Huang M-J, Wang L, Huang Y-H, Wang J-P. Application of GORE-TEX dual mesh fixing into peritoneum in sigmoid-colostomy to prevent peristomal hernia. Zhonghua Wei Chang Wai Ke Za Zhi. 2009;12(5):480–2.
59. Vierimaa M, Klintrup K, Biancari F, Victorzon M, Carpelan-Holmström M, Kössi J, et al. Prospective, randomized study on the use of a prosthetic mesh for prevention of parastomal hernia of permanent colostomy. Dis Colon Rectum. 2015;58(10):943–9.
60. Lambrecht JR, Larsen SG, Reiertsen O, Vaktskjold A, Julsrud L, Flatmark K. Prophylactic mesh at end-colostomy construction reduces parastomal hernia rate: a randomized trial. Color Dis. 2015;17(10):O191–7.
61. López-Cano M, Serra-Aracil X, Mora L, Sánchez-García JL, Jiménez-Gómez LM, Martí M, et al. Preventing parastomal hernia using a modified Sugarbaker technique with composite mesh during laparoscopic abdominoperineal resection: a randomized controlled trial. Ann Surg. 2016;264(6):923–8.

38 Transanal Endoscopic Surgery for Benign Rectal Lesions: Preparation and Surgical Techniques

Teresa deBeche-Adams

Introduction and Rationale

Local excision of rectal lesions has increased in appeal because of the obvious benefits of decreased postoperative morbidity, improved functional outcomes, and the avoidance of a stoma. Standard transanal excision (TAE) is reserved for tumors smaller than 4 cm in diameter within 6–8 cm of the anal verge. This approach is limited by anal retractors that can be quite cumbersome, sometimes satisfactory for pedunculated tumors, but often difficult for sessile lesions providing limited visualization. With the lack of precision and visual clarity, specimens often end up fragmented and with positive margins [1].

These techniques together (TEM, TAMIS, and TEO) form a generalized classification of transanal endoscopic surgery (TES) comprised of several different reusable and disposable platforms for transanal surgery. This will be discussed for use in the context of resection of benign rectal lesions for both submucosal and full-thickness excisions.

TEM

The transanal endoscopic microsurgery (TEM) platform (Richard Wolf, Knittlingen, Germany), introduced in the 1980s by Dr. Gerhard Buess, was the first TES platform to be introduced. It has demonstrated to be superior to standard TAE for treating benign and malignant rectal lesions [2–5]. This is likely due to its ability to perform high-quality resections with enhanced optics, instruments, and a specialized insufflation system. This allows for decreased incidence in fragmentation of the rectal specimen and subsequently lower recurrence rates [6, 7]. Little has changed in the system in over 30 years, proving its advanced technology

T. deBeche-Adams (✉)
AdventHealth Orlando, Colorectal Surgery, Orlando, FL, USA

P. Sylla et al. (eds.), *The SAGES Manual of Colorectal Surgery*,
https://doi.org/10.1007/978-3-030-24812-3_38

for the time, though widespread application of TEM has been slow. This could be due to several barriers, most notably its steep learning curve and expensive equipment [8, 9].

TEO

The transanal endoscopic operation (TEO®) system (Karl Storz, Tuttlingen, Germany), which is similar to the TEM platform, was designed to utilize standard laparoscopic equipment with a stable reusable transanal platform. Both include a 40 mm proctoscope, faceplate, and support arm allowing the surgeon to work autonomously without the need for an assistant to drive the camera. TEO offers varying rectoscope lengths of 7.5, 15, and 20 cm and an option to use a conventional 5 mm laparoscope. Its benefit includes the fact that the platform and specialized instrumentation are reusable and can be combined with additional disposable instrumentation as needed.

TAMIS

Transanal minimally invasive surgery (TAMIS) is a technique that was originally developed in 2009 as a hybrid between TEM and single-site laparoscopy for resection of rectal lesions [10]. It was developed out of the need for a practical alternative to TEM, capitalizing on the availability of current single-site access ports, which proved to be both technically feasible and affordable without purchase of specialized equipment. TAMIS is categorized by the use of a single-site port transanally in combination with conventional laparoscopic instruments, a laparoscopic camera lens, and a standard laparoscopic CO_2 insufflator for the purpose of performing endoluminal rectal surgery. It was originally described using the single-incision laparoscopic surgery port (SILS™ Port; Covidien, Mansfield, MA, USA) noting that its upper border anchored nicely at the anorectal ring. The GelPOINT® path transanal access platform (Applied Medical, Rancho Santa Margarita, CA, USA) was specifically designed for transanal access building on their previous single-site devices. Both are the only commercially available ports approved by the Food and Drug Administration (FDA) in the United States, with multiple other platforms available from other companies worldwide.

Comparable results have been reported with TAMIS in terms of fragmentation rate, margin positivity, and recurrence rate when compared to TEM [11, 12]. Advantages of TAMIS over TEM include rapid setup time, increased field of view within the rectal lumen, ability to adapt existing laparoscopic instruments already in the hospital, and the ease of patient positioning within the operating room [13–17].

Indications and Contraindications

This chapter will focus on recommendations for benign rectal lesions and suspected benign lesions, considering that occult cancers are occasionally discovered on final pathology of these polyps. A general rule of thumb is that if the lesion can be fully visualized with a rigid proctoscope, it is likely amenable to resection with TES. Lesions extending more proximal than what is easily visualized in the office may prove to be too difficult for local excision. Conversely, very distal lesions may reveal frustration during dissection due to difficulty placing the transanal access device, especially using TAMIS technique. In this situation, a hybrid approach may be used which will be described later.

The most common application for TES, as originally described by Buess, is the resection of rectal adenomas [2]. Farther reaching than TAE, this has expanded to include large or sessile lesions or endoscopically unresectable adenomas or those that are recurrent. Multiple large series with hundreds of patients have reported low recurrence rates ranging from 4 to 7.6% after TES for benign polyps [6, 18, 19]. In addition, small carcinoid tumors less than 2 cm are well suited for local excision via TES. The risk of metastases from these small carcinoid tumors is low and provides a reasonable alternative in the absence of metastases on preoperative imaging. Several institutions have reported resections of small rectal neuroendocrine tumors widely used using TEM with no evidence recurrence [20, 21].

Most contraindications are relative. When beginning these techniques, it is best to attempt resections of lesions in the mid and distal rectum (10 cm or below). Those more proximal than 10 cm risk peritoneal entry and can be difficult to manage without the necessary skill set. Large bulky lesions are also difficult given the limited space inherent to operating within the rectal lumen. Caution should be used when deciding to resect these lesions transanally as the surgeon should not compromise the margins of resection or inadvertently subject a patient to local excision when there is a chance an occult malignancy is present within the specimen. Lesions that are firm and fixed should be assumed to harbor a malignancy and therefore not be resected in the submucosal plane.

As the surgeon's comfort level with these techniques improves, larger polyps and more difficult dissections will become possible [14]. Even circumferential lesions are not a contraindication, as the transanal platform allows more precise dissection in the full thickness and submucosal planes and the ability to perform a handsewn anastomosis to maintain intestinal continuity [15].

Principles and Quality Benchmarks of the Approach

As with any local excision, the expectation of a complete, en bloc resection without fragmentation of the specimen with negative margins is the goal. For benign lesions, a 5 mm margin should be marked out prior to beginning dissection to ensure a negative margin. Benign lesions may be dissected in the submucosal plane, though it is generally recommended that a full-thickness excision be performed in the event that an occult malignancy is identified on pathologic review. For more details on the management of malignant rectal lesions, please refer to the Chap. 39 on TES for rectal cancer.

Preoperative Planning, Patient Workup, and Optimization

Orientation and Location of the Lesion

When a rectal lesion is identified on digital rectal exam, careful observation of its characteristics should be noted, including location from the anal verge and the anorectal junction, positional orientation within the rectal lumen, size, and whether it is soft or firm and mobile or fixed. Video endoscopy or office proctosigmoidoscopy should be repeated by the operating surgeon to confirm the impression and allow for operative planning. It is imperative to adequately identify the location and orientation of the lesion as this will guide the preoperative planning including intraoperative positioning of the patient.

Notation must be made of the height of the tumor in the rectum as divided by the valves of Houston into low (0–5 cm), mid (6–10 cm), and upper (11–15 cm) rectum. Also, whether the lesion is anterior or posterior and right or left sided will dictate if the patient will be positioned in lithotomy, prone, or decubitus position. Especially with the TEM platform, the exact spatial orientation of the lesion (anterior vs. posterior, right vs. left) must be determined to allow correct positioning in the operative theater.

Workup

A colonoscopy should be performed to rule out any synchronous lesions and to further characterize the rectal mass. Targeted biopsies of the rectal lesion may be taken of areas showing suspicion for malignancy. These may be more informative than random superficial biopsies which are subject to sampling error and might be misleading.

Imaging of the lesion may prove beneficial if there is still question of possible malignancy. The preferred imaging modalities for a rectal lesion include rectal MRI or endorectal ultrasound (EUS). Using one or both is acceptable and should be dependent upon institutional availability and expertise. Some data suggest MRI may over-stage rectal villous adenomas more than 50% of the time, recommending that EUS is the preferred method for preoperative evaluation of villous adenomas [22]. Other data suggest that preoperative imaging may not be necessary for clinically benign lesions before local excision. A dual institution study recently published a series of 620 patients of which 272 underwent preoperative imaging and 348 were without. There was no difference in the incidence of malignancy on final pathology in patients with preoperative imaging vs. those without (17% vs. 15%). In addition, the incidences of margin involvement and the need for salvage operation for the two groups were similar, concluding that if the important end results of local excision are not affected by preoperative imaging, then it may not be necessary [23]. Lastly, chest, abdomen, and pelvis staging CT scans for benign lesions are not commonly indicated.

Ambulatory Surgery Versus Admission

TES is generally viewed as safe and able to be performed as an outpatient procedure. Depending on comorbidities of the patient, the option to admit for 23-hour observation with discharge on the first postoperative day is also reasonable. Several centers have looked at details for admission and readmission after these procedures. Common reasons for admission include surgeon's discretion for further monitoring, urinary retention, bleeding, and breach of the peritoneal cavity. Some factors that may dictate whether a patient requires admission have been found to include tumor height, prolonged operative time, unsutured surgical defect, and surgeon experience. There are other risk factors for complications including tumor size >6 cm and antiplatelet medication. The most common reasons for readmission were hemorrhage, pain, and infection [24, 25]. It is helpful if patients are counseled on the potential need for admission during their preoperative consultation.

Preoperative Preparation

Perioperative protocols should follow the standards for colorectal surgery, including preoperative antibiotics and DVT prophylaxis. Some form of a bowel preparation is needed to ensure adequate visualization of the lesion, but the type can be left up to the operating surgeon's preference. Full mechanical bowel preparations are often used and would consist of an osmotic laxative such as polyethylene glycol or similar used for colonoscopy. This will produce clear visualization but may lead to constant inflow of liquid bowel contents in the surgical field. A flexible sigmoidoscopy preparation (dose of oral laxative and two enemas) may also be used and is more than adequate for visualization in most patients. If solid fecal matter is still present within the rectum, it can be easily pushed proximal to the lesion with a small surgical sponge. The former is likely more advantageous with more proximal lesions and the latter for distal lesions.

Routine placement of a Foley catheter is not mandatory but can be considered, especially in cases that are expected to take considerable time. Another scenario where Foley placement is beneficial is when resecting anterior lesions in a male patient. The catheter can be used as an indicator of injury to the urethra or can be used to manipulate the prostate (gentle tugging on the catheter) for orientation before an injury occurs.

Anesthesia

One important caveat to consider when operating within the insufflated rectum is that forceful diaphragmatic breathing may collapse the operative field. With the use of general endotracheal anesthesia, the patient can be paralyzed and negate the ill effects of this. Most TES procedures have been described and are performed under general anesthesia [1, 2]. Under special circumstances, spinal anesthetic can also be used and has been described as being safe and feasible by several institutions [26].

Operative Setup

Positioning and Setup

TEM procedures require slightly more operative setup time given the complexity of the equipment. Patients are usually positioned so that the lesion to be resected is in the downward orientation, e.g., lithotomy for a posterior lesion or prone jackknife with spread legs for an anterior lesion. This may require patients to be placed on their side for lateral lesions, in which case they can easily be secured with a bean bag. Conversely, TEO procedures can usually be performed in lithotomy position except for anterior lesions where peritoneal entry is anticipated. Both TEM and TEO equipment require the use of a U-shaped arm to secure the operating scope to the bed; however, this negates the need for an assistant to hold the camera.

For TAMIS procedures, lithotomy positioning can be used in all patients regardless of the lesion location. This expedites setup time in the operating room. Allen or candy cane stirrups may be used based on their availability. In contrast to what is mentioned above, TAMIS requires a designated camera driver to assist in the procedure.

If there is any question that abdominal access may be required, such as anticipated peritoneal entry for anterior proximal lesions, Allen stirrups are preferred so that the legs may be repositioned for the abdominal portion of the procedure. The disadvantage of having to reposition the patient in the case of peritoneal entry must be considered.

Both procedures should position patients low enough on the table to enable transanal access. Slight Trendelenburg position can be added as needed. A video monitor placed over the patient's torso and positioned between the legs provides the most ergonomic position for the operating surgeon and assistant (Fig. 38.1). Patients can then be prepped and draped in the normal fashion. If peritoneal entry is anticipated, the abdomen can be prepped preemptively as well.

Equipment

TEM and TEO

TEM equipment consists of a rigid operating rectoscope anchored to the operating table using an adjustable jointed U-shaped arm, specialized insufflation allowing consistent pneumorectum, 3D angled stereoscopic endoscope, and specialized

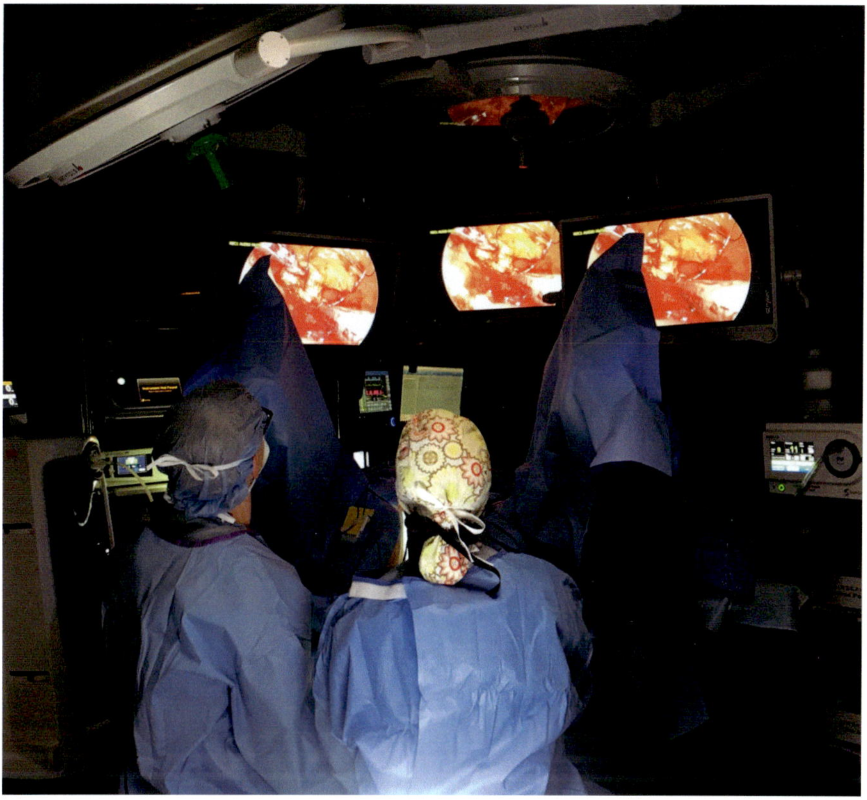

Fig. 38.1 TAMIS setup. Surgeon and assistant are seated facing the perineum with monitors placed above patient for ergonomic viewing while operating

angled instrumentation for dissection (Fig. 38.2a–c). The commercially available rectoscopes are ~4 cm in diameter and come in both beveled and straight configurations. Different lengths of 12 or 20 cm rectoscopes are also available. The longer versions greatly increase the ease of operating in the proximal rectum. The specialized insufflators allow for variability in intrarectal pressure during irrigation and suctioning to prevent loss of visualization during the operation. The external end of the rectoscope is covered with a sealed facepiece with an air tight rubber seal and sealed working ports to maintain insufflation. At the beginning of the procedure, the rectoscope is inserted up to the lesion under direct vision using manual insufflation. The scope is then secured to the operating table with the U-shaped arm. The scope produces a 40 degree downward view and does limit some of the operator's lateral field of vision. Because of this limitation, the scope may be repositioned several times during the course of the dissection to keep the operative field in the center of view. Angled instruments for grasping, retraction, and cautery, as well as self-righting needle drivers, are inserted through the working ports. "Silver bullets" may be applied to the ends of the suture to forego knot tying.

TEO is a less expensive rigid platform permitting use of standard laparoscopic instrumentation and a 5 mm 30 degree laparoscope (Fig. 38.3). The rectoscope is

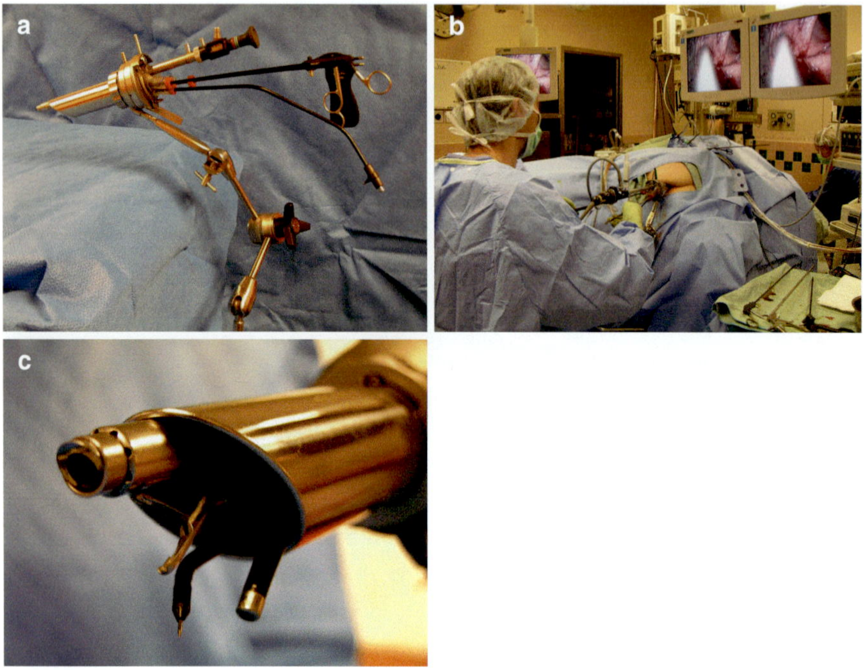

Fig. 38.2 (**a**–**c**) TEM setup. (**a**) TEM system (Robert Wolf, Knittlingen, Germany). (**b**) Patient is placed in right lateral decubitus position for a right-sided lesion. Once the operating rectoscope is positioned at the level of the lesion, it is secured to the bed with a Martin arm. (**c**) Specialized instruments can then be inserted through the rectoscope for resection of the lesion. (All: Copyright retained by Mark H. Whiteford, MD)

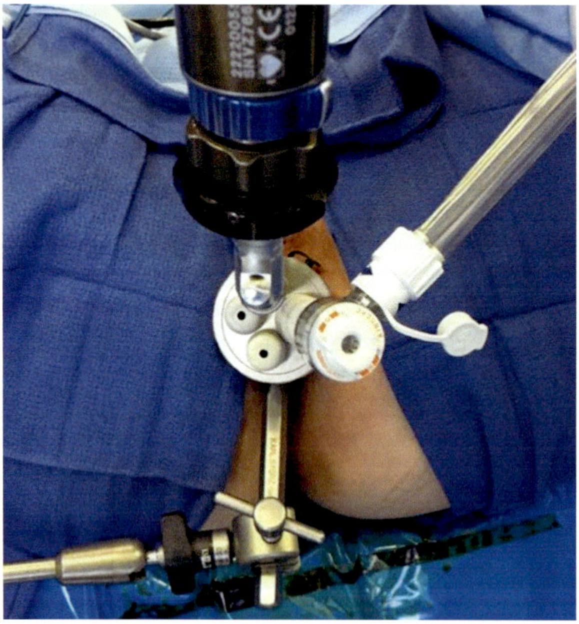

Fig. 38.3 TEO® (Karl Storz, Tuttlingen, Germany) with Airseal® insufflation system (AirSeal®, ConMed, Utica, NY, USA). (Courtesy of Patricia Sylla, MD)

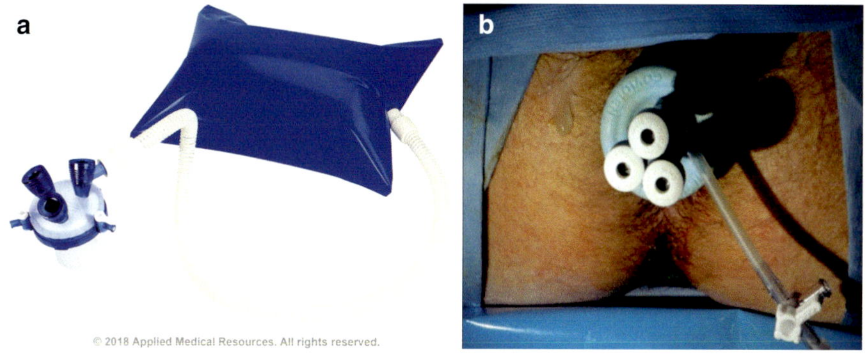

Fig. 38.4 (**a**, **b**) Currently available ports in the United States for TAMIS. (**a**) GelPOINT® path (used with permission of Applied Medical, Rancho Santa Margarita, CA, USA). (**b**) SILS™ port (Medtronic, Minneapolis, MN, USA)

also secured to the table with the multijointed U-shaped arm allowing the surgeon to operate autonomously without an assistant to hold the camera, similar to TEM. It also comes in straight or beveled ends but has 3 different lengths to the rectoscope: 7.5, 15, and 20 cm. The channels of the scope can accommodate instruments from 3 to 14 mm including endoscopic staplers. It also differs from TEM in that the insufflation system is not specialized and standard laparoscopic insufflators are used. It can be combined with specialized high-flow insufflators.

TAMIS

TAMIS can be performed using commercially available access ports including disposable and reusable options (Fig. 38.4a, b). Most allow insufflation through a separate channel, and some provide an additional separate channel for smoke evacuation to maintain clear visualization throughout the procedure. To combat the limitations of standard insufflators' slow cycling and inability to maintain pneumorectum during suctioning, several modifications have been designed or adapted for the available ports. These work with varying degrees of success and include high-flow insufflation using a valveless trocar system and an attachable bag that serves as a reservoir to prevent fluctuations in insufflation pressure. The remaining equipment is standard instrumentation found in the operating room, usually from a rectal tray and a laparoscopic cholecystectomy tray. A 30 or 45 degree angled laparoscope is preferred over 0 degree scopes, ideally with inline or right-angled optical cables. Bariatric length laparoscopes can also be used to vary the length of instruments to prevent collision. Maryland graspers, or similar, may be used for retraction. Monopolar electrosurgery is generally adequate for dissection and can be chosen from a variety of handheld options. Closure of the defect is accomplished with simple laparoscopic suturing techniques using standard needle drivers.

Accessory Equipment

Advanced devices can also be used for TES procedures but will add expense to the operation. Overall procedural costs, equipment availability, and lesion complexity should be considered prior to using these devices routinely. Advanced insufflation systems (AirSeal®, ConMed, Utica, NY, USA) can provide stable insufflation and smoke evacuation for TEO and TAMIS procedures as opposed to standard insufflation towers [27]. Advanced bipolar energy dissectors would be excessive for a submucosal dissection but may simplify a full-thickness resection and aid in hemostasis. There are several commercially available advanced laparoscopic closure devices that may speed up closure of the defect and therefore decrease operative times.

Operative Technique: Surgical Steps

Insufflation

Initial pressure settings for insufflation should be 8–15 mmHg and can be increased in a stepwise fashion if there is difficulty maintaining distention of the rectum. CO_2 insufflation has been described as providing a natural "pneumo-dissection" which helps expose the planes of dissection [10, 28].

Marking Out the Lesion

Standard principles used in transanal resection should be followed for TES resections. Electrocautery set on 30–40 watts used on the coagulation setting is sufficient for dissection and to permit hemostasis. It is recommended that the lesion be marked with dots of cautery around its circumference to ensure an adequate margin prior to beginning the dissection. For benign lesions, a 5 mm margin is sufficient (Fig. 38.5). For those with high suspicion of having a malignancy, a 10 mm margin is preferred when feasible. Gentle handling of tissues and avoidance of directly grasping the lesion will help to preserve the specimen.

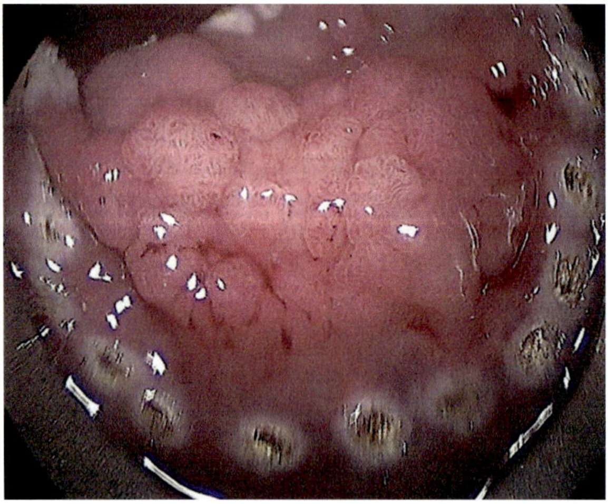

Fig. 38.5 Benign lesion with cautery marks outlining the resection margin prior to beginning dissection

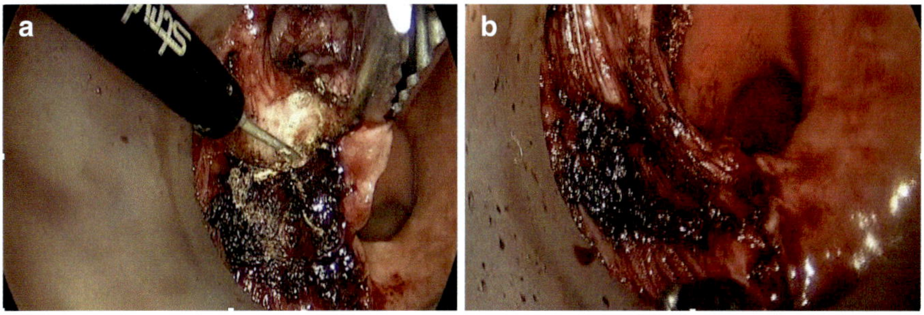

Fig. 38.6 (**a**, **b**) Submucosal plane of dissection for a benign rectal polyp. (**a**) Note the muscularis layer being separated from the mucosa. (**b**) Completed resection showing the muscularis layer intact within the wound bed. These defects can be left open since there is not a full-thickness defect through the rectal wall

Submucosal Dissection

As mentioned previously, benign lesions such as adenomas may be excised in the submucosal plane with a negative margin. When starting the dissection, the surgeon will note division of the mucosa with entry into the submucosal plane and may begin to see underlying muscle fibers from the muscularis layer deep to the submucosa (Fig. 38.6a, b). Careful dissection of these muscle fibers away from the submucosal layer with short bursts of cautery will maintain the plane of dissection. The tissue around the lesion will be quite thin and should be handled gently to prevent tearing or "button-hole" defects in the pathologic specimen.

Full-Thickness Excision

Most high-volume centers would endorse full-thickness excision to prevent the inadvertent under treatment of an occult malignancy. For full-thickness excisions, it is very important to remain perpendicular to the tumor so as not to compromise the deep margin. After division of the mucosa, the surgeon will continue through the circular and longitudinal muscle fibers before breaching the entire rectal wall and noting the areolar tissue at the interface of the mesorectum (Fig. 38.7a–c). This plane is ideal for the dissection to continue as it is fairly avascular. It may prove slightly more difficult to identify anteriorly as the anterior mesorectal fat is oftentimes thin if not nonexistent. If a nodal harvest is desired, dissection into the mesorectum can yield several nodes for sampling. This is more easily performed posteriorly. For posterior tumors, care must be taken not to disturb the mesorectal envelope in the event that unfavorable pathology is discovered unexpectedly. This would still allow a rescue TME to be performed without violating oncologic principles [29].

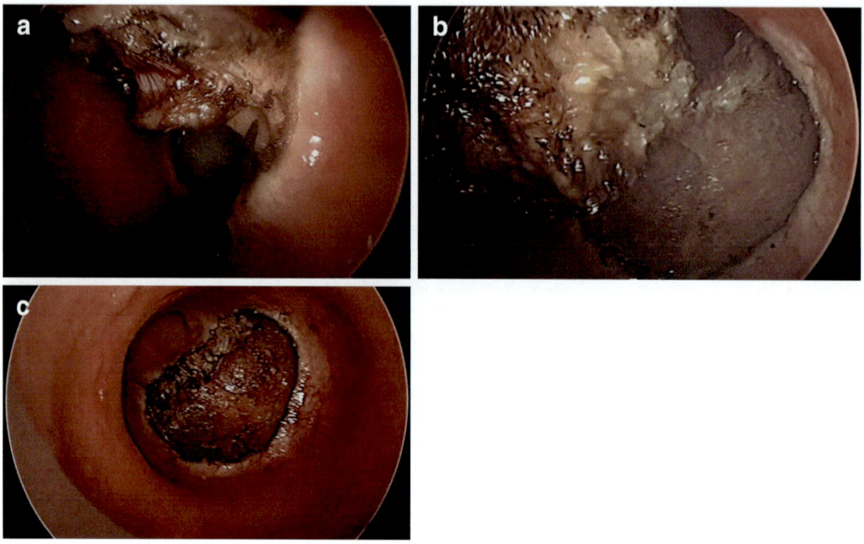

Fig. 38.7 (**a**–**c**). Full-thickness resection of a rectal lesion. (**a**) Note visualization of the mesorectal fat once the rectal wall has been divided. Dissection in this plane is fairly avascular and can proceed quickly with the aid of insufflation to develop the areolar plane. (**b**) A small portion of mesorectal fat can be seen on the deep side of the specimen. This will allow for preservation of the deep margin for pathologic evaluation in the event an unsuspecting malignancy is identified in the specimen. (**c**) Resected bed after a full-thickness excision with clearly visible mesorectal fat

Closure

Closure of the defect is one of the more difficult and time-consuming portions of the procedure. Submucosal resections can usually be left open as these are not full-thickness defects. Full-thickness defects located distal to the peritoneal reflection can technically be left open as they are extraperitoneal; however, it is highly recommended to close all defects as it is good practice for the necessary skills needed to close defects of the peritoneal cavity when they occur.

After resection of the specimen, defects will always appear larger than expected because of continuous insufflation stenting the rectum open. The insufflation pressure can be decreased to 8–10 mmHg allowing the edges to come in closer proximity for closure.

Defects are closed transversely so as not to narrow the lumen of the rectum. This can be accomplished in an interrupted fashion with multiple figure-of-eight sutures or with a running suture (Fig. 38.8a, b). It is quite difficult to tie intracorporeally within the limited confines of the rectal lumen. To overcome this, intraluminal knot tying can be facilitated with the use of a knot pusher or suture clips. Advanced laparoscopic suturing devices can fasten closure, thereby decreasing operative times. If closure is attempted in an interrupted fashion, it is easiest to bisect the defect at the center and continue in this manner until the entire defect is

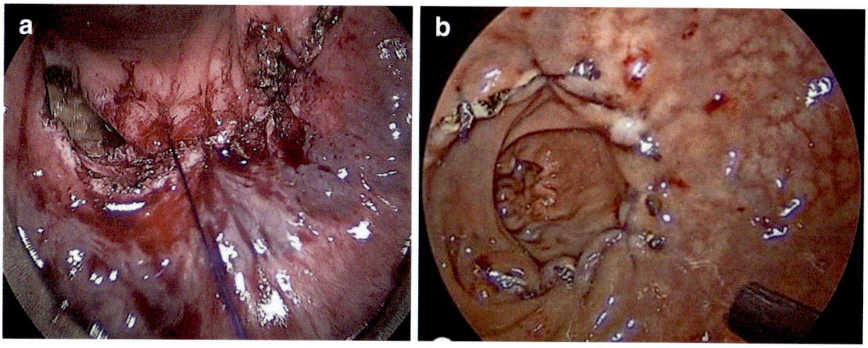

Fig. 38.8 (a) Closure of the full-thickness defect with interrupted sutures. (b) Completed closure of the defect

closed. Barbed suture is advantageous to use when running the defect closed as it obviates the need for knot tying.

Very distal defects may require closure with standard transanal equipment due to the access channel obscuring the distal edge. A useful trick is to place a suture at the proximal midsection of the defect endoscopically before removing the transanal platform. This will allow the surgeon to have a traction and reference point to continue the closure.

In patients who were previously radiated, higher incidences of wound dehiscence have been reported [30]. This is likely to produce pain, bleeding, and drainage. Many experts would recommend leaving these defects open or reapproximating them loosely with just a few interrupted sutures. Patients should be counseled preoperatively about this complication and managed expectantly through their discomfort.

Pitfalls and Troubleshooting

Loss of Insufflation

The most troublesome and disruptive occurrence during TES procedures is loss of pneumorectum and collapse of the operative visual field. The first step is to check the system for any obvious air leaks. This may require repositioning of access channels, seals, and tubing to prevent CO_2 from escaping the system. Another beneficial maneuver is to ensure that the patient is fully paralyzed if under general anesthesia. Excursional diaphragmatic breathing can overcome insufflation pressures and cause the rectum to collapse. Patients with visceral obesity may pose a similar challenge and may be tilted slightly so that the weight of the abdomen is not directly in the midline. It will take longer in these patients to overcome the resistance from a heavy abdominal wall, distend the colon fully, and establish adequate pneumorectum.

Lesions in the Distal Rectum

For very distal lesions at or just above the dentate line, a hybrid approach may be employed to facilitate resection, especially when using the TAMIS platform [31]. In this instance, the distal margin incision is begun using standard transanal retractors and electrocautery. Once the distal edge of the resection is developed, the transanal access channel can be inserted to use for the remainder of the lateral and proximal dissection. This allows improved visualization of the proximal extent of the lesion and less fragmentation of the specimen. Closing these distal defects is easier, as a single suture can be placed on the proximal edge of the excision site in the midline and used to reapproximate to the distal edge via the standard transanal approach [32, 33].

Peritoneal Entry

Full-thickness excision of lesions located in the middle or upper third of the rectum, notably anterior lesions, is associated with a higher risk of peritoneal entry. This is likely due to a lower peritoneal reflection on the anterior and lateral surfaces of the rectum, especially in the female pelvis. Studies have shown no increase in complication rates with peritoneal breach and surmise that proximal lesions should not be excluded from TES because of the chance of peritoneal entry. Current data reveal an occurrence rate between 1% and 15% [32, 34–37].

If intraperitoneal entry does take place, it may be initially noticed by an obvious defect into the abdominal cavity. The best next step is to stop dissection immediately and grasp the edge of the defect while still visible. This will allow prompt closure of the peritoneum to re-establish insufflation and continue on with the surgery. Sometimes entry is not this obvious, and the initial impression is loss of pneumorectum with leakage of insufflation into the abdominal cavity. Pausing for a few moments may allow the two cavities to equilibrate and the surgeon to regain visualization. Increasing the insufflation pressure may also aid in restoring pneumorectum. If the pressure from the abdomen is too great, it can be decompressed with a Veress needle or trocar in the abdomen.

The patient should be placed in Trendelenburg position to allow the abdominal contents to fall out of the pelvis so as not to injure the adjacent bowel during rectal wall closure. Though many peritoneal entries can be closed via the transanal approach, it can occasionally be difficult to maintain adequate visualization due to loss of pneumorectum. If this occurs, there are two viable options. First, if available, consider changing the transanal access to a longer channel. This may stent the rectum open closer to the peritoneal defect to allow visualization and closure. If this is not available or unsuccessful, converting to a laparoscopic assisted approach to aid in closure of the defect should not be delayed [38]. A Gastrografin enema study may be considered prior to discharge and is especially necessary if the patient is showing clinical signs of a leak after repair.

Learning Curve

Although TEM offers the potential for more precise excision, it has a steep learning curve and requires costly equipment [7, 9]. Specialized training courses are required before implementing it in a surgical program. Conversely, TAMIS has proven to be easier to adapt to, though not without its own learning curve [39]. It is still considered a complex procedure that requires a minimum of 14–24 cases to reach an acceptable R1 resection rate and lower operative duration [40].

Outcomes

TAE Versus TES

Unsurprisingly, there is a paucity of randomized controlled trials comparing TAE to TES, though current evidence continues to show a benefit to resecting rectal lesions with through advanced endoscopic platforms. The large majority of data stems from the TEM literature and portends an improved outcome in terms of microscopic margin positivity rates, specimen fragmentation rates, and recurrence rates [1, 6, 7]. Even for benign lesions, this should relay benefit to patients undergoing local resection while providing lower morbidity and reduced rates of stoma creation (Table 38.1) [12, 18, 19, 34, 35, 41–43]. The TAMIS data are relatively sparser but has thus far proven equivalent results to TEM, likely proving that the enhanced visualization with pneumorectum is likely what differentiates the two from TAE (Table 38.2) [11, 12, 31, 32, 44].

Complications

Intraoperative complications are mostly related to bleeding and peritoneal entry. As mentioned previously, peritoneal entry is often expected with resection of certain lesions and can be closed through a transanal approach the majority of the time. Less common intraoperative events include retroperitoneal, intraperitoneal, and subcutaneous emphysema, vaginal entry, and prostatic-urethral injury.

Postoperative complications associated with TES include bleeding, urinary retention, wound dehiscence, pain, infection, rectal stenosis, and transient fecal

Table 38.1 Largest TEM/TEO series results

Study	Benign etiology	Fragmentation (%)	Positive margins (%)	Recurrence (%)	Complications (%)	Peritoneal entry (%)	Stoma (%)
Lee et al. [12]	156	3[a]	5[a]	–	10[a]	3[a]	0.7[a]
Ramkumar et al. [34]	335	–	18[a]	–	7.1[a]	7.5	0.2[a]
Mege et al. [35]	123	–	10.8[a]	2.4	24.7[a]	17.9	2[a]
Guerrieri et al. [18]	366	–	–	4	7[a]	3.2[a]	0.5
Ramirez et al. [19]	149	–	5.8[a]	6	14	4[a]	–
Tsai et al. [41]	158	–	–	5	21[a]	6.7[a]	–
Saget et al. [42]	80	5.4[a]	11.9[a]	7[a]	24[a]	14	2.4[a]
Allaix et al. [43]	184	0	–	6	7.6[a]	4.3[a]	0

[a]Data reflect total rate for benign and malignant cases

Table 38.2 TAMIS series results

Study	Benign etiology	Fragmentation (%)	Positive margins (%)	Recurrence (%)	Complications (%)	Peritoneal entry (%)	Stoma (%)
Lee et al. [12]	228	4[a]	7[a]	–	9[a]	3[a]	0
Martin-Perez et al. [32]	152	4.1	4.4[a]	2.7[a]	8.7[a]	1[a]	–
Lee et al. [44]	90	3	6	3	7	6	0
Keller et al. [31]	50	1.3	0	0	4[a]	4[a]	2.6[a]
Albert et al. [11]	25	4[a]	8	4	8[a]	4	–

[a]Data reflect total rate for benign and malignant cases

incontinence (Table 38.3) [11, 12, 18, 19, 34, 35, 44]. TES results in minimal anal sphincter dysfunction [45, 46]. Older age may herald a worse prognosis with regard to fecal incontinence; however, this may prove to be temporary and reversible on the patient's quality of life after 1-year follow-up [47, 48]. Rectovaginal fistula has also been described and should be cautiously considered in female patients, as well as rectourethral and rectovesicular fistulae in men [25, 31]. The incidence of these will rise with prior radiation to the pelvis, especially the prostate, and requires counseling with the patient, particularly before resection of anterior lesions. Alternatively, TES may be used as a platform to correct rectovaginal and rectourethral fistulae [49].

Additional Uses

TES has also been described for resection of benign rectal lesions other than adenomas. Case reports of successful resection of endometriomas, perirectal dermoid cysts, perirectal myxoid pseudocysts, rectal schwannomas, and rectal GIST can be found in the literature [50–55]. In addition, TES can be used for diagnostic purposes, such as resection of a post-polypectomy scar to ensure no residual dysplasia or even early cancer is present at the site.

Table 38.3 Complication rates

Study	Bleeding (%)	Urinary retention (%)	Wound dehiscence (%)	Pain (%)	Infusion (%)	Rectal stenosis (%)	Fecal incontinence (%)	Rectovaginal fistula (%)	Rectourethral fistula (%)	Bladder fistula (%)
Albert et al. [11]	2[a]	0	0	–	0	0	–	–	–	–
Lee et al. [12]	3.9[a]	3.1[a]	–	2.5[a]	–	–	–	–	–	–
Keller et al. [31]	1.3[a]	–	–	–	–	1.3[a]	–	1.3[a]	–	–
Martin-Perez et al. [32]	2.8[a]	1.3[a]	0.5[a]	–	–	–	–	–	–	–
Ramkumar et al. [34]	2.6[a]	2.7[a]	–	–	–	–	–	–	–	0.3[a]
Mege et al. [35]	12.4[a]	3.1[a]	–	2.1[a]	–	7.2[a]	0	–	–	–
Lee et al. [44]	3.3	1.1	0	0	–	–	1.1	1.1	–	–
Guerrieri et al. [18]	1.5[a]	–	4.5[a]	3.7[a]	0.5[a]	0.2[a]	1[a]	0.2[a]	–	–
Ramirez et al. [19]	8[a]	2.3[a]	–	–	1.2[a]	1.7[a]	–	1.2[a]	–	–
Tsai et al. [41]	1.5[a]	10.8[a]	1.5[a]		0.7[a]	0	4.1[a]	0	0	0
Saget et al. [42]	5[a]	–	–	–	–	8[a]	–	–	–	–
Allaix et al. [43]	3.7[a]	0	1.7[a]	–	1.7[a]	–	0.3[a]	1.3[a]	–	0.3[a]

[a]Data reflect total rate for benign and malignant cases

Conclusions

Transanal endoscopic surgery is a safe and effective means of local resection for benign rectal lesions following adequate workup. Evidence shows increased quality of specimens using TES, resulting in lower rates of margin positivity, fragmentation of specimen, and recurrence. Amid improved results compared to TAE, superior functional outcomes over radical resection and equivalent results between TEM and TAMIS, surgeons will continue to use these techniques to improve patient care.

References

1. Clancy C, Burke JP, Albert MR, O'Connell PR, Winter DC. Transanal endoscopic microsurgery versus standard transanal excision for the removal of rectal neoplasms: a systematic review and meta-analysis. Dis Colon Rectum. 2015;58(2):254–61.
2. Buess G, Theiss R, Günther M, Hutterer F, Pichlmaier H. Transanal endoscopic microsurgery. Leber Magen Darm. 1985;15(6):271–9.
3. Saclarides TJ, Smith L, Ko ST, Orkin B, Buess G. Transanal endoscopic microsurgery. Dis Colon Rectum. 1992;35(12):1183–91.
4. Lev-Chelouche D, Margel D, Goldman G, Rabau MJ. Transanal endoscopic microsurgery: experience with 75 rectal neoplasms. Dis Colon Rectum. 2000;43(5):662–7; discussion 667–8
5. Cataldo PA. Transanal endoscopic microsurgery. Surg Clin North Am. 2006;86(4):915–2.
6. de Graaf EJ, Burger JW, van Ijsseldijk AL, Tetteroo GW, Dawson I, Hop WC. Transanal endoscopic microsurgery is superior to transanal excision of rectal adenomas. Color Dis. 2011;13(7):762–7.
7. Moore JS, Cataldo PA, Osler T, Hyman NH. Transanal endoscopic microsurgery is more effective than traditional transanal excision for resection of rectal masses. Dis Colon Rectum. 2008;51(7):1026–30; discussion 1030–1
8. Maslekar S, Pillinger SH, Sharma A, Taylor A, Monson JR. Cost analysis of transanal endoscopic microsurgery for rectal tumours. Color Dis. 2007;9(3):229–34.
9. Koebrugge B, Bosscha K, Ernst MF. Transanal endoscopic microsurgery for local excision of rectal lesions: is there a learning curve? Dig Surg. 2009;26(5):372–7.
10. Atallah S, Albert M, Larach S. Transanal minimally invasive surgery: a giant leap forward. Surg Endosc. 2010 Sep;24(9):2200–5.
11. Albert MR, Atallah SB, deBeche-Adams TC, Izfar S, Larach SW. Transanal minimally invasive surgery (TAMIS) for local excision of benign neoplasms and early-stage rectal cancer: efficacy and outcomes in the first 50 patients. Dis Colon Rectum. 2013;56(3):301–7.
12. Lee L, Edwards K, Hunter IA, Hartley JE, Atallah SB, Albert MR, et al. Quality of local excision for rectal neoplasms using Transanal endoscopic microsurgery versus Transanal minimally invasive surgery: a multi-institutional matched analysis. Dis Colon Rectum. 2017;60(9):928–35.
13. Melin AA, Kalaskar S, Taylor L, Thompson JS, Ternent C, Langenfeld SJ. Transanal endoscopic microsurgery and transanal minimally invasive surgery: is one technique superior? Am J Surg. 2016;212(6):1063–7.
14. Lim SB, Seo SI, Lee JL, Kwak JY, Jang TY, Kim CW, et al. Feasibility of transanal minimally invasive surgery for mid-rectal lesions. Surg Endosc. 2012;26(11):3127–32.
15. Barendse RM, Doornebosch PG, Bemelman WA, Fockens P, Dekker E, de Graaf EJ. Transanal employment of single access ports is feasible for rectal surgery. Ann Surg. 2012;256(6):1030–3.
16. Khoo RE. Transanal excision of a rectal adenoma using single-access laparoscopic port. Dis Colon Rectum. 2010;53(7):1078–9.

17. Watts ES, Peacock O, Gupta A, Speake WJ, Lund JN. Anyone for TAMIS? Tech Coloproctol. 2013;17(2):253–5.
18. Guerrieri M, Baldarelli M, de Sanctis A, Campagnacci R, Rimini M, Lezoche E. Treatment of rectal adenomas by transanal endoscopic microsurgery: 15 years' experience. Surg Endosc. 2010;24(2):445–9.
19. Ramirez JM, Aguilella V, Gracia JA, Ortego J, Escudero P, Valencia J, et al. Local full-thickness excision as first line treatment for sessile rectal adenomas: long-term results. Ann Surg. 2009;249(2):225–8.
20. Kinoshita T, Kanehira E, Omura K, Tomori T, Yamada H. Transanal endoscopic microsurgery in the treatment of rectal carcinoid tumor. Surg Endosc. 2007;21(6):970–4.
21. Chen WJ, Wu N, Zhou JL, Lin GL, Qiu HZ. Full-thickness excision using transanal endoscopic microsurgery for treatment of rectal neuroendocrine tumors. World J Gastroenterol. 2015;21(30):9142–9.
22. Nascimbeni R, Burgart LJ, Nivatvongs S, Larson DR. Risk of lymph node metastasis in T1 carcinoma of the colon and rectum. Dis Colon Rectum. 2002 Feb;45(2):200–6.
23. Lee L, Arbel L, Albert M, Atallah S, Hill J, Monson JRT. Radiologic evaluation of clinically benign rectal neoplasms may not be necessary before local excision. Dis Colon Rectum. 2018;61(10):1163–9.
24. Serra-Aracil X, Labró-Ciurans M, Rebasa P, Mora-López L, Pallisera-Lloveras A, Serra-Pla S, et al. Morbidity after transanal endoscopic microsurgery: risk factors for postoperative complications and the design of a 1-day surgery program. Surg Endosc. 2019;33(5):1508–17.
25. Brown CJ, Gentles JQ, Phang TP, Karimuddin AA, Raval MJ. Transanal endoscopic microsurgery as day surgery - a single-centre experience with 500 patients. Color Dis. 2018;20(10):310–5.
26. Arezzo A, Cortese G, Arolfo S, Bullano A, Passera R, Galietti E, et al. Transanal endoscopic operation under spinal anaesthesia. Br J Surg. 2016;103:916–20.
27. Bislenghi G, Wolthuis AM, de Buck van Overstraeten A, D'Hoore A. AirSeal system insufflator to maintain a stable pneumorectum during TAMIS. Tech Coloproctol. 2015;19(1):43–5.
28. McLemore EC, Weston LA, Coker AM, Jacobsen GR, Talamini MA, Horgan S, et al. Transanal minimally invasive surgery for benign and malignant rectal neoplasia. Am J Surg. 2014;208(3):372–81.
29. Coton C, Lefevre JH, Debove C, Creavin B, Chafai N, Tiret E, et al. Does trans-anal local resection increase morbidity for subsequent total mesorectal excision for early rectal cancer? Color Dis. 2019;21(1):15–22.
30. Marks JH, Valsdottir EB, DeNittis A, Yarandi SS, Newman DA, Nweze I, et al. Transanal endoscopic microsurgery for the treatment of rectal cancer: comparison of wound complication rates with and without neoadjuvant radiation therapy. Surg Endosc. 2009;23(5):1081–7.
31. Keller DS, Tahilramani RN, Flores-Gonzalez JR, Mahmood A, Haas EM. Transanal minimally invasive surgery: review of indications and outcomes from 75 consecutive patients. J Am Coll Surg. 2016;222(5):814–22.
32. Martin-Perez B, Andrade-Ribeiro GD, Hunter L, Atallah S. A systematic review of transanal minimally invasive surgery (TAMIS) from 2010 to 2013. Tech Coloproctol. 2014;18(9):775–88.
33. deBeche-Adams T, Hassan I, Haggerty S, Stefanidis D. Transanal minimally invasive surgery (TAMIS): a clinical spotlight review. Surg Endosc. 2017;31(10):3791–800.
34. Ramkumar J, Karimuddin AA, Phang PT, Raval MJ, Brown CJ. Peritoneal perforation during transanal endoscopic microsurgery is not associated with significant short-term complications. Surg Endosc. 2019;33(3):849–53.
35. Mege D, Petrucciani N, Maggiori L, Panis Y. Peritoneal perforation is less a complication than an expected event during transanal endoscopic microsurgery: experience from 194 consecutive cases. Tech Coloproctol. 2017;21(9):729–36.
36. Gavagan JA, Whiteford MH, Swanstrom LL. Full-thickness intraperitoneal excision by transanal endoscopic microsurgery does not increase short-term complications. Am J Surg. 2004;187:630–4.

37. Marks JH, Frenkel JL, Greenleaf CE, D'Andrea AP. Transanal endoscopic microsurgery with entrance into the peritoneal cavity: is it safe? Dis Colon Rectum. 2014;57(10):1176–82.
38. Issa N, Fenig Y, Yasin M, Schmilovitz-Weiss H, Khoury W, Powsner E. Laparoscopy following peritoneal entry during transanal endoscopic microsurgery may increase the safety and maximize the benefits of the transanal excision. Tech Coloproctol. 2016;20(4):221–6.
39. Rimonda R, Arezzo A, Arolfo S, Salvai A, Morino M. TransAnal Minimally Invasive Surgery (TAMIS) with SILS™ port versus Transanal Endoscopic Microsurgery (TEM): a comparative experimental study. Surg Endosc. 2013;27(10):3762–8.
40. Lee L, Kelly J, Nassif GJ, Keller D, Debeche-Adams TC, Mancuso PA, et al. Establishing the learning curve of transanal minimally invasive surgery for local excision of rectal neoplasms. Surg Endosc. 2018;32(3):1368–76.
41. Tsai BM, Finne CO, Nordenstam JF, Christoforidis D, Madoff RD, Mellgren A. Transanal endoscopic microsurgery resection of rectal tumors: outcomes and recommendations. Dis Colon Rectum. 2010;53(1):16–23.
42. Saget A, Maggiori L, Petrucciani N, Ferron M, Panis Y. Is there a limit to transanal endoscopic surgery? A comparative study between standard and technically challenging indications among 168 consecutive patients. Color Dis. 2015;17(7):O155–60.
43. Allaix ME, Arezzo A, Caldart M, Festa F, Morino M. Transanal endoscopic microsurgery for rectal neoplasms: experience of 300 consecutive cases. Dis Colon Rectum. 2009;52:1831–6.
44. Lee L, Burke JP, deBeche-Adams T, Nassif G, Martin-Perez B, Monson JRT, et al. Transanal minimally invasive surgery for local excision of benign and malignant rectal neoplasia: outcomes from 200 consecutive cases with midterm follow up. Ann Surg. 2018;267(5):910–6.
45. Karakayali FY, Tezcaner T, Moray G. Anorectal function and outcomes after transanal minimally invasive surgery for rectal tumors. J Minim Access Surg. 2015;11(4):257–62.
46. Verseveld M, Barendse RM, Gosselink MP, Verhoef C, de Graaf EJ, Doornebosch PG. Transanal minimally invasive surgery: impact on quality of life and functional outcome. Surg Endosc. 2016;30(3):1184–7.
47. Jakubauskas M, Jotautas V, Poskus E, Mikalauskas S, Valeikaite-Tauginiene G, Strupas K, et al. Fecal incontinence after transanal endoscopic microsurgery. Int J Color Dis. 2018;33(4):467–72.
48. Hompes R, Ashraf SQ, Gosselink MP, van Dongen KW, Mortensen NJ, Lindsey I, et al. Evaluation of quality of life and function at 1 year after transanal endoscopic microsurgery. Color Dis. 2015;17(2):54–61.
49. Atallah S, Albert M, Debeche-Adams T, Larach S. Transanal minimally invasive surgery (TAMIS): applications beyond local excision. Tech Coloproctol. 2013;17(2):239–43.
50. Ferrer-Márquez M, Rubio-Gil F, Ortega-Ruiz S, Blesa-Sierra I, Álvarez-García A, Jorge-Cerrudo J, et al. Transanal endoscopic microsurgery for the treatment of uncommon rectal lesions. Cir Esp. 2017;95(6):335–41.
51. Clerico G, Gallo G, Realis Luc A, Trompetto M. Transanal endoscopic microsurgery for perirectal dermoid cysts. Tech Coloproctol. 2017;21(4):319–20.
52. Gallo G, Clerico G, Luc AR, Trompetto M. Perirectal myxoid pseudocyst removed by transanal endoscopic microsurgery. Tech Coloproctol. 2016;20(11):801–3.
53. Banky B, Saleki M, Gill TS. Transanal endoscopic microsurgery in the management of rectal wall endometriosis. BMJ Case Rep. 2016;2016.
54. Suzuki T, Suwa K, Hada T, Okamoto T, Fujita T, Yanaga K. Local excision of rectal schwannoma using transanal endoscopic microsurgery: a case report. Int J Surg Case Rep. 2014;5(12):1193–6.
55. Liu Q, Zhong G, Zhou W, Lin G. Initial application of transanal endoscopic microsurgery for high-risk lower rectal gastrointestinal stromal tumor after imatinib mesylate neoadjuvant chemotherapy: a case report. Medicine (Baltimore). 2017;96(29):e7538.

Transanal Endoscopic Surgery for Rectal Cancer: Indications, Staging, and Perioperative Considerations

39

Mark H. Whiteford

Introduction and Rationale

The primary goal in the treatment of rectal cancer is curative therapy, best obtained through multidisciplinary care and the stage-appropriate use of three complementary modalities: total mesorectal excision surgery (TME), radiation therapy, and chemotherapy. Through en bloc resection of the rectal tumor and mesorectal lymph nodes, TME affords the highest chance of cure. However, TME is also associated with significant morbidity including a weeklong hospital stay, prolonged postoperative convalescence, risks of infections, and urinary, sexual, and defecatory dysfunction. TME is also accompanied by a temporary and occasionally permanent ostomy. Morbidity following TME in recent randomized trials ranges from 37 to 58%, and 30-day mortality is around 1% [1, 2].

It is from these concerns that surgeons have sought to identify patients that could be candidates for rectal sparing transanal local excision. Preservation of the rectum can avoid the significant morbidity and mortality of radical surgery and better maintain defecatory function. Unfortunately there is no single modality, histologic feature, radiographic study, and size and location of tumor that can predict with consistent accuracy whether the tumor extends beyond the rectal or has spread to regional lymph nodes.

In an ideal world, if we could accurately predict that there was no tumor in the lymph nodes and that complete local excision could be achieved, then local excision surgery would be curative. Conventional transanal excision (TAE) relies upon self-retaining and handheld retractors, stay sutures used to prolapse the rectal tissue into view, and extracorporeal lighting and viewing. In theory, transanal excision sounds straightforward; however, in practice, the surgeon faces significant challenges such

M. H. Whiteford (✉)
The Oregon Clinic, PC, Gastrointestinal and Minimally Invasive Surgery Division, Providence Cancer Institute, Oregon Health and Science University, Portland, OR, USA
e-mail: mwhiteford@orclinic.com

P. Sylla et al. (eds.), *The SAGES Manual of Colorectal Surgery*,
https://doi.org/10.1007/978-3-030-24812-3_39

as limited reach and retraction, poor lighting, and suboptimal exposure. Because of these physical limitations, TAE has been limited to benign lesions and malignant lesions less than 4 cm in maximum diameter and within 8 cm of the anal verge. Lesions exceeding these criteria were felt to require radical surgery.

Indications and Contraindications

The most common indication for transanal endoscopic surgery (TES) is for submucosal and full-thickness resection of benign lesions not otherwise resectable using standard colonoscopy. For more details, please refer to the Chap. 38 on TES for benign rectal lesions. With respect to rectal cancer, TES does not remove the at-risk mesorectal lymph nodes and, therefore, should be limited to selected early cancers with no evidence of local regional disease on imaging and have a low risk of occult lymph node metastasis. TES for rectal cancer might also be appropriate for more advanced tumors in patients who are unfit or unwilling to undergo radical surgery. The primary mode of determining increased risk of nodal metastasis remains in the domain of standard histologic evaluation. Unfortunately, this remains an imprecise science. No single histologic characteristic can predict lymph node metastasis in isolation; however, histologic factors that are associated with an increased chance of lymph node metastasis and local recurrence include T1SM3 and T2 depth of invasion, grade 3 histology, lymphovascular invasion, and positive margin status [3]. There are also not any currently available genetic, molecular, or immunologic markers that have increased diagnostic accuracy.

Principles and Quality Benchmarks

For malignant rectal lesions, the goal of transanal excision is complete en bloc resection without fragmentation of the specimen and negative margins. For rectal cancer, a 10 mm margin should be marked out prior to beginning dissection to ensure a negative margin. Submucosal dissection is not recommended for lesions harboring a known focus of invasive carcinoma.

Histologic Factors for Predicting Risk of Lymph Node Metastasis

Following full-thickness excisional biopsy via TES, histology slides should be reviewed, ideally at a multidisciplinary tumor board, to assess depth of invasion, margin status, and tumor histology. Patients that are identified as having adverse histologic features or have positive or indeterminate margins are at higher risk for local recurrence and should be treated with TME to ensure adequate staging and treatment (Table 39.1). There is also an additive relationship between increased number of adverse risk factors and incidence of lymph node metastasis [4, 5]. Figure 39.1 illustrates the odds ratios for the individual histologic risk factors [6].

Table 39.1 Local recurrence rates (percentage) at 36 months following TEM excision of rectal cancer

		Maximum tumor diameter (cm)					
Depth of invasion	Lymphatic invasion	≤1	1.1–2	2.1–3	3.1–4	4.1–5	≥5.1
pT1 SM1	No	3.0	3.6	4.4	5.4	6.6	8.1
	Yes	5.2	6.4	7.7	9.4	11.4	13.7
pT1 SM2–3	No	10.5	12.7	15.3	18.5	22.1	26.4
	Yes	17.8	21.4	25.5	30.3	35.7	41.8
pT2	No	9.8	11.9	14.3	17.3	20.7	24.7
	Yes	16.7	20.0	23.9	28.5	33.7	39.5
pT3	No	19.7	23.6	28.0	33.2	39.0	45.4
	Yes	32.2	37.9	44.1	51.0	58.3	65.7

Used with permission of John Wiley and Sons from Bach et al. [4]
pT pathological tumor stage, *SM1 and SM2–3* Kikuchi submucosal stage

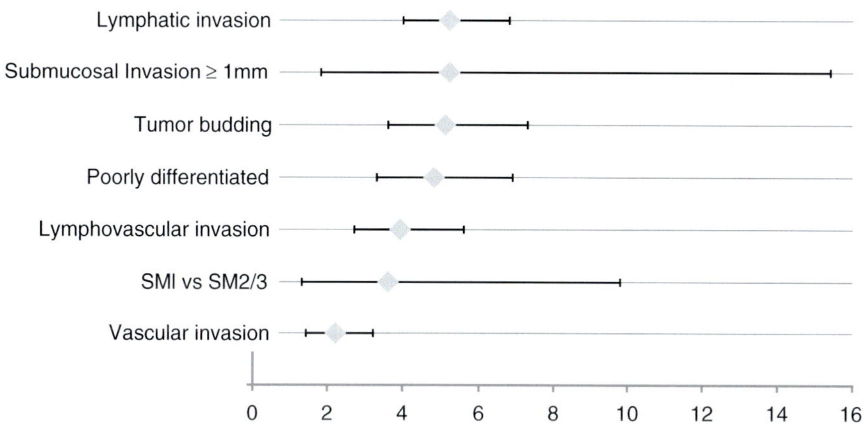

Fig. 39.1 Relative risk (95% confidence intervals) of lymph node metastasis in pT1 rectal cancers. SM1, invasion into superficial third of submucosa. SM2/SM3, invasion into middle and deep third of the submucosa. (Used with permission of Georg Thieme Verlag KG from Bosch et al. [6])

Depth of Invasion

When considering adverse histologic features for early rectal cancer, depth of tumor invasion is the most familiar and commonly referenced factor. T1 cancers are associated with a 10–15% incidence of occult lymph node metastases, and T2 cancers are associated with a 20–28% risk of lymph node metastasis [7–10]. Kikuchi and coauthors demonstrated the importance of depth of invasion within subclasses of submucosa invasion on the node metastasis and local recurrence in T1 cancers. By dividing submucosal invasion in the upper, middle, and lower thirds of the submucosa (SM1, SM2, SM3), an incremental increase in the risk of nodal metastases with a deeper depth of invasion is observed. SM3 level of invasion conferred a similar risk of nodal metastases as did a T2 cancer [11, 12]. Ding and coauthors described a similar phenomenon for T2 cancers whereby risk of lymph node metastasis increases with deeper penetration of the tumor into the muscularis propria [13].

Colonoscopic polypectomy specimens are usually partial thickness, so without the complete submucosal layer to visualize, the Kikuchi submucosal level of invasion cannot be determined. Under these circumstances, another predictive measurement system for depth submucosal invasion is needed. A Japanese collaborative study led by Kitajima reported that sessile polyps with depth of invasion <1 mm, as measured from the muscularis propria, and pedunculated polyps with <3 mm submucosal invasion into the polyp neck predicted for a very low risk of lymph node metastasis [14, 15].

Tumor Budding

There is increased recognition that tumor budding, defined as small nests of five or more cancer cells along the invasive front of the tumor, is a strong predictor of lymph node metastasis in colon and rectal cancer. Tumor budding is present in 16–25% of T1 cancers [16–18] and has an odds ratio of 5.1–5.8 at predicting lymph node metastases [6, 8].

Lymphovascular Invasion

Lymphovascular invasion (LVI) is present in 12–32% of T1 rectal cancers [7, 17]. LVI has long been recognized a predictor of lymph node metastasis with a reported odds ratio between 3.0 and 11.5 [6–8, 19].

Poor Differentiation

Poorly differentiated tumor histology has also long been a predictor of lymph node metastasis in early rectal cancer. However, this feature is seen rather infrequently and is only present in 2–4% of early rectal cancers [5, 6, 8, 20].

Preoperative Planning, Patient Workup, and Optimization

Once a patient has been diagnosed with rectal cancer, a standardized workup is initiated to exclude synchronous colorectal neoplasm and assess for locally advanced and metastatic disease [3]. Synchronous neoplasm is excluded via screening colonoscopy. Metastatic disease is evaluated using CT scan of the chest, abdomen, and pelvis. Local regional disease is evaluated using rectal cancer protocol MRI or endorectal ultrasound (EUS). EUS is useful in evaluating candidates for local excision, as it is better than MRI and CT in visualizing the individual layers of the bowel wall and differentiating superficial T1 and T2 rectal cancers [19]. Rectal cancer protocol MRI is a useful adjunct in assessment and surveillance of mesorectal lymph nodes [21].

For optimal surgical planning, preoperative rigid or flexible sigmoidoscopy is necessary to assess the location and extent of the rectal tumor, the tumor height from the anal verge, anterior/posterior/lateral location, tumor bulk, extent of circumferential involvement, or other features which might hinder access to the proximal border of the tumor. This can affect choice of patient positioning, planned complexity and length of surgery, risk of intraperitoneal entry, and plan for closure strategy.

Sometimes a "rectal" tumor is found up in the sigmoid, beyond the reach of transanal instruments.

Standard transanal excision has typically been restricted to tumors that are less than 40% of the circumference of the rectum and tumors within 8 cm of the anal verge. These limitations, however, arose not because these dimensions portend high risk of recurrence, but rather, they represented the restricted reach and visibility afforded through standard transanal instrumentation. TES – through improved lighting, visualization, advanced instrumentation, and the benefit of a stable pneumorectum – overcomes these size and location restrictions such that they are no longer considered a contraindication, provided the tumor can be removed en bloc with negative margins.

Operative Setup and Technique

The requisite equipment for transanal endoscopic surgery involves an operating transanal platform, laparoscopic or modified laparoscopic instruments, CO_2 insufflation unit, laparoscope and light source, suction device, and monopolar and/or bipolar energy sources and handpieces depending on the surgeons' preferences and a method to close the rectal wall defect such as suture or laparoscopic suture devices. Each TES platform will require a greater or lesser amount of disposable and reusable equipment. The initial TES platforms used rigid, reusable proctoscopes, transanal endoscopic microsurgery (TEM, Richard Wolf Medical Instruments, Knittlingen, Germany), and transanal endoscopic operating system (TEO®, Karl Storz, Tuttlingen, Germany). Transanal minimally invasive surgery (TAMIS), introduced in 2010, utilizes a disposable single-port platform placed transanally. The most common TAMIS platform is the GelPOINT® Path (Applied Medical, Rancho Santa Margarita, CA, USA).

As with all major surgeries, patient comorbidities and nutritional and smoking status should be optimized prior to elective surgery. Preoperative preparation involves a bowel preparation to ensure the rectal lumen and surgical field remain as clear as possible during the procedure. Most surgeons advocate for a full mechanical bowel preparation to achieve this goal, and some centers report clearance with enemas alone. Colorectal surgery prophylactic preprocedural intravenous antibiotics are administered in the operating room. Since spontaneous patient breathing can compromise adequate pneumorectum, general anesthesia with muscular relaxation is the preferred anesthetic modality.

Patient positioning is based on surgeon preference and surgical platform. TAMIS, using the disposable platform with straight instruments, can universally be done in lithotomy position. This also permits easy access to the abdomen for laparoscopy in the event of intraperitoneal entry and need for laparoscopic closure. TEM and TEO reusable platforms have beveled proctoscopes and angled instruments that facilitate operating on tumors located in the down position. Hence, patients with anterior tumors can be positioned prone split leg, posterior tumors in lithotomy, and lateral tumors in decubitus hip flex position. Intraperitoneal entry with TEM and TEO can usually be repaired transanally. Since TES patients have minimal postoperative discomfort, they can be managed as an outpatient or a 23-hour overnight stay.

Technique for TEM and TEO

Following positioning, the anus is gently dilated to facilitate insertion of the 4-cm-diameter proctoscope. The proctoscope is secured to the table with a U-shaped mounting arm. An airtight faceplate is secured, and tubing is connected to the suction insufflator unit. Pneumorectum is established and the video laparoscope adjusted to view the target lesion. Three instrument ports are available for use of the modified angled TEM/TEO laparoscopic instruments.

Needle tip electrocautery is utilized to demarcate a 10 mm margin around a cancer. Full-thickness dissection is then initiated and carried into the mesorectal fat (Fig. 39.2). Partial en bloc resection of the adjacent mesorectum has also been described for T1 lesions with unfavorable histology and T2 lesions [22]. The risk of bleeding is higher when operating on larger lesions and in the mesorectum where larger vessels are encountered. Bipolar or ultrasonic energy devices should be used or on standby for these situations. Continuous suction functions to clear the cautery smoke during the procedure. The integrated suction-insufflation unit prevents loss of pneumorectum from suctioning.

Following specimen removal, the defect is closed transversely using a running absorbable suture. A metal clip is locked at each end of the suture in lieu of intracorporeal knot tying. Alternative closing techniques include use of barbed sutures or laparoscopic suturing device. Closure of large resection defects is facilitated by starting the closure with a bisecting suture in the middle of the defect, thereby converting one large defect into two small defects (Figs. 39.3 and 39.4). With the increased proximal reach of TEM/TEO, intraperitoneal entry occasionally occurs and, in experience hands, can safely be closed via the TEM/TEO instrumentation [23–25]. TEM/TEO suffers from technical limitations of the rigid proctoscope causing significant instrument conflict and has a longer learning curve for both technique and instrument troubleshooting compared to other transanal techniques.

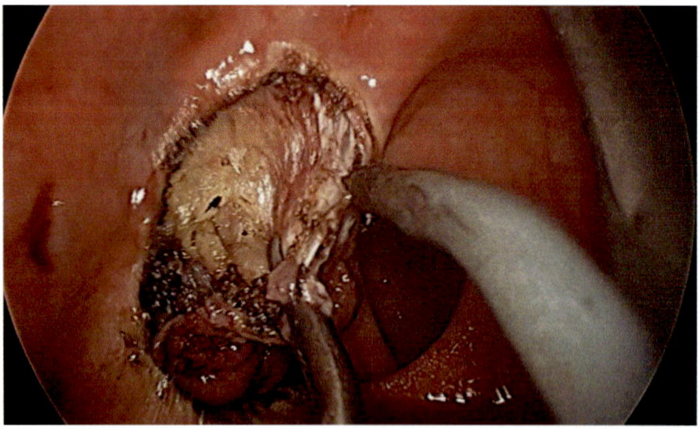

Fig. 39.2 Full-thickness resection into the mesorectal fat following dissection through the TEM platform. (Copyright retained by Mark H. Whiteford, MD)

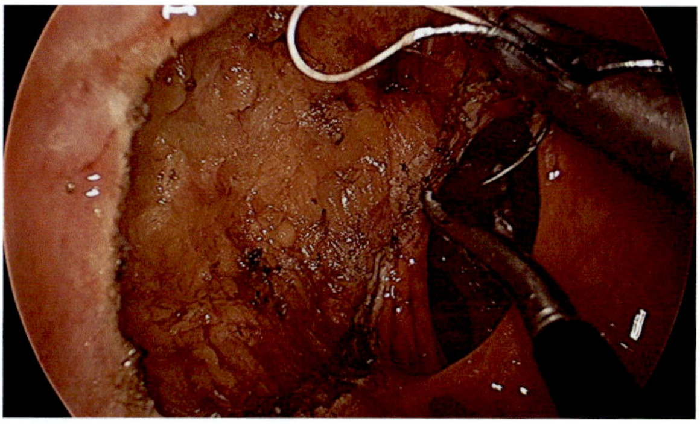

Fig. 39.3 Large full-thickness defect. (Copyright retained by Mark H. Whiteford, MD)

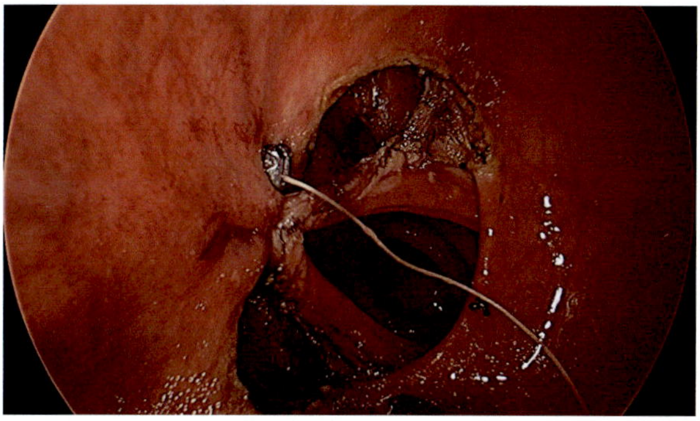

Fig. 39.4 Large defect bisected with suture closure. (Copyright retained by Mark H. Whiteford, MD)

Technique for TAMIS

TAMIS is a modification of TEM whereby the reusable rigid 4-cm-diameter operating proctoscope is replaced by a flexible, disposable single-port laparoscopic platform (Fig. 39.5). Standard laparoscopic instruments are utilized. Insufflation and smoke evacuation are accomplished using specialized high-flow insufflators such as the AirSeal® insufflator (ConMed, Utica, NY, USA), to avoid bellowing of the pneumorectum from standard laparoscopic insufflators. A 1 cm and full-thickness resection principles are identical to those mentioned above for TEM/TEO. Defect closure techniques vary among authors and include the use of different laparoscopic suturing devices or barbed sutures (Fig. 39.6) [26]. Intraperitoneal entry during TAMIS is more likely to require laparoscopic assistance for defect closure due to loss of rectum and visualization of the defect via the transanal device [27].

Oncologic Outcomes

The oncologic results following local excision of rectal cancer are mostly derived from case series and phase 2 trials. Many of these studies are subject to selection bias, include patients who had malignant polyps excised colonoscopically, or only

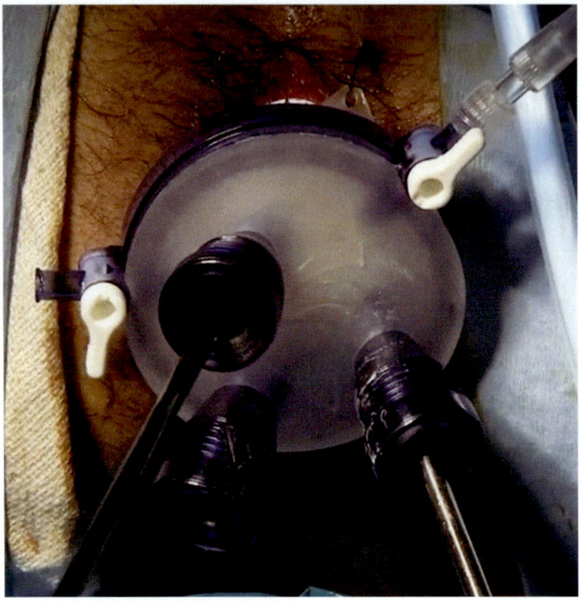

Fig. 39.5 TAMIS platform inserted transanally for TES. (Courtesy of Dr. Daniel Popowich)

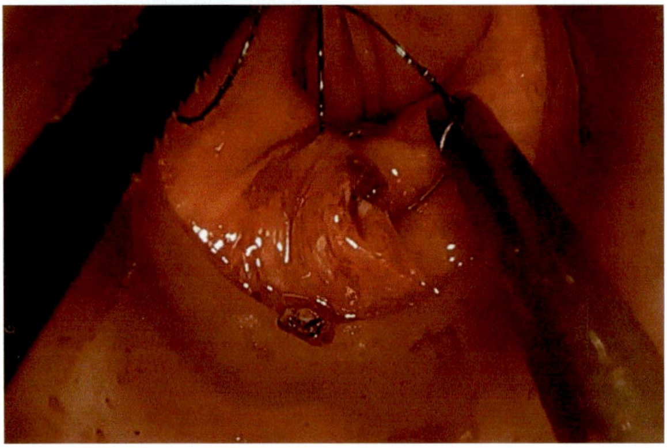

Fig. 39.6 Transanal endoscopic suturing of a full-thickness rectal defect through a TAMIS platform using a barbed suture. (Courtesy of Dr. Daniel Popowich)

track patients with favorable histology and negative margins. It is therefore difficult to make high-probability predictions for this heterogeneous disease process.

Clinical T1Nx Cancer

CALGB 8984 was a multicenter phase 2 trial examining long-term outcomes of local excision for early rectal cancer. One hundred seventy-seven patients with early-stage low rectal cancer underwent transanal excision. T1 cancers with negative margins (n = 59) were followed with no further treatment. T2 cancers with negative margins (n = 51) underwent adjuvant long-course chemoradiotherapy

Table 39.2 Long-term oncologic results comparing transanal endoscopic surgery and radical total mesorectal excision for favorable T1 rectal cancer

Series (year)	Number of patients	Follow-up (months)	5-year local recurrence	5-year disease-free survival	5-year overall survival
Winde	24 TEM	41	4.1%	–	96%
(1996) [33]	26 TME	46	0%	–	96%
Heintz	46 TEM	52	4.3%	–	79%
(1998) [34]	34 TME	52	2.9%	–	81%
Lee (2003)	52 TEM	–	4.1%	95%	100%
[35]	17 TME	–	0%	94%	93%
Ptok (2007)	105	43	6.0%	91%	84%
[36]	TAE + TEM				
	312 TME	42	2.0%	92%	92%
De Graaf	80 TEM	42	24%	90%	75%
(2009) [37]	75 TME	84	0%	87%	77%

TEM transanal endoscopic microsurgery, *TME* total mesorectal excision, *TAE* transanal excision

(5400 cGy, 5-fluorouracil). The 6-year local failure-free survival was 83% for T1 [28]. These optimistic results, however, were tempered by multiple subsequent single-institution reports demonstrating recurrence rates from 7% to 18% following transanal excision for favorable T1 cancers [29–32].

There are limited quality data comparing oncologic outcomes between TES and radical surgery for favorable T1 rectal cancer. Five of the larger studies are summarized in Table 39.2 [33–37]. Winde and coauthors published the only randomized trial comparing TEM to low anterior resection; however, this study was underpowered by only including 50 patients. Taken together, these studies demonstrate that TEM has a higher incidence of local recurrence relative to radical surgery; however, because of salvage radical surgery, 5-year tumor-specific survival and overall survival between the two techniques are not statistically different.

There are no long-term oncologic data comparing TAMIS to radical surgery. There is one large multi-institution cohort study comparing medium-term (14 months) follow-up of TAMIS ($n = 181$) to long-term (42 months) follow-up for TEM ($n = 247$) for benign and malignant rectal neoplasms. All stage (Tis, T1, T2, T3) local recurrence and 5-year disease-free survival for TAMIS and TEM were similar at 7% and 78% vs 7% and 80%, respectively [38].

Clinical T2Nx Cancer

Local recurrence following transanal excision alone for T2 rectal cancer is severalfold higher than that following radical surgery. To compensate for this, radiation therapy has been added to local excision of T2 rectal cancer to reduce the rate of local recurrence. The abovementioned CALGB 8984 trial reported a 71% 6-year failure-free survival for T2 cancers treated with adjuvant radiation therapy [28]. Lezoche and coauthors enrolled 100 patients in a single-institution randomized trial comparing neoadjuvant chemoradiotherapy followed by TES vs neoadjuvant chemoradiotherapy followed by laparoscopic TME for favorable ultrasound-staged uT2 N0 low rectal tumors. There was no difference in the probability of local recurrence or cancer-related survival at 5 years [22].

The American College of Surgeons Oncology Group Z6041 phase 2 multicenter trial enrolled 90 patients with uT2 N0 rectal cancer to undergo preoperative chemoradiotherapy with capecitabine plus oxaliplatin followed by local excision. A total of 77 patients completed treatment of which 98% had a negative resection margin, and 64% of tumors were downstaged (ypT0–T1), of which 44% had a pathologic complete response. There was no treatment-related mortality, and at a median follow-up of 56 months, 3-year disease-free survival was 88%, and overall survival was 95%. Bowel function and quality of life returned to baseline by 12 months [39].

Pitfalls and Troubleshooting

TES complications are similar to those of other anorectal surgeries and tend to be of low severity and of short duration. Mortality is rare [40, 41].

Intraoperative Complications

Intraoperative hemostasis is a surgical norm. TES is no different in this regard; however, the surgeon needs to develop the important balance between adequate suctioning to visualize the site of bleeding and excessive suctioning which results in loss of pneumorectum and needed exposure. Typical bleeding sites include the muscularis propria of the rectal wall and the mesorectal vessels. Bulky lesions also tend to have more robust blood supply and are more prone for brisk bleeding. Most bleeding can be controlled with monopolar cautery. Additional techniques include graspers connected to cautery, bipolar or ultrasonic energy devices, epinephrine injection, laparoscopic clips, suture ligation, and, rarely, packing.

Most of the rectum lies in an extraperitoneal location and is surrounded by a fatty mesorectum. TES excision into this extraperitoneal space rarely causes significant infection or morbidity. The anterior and lateral upper rectum, however, becomes an intraperitoneal organ whereby full-thickness transgression can result in intraperitoneal defect which mandates secure closure. Once considered a complication requiring laparoscopy/laparotomy and transabdominal repair, in the hands of experienced surgeons with a transanal laparoscopic suturing skill set, intraperitoneal entry and defect closure have been demonstrated to be safe using the rigid platforms [23–25]. At the time of intraperitoneal entry, CO_2 pneumorectum escapes into the abdominal cavity with resultant loss in pneumo-distention of the rectum and potential collapse of the working space. The rigid reusable TES platforms are able to maintain exposure to the intraperitoneal defect which permits transanal suturing to be completed. The TAMIS platform, however, does not stent the rectal lumen open, so complicated intraperitoneal entry using this device is often managed by converting to a laparoscopic approach for suture repair of the rectal defect [27]. Until a TES surgeon has acquired adequate endoluminal suturing skills to securely close an intraperitoneal entry, it is best to avoid upper rectal and anterior lesions early in their experience.

Postoperative Complications

Most common complication following TES surgery is urinary retention which occurs in 5–10% of cases [40, 41]. Like other anorectal surgeries, this is usually a self-limiting event which might require short-term urinary catheterization.

Small amounts of rectal bleeding and spotting are to be expected following transanal surgery. Major bleeding resulting in readmission or return to the operating room is infrequent. These events typically occur several days postoperatively related to a suture line disruption or later when patients restart their anticoagulation. Treatment is based on the severity and the clinical condition of the patient. Often the bleeding stops spontaneously; otherwise, a return to the operating room is necessary to obtain hemostasis using whatever combination of techniques deemed necessary, transanal endoscopic surgery, traditional transanal instrumentations, or flexible endoscopic techniques.

Suture line dehiscence is suspected when patients report increased bloody and mucous drainage, constant pelvic pain, and perhaps fevers and night sweats, usually several days to a week following surgery. It is more common following excision of low tumors and in patients that have received neoadjuvant radiation. True pelvic sepsis and fistulas are rare complications as is the need for urgent fecal diversion, but this must be considered where clinically appropriate.

Conclusion

The standard surgical treatment for early rectal cancer is total mesorectal excision. Oncologic equivalence between transanal endoscopic surgery and total mesorectal excision has not yet been demonstrated in the scientific literature so must still be considered a compromise. That said, many patients unfit for or unwilling to undergo radical surgery for early rectal cancer will choose organ sparing transanal endoscopic surgery for their treatment. Like all rectal cancer surgery, TES for early rectal cancer should be part of a multidisciplinary team to assure proper preoperative staging and interpretation, thoughtful patient selection, sound technical performance to obtain en bloc resection with negative margins, and careful histologic evaluation of the resection specimen. Tumors with unfavorable histology, including tumor budding, lymphovascular invasion, and deep submucosal invasion, have a high risk of occult lymph node metastasis and subsequent local recurrence. These patients should be steered toward radical surgery, be considered for adjuvant radiation, or be offered close surveillance follow-up.

References

1. van der Pas MH, Haglind E, Cuesta MA, Fürst A, Lacy AM, Hop WC, et al. Laparoscopic versus open surgery for rectal cancer (COLOR II): short-term outcomes of a randomised, phase 3 trial. Lancet Oncol. 2013;14(3):210–8.
2. Fleshman J, Branda M, Sargent DJ, Boller AM, George V, Abbas M, et al. Effect of laparoscopic-assisted resection vs open resection of stage II or III rectal cancer on pathologic outcomes: the ACOSOG Z6051 randomized clinical trial. JAMA. 2015;314(13):1346–55.

3. NCCN Clinical practice guidelines in oncology, Rectal Cancer, version 3.2018, August 7, 2018. NCCN.org.
4. Bach SP, Hill J, Monson JR, Simson JN, Lane L, Merrie A, Warren B, Mortensen NJ, Association of Coloproctology of Great Britain and Ireland Transanal Endoscopic Microsurgery (TEM) Collaboration. A predictive model for local recurrence after transanal endoscopic microsurgery for rectal cancer. Br J Surg. 2009;96(3):280–90.
5. Ha RK, Han KS, Sohn DK, Kim BC, Hong CW, Chang HJ, et al. Histopathologic risk factors for lymph node metastasis in patients with T1 colorectal cancer. Ann Surg Treat Res. 2017;93(5):266–71.
6. Bosch SL, Teerenstra S, de Wilt JH, Cunningham C, Nagtegaal ID. Predicting lymph node metastasis in pT1 colorectal cancer: a systematic review of risk factors providing rationale for therapy decisions. Endoscopy. 2013;45(10):827–34.
7. Chang HC, Huang SC, Chen JS, Tang R, Changchien CR, Chiang JM, et al. Risk factors for lymph node metastasis in pT1 and pT2 rectal cancer: a single-institute experience in 943 patients and literature review. Ann Surg Oncol. 2012;19(8):2477–84.
8. Glasgow SC, Bleier JI, Burgart LJ, Finne CO, Lowry AC. Meta- analysis of histopathological features of primary colorectal cancers that predict lymph node metastases. J Gastrointest Surg. 2012;16(5):1019–28.
9. Blumberg D, Paty PB, Guillem JG, Picon AI, Minsky BD, Wong WD, et al. All patients with small intramural rectal cancers are at risk for lymph node metastasis. Dis Colon Rectum. 1999;42(7):881–5.
10. Salinas HM, Dursun A, Klos CL, Shellito P, Sylla P, Berger D, et al. Determining the need for radical surgery in patients with T1 rectal cancer. Arch Surg. 2011;146(5):540–4.
11. Kikuchi R, Takano M, Takagi K, Fujimoto N, Nozaki R, Fujiyoshi T, et al. Management of early invasive colorectal cancer. Risk of recurrence and clinical guidelines. Dis Colon Rectum. 1995;38(12):1286–95.
12. Nascimbeni R, Burgart LJ, Nivatvongs S, Larson DR. Risk of lymph node metastasis in T1 carcinoma of the colon and rectum. Dis Colon Rectum. 2002;45(2):200–6.
13. Ding PR, An X, Cao Y, Wu XJ, Li LR, Chen G, et al. Depth of tumor invasion independently predicts lymph node metastasis in T2 rectal cancer. J Gastrointest Surg. 2011;15:130–6.
14. Kitajima K, Fujimori T, Fuji S, Takeda J, Ohkura Y, Kawamata H, et al. Correlations between lymph node metastasis and depth of submucosal invasion in submucosal invasive colorectal carcinoma: a Japanese collaborative study. J Gastroenterol. 2004;39:534–43.
15. Watanabe T, Muro K, Ajioka Y, Hashiguchi Y, Ito Y, Saito Y, et al. Japanese Society for Cancer of the Colon and Rectum Japanese Society for Cancer of the Colon and Rectum (JSCCR) guidelines 2016 for the treatment of colorectal cancer. Int J Clin Oncol. 2018;23:1–34.
16. Hase K, Shatney C, Johnson D, Trollope M, Vierra M. Prognostic value of tumor "budding" in patients with colorectal cancer. Dis Colon Rectum. 1993;36:627–35.
17. Okuyama T, Oya M, Ishikawa H. Budding as a risk factor for lymph node metastasis in pT1 or pT2 well-differentiated colorectal adenocarcinoma. Dis Colon Rectum. 2002;45(5):628–34.
18. Wang HS, Liang WY, Lin TC, Chen WS, Jiang JK, Yang SH, et al. Curative resection of T1 colorectal carcinoma: risk of lymph node metastasis and long-term prognosis. Dis Colon Rectum. 2005;48:1182–92.
19. Morino M, Risio M, Bach S, Beets-Tan R, Bujko K, Panis Y, et al. Early rectal cancer: the European Association for Endoscopic Surgery (EAES) clinical consensus conference. Surg Endosc. 2015;29(4):755–73.
20. Kobayashi H, Mochizuki H, Kato T, Mori T, Kameoka S, Shirouzu K, et al. Is total mesorectal excision always necessary for T1–T2 lower rectal cancer? Ann Surg Oncol. 2010;17:973–80.
21. Beets-Tan RG, Lambregts DM, Maas M, Bipat S, Barbaro B, Caseiro-Alves F, et al. Magnetic resonance imaging for the clinical management of rectal cancer patients: recommendations from the 2012 European Society of Gastrointestinal and Abdominal Radiology (ESGAR) consensus meeting. Eur Radiol. 2013;23(9):2522–31.
22. Lezoche E, Baldarelli M, Lezoche G, Paganini AM, Gesuita R, Guerrieri M. Randomized clinical trial of endoluminal locoregional resection versus laparoscopic total mesorectal excision for T2 rectal cancer after neoadjuvant therapy. Br J Surg. 2012;99:1211–8.

23. Gavagan JA, Whiteford MH, Swanstrom LL. Full-thickness intraperitoneal excision by transanal endoscopic microsurgery does not increase short-term complications. Am J Surg. 2004;187(5):630–4.
24. Ramwell A, Evans J, Bignell M, Mathias J, Simson J. The creation of a peritoneal defect in transanal endoscopic microsurgery does not increase complications. Color Dis. 2009;11(9):964–6.
25. Morino M, Allaix ME, Famiglietti F, Caldart M, Arezzo A. Does peritoneal perforation affect short- and long-term outcomes after transanal endoscopic microsurgery? Surg Endosc. 2013;23(1):181–8.
26. Albert MR, Atallah SB, deBeche-Adams TC, Izfar S, Larach SW. Transanal minimally invasive surgery (TAMIS) for local excision of benign neoplasms and early-stage rectal cancer: efficacy and outcomes in the first 50 patients. Dis Colon Rectum. 2013;56(3):301–7.
27. Hahnloser D, Cantero R, Salgado G, Dindo D, Rega D, Delrio P. Transanal minimal invasive surgery for rectal lesions: should the defect be closed? Color Dis. 2015;17(5):397–402.
28. Steele GD Jr, Herndon JE, Bleday R, Russell A, Benson A III, Hussain M, et al. Sphincter-sparing treatment for distal rectal adenocarcinoma. Ann Surg Oncol. 1999;6(5):433–41.
29. Mellgren A, Sirivongs P, Rothenberger DA, Madoff RD, García-Aguilar J. Is local excision adequate therapy for early rectal cancer? Dis Colon Rectum. 2000;43:1064–71.
30. Paty PB, Nash GM, Baron P, Zakowski M, Minsky BD, Blumberg D, et al. Long-term results of local excision for rectal cancer. Ann Surg. 2002;236(4):522–9.
31. Nascimbeni R, Nivatvongs S, Larson DR, Burgart LJ. Long-term survival after local excision for T1 carcinoma of the rectum. Dis Colon Rectum. 2004;47:1773–9.
32. Madbouly KM, Remzi FH, Erkek BA, Senagore AJ, Baeslach CM, Khandwala F, et al. Recurrence after transanal excision of T1 rectal cancer: should we be concerned? Dis Colon Rectum. 2005;48(4):711–9.
33. Winde G, Nottberg H, Keller R, Schmid KW, Bünte H. Surgical cure for early rectal carcinomas (T1). Transanal endoscopic microsurgery vs anterior resection. Dis Colon Rectum. 1996;39(9):969–76.
34. Heintz A, Mörschel M, Junginger T. Comparison of results after transanal endoscopic microsurgery and radical resection for T1 carcinoma of the rectum. Surg Endosc. 1998;12(9):1145–8.
35. Lee W, Lee D, Choi S, Chun H. Transanal endoscopic microsurgery and radical surgery for T1 and T2 rectal cancer. Surg Endosc. 2003;17(8):1283–7.
36. Ptok H, Marusch F, Meyer F, Schubert D, Koeckerling F, Gastinger I, et al. Oncological outcome of local vs radical resection of low-risk pT1 rectal cancer. Arch Surg. 2007;142(7):649–55.
37. De Graaf EJ, Doornebosch PG, Tollenaar RA, Meershoek-Klein Kranenbarg E, de Boer AC, et al. Transanal endoscopic microsurgery versus total mesorectal excision of T1 rectal adenocarcinomas with curative intention. Eur J Surg Oncol. 2009;35(12):1280–5.
38. Lee L, Edwards K, Hunter IA, Hartley JE, Atallah SB, Albert MR, et al. Quality of local excision for rectal neoplasms using transanal endoscopic microsurgery versus transanal minimally invasive surgery: a multi-institutional matched analysis. Dis Colon Rectum. 2017;60(9):928–35.
39. Garcia-Aguilar J, Renfro LA, Chow OS, Shi Q, Carrero XW, Lynn PB, et al. Organ preservation for clinical T2N0 distal rectal cancer using neoadjuvant chemoradiotherapy and local excision (ACOSOG Z6041): results of an open-label, single-arm, multi-institutional, phase 2 trial. Lancet Oncol. 2015;16:1537–46.
40. Kumar AS, Coralic J, Kelleher DC, Sidani S, Kolli K, Smith LE. Complications of transanal endoscopic microsurgery are rare and minor: a single institution's analysis and comparison to existing data. Dis Colon Rectum. 2013;56(3):295–300.
41. Tsai BM, Finne CO, Nordenstam JF, Christoforidis D, Madoff RD, Mellgren A. Transanal endoscopic microsurgery resection of rectal tumors: outcomes and recommendations. Dis Colon Rectum. 2010;53:16–23.

40 Advanced Techniques for Specimen Extraction During Laparoscopic Colorectal Surgery

Albert M. Wolthuis

Introduction and Rationale

Over the last 20 years, laparoscopic colorectal surgery has shown equal efficacy in cancer treatment as open surgery [1]. In comparison to open colorectal surgery, a laparoscopic approach reduces postoperative morbidity and shortens hospital stay [2]. With the introduction of enhanced recovery protocols, hospital stay after a laparoscopic colorectal resection has been further reduced [3–5]. Fast-track programs or so-called enhanced recovery after surgery (ERAS) protocols, pioneered by Kehlet and colleagues, were developed to reduce the surgical stress response, organ dysfunction, and morbidity.

Postoperative recovery is enhanced by a multimodality set of measures proposed by the various stakeholders in postoperative care [3]. However, a laparoscopic approach still has inherent drawbacks, such as incision-related complications (wound infection/incisional hernia) and postoperative morbidity. Because the length of the abdominal incision is directly related to the incisional hernia rate [6], avoiding a laparotomy might influence the rate of postoperative wound complications. In the quest to optimize outcomes after laparoscopic colorectal surgery, reduction of access trauma could be a way to improve recovery. In the early 1990s, Franklin and coauthors developed the concept of a totally laparoscopic approach for a sigmoid resection, which was later called NOSE-colectomy [7]. With NOSE, the specimen is delivered via a natural orifice, and the anastomosis is created intracorporeally. Natural orifice specimen extraction (NOSE) during laparoscopic colorectal surgery has the potential advantage of decreasing surgical trauma to the abdominal wall, resulting in a lower complication rate, faster recovery, and shorter length of hospital stay.

A. M. Wolthuis (✉)
University Hospital Leuven, Department of Abdominal Surgery, Catholic University Leuven, Leuven, Belgium
e-mail: Albert.wolthuis@uzleuven.be

P. Sylla et al. (eds.), *The SAGES Manual of Colorectal Surgery*,
https://doi.org/10.1007/978-3-030-24812-3_40

In 2008, Sylla and coauthors explored the feasibility of natural orifice transluminal endoscopic surgery (NOTES) transanal rectosigmoid resection with and without transgastric endoscopic assistance in a porcine model [8]. Preclinical studies clearly indicated the need for a hybrid transanal procedure to allow proximal vascular control and splenic flexure mobilization. The efforts have resulted in the first hybrid NOTES transanal total mesorectal excision (taTME) [9]. During the last few years, taTME was developed by merging different concepts of transanal minimally invasive surgery: laparoscopic transanal abdominal transanal (TATA) resection [10, 11], transanal endoscopic surgery (TES) [12], and natural orifice specimen extraction (NOSE) [13]. As such, when the specimen is extracted transanally – after completion of TME – this could be considered a NOSE-procedure as well, because an extraction site incision can be avoided. The specimen is extracted through the anal canal (transanal NOSE), in contrast with transrectal NOSE-colectomy when the specimen is extracted through the intact rectum and anal canal (e.g., this could be performed during a sigmoid or high anterior resection). In this chapter, the distinction is made between transanal and transrectal NOSE-techniques. Transvaginal specimen extraction during laparoscopic resection could also be considered a NOSE-technique. The main advantage of transvaginal NOSE is the possibility to extract large specimens following both right-sided and left-sided colonic resections, but this approach is only applicable to female patients with a non-intact hymen who give informed consent for this approach. Therefore, this technique will not be discussed in this chapter.

Indications and Contraindications

Transrectal NOSE

Before laparoscopic NOSE-colectomy can be introduced as an alternative to conventional laparoscopic colectomy, safety and feasibility were studied prospectively in a large cohort of consecutive patients [14]. Patient selection appears to be of paramount importance, and contraindications for transrectal NOTES include a body mass index (BMI) >35 kg/m^2, a bulky mesocolon, large tumors, the presence of a rectal stricture, and proximal diverticular disease [15]. Relative contraindications include immunosuppression, abnormal blood coagulation, peritoneal dialysis, a history of anal surgery, prior laparotomy, and any other condition that would preclude laparoscopy. Pathology-specific exclusion criteria include diverticulitis of the proximal sigmoid colon, acute diverticulitis including Hinchey stages I to IV, and advanced stage colon carcinoma, defined as clinically staged T3 or T4 tumors (cT3 or cT4). Transrectal NOSE-procedures can be considered after so-called high anterior resection, when the rectum remains intact and the top of the rectum is opened for specimen extraction.

Moreover, laparoscopic partial mesorectal excisions (PME) could also be amendable for transrectal NOSE. This procedure could only be done for lesions above the peritoneal reflection, because rectal opening and cross-stapling will become more difficult when dissection proceeds toward the pelvic floor.

Transanal NOSE

In 1984, Gerald Marks developed the technique of transanal abdominal transanal (TATA) proctosigmoidectomy with coloanal anastomosis for low rectal cancer after preoperative radiation therapy [16]. This technique was later performed in a minimally invasive way and popularized by his son John Marks [10]. In 1997, Teramoto and colleagues described a new technique of laparoscopic TME with intersphincteric dissection and "per anum" specimen retrieval. From that same group, data from a small cohort of patients were reported by Watanabe and coauthors [17, 18]. In 2003, Rullier and coauthors added coloplasty to this technique [19], and Person and coauthors described the original technique for totally laparoscopic low anterior resection with transperineal hand-sewn colonic J-pouch anastomosis for low rectal cancer [11]. Obviously, transanal NOSE is only possible after TME either performed using the TATA or the taTME technique. Therefore, the main indication for transanal NOSE is rectal cancer of the distal third of the rectum in patients requiring a low coloanal anastomosis. Indications vary among authors, but the following criteria should be taken into account when considering transanal NOSE: gender, BMI, neoadjuvant chemoradiation, tumor distance from the anorectal ring, tumor stage and size, anal sphincter function, and type of planned coloanal anastomosis [10, 20].

Principles and Quality Benchmarks

Both transanal NOSE and transrectal NOSE involve opening of the colon and/or rectum during surgery to facilitate specimen dissection, transection, and specimen extraction.

Complications relate to the potential contamination of the abdominal cavity or the pelvis with subsequent infection. The bacteriological impact of both rectotomy and proximal colotomy for anvil insertion and specimen extraction with possible intracorporeal soiling includes a heightened inflammatory response [21]. Intuitively, one would expect higher CRP levels and more positive cultures in patients undergoing NOSE-colectomy, because the colon and rectum are opened intraperitoneally with bacterial contamination of the peritoneal cavity [21]. Therefore, in order to justify the use of NOTES, the risk of infectious complications and inflammatory response should not exceed the potential advantages of this approach. Moreover, when dealing with malignant disease, tumor seeding and tumor cell implantation must be avoided. Anorectal washout and protection of the rectum and anal canal by the use of plastic sleeves or bags are essential in order to minimize leakage of fecal material and tumor cells during specimen extraction. A wound protector is typically inserted into the anal canal during transanal NOSE.

Other technical considerations include the creation of a well-vascularized proximal conduit which can be facilitated by the use of near-infrared imaging for perfusion assessment and tension-free colorectal anastomosis which can be facilitated by splenic flexure mobilization [22]. It is strongly recommended that the splenic flexure be completely mobilized when transanal NOSE is considered in order to achieve transanal specimen extraction without tension. Of note, it can be difficult to extract a bulky specimen through the anal canal. Therefore, full muscle relaxation should be obtained and provided by the anesthesia team.

Moreover, the relative size of the specimen in relation to that of the pelvis should be taken into consideration when considering transanal NOSE. In a male with a narrow pelvis (in combination with an enlarged prostate), extraction of a bulky specimen through the anal canal may be impeded. It should be stressed that specimen disruption should be avoided at all costs, so if the specimen cannot safely be extracted by gentle pulling without risk, an alternative abdominal extraction site must be selected.

Preoperative Planning, Patient Workup, and Optimization

For patients with rectal cancer, tumors should be staged by CT scan and pelvic magnetic resonance imaging (MRI). The decision regarding the use of neoadjuvant therapy should be discussed at local multidisciplinary team meetings according to standard NCCN guidelines.

On the day prior to surgery, patients undergo mechanical bowel preparation in combination with oral antibiotics. Although mechanical bowel preparation is not recommended for colectomy in ERAS protocols, it can be used in patients undergoing laparoscopic NOSE-colectomy, because of concerns of perioperative peritoneal contamination with solid stool. In our current practice, we abandoned bowel preparation, and patients administer enemas on the day of surgery. With respect to operative preparation, the patient is placed in modified Lloyd-Davies position on a moldable beanbag to allow a steep Trendelenburg position (Fig. 40.1a, b).

The surgeon should plan their operative strategy – i.e., site of specimen extraction, site of rectal transection, and creation of a well-perfused and tension-free anastomosis – based on tumor height from the anal verge. If the tumor is low but with enough of an anorectal cuff to create a low-stapled anastomosis, the surgeon should be prepared to suture close the rectal stump with a distal purse string in order to allow single-stapling (please see next section for technical considerations).

Operative Technique: Surgical Steps

Transrectal NOSE

A step-by-step approach of laparoscopic NOSE sigmoid colectomy was published in 2011 [23]. After administration of preoperative intravenous antibiotic prophylaxis (cefuroxime 2 g and metronidazole 1.5 g), general anesthesia is induced. The peritoneal cavity is entered in the left subcostal region with a Veress needle, and pneumoperitoneum is established to a pressure of 15 mmHg. A standardized 4-port

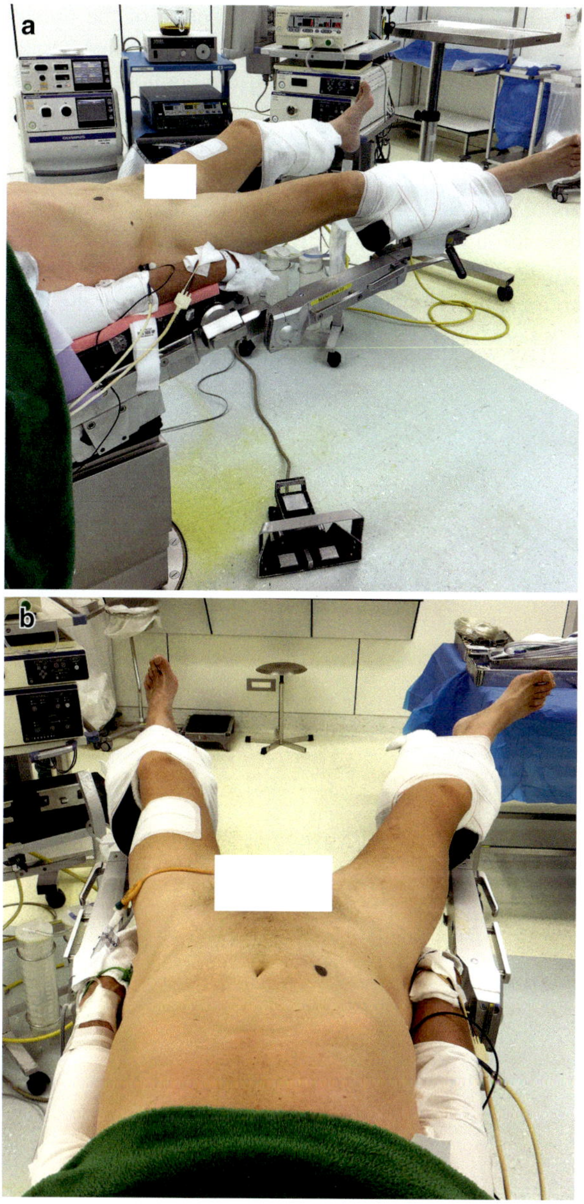

Fig. 40.1 (**a**, **b**) Patient positioning: modified Lloyd-Davies position

laparoscopic technique is used, and a conventional medial-to-lateral approach is performed with straight laparoscopic instruments and a 30° 5-mm laparoscope. The inferior mesenteric artery (IMA) and inferior mesenteric vein (IMV) can be clipped and divided (depending on whether this is an oncologic resection or not), safeguarding the left ureter, the gonadal vessels, and the autonomic hypogastric nerves. The sigmoid colon is mobilized by incising Toldt's fascia, a partial mesorectal excision

(PME) with division of the mesorectum of the upper rectum, allowing the rectal ampulla and reservoir function to be preserved. After the proximal and distal colonic margins have been established, the sigmoid mesentery is divided with a vessel-sealing device. The devascularized specimen is isolated, and both the proximal sigmoid colon and proximal rectum are tied off with a nonabsorbable suture. A rectotomy is then performed to deliver the anvil from a circular stapler into the abdominal cavity (Fig. 40.2a–e). The spike from the circular stapler has a built-in hole through which a suture is attached and used to manipulate the anvil. A colotomy is made at the level of the transition between descending and proximal sigmoid colon, the anvil is introduced into the lumen of the descending colon, and the spike

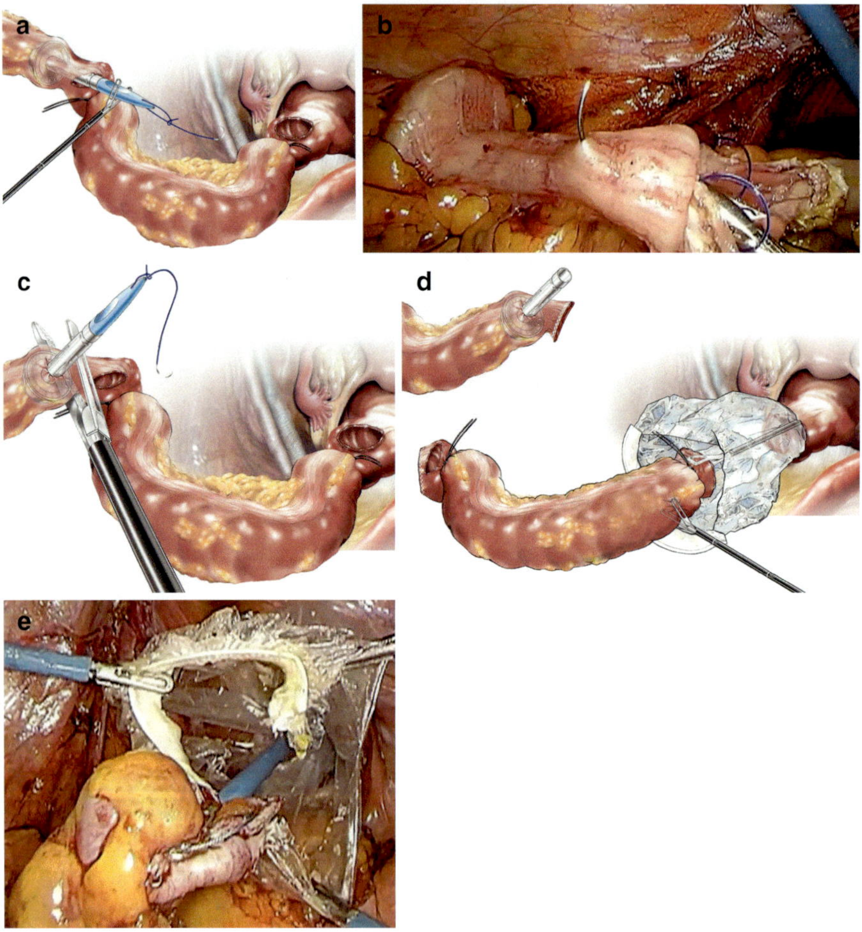

Fig. 40.2 (**a**) Anvil insertion into the descending colon. (**b**, **c**) Anvil retrieval by pulling on the suture placed along the antimesenteric colon, with division of the proximal bowel with a 60-mm endoscopic linear stapler. (**d**, **e**) Transrectal NOSE via a protected rectum. (Used with permission of Springer Nature from Wolthuis [42])

is pulled out along the antimesenteric aspect of the colon above the colotomy. The spike is disconnected from the anvil and extracted. The colon containing the enterotomy is transected with an endoscopic linear stapler. Now, the proximal colon is ready for anastomosis. The rectum is transected with laparoscopic endoshears, and the colonic specimen is placed in a plastic pouch and extracted transrectally. The rectal stump is closed with the endoscopic stapler, and the rim of proximal rectum is extracted through the 12-mm trocar. A functional end-to-end stapled intracorporeal colorectal anastomosis is created using the circular stapler, and an air leak test is routinely performed.

Transanal NOSE

Transanal NOSE could be a step during taTME. First, taTME is performed with a one- or two-team approach as described elsewhere [24–26]. If the rectosigmoid specimen and left colon are mobilized completely, a commercially available wound protector should be inserted into the anal canal for protection and to facilitate of specimen extraction (Fig. 40.3a, b). The procedure continues with specimen and colon that will be used for reconstruction being brought out through the anus. It should be stressed that this is not feasible in every patient, because of specimen size, tumor measurements, and pelvic dimensions. As such, it is left to the surgeon to decide whether specimen extraction should be done transanally or transabdominally. In general, large tumors (>3 cm), higher BMI (>35 kg/m^2), and a narrow pelvis are suboptimal conditions for transanal NOSE. Procedures are usually technically easier to perform in female patients, given a wider pelvis. Adequate colon length should be obtained via mobilization of the splenic flexure. It is essential that the IMV be transected proximally, and this is best achieved by dividing it immediately inferior to the inferior border of the pancreas. Care should be taken not to

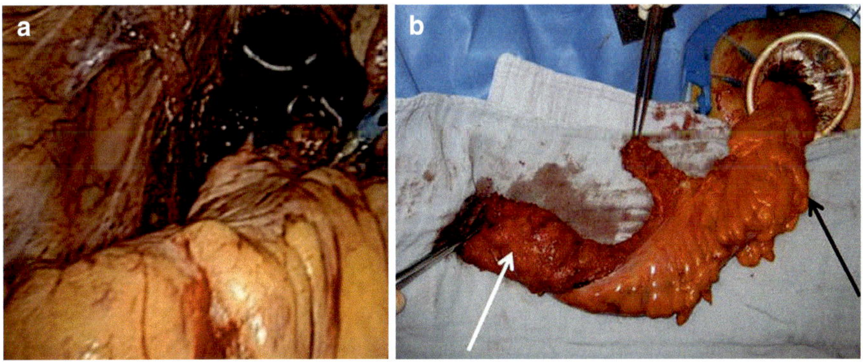

Fig. 40.3 (**a**) After laparoscopic-assisted taTME, a wound protector is inserted into the anal canal, and the specimen can be extracted transanally with a laparoscopic grasper. (**b**) Transanal NOSE. Exteriorized TME specimen with its vascular pedicle (white arrow) and proximal colon used for the reconstruction (black arrow)

damage the marginal artery by tearing and putting too much traction on the specimen.

Following specimen extraction, the colon is transected transanally, and the anvil is inserted in the proximal colon. Either hand-sewn or low single stapled, anastomosis can be performed. For a hand-sewn anastomosis, after transection of the specimen, the colon should be gently pushed into the anal canal, and laparoscopy can be performed to confirm that there is no twisting of the colon or its mesentery. If oncologically safe, a low stapled anastomosis should be performed, because it tends to result in better functional outcomes. For a stapled anastomosis, a double purse-string technique is necessary. The open rectal stump should be closed with a carefully placed purse-string suture. It is necessary to take full-thickness bites but to avoid taking the vaginal wall. Moreover, gaps should be avoided, because this will potentially lead to an anastomotic leak. When the anvil is sutured in place and the distal purse string is completed, three different stapling techniques can be used to create a stapled coloanal anastomosis [27].

Pitfalls and Troubleshooting

Technically, the leap from conventional laparoscopic colectomy to laparoscopic NOSE-colectomy is substantial in comparison to the presumed benefit. Indeed, presumed short-term advantages are less morbidity and less postoperative pain leading to a decrease in stress response and length of hospital stay. However, advanced technical skills are required with experience in laparoscopic colorectal surgery, NOSE-techniques, and familiarity with creating an intracorporeal anastomosis.

Specimen extraction without rectal protection is an option for benign disease, but this can be difficult, because the specimen can become stuck in the rectum [28, 29]. Originally, transrectal specimen retrieval involved a specimen-retrieval pouch, but positional changes of the specimen and air trapping in the bag often hampered extraction. Moreover, the specimen can bunch up and become impossible to extract. To solve this problem and expand the indications for NOSE-colectomy with transrectal specimen extraction, a plastic sleeve can be inserted through the anorectum to protect the rectal lumen, so that the specimen can be extracted in a straight rather than coiled up configuration. Specimen extraction is either performed with a long laparoscopic grasper or a long ring forceps.

Drawbacks of this modified technique include the fact that the end of the sleeve is left open, so that the rectum more or less is protected by a "plastic tunnel" instead of a hermetically closed bag. Most authors recommend rectal protection during specimen extraction, especially when resections are performed for malignant disease. This can be accomplished with a specimen-retrieval pouch or by inserting a rigid rectoscope normally used during transanal endoscopic microsurgery (TEM). Insertion of a rigid rectoscope requires anal dilation, and the inner diameter of the rectoscope will determine the maximum size of the specimen to be retrieved. Therefore, larger specimens should be extracted in a retrieval pouch, which is impermeable to fluids, thus minimizing the risk of tumor cell dissemination. Because colorectal anastomosis is made using a triple-stapling technique, proximal diverticular disease could lead to an anastomotic leak, due to inadvertent diverticulum cross-stapling. This should be assessed on preoperative CT scanning and avoided at operation.

Outcomes

It is difficult to report postoperative outcomes including morbidity and length of hospital stay following transanal and transrectal NOSE, because of heterogeneity between studies (Table 40.1). Differences in technique, such as the number of abdominal ports (three to five ports), rectal protection (none, rigid rectoscope, camera sleeve, or retrieval bag), and anastomotic technique (double stapled and triple stapled), will impact outcomes. In general, it is accepted that laparoscopic NOSE-colectomy is as safe as conventional laparoscopic resection with an anastomotic leak rate ranging 2–5% [23, 30]. Although anastomotic leakage is the most serious complication, intraluminal bleeding remains a concern with an incidence around 4.5% [14]. If anastomotic bleeding occurs, it can be controlled endoscopically without significant impact on recovery. Transrectal NOSE is a valid option for specimen extraction and the creation of a colorectal anastomosis because of its applicability in both male and female patients and for a wide range of left-sided colonic pathologies including diverticulitis, endometriosis, adenoma, and carcinoma. Moreover, the direct access to the peritoneal cavity provided by the transrectal route further contributes to the feasibility of this approach.

Among the few studies reporting outcomes of transanal NOSE-procedures, most combined laparoscopic TME with either transabdominal or transanal specimen extraction (Table 40.1). Moreover, with the recent introduction of taTME-techniques, studies described outcomes of a combined laparoscopic and transanal approach for TME, of which transanal extraction is only one of the many steps. Transanal NOSE was demonstrated to be feasible. No randomized studies are available, but a comparative study of transanal NOSE versus transabdominal specimen extraction showed no detrimental impact on oncological and functional outcome when transanal NOSE was performed [20]. This retrospective study included 220 patients with low rectal cancer, who underwent laparoscopic TME with hand-sewn coloanal anastomosis. Transanal NOSE was performed in 122 patients, and in 98 patients the specimen was extracted transabdominally. There was no difference in circumferential resection margin positivity, mesorectal grade, local recurrence, and disease-free survival rate between the two groups.

Table 40.1 Studies that describe outcome of transrectal and transanal NOSE-procedures

Author	Year	Type of study	N	Indication	Ports (N)	Protection	Anastomosis	Mean OR time (min)	Morbidity (N, Clavien-Dindo grade)	Median LOS (days)
Transrectal NOSE										
Franklin [31]	2013	Case series	277	Benign and malignant	4	Retrieval bag	TS	164.7	Leakage (3, 3b)	6.9[a]
Han [32]	2013	Case series	34	Malignant	5	TEM and bag	DS	151.6	Leakage (6, 3b)	9
Leung [33]	2013	RCT	35	Malignant	4	TEO	DS	105[b]	None	5
Zhang [34]	2014	Case-matched	65	Malignant <6 cm	4	Soft tissue retractor	TS	111.6	Leakage (2, 3b)	9[a]
Wolthuis [14]	2015	Case series	110	Benign and malignant <4 cm	4	Retrieval bag	TS	90[b]	Leakage (1, 3b), LGIB (2, 3b)	4
Lamm [35]	2015	Case series	40	Benign	5	Soft tissue retractor	DS/TS	173[b]	Peritonitis (1, 3b), LGIB (2, 3b), leakage (1, 4a)	6
Huang [36]	2016	Case series	32	Malignant <6.5 cm	4	TEO	TS	192	SSI (1), ileus (2)	6.5[a]
Saurabh [37]	2017	Case-matched	82	Malignant <5 cm	4	TEO	SS	227.9	Leakage (2, 3b)	4.8[a]
Shimizu [38]	2017	Case series	40	Malignant <3 cm	NA	NA	NA	223.8	Leakage (1, 3a)	10.2[a]
Transanal NOSE										
Rullier [19]	2003	Case series	32	Malignant	NA	None	Hand-sewn	420[b]	22% major	9
Marks [10]	2010	Case series	79	Malignant	3–6	None	Hand-sewn	NA	19% minor, 11% major	5
Kang [39]	2012	Comparative	53	Malignant	5(6)	Retrieval bag	SS	357	Leakage (4), abscess (2)	9
Bie [40]	2013	Case series	131	Malignant	NA	None	SS	166[b]	None	10
Denost [20]	2015	Comparative	122	Malignant	5	None	Hand-sewn	NA	15% major	9
Rasulov [41]	2016	Case series	30	Malignant	4	None	Stapled/hand-sewn	320[b]	27% minor	8

Note: Only studies with a sample size >30 patients are shown

DS double stapled, *LGIB* low gastrointestinal bleeding, *LOS* length of stay, *NA* not available, *N* number of patients, *OR* operating room, *RCT* randomized controlled trial, *TEA* transanal endoscopic applicator, *TEM* transanal endoscopic microsurgery, *TEO* transanal endoscopic operation, *SS* single stapled, *TS* triple stapled

[a]Mean LOS

[b]Median OR time

Conclusions

One of the goals of modern minimally invasive laparoscopic colorectal surgery is reduction of incision-related morbidity. NOSE-procedures could be the next step in bridging conventional laparoscopic surgery to pure human NOTES procedures by minimizing abdominal access trauma.

References

1. Kuhry E, Schwenk WF, Gaupset R, Romild U, Bonjer HJ. Long-term results of laparoscopic colorectal cancer resection. Cochrane Database Syst Rev. 2008;(2):CD003432.
2. Schwenk W, Haase O, Neudecker J, Muller JM. Short term benefits for laparoscopic colorectal resection. Cochrane Database Syst Rev. 2005;(3):CD003145.
3. Kehlet H. Fast-track colorectal surgery. Lancet. 2008;371(9615):791–3.
4. Spanjersberg WR, Reurings J, Van Laarhoven CHJM. Fast track surgery versus conventional recovery strategies for colorectal surgery. Cochrane Database Syst Rev 2009(2): CD007635.
5. Vlug MS, Wind J, Hollmann MW, Ubbink DT, Cense HA, Engel AF, et al. Laparoscopy in combination with fast track multimodal management is the best perioperative strategy in patients undergoing colonic surgery: a randomized clinical trial (LAFA-study). Ann Surg. 2011;254(6):868–75.
6. Laurent C, Leblanc F, Bretagnol F, Capdepont M, Rullier E. Long-term wound advantages of the laparoscopic approach in rectal cancer. Br J Surg. 2008;95(7):903–8.
7. Franklin ME Jr, Ramos R, Rosenthal D, Schuessler W. Laparoscopic colonic procedures. World J Surg. 1993;17(1):51–6.
8. Sylla P, Willingham FF, Sohn DK, Gee D, Brugge WR, Rattner DW. NOTES rectosigmoid resection using transanal endoscopic microsurgery (TEM) with transgastric endoscopic assistance: a pilot study in swine. J Gastrointest Surg. 2008;12(10):1717–23.
9. Sylla P, Rattner DW, Delgado S, Lacy AM. NOTES transanal rectal cancer resection using transanal endoscopic microsurgery and laparoscopic assistance. Surg Endosc. 2010;24(5):1205–10.
10. Marks J, Mizrahi B, Dalane S, Nweze I, Marks G. Laparoscopic transanal abdominal transanal resection with sphincter preservation for rectal cancer in the distal 3 cm of the rectum after neoadjuvant therapy. Surg Endosc. 2010;24(11):2700–7.
11. Person B, Vivas DA, Wexner SD. Totally laparoscopic low anterior resection with transperineal handsewn colonic J-pouch anal anastomosis for low rectal cancer. Surg Endosc. 2006;20(4):700–2.
12. Albert MR, Atallah SB, deBeche-Adams TC, Izfar S, Larach SW. Transanal minimally invasive surgery (TAMIS) for local excision of benign neoplasms and early-stage rectal cancer: efficacy and outcomes in the first 50 patients. Dis Colon Rectum. 2013;56(3):301–7.
13. D'Hoore A, Wolthuis AM. Laparoscopic low anterior resection and transanal pull-through for low rectal cancer: a Natural Orifice Specimen Extraction (NOSE) technique. Color Dis. 2011;13(Suppl 7):28–31.
14. Wolthuis AM, de Buck van Overstraeten A, Fieuws S, Boon K, D'Hoore A. Standardized laparoscopic NOSE-colectomy is feasible with low morbidity. Surg Endosc. 2014;29(5):1167–73.
15. Wolthuis AM, Van Geluwe B, Fieuws S, Penninckx F, D'Hoore A. Laparoscopic sigmoid resection with transrectal specimen extraction: a systematic review. Color Dis. 2012;14(10):1183–8.
16. Marks G, Mohiuddin M, Rakinic J. New hope and promise for sphincter preservation in the management of cancer of the rectum. Semin Oncol. 1991;18(4):388–98.
17. Teramoto T, Watanabe M, Kitajima M. Per anum intersphincteric rectal dissection with direct coloanal anastomosis for lower rectal cancer: the ultimate sphincter-preserving operation. Dis Colon Rectum. 1997;40(10 Suppl):S43–7.

18. Watanabe M, Teramoto T, Hasegawa H, Kitajima M. Laparoscopic ultralow anterior resection combined with per anum intersphincteric rectal dissection for lower rectal cancer. Dis Colon Rectum. 2000;43(10 Suppl):S94–7.
19. Rullier E, Sa Cunha A, Couderc P, Rullier A, Gontier R, Saric J. Laparoscopic intersphincteric resection with coloplasty and coloanal anastomosis for mid and low rectal cancer. Br J Surg. 2003;90(4):445–51.
20. Denost Q, Adam JP, Pontallier A, Celerier B, Laurent C, Rullier E. Laparoscopic total mesorectal excision with coloanal anastomosis for rectal cancer. Ann Surg. 2015;261(1):138–43.
21. Zattoni D, Popeskou GS, Christoforidis D. Left colon resection with transrectal specimen extraction: current status. Tech Coloproctol. 2018;22(6):411–23.
22. Ris F, Liot E, Buchs NC, Kraus R, Ismael G, Belfontali V, et al. Multicentre phase II trial of near-infrared imaging in elective colorectal surgery. Br J Surg. 2018;105(10):1359–67.
23. Wolthuis AM, Penninckx F, D'Hoore A. Laparoscopic sigmoid resection with transrectal specimen extraction has a good short-term outcome. Surg Endosc Other Interv Tech. 2011;25(6):2034–8.
24. Wolthuis AM, Bislenghi G, de Buck van Overstraeten A, D'Hoore A. Transanal total mesorectal excision: towards standardization of technique. World J Gastroenterol. 2015;21(44):12686–95.
25. Wolthuis AM, Cini C, Penninckx F, D'Hoore A. Transanal single port access to facilitate distal rectal mobilization in laparoscopic rectal sleeve resection with hand-sewn coloanal anastomosis. Tech Coloproctol. 2012;16(2):161–5.
26. Wolthuis AM, de Buck van Overstraeten A, D'Hoore A. Dynamic article: transanal rectal excision: a pilot study. Dis Colon Rectum. 2014;57(1):105–9.
27. Penna M, Knol JJ, Tuynman JB, Tekkis PP, Mortensen NJ, Hompes R. Four anastomotic techniques following transanal total mesorectal excision (TaTME). Tech Coloproctol. 2016;20(3):185–91.
28. Akamatsu H, Omori T, Oyama T, Tori M, Ueshima S, Nishida T, et al. Totally laparoscopic low anterior resection for lower rectal cancer: combination of a new technique for intracorporeal anastomosis with prolapsing technique. Dig Surg. 2009;26(6):446–50.
29. Leroy J, Costantino F, Cahill RA, D'Agostino J, Morales A, Mutter D, et al. Laparoscopic resection with transanal specimen extraction for sigmoid diverticulitis. Br J Surg. 2011;98(9):1327–34.
30. Wolthuis AM, Meuleman C, Tomassetti C, D'Hooghe T, Fieuws S, Penninckx F, et al. Laparoscopic sigmoid resection with transrectal specimen extraction: a novel technique for the treatment of bowel endometriosis. Hum Reprod. 2011;26(6):1348–55.
31. Franklin ME, Jr., Liang S, Russek K. Natural orifice specimen extraction in laparoscopic colorectal surgery: transanal and transvaginal approaches. Tech Coloproctol. 2013;17 Suppl 1(1):S63–7.
32. Han Y, He YG, Zhang HB, Lv KZ, Zhang YJ, Lin MB, et al. Total laparoscopic sigmoid and rectal surgery in combination with transanal endoscopic microsurgery: a preliminary evaluation in China. Surg Endosc. 2013;27(2):518–24.
33. Leung AL, Cheung HY, Fok BK, Chung CC, Li MK, Tang CN. Prospective randomized trial of hybrid NOTES colectomy versus conventional laparoscopic colectomy for left-sided colonic tumors. World J Surg. 2013;37(11):2678–82.
34. Xingmao Z, Haitao Z, Jianwei L, Huirong H, Junjie H, Zhixiang Z. Totally laparoscopic resection with natural orifice specimen extraction (NOSE) has more advantages comparing with laparoscopic-assisted resection for selected patients with sigmoid colon or rectal cancer. Int J Color Dis. 2014;29(9):1119–24.
35. Lamm SH, Zerz A, Efeoglou A, Steinemann DC. Transrectal rigid-hybrid natural orifice translumenal endoscopic sigmoidectomy for diverticular disease: a Prospective Cohort Study. J Am Coll Surg. 2015;221(4):789–97.
36. Huang CC, Chen YC, Huang CJ, Hsieh JS. Totally laparoscopic colectomy with intracorporeal side-to-end colorectal anastomosis and transrectal specimen extraction for sigmoid and rectal cancers. Ann Surg Oncol. 2016;23(4):1164–8.

37. Saurabh B, Chang SC, Ke TW, Huang YC, Kato T, Wang HM, et al. Natural orifice specimen extraction with single stapling solorectal anastomosis for laparoscopic anterior resection: feasibility, outcomes, and technical considerations. Dis Colon Rectum. 2017;60(1):43–50.
38. Shimizu H, Adachi K, Ohtsuka H, Osaka I, Takuma K, Takanishi K, et al. Totally laparoscopic resection for low sigmoid and rectal cancer using natural orifice specimen extraction techniques. Surg Laparosc Endosc Percutan Tech. 2017;27(4):e74–e9.
39. Kang J, Min BS, Hur H, Kim NK, Lee KY. Transanal specimen extraction in robotic rectal cancer surgery. Br J Surg. 2012;99(1):133–6.
40. Bie M, Wei ZQ. A new colorectal/coloanal anastomotic technique in sphincter-preserving operation for lower rectal carcinoma using transanal pull-through combined with single stapling technique. Int J Color Dis. 2013;8:8.
41. Rasulov AO, Mamedli ZZ, Gordeyev SS, Kozlov NA, Dzhumabaev HE. Short-term outcomes after transanal and laparoscopic total mesorectal excision for rectal cancer. Tech Coloproctol. 2016;20(4):227–34.
42. Wolthuis A. Transrectal specimen extraction: should this be catching on? In: Schlachta CM, Sylla P, editors. Current common dilemmas in colorectal surgery. Cham: Springer International Publishing; 2018. p. 227–37.

Index

P. Sylla et al. (eds.), *The SAGES Manual of Colorectal Surgery*,
https://doi.org/10.1007/978-3-030-24812-3

D

N

FSC
www.fsc.org
MIX
Papier aus verantwortungsvollen Quellen
Paper from responsible sources
FSC® C105338

If you have any concerns about our products,
you can contact us on
ProductSafety@springernature.com

In case Publisher is established outside the EU,
the EU authorized representative is:
Springer Nature Customer Service Center GmbH
Europaplatz 3, 69115 Heidelberg, Germany

Printed by Libri Plureos GmbH
in Hamburg, Germany